Foot and Ankle Disorders

Emilio Wagner Hitschfeld
Pablo Wagner Hitschfeld

Editors

Foot and Ankle Disorders

A Comprehensive Approach in Pediatric
and Adult Populations

Volume I

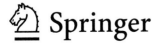 Springer

Editors
Emilio Wagner Hitschfeld
Orthopedic Surgery Department
Clínica Alemana de Santiago - Universidad
del Desarrollo
Santiago, RM - Santiago, Chile

Pablo Wagner Hitschfeld
Orthopedic Surgery Department
Clínica Alemana de Santiago - Universidad
del Desarrollo, Hospital Militar de
Santiago – Universidad de los Andes
Santiago, RM - Santiago, Chile

ISBN 978-3-030-95740-7   ISBN 978-3-030-95738-4   (eBook)
https://doi.org/10.1007/978-3-030-95738-4

This Springer imprint is published by the registered company Springer Nature Switzerland AG
The registered company address is: Gewerbestrasse 11, 6330 Cham, Switzerland

This book is gratefully dedicated to our mom and dad, Sonia and Rodolfo, for their life guidance, support, unconditional love, patience, and continuous teachings. Parents are the unsung heroes of every life. Thank you for everything.

Emilio and Pablo

Foreword

On so many levels, it is an extraordinary pleasure to review this book. Foot and ankle surgeons globally have benefited from the incredible insight, creativity, and innovation of Emilio and Pablo Wagner, and I now have the privilege to review work not only of good friends but also surgeons who I admire very much.

All textbooks carry a unique message which conveys the philosophy not only of the editors but also of the carefully selected contributors, and this is clearly evident here. The contributors are all world renowned in our field, giving this book tremendous credibility. There is a preponderance of contributors from Latin America which makes this book very appealing. While we may strive for global standardization of approaches to treatment of foot and ankle deformities, this is unrealistic. Treatments are determined by our training and experiences, the cultural and regional context in which patients are examined, as well as materials and availability of implants. The inclusion of regional experts each with a very different focus of foot and ankle treatment presents the reader with an excellent overview of the most important pathologies.

The book has been organized into different important sections including principles of foot and ankle evaluation, pediatric conditions, adult deformities, and trauma. The inclusion of a very comprehensive section on pediatric foot and ankle deformities is outstanding. These chapters cover all the essentials and are an outstanding additional contribution to our understanding of childhood deformities. All too often, foot and ankle surgery textbooks focus on the adult, ignoring the pathogenesis, principles, and evolution of deformity. A good example and a wonderful chapter to read is on the clubfoot by Dalia Sepúlveda. It is extraordinarily thorough, extremely well illustrated, and not only focuses on the Ponseti method of treatment but also provides a very good overview of the kinematics of the subtalar joint and principles of treatment. The chapter by another world leader, Vince Mosca, is a must read for any surgeon interested in foot and ankle with a focus on principles of evaluation and treatment, so well-stated "techniques change, but principles are forever."

When I read the book in preparation for writing this preface, I was obviously drawn to those topics in which I myself have a specific interest, and the chapter by Emilio and Pablo Wagner on localized osteoarthritis of the ankle is a great example.

It is incredibly well illustrated, and the thoughtful approach to supramalleolar oste-otomies is one of the best overviews of this subject that I have ever read. The inclu-sion of three chapters on the management of ankle arthritis is a good reflection of the editors' interest in this topic, and each one thoughtfully presented by great authorities on this subject.

This textbook is a wonderful compilation of topics which are germane to our practice, written by global leaders in the field, and will be an excellent resource for all of us.

Mark S. Myerson
University of Colorado
Boulder, CO, USA

Steps2Walk
Greenwood Village, CO, USA

Preface

Foot and ankle orthopedics and traumatology is a fascinating subspecialty within general orthopedics which has been receiving increased attention in the world in the last 20 years. Enormous development in understanding its complex biomechanics, joint pathology, soft tissue stress pathology, and trauma has pushed this subspecialty to unknown levels of interest worldwide. More orthopedic centers around the world now focus their attention on foot and ankle lesions, training orthopedic surgeons in this area, forming fellowship training groups, and generating basic and clinical science studies.

As our general understanding in foot and ankle trauma and orthopedics in adult population has improved, simultaneous interest and development has been seen in pediatric literature, where a unique approach is currently followed with significant differences from adult approach. As any medical specialty with an ever-expanding field of basic science, diagnosis, and treatment options, it is difficult to find a common place for a focused approach to foot and ankle pathology in adult and pediatric population. This difficulty is seen in residency and fellowship programs where our residents and fellows need a text to base their knowledge.

This book tries to fill the gap of information and interconnection between adult and pediatric foot and ankle lesions, describing, analyzing, and offering treatment alternatives for the most common topics in both groups of patients. Written by recognized experts in their respective fields from 14 different countries, this book provides information about foot and ankle biomechanics, soft tissue lesions, trauma and sports lesions, orthopedic deformities, and systemic disorders. Every chapter is written with a focused approach, allowing the reader to fully understand from the basics up to the most current surgical or conservative treatment for each problem. Lower limb reconstruction concepts are also included, such as tibial posttraumatic deformities, tibial osteomyelitis, and tibial bone defects reconstruction techniques.

We are sure that this book will serve as a guide for orthopedic surgeons, foot and ankle fellowship programs, and any orthopedic surgeon who wants to know more about this incredible subspecialty.

Santiago, RM - Santiago, Chile   Emilio Wagner Hitschfeld
Santiago, RM - Santiago, Chile   Pablo Wagner Hitschfeld

Acknowledgment

We would like to acknowledge the extraordinary work of all authors present in this book. They all did an outstanding work with their respective chapters, giving the reader updated information.

We would as well like to recognize and thank our mentors, John Gould, Mark Myerson, John Herzenberg, and Beat Hintermann. Without their influence in our lives, neither this book nor our current practice would exist.

Contents

Volume I

Part I   Basic Science and General Considerations

Foot and Ankle Biomechanics Gait Analysis 3
Manuel Monteagudo and Pilar Martínez de Albornoz

Imaging in Ankle and Foot................................... 25
Nicolas Zilleruelo V.

Open vs Minimally Invasive Surgery: Advantages and Disadvantages.. 43
Mariano De Prado, Manuel Cuervas-Mons, and Virginia De Prado

Tumors of the Foot and Ankle 71
Eduardo Botello and Tomas Zamora

**Care and Management of Surgical Wounds, Wounds Dehiscence,
and Scars** 89
Leonardo Parada and Günther Mangelsdorff

Part II   Pediatric Orthopaedics and Traumatology

**Biomechanics, Assessment, and Management Principles
for Pediatric Foot Deformities** 115
Vincent S. Mosca

Clubfoot 133
Dalia Sepúlveda Arriagada and Nicolas Valdivia Rojo

Pediatric Metatarsus Adductus and Cavovarus Foot 157
Maryse Bouchard

Pediatric Flexible and Rigid Flatfoot 179
Kyle M. Natsuhara and Jacob R. Zide

xiii

Foot Osteochondrosis   197
Pablo J. Echenique Díaz and Pablo Schaufele Muñoz

Fibular Hemimelia: Principles and Techniques of Management   213
Philip K. McClure and John E. Herzenberg

**Brachymetatarsia: Surgical Management with Internal
and External Fixation**   273
Noman A. Siddiqui

Lesser Toe Deformities   291
Carlos Pargas and Pablo Wagner Hitschfeld

Neurologic Foot   313
Gino Martínez and Gonzalo Chorbadjian

Pediatric Diaphyseal Tibia and Distal Tibia Fractures   335
Cristian Olmedo Gárate and Cristian Artigas Preller

Ankle Transitional Fractures   351
Matias Sepulveda and Estefania Birrer

Part III   Adult Orthopaedics: Forefoot

Hallux Valgus   371
Pablo Wagner Hitschfeld and Emilio Wagner Hitschfeld

Hallux Rigidus: A Comprehensive Review   409
Gaston Slullitel and Valeria Lopez

Sesamoiditis   427
Florencia Pacheco Martinez and Eduardo Fuentes Morales

Metatarsalgia   443
Pilar Martinez de Albornoz and Manuel Monteagudo

Deformity of the Lesser Toes   467
Pablo Sotelano and Daniel Sebastián Villena

Morton's Neuroma   493
Rodrigo Melo Grollmus and Cristián Ortiz Mateluna

Bunionette   517
Manuel Resende Sousa, Daniel Ribeiro Mendes, and João Vide

Part IV   Adult Orthopaedics: Midfoot, Rearfoot and Ankle

Progressive Collapsing Foot Deformity – Flatfoot   537
Jaeyoung Kim and Jonathan T. Deland

**Latest Trends in Flatfoot Management: Contributions
of the Spring Ligament Complex and the Deltoid Ligament**   555
Brian T. Sleasman and Anish R. Kadakia

Cavus Foot 567
Mark S. Myerson and Shuyuan Li

"Management of Severe Untreated and Recurrent Clubfoot
Deformity in the Child and Adult" 593
Mark S. Myerson and Shuyuan Li

Muller Weiss Disease 615
Manuel Monteagudo and Ernesto Maceira

Surgical Techniques for Peritalar Osteoarthrosis:
Talonavicular, Subtalar, Calcaneocuboid, and Midfoot 637
José Antônio Veiga Sanhudo and Marco Túlio Costa

Forefoot-Driven Hindfoot Deformity: Coupled Deformity 669
Norman Espinosa and Georg Klammer

Localized Osteoarthritis of the Ankle 691
Emilio Wagner Hitschfeld and Pablo Wagner Hitschfeld

Diffuse Ankle Osteoarthritis 723
Markus Knupp

Volume II

Part V   Adult Orthopaedics: Tibial Reconstruction

Tibial Post-traumatic Deformity 745
Arnd F. Viehöfer and Stephan H. Wirth

Septic Ankle Arthritis and Tibial Osteomyelitis. 759
Pablo Mery and Joaquín Palma

Tibial Bone Defect Reconstruction Techniques 801
Gonzalo F. Bastías and Gregorio Verschae

Below-Knee Amputations. 817
Roberto Muñoz Molina and Octavio Polanco Torres

Part VI   Adult Orthopaedics: Tendinopathy, Soft Tissue Pathology
            and Systemic Diseases

Insertional Achilles Tendinopathy: Diagnosis and Treatment 841
Giovanni Carcuro and Manuel J. Pellegrini P.

Non-insertional Achilles Tendinopathy. 855
Rocco Aicale and Nicola Maffulli

Achilles Lengthening 869
Manuel Resende Sousa, Daniel Ribeiro Mendes, and João Vide

Plantar Fasciitis. 885
Mario Abarca and Jorge Filippi

Foot and Ankle Tendon Transfers: Surgical Techniques 901
Jose Carlos Cohen

Diabetic Foot 941
Alexandre Leme Godoy-Santos and Rafael Barban Sposeto

Rheumatoid Foot 955
Sergio Fernandez C. and Hugo Henriquez

Charcot Neuroarthropathy 985
Rafael Barban Sposeto and Alexandre Leme Godoy-Santos

Nerve Entrapment Syndromes of the Lower Limbs 1005
Marcelo Pires Prado and Guilherme Honda Saito

Part VII   Adult Sports Lesions and Traumatology

Peroneal Tendon Tears: Evaluation and Treatment 1023
James W. Brodsky and Daniel D. Bohl

Anterior Ankle Impingement and Ankle Instability 1045
Jordi Vega and Miki Dalmau-Pastor

**Diagnosis and Treatment of Talus Osteochondral Lesions:
Current Concepts** 1065
Caio Nery and Marcelo Pires Prado

Posterior Ankle Impingement 1107
Daniel Baumfeld and Tiago Baumfeld

Common Stress Fractures Around the Foot and Ankle 1119
Roberto Zambelli and Nacime Salomão Barbachan Mansur

Achilles Tendon Ruptures 1137
Diego Zanolli and Rubén Radkievich

Ankle Fractures 1165
Guillermo Arrondo and Florencio Pablo Segura

Tibial Pilon Fracture 1207
Christian Bastias and Leonardo Lagos

Calcaneus Fractures 1225
Stefan Rammelt and Christine Marx

Talus Fracture 1253
Florencio Pablo Segura and Guillermo Arrondo

Midfoot Injuries 1281
Leandro Casola and German Joannas

Diaphyseal and Distal Tibia Fractures 1315
Rodrigo Pesántez and Eduardo José Burgos

Metatarsal Fractures 1329
Gabriel Khazen

Compartment Syndrome of the Leg and Foot 1361
Omar Ituriel Vela Goñi and Luis Felipe Hermida Galindo

Index. 1385

Contributors

Mario Abarca Hospital Sótero del Río, Santiago, Chile

Rocco Aicale Department of Musculoskeletal Disorders, Faculty of Medicine and Surgery, University of Salerno, Baronissi, Italy

Clinica Ortopedica, Ospedale San Giovanni di Dio e Ruggi D'Aragona, Salerno, Italy

Gonzalo Chorbadjian Clínica Alemana – Universidad del Desarrollo, Santiago, Chile

Hospital Clínico San Borja Arriarán, Santiago, Chile

Dalia Sepúlveda Arriagada Private Practice, COTI Chile, Santiago, Chile

Guillermo Arrondo Instituto Dupuytren, Ciudad Autónoma de Buenos Aires, Argentina

Department of Leg, Ankle and Foot, Dupuytren Institute, Ciudad Autónoma de Buenos Aires, Argentina

Christian Bastias Hospital Mutual de Seguridad C. Ch. C., Clínica Santa Maria, Santiago, Chile

Gonzalo F. Bastías Clínica las Condes, Santiago, Chile

Hospital del trabajador de Santiago, Santiago, Chile

Daniel Baumfeld Federal University of Minas Gerais, Felicio Rocho Hospital, Belo Horizonte, MG, Brazil

Tiago Baumfeld Felicio Rocho Hospital, Belo Horizonte, MG, Brazil

Estefania Birrer Universidad Austral de Chile, Valdivia, Chile

Hospital Base de Valdivia, Valdivia, Chile

Daniel D. Bohl Baylor University Medical Center, Dallas, TX, USA

Eduardo Botello Orthopaedic Oncology and Lower Limb Reconstructive Surgery, Orthopaedic Surgery Department, Pontificia Universidad Católica de Chile, , Santiago, Chile

Maryse Bouchard The Hospital for Sick Children, Division of Orthopaedic Surgery, University of Toronto, Toronto, ON, Canada

James W. Brodsky Baylor University Medical Center, Dallas, TX, USA

Eduardo José Burgos Hospital Universitario Fundación Santa Fé, Bogotá, Colombia

Giovanni Carcuro University of the Andes Clinic, Las Condes, Chile

Leandro Casola Foot and Ankle Division, Dupuytren Institute, Ciudad Autónoma de Buenos Aires (CABA), Argentina

Jose Carlos Cohen Foot and Ankle Surgery, Federal University Hospital of Rio De Janeiro/Brazil (UFRJ/ HUCFF), Rio De Janeiro, Brazil

Marco Túlio Costa Hospital Santa Casa de Misericórdia de São Paulo, São Paulo, Brazil

Manuel Cuervas-Mons Orthopedic Surgery and Traumatology Service, Hospital General Universitario Greogrio Marañon, Madrid, Madrid, Spain

Miki Dalmau-Pastor Laboratory of Arthroscopic and Surgical Anatomy, Department of Pathology and Experimental Therapeutics (Human Anatomy Unit), University of Barcelona, Barcelona, Spain

MIFAS by GRECMIP, Merignac, France

Martinez de Albornoz Pilar Quiron salud University Hospital Madrid, Madrid, Spain

Pilar Martínez de Albornoz Orthopaedic Foot and Ankle Unit, Orthopaedic and Trauma Department, Hospital Universitario Quirónsalud Madrid, Madrid, Spain

Jonathan T. Deland Hospital for Special Surgery, New York, NY, USA

Mariano De Prado Service of Orthopedic Surgery and Traumatology, Hospital Quironsalud Murcia, Murcia, Spain

Virginia De Prado Podiatry Service, Hospital Quironsalud Murcia, Murcia, Spain

Pablo J. Echenique Díaz Universidad Austral de Chile, Valdivia, Chile

Hospital Base Valdivia, Los Ríos, Chile

Norman Espinosa Institute for Foot and Ankle Reconstruction Zurich, FussInstitut Zurich, Zurich, Switzerland

Sergio Fernandez C. Clínica Santa María, Servicio de Ortopedia y Traumatología, Equipo de Pie y Tobillo, Santiago, Chile

Jorge Filippi Clínica Las Condes, Santiago, Chile

Hospital del Trabajador, Santiago, Chile

Luis Felipe Hermida Galindo ABC Medical Center, Santa Fe Campus, Ciudad de México, México

Cristian Olmedo Gárate Clinica Alemana de Santiago, Santiago, Chile

Hospital Clínico San Borja Arriarán, Santiago, Chile

Hospital Padre Hurtado, Santiago, Chile

Alexandre Leme Godoy-Santos University of São Paulo/Hospital Israelita Albert Einstein, São Paulo, Brazil

Omar Ituriel Vela Goñi Orthopaedics and Traumatology Institute at Zambrano Hellion Hospital, San Pedro Garza García, Nuevo León, México

Rodrigo Melo Grollmus Department of Orthopedic Surgery, Foot and Ankle Unit, Clinica Las Condes, Santiago, Chile

Department of Orthopedic Surgery, Foot and Ankle Unit, Hospital Militar de Santiago, Santiago, Chile

Hugo Henriquez Clínica Santa María, Servicio de Ortopedia y Traumatología, Equipo de Pie y Tobillo, Santiago, Chile

Instituto Traumatológico de Santiago, Equipo de Pie y Tobillo, Santiago, Chile

John E. Herzenberg International Center for Limb Lengthening, Rubin Institute for Advanced Orthopedics, Sinai Hospital of Baltimore, Baltimore, MD, USA

German Joannas Foot and Ankle Division "CEPP", Dupuytren Institute, Ciudad Autónoma de Buenos Aires (CABA), Argentina

Foot and Ankle Division, Centro Artroscópico Jorge Batista SA, Ciudad Autónoma de Buenos Aires (CABA), Argentina

Foot and Ankle Division, Barrancas Institute, Buenos Aires, Argentina

Anish R. Kadakia Northwestern University – Feinberg School of Medicine, Northwestern Memorial Hospital, Department of Orthopedic Surgery, Chicago, IL, USA

Gabriel Khazen Hospital de Clinicas Caracas, Caracas, Venezuela

Jaeyoung Kim Hospital for Special Surgery, New York, NY, USA

Georg Klammer Institute for Foot and Ankle Reconstruction Zurich, FussInstitut Zurich, Zurich, Switzerland

Markus Knupp University of Basel, Mein Fusszentrum Basel, Basel, Switzerland

Leonardo Lagos Hospital Mutual de Seguridad C. Ch. C., Clínica Santa Maria, Santiago, Chile

Shuyuan Li, MD, PhD Department of Orthopaedics, University of Colorado Anschutz Medical Campus, Aurora, CO, USA

Steps2Walk, Greenwood Village, CO, USA

Valeria Lopez Instituto de Ortopedia y Traumatología Dr. Jaime Slullitel, Rosario, Santa Fe, Argentina

Ernesto Maceira Orthopaedic Foot and Ankle Unit, Complejo Hospitalario La Mancha Centro, Alcázar de San Juan, Ciudad Real, Spain

Nicola Maffulli Department of Musculoskeletal Disorders, Faculty of Medicine and Surgery, University of Salerno, Baronissi, Italy

Clinica Ortopedica, Ospedale San Giovanni di Dio e Ruggi D'Aragona, Salerno, Italy

Queen Mary University of London, Barts and the London School of Medicine and Dentistry, Centre for Sports and Exercise Medicine, Mile End Hospital, London, UK

Keele University, Faculty of Medicine, School of Pharmacy and Bioengineering, Guy Hilton Research Centre, Hartshill, Stoke-on-Trent, UK

Günther Mangelsdorff Department of Plastic Surgery and Burns, Hospital del Trabajador, Santiago, Chile

Department of Plastic Surgery, Clínica Santa Maria, Santiago, Chile

Nacime Salomão Barbachan Mansur Grupo de Medicina e Cirurgia do Pé e Tornozelo, Departamento de Ortopedia e Traumatologia, Escola Paulista de Medicina, Universidade Federal de São Paulo, São Paulo, SP, Brazil

Florencia Pacheco Martinez Instituto de Seguridad del Trabajo Viña del Mar, Clínica Ciudad del Mar, Viña del Mar, Chile

Christine Marx University Center for Orthopaedics, Trauma and Plastic Surgery, University Hospital Carl Gustav Carus at TU Dresden, Dresden, Germany

Cristián Ortiz Mateluna Department of Orthopedic Surgery, Foot and Ankle Unit, Clinica Universidad de los Andes, Santiago, Chile

Philip K. McClure International Center for Limb Lengthening, Rubin Institute for Advanced Orthopedics, Sinai Hospital of Baltimore, Baltimore, MD, USA

Daniel Ribeiro Mendes Foot and Ankle Unit at Hospital Cuf Tejo, Lisbon, Portugal

Pablo Mery Pontificia Universidad Católica de Chile, Santiago, Chile

Roberto Muñoz Molina Clínica Bupa Antofagasta, Universidad de Antofagasta, Antofagasta, Chile

Manuel Monteagudo Quironsalud University Hospital Madrid, Madrid, Spain

Eduardo Fuentes Morales Instituto de Seguridad del Trabajo Viña del Mar, Clínica Ciudad del Mar, Viña del Mar, Chile

Vincent S. Mosca Orthopedics, University of Washington School of Medicine, Seattle, WA, USA

Pediatric Orthopedic Surgeon, Seattle Children's Hospital, Seattle, WA, USA

Pablo Schaufele Muñoz Universidad de Concepción, Concepción, Chile

Hospital Clínico Regional de Concepción Dr. Guillermo Grant Benavente, Biobío, Chile

Mark S. Myerson, MD Department of Orthopaedics, University of Colorado Anschutz Medical Campus, Aurora, CO, USA

Steps2Walk, Greenwood Village, CO, USA

Kyle M. Natsuhara Department of Orthopaedic Surgery, Baylor University Medical Center, Dallas, TX, USA

Caio Nery Hospital Israelita Albert Einstein, São Paulo, Brasil

Joaquín Palma Pontificia Universidad Católica de Chile, Complejo Asistencial Dr. Sótero del Río, Santiago, Chile

Leonardo Parada Department of Plastic Surgery and Burns, Hospital del Trabajador, Santiago, Chile

Department of Plastic Surgery, Clínica Las Condes, Santiago, Chile

Carlos Pargas Sinai Hospital of Baltimore, Baltimore, MD, USA

Manuel J. Pellegrini P. University of the Andes Clinic, Las Condes, Chile

Clinical Hospital of the University of Chile, Santiago, Chile

Rodrigo Pesántez Hospital Universitario Fundación Santa Fé, Universidad de Los Andes, Bogota, Colombia

Marcelo Pires Prado Department of Orthopaedics, Hospital Israelita Albert Einstein, Sao Paulo, SP, Brazil

Hospital Israelita Albert Einstein, Foot and Ankle Department, Sao Paulo, SP, Brazil

Cristian Artigas Preller Universidad de Chile, Santiago, Chile

Hospital de Niños Roberto del Río, Santiago, Chile

Rubén Radkievich Clínica Alemana, Santiago, Chile

Hospital DIPRECA, Santiago, Chile

Stefan Rammelt University Center for Orthopaedics, Trauma and Plastic Surgery, University Hospital Carl Gustav Carus at TU Dresden, Dresden, Germany

Nicolas Valdivia Rojo Servicio de Salud Bio bio, Concepción, Chile

Hospital Base Los Angeles, Concepción, Chile

Sanatorio Alemán, Concepción, Chile

Guilherme Honda Saito Department of Orthopaedics, Hospital Sírio Libanês, Sao Paulo, SP, Brazil

José Antônio Veiga Sanhudo Hospital Moinhos de Vento de Porto Alegre, Porto Alegre, RS, Brazil

Florencio Pablo Segura Universidad Nacional de Córdoba, Nuevo Hospital San Roque, Ciudad de Córdoba, Argentina

Centro Privado de Ortopedia y Traumatología, Ciudad de Córdoba, Argentina

O. Matías Sepúlveda Universidad Austral de Chile, Valdivia, Chile

Hospital Base de Valdivia, Valdivia, Chile

AO Foundation, PAEG Expert Group, Davos, Switzerland

Noman A. Siddiqui International Center for Limb Lengthening/Rubin Institute for Advanced Orthopedics, Sinai Hospital of Baltimore, Baltimore, MD, USA

Brian T. Sleasman Northwestern University – Feinberg School of Medicine, Northwestern Memorial Hospital, Department of Orthopedic Surgery, Chicago, IL, USA

Gaston Slullitel Instituto de Ortopedia y Traumatología Dr. Jaime Slullitel, Rosario, Santa Fe, Argentina

Pablo Sotelano Hospital Italiano de Buenos Aires, Buenos Aires, Argentina

Gino Martínez Clínica Universidad de Los Andes, Santiago, Chile

Instituto Teletón, Santiago, Chile

Manuel Resende Sousa Foot and Ankle Unit at Hospital da Luz, Lisbon, Portugal

Department of Youth Football at Sport Lisboa e Benfica, Lisbon, Portugal

Rafael Barban Sposeto University of São Paulo, São Paulo, Brazil

Octavio Polanco Torres Hospital Regional Talca, Universidad Católica del Maule, Talca, Chile

Jordi Vega Laboratory of Arthroscopic and Surgical Anatomy, Department of Pathology and Experimental Therapeutics (Human Anatomy Unit), University of Barcelona, Barcelona, Spain

Foot and Ankle Unit, iMove Traumatology-Clinica Tres Torres, and Hospital Quirón Barcelona, Barcelona, Spain

MIFAS by GRECMIP, Merignac, France

Foot and Ankle Consultant, Clinique Montchoisi, Lausanne, Switzerland

Gregorio Verschae Clinica Redsalud, Santiago, Chile

João Vide Foot and Ankle Surgeon at Hospital da Luz, Lisbon, Portugal

Foot and Ankle Surgeon at Hospital Particular do Algarve, Faro, Portugal

Arnd F. Viehöfer University Hospital Balgrist, Zurich, Switzerland

Daniel Sebastián Villena Hospital Italiano de Buenos Aires, Buenos Aires, Argentina

Emilio Wagner Hitschfeld Orthopedic Surgery Department, Clínica Alemana de Santiago - Universidad del Desarrollo, Santiago, RM - Santiago, Chile

Pablo Wagner Hitschfeld Orthopedic Surgery Department, Clínica Alemana de Santiago - Universidad del Desarrollo, Hospital Militar de Santiago – Universidad de los Andes, Santiago, RM - Santiago, Chile

Stephan H. Wirth University Hospital Balgrist, Zurich, Switzerland

Roberto Zambelli Serviço de Ortopedia da Rede Mater Dei de Saúde, Belo Horizonte, MG, Brazil

Faculdade de Ciências Médicas de Minas Gerais, Belo Horizonte, MG, Brazil

Tomas Zamora Orthopaedic Oncology and Lower Limb Reconstructive Surgery, Orthopaedic Surgery Department, Pontificia Universidad Católica de Chile, Santiago, Chile

Diego Zanolli Clínica Alemana, Santiago, Chile

Hospital Militar, Santiago, Chile

Jacob R. Zide Department of Orthopaedic Surgery, Baylor University Medical Center, Dallas, TX, USA

Department of Orthopaedic Surgery, UT Southwestern Medical School, Dallas, TX, USA

Department of Surgery, Texas A&M Health Science Center College of Medicine, Dallas, TX, USA

Nicolas Zilleruelo V. Musculoskeletal Radiologist, Clinica Alemana de Santiago, Santiago, Chile

Part I
Basic Science and General Considerations

Foot and Ankle Biomechanics Gait Analysis

Manuel Monteagudo and Pilar Martínez de Albornoz

1   Introduction and History

Biomechanics is the study of mechanical engineering, specifically Newton's laws, applied to the musculoskeletal system. Understanding the biomechanics of the foot and ankle allows us to appreciate the intrinsic and extrinsic function of the components of the system, their mutual relationships, and helps us to understand the pathology, to propose an orthopedic (mechanical) treatment and also a surgical indication. The potential impact of a surgery can be intuited after a biomechanical study of a pathology, and the outcome can be evaluated postoperatively with quantitative and qualitative means. Although the focus of this chapter and this book is the foot and ankle, these body segments cannot be considered as isolated elements but as a kinetic chain that can function in an open and closed manner. The biomechanics of the foot and ankle are intimately related to the knee, hip, and spine.

Gait analysis is the systematic study of the human gait. Since gait is a mechanical process within a biological system, gait analysis allows us to put the knowledge of foot and ankle biomechanics to practical use. We cannot understand or interpret gait without knowing its mechanics. In recent years, gait analysis has gained popularity for its applications in footwear and insole design.

The observation of human gait dates back to the very origin of man. Aristotle, around 340 BC, is credited with the first comments on human gait [1]. However, it was not until the Renaissance that the first systematic studies appeared. Giovanni

M. Monteagudo (✉)
Quironsalud University Hospital Madrid, Madrid, Spain

P. Martínez de Albornoz
Orthopaedic Foot and Ankle Unit, Orthopaedic and Trauma Department, Hospital Universitario Quirónsalud Madrid, Madrid, Spain

E. Wagner Hitschfeld, P. Wagner Hitschfeld (eds.), *Foot and Ankle Disorders*,
https://doi.org/10.1007/978-3-030-95738-4_1

3

Alfonso Borelli was a physicist and mathematician who made notable contributions to medicine as a pioneer in the school of iatromechanics [2]. Iatrophysics or iatro-mechanics was a current in the medical sciences that developed in the seventeenth century and sought the application of physics to provide an answer to the questions of human physiology and pathology. The explanation of biological phenomena was based on the assumption that living beings functioned as if they were machines. In his work *De Motu Animalium*, published in 1680, Borelli measured the center of gravity of the human body and described how we maintain our balance during walking with the constant forward movement of the support zone provided by the feet. Other Renaissance classics such as Leonardo da Vinci, Galileo, and Newton also gave us useful descriptions of human gait [1]. In 1836, the Weber brothers in Germany gave us the first clear description of gait and made precise measurements of the gait times and pendulum swing of a cadaver leg [1].

Two pioneers of kinematic gait measurements worked in the 1870s, far apart geographically. In Paris, Marey published a study of human limb movements in 1873 and plotted the body's center of gravity and the pressures recorded in the feet [3]. In 1878, Muybridge made a name for himself in California by demonstrating that, when a horse trotted, there were times when all four legs were in the air. Measurements were made using 24 cameras that were triggered in rapid succession as the horse touched fine threads placed on the race track. Muybridge also conducted studies of naked human bodies walking, running, and performing other kinds of amazing activities [3].

In 1895, Braune and Fischer's knowledge of three-dimensional trajectories, velocities, and accelerations of different body segments were incorporated in the book *Der Gang des Menschen* [4]. In the 1930s, Bernstein studied in Moscow the center of gravity of each segment of the lower limbs and of the whole body [1]. Amar in 1924 and Elftman in 1938 developed the first gait platforms that contributed significantly to the scientific study of gait [1]. In the 1940s, Scherb in Switzerland studied the musculature and its activation during gait with the use of electromyography [2]. In the 1950s, a group of researchers at the University of California led by Inman and Eberhart integrated many of the existing studies and eventually published *Human Walking*, one of the universal reference books in the study of gait [5]. Sutherland and Perry pioneered the clinical applications of gait analysis in America and Rose and Baumann in Europe [6, 7]. Gage developed in recent decades the study of gait in neurological diseases, with modern imaging techniques in his laboratory [8, 9]. Kirtley wrote one of the reference works – *Clinical Gait Analysis* – for understanding the latest advances in gait analysis and has developed numerous Internet resources for the study of gait mechanics [3]. The development of computer engineering with modern computers has universalized gait studies in recent years.

2   Human Gait

Human gait is a form of bipedal locomotion, with alternating activity of the lower limbs and maintenance of dynamic balance [10]. The phasic action of the lower limbs is described in terms of a series of events that occur repeatedly, constituting the so-called gait cycle [6]. In an arbitrary manner (an easily recorded event), the start of the gait cycle is taken as the contact of a limb with the ground, so that the end of the cycle is reached when the same limb contacts the ground again [6]. During this time interval, a series of events will allow the cycle to be divided into distinct phases and periods (Fig. 1). The first consideration in understanding these divisions is whether or not the limb contacts the ground. The phases of stance (60%) and swing (40%) are thus defined. The activity of the opposite limb in normal gait is similar to that of the reference limb but offset by half a cycle as the stance period is longer than the swing period. There will thus be two subphases of simultaneous support of the two limbs: the initial double support (braking double support) and the final double support (thrusting double support), each of which will account for around 10% of the cycle and determine the loading response and pre-swing periods, respectively [11]. From the above it can be deduced that during gait there is always contact of at least one foot with the ground. However, in other forms of locomotion such as running, there are periods of flight in which none of the lower limbs contact the ground. Running is a succession of jumps [12]. In race walking, disqualification from sport occurs when the participant moves forward without maintaining contact with the ground [13].

Under normal conditions, the initial contact with the ground is made with the heel, and the rest of the foot descends progressively to a plantigrade position. This position is reached approximately when the opposite limb lifts off the ground. During this interval, which coincides with the initial double stance, the lower supporting limb takes the heel as a fulcrum. When the foot is plantigrade, and until the heel separates from the ground, the ankle becomes the pivot fulcrum, which defines the intermediate stance period (midstance) that occupies between 10% and 30% of the gait cycle. As soon as the heel is no longer in contact with the ground, the forefoot becomes the fulcrum on which the supporting limb progresses. The interval during which the only contact of the body with the ground is the forefoot of the reference limb is known as the terminal stance period (30–50% of the cycle) and ends when the

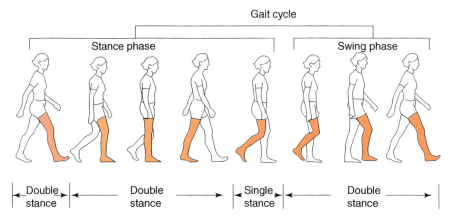

Fig. 1 The gait cycle with its different phases of stance (60%), swing (40%), and rockers

double push-off begins, i.e., when the opposite foot contacts the ground. From this moment on, although from a descriptive point of view the limb under study continues to be in stance phase with the forefoot as fulcrum, preparing for the next flight when it is freed from the support of the body weight. The opposite limb progressively assumes this load, which is why the interval between the contact of the opposite foot and the take-off of the homolateral foot (final double support or push-off) is also known as the pre-balance period (50–60%) [14].

In gait analysis terminology, the periods of stance during which the anterograde rotation of the tibia occurs on each of these three fulcrums are known as rockers [6]. Each of these rockers requires active muscular control to effectively ensure the coexistence of two phenomena that are in principle difficult to reconcile: the achievement of a stable stance and the maintenance of progression. From a mechanical point of view, the rockers are responsible for controlling the point of application of the ground reaction force vector (GRF) which, under normal conditions, progressively advances from the heel towards the forefoot on the first ray. The representation of each of the ground reaction force vectors throughout the stance period gives rise to a diagram that has been compared to the wings of a butterfly. Each of these vectors is applied more distally each time than the previous one and points towards the instantaneous position of the body center of mass. This is with the exception of the first recordings, in which the first vectors do not point towards the center of mass at the initial contact, but in a vertical direction, revealing the character of the free fall experienced after the swing. Jacqueline Perry divided the gait cycle into three rockers to explain the different leg-foot-floor interactions [6].

First rocker: The control of the first rocker is due to the ankle dorsiflexor muscles (L5 root) which work in eccentric action (during their contraction their points of origin and insertion move away). Our muscles are more effective when working in eccentric action than when working in concentric action and resist isometric action very well. The main ankle dorsiflexor is the tibialis anterior, assisted by the extensor digitorum longus and modulated by the extensor hallucis longus and peroneus tertius (Fig. 2). Functional failure of the extensor digitorum longus leads to persistent

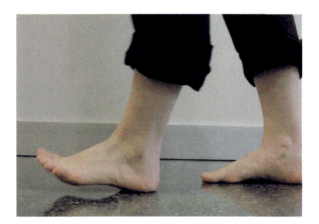

Fig. 2 First rocker ("heel rocker"). Photograph at slow shutter speed showing the descent of the foot and heel contact. The extensor digitorum longus, along with the peroneus tertius, modulates the Achilles tendon and extensor hallucis longus during swing and initial contact

abnormal foot roll in inversion, especially if the peroneal tertius is missing, which occurs in about 10% of the normal population [15]. Global failure of the dorsiflexors, whether primary (flaccid paralysis of the dorsiflexors) or secondary (spastic triceps paralysis or passive block to ankle dorsiflexion), will produce an abnormal first rocker, which may be shortened in time (abrupt and uncontrolled descent of the sole of the foot) producing an "audible clap" as the foot slumps to the ground, or even not present at all. The absence of the first rocker obviously occurs when the initial contact is made with the forefoot (severe equinus) or with the entire sole (moderate equinus) (Fig. 3). There is another form of mild or subclinical equinus in which the initial contact is made with the heel but the relative duration of the first rocker is reduced; its clinical importance lies in the tendency of the subtalar joint to compensate for the lack of ankle dorsiflexion with persistent eversion to achieve a "pseudodorsiflexion" of the foot, which can end up producing a plano-valgus deformity and/or metatarsalgia of the central rays due to insufficiency of the first when the plantar aponeurosis and the peroneus longus are unable to stabilize the first metatarsal against the ground.

Second rocker: The second roll, known as the ankle rocker, occurs while the foot under study adopts a plantigrade stance (Fig. 4). The rotation of the lower limb that allows the progression of the body's center of mass is performed by taking the

Fig. 3 Neurological equinus. Absence of conventional first rocker. The first rocker is over the forefoot

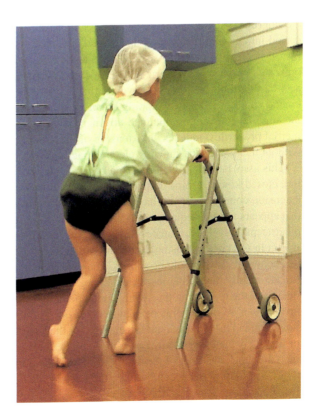

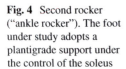

Fig. 4 Second rocker ("ankle rocker"). The foot under study adopts a plantigrade support under the control of the soleus

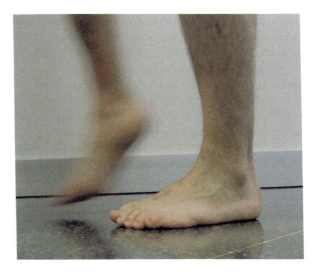

"supra-ankle" joint as the fulcrum. Its control is due to the soleus (S1 root), the monoarticular element of the triceps suralis, which brakes the advancement of the tibia over the talus. The muscle undergoes a remarkable electromyographic activation, just as soon as the center of mass moves forward with respect to the vertical to the fulcrum. This reference makes it possible to subdivide the intermediate stance period into an initial subphase and a final subphase. In the latter, the tibia is tilted forward with respect to the vertical to the ankle axis, and the activation of the soleus brakes its advance in eccentric action. In classical anatomy, it is stated that a muscle acts on the joints it crosses. However, the eccentric action of the soleus in closed kinetic chain produces a whipping effect on the knee so that, by braking the tibia, the simultaneous and maintained advance of the body center of mass (due to its inertial properties) induces an extension of the knee during the intermediate stance without the quadriceps showing electrical activity.

This association of plantar flexion of the ankle (made impossible by the ground in a closed kinetic chain) with knee extension is known as the ankle-flexion/knee-extension couple [6, 8] and has its pathological expression in the knee recurvatum that appears as a consequence of rigid equinus deformities of the foot and ankle. The quadriceps actively participates just before the initial contact, to collaborate with the inertia in the knee extension at the end of the swing. Should the quadriceps not do this action, the step would be shorter. The extension of the knee during the swing is fundamentally due to the inertia of the leg-foot segments that produces the active flexion of the hip during the swing (fundamentally by the action of the psoas). The involvement of the quadriceps in knee extension is a matter of velocity: the inertial forces extend the knee, but not fast enough for the knee to be extended at the moment of initial contact. The quadriceps is also still active during the initial contact, being then the shock absorber of the first peak of knee flexion. But the quadriceps is inactive when, during the second rocker, the knee is extended to functionally lengthen the supporting limb.

Fig. 5 Third rocker ("forefoot rocker"). The generation of power at the ankle pushes up the body's center of mass and allows the foot to take off

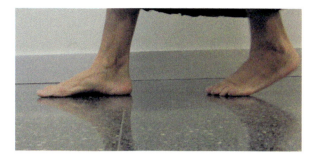

Third rocker: The third rocker, or forefoot rocker, comprises 30% of the total cycle (30–60%) and 50% of the stance period. Maintenance of gait progression is executed with a roll over the metatarsophalangeal "break point" (Fig. 5). The knee, which during the intermediate period had been extended, initiates its second peak of flexion when the opposite limb contacts the ground. The control of the third rocker is no longer due only to the soleus but to the entire triceps suralis including its biarticular component, the gastrocnemius. During the initial two thirds of the third rocker (30–50% of the cycle: period of final support or terminal stance), contact with the ground is exclusive to the homolateral limb, with the greatest degree of muscular activity being registered in the calf, with a peak of power generation in the ankle (concentric action). When the opposite limb contacts the ground (50% of the cycle), the homolateral limb begins to unload, preparing for the swing (pre-swing), and knee flexion accelerates, reaching its peak in the swing. This can be seen in the curve of the kinematic record of the knee in the sagittal plane. The double hump of a camel corresponds to the first peak of flexion as a damping mechanism (resisted by the monoarticular components of the quadriceps in eccentric action) and to the second which ensures the advancement of the limb and the clearance of the foot from the ground. The active flexion of the hip by the psoas is determinant for the achievement of the second peak of knee flexion. This situation is possible by making use of the inertial properties of a body segment, in this case, the leg. This led authors as relevant in the study of gait analysis as J Perry, to consider the end of stance phase as a pull-off rather than a push-off (Fig. 6) [1]. The power generation peak at the ankle is a true push-off that raises the body center of mass at final stance, increasing its potential energy to the detriment of its kinetic component. But the hip drag component during pre-swing is also indisputable [8].

Normal gait has five attributes that must be considered and kept in mind in order to judge whether it is pathological or not: [9]

1. Stability during stance.
2. Clearance of the foot from the ground during the swing.
3. Proper stride length.
4. Correct prepositioning of the foot for initial contact.
5. Conservation of energy.

Fig. 6 Posterior view of a normal foot in third rocker, already in pre-balance phase. Note the inversion of the heel and the correct functioning of the windlass mechanism. At this point, the length of the metatarsals (especially relative among them) is important as a factor in generating overload

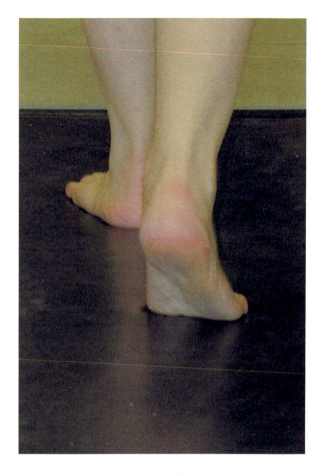

3 Mechanical Functioning of the Ankle and Foot During Gait

It is very important for the clinician to be aware of the relative foot-floor position – the contact pattern – during each of the three rockers and to understand what the mission of the foot is during each of these three periods of gait.

The first rocker involves heel contact with the ground, and its primary function is to cushion impact. The entire lower limb, together with the axial skeleton, participates in this cushioning effect. The trunk erector muscles, the hip flexors, the extensor apparatus of the knee, and the viscoelastic properties of the plantar fibroadipose tissue contribute to the cushioning of the initial contact. In the foot there is a very peculiar shock absorption mechanism, which uses the phenomenon of the variable configuration of the plantar vault. This mechanism provided by the tarsal joints in response to load is due to tarsal pronation. Pronation is passive, and occurs because the point of contact of the heel with the ground is slightly outside the projection of the axis of the leg. If it coincided exactly with it, no movement would be produced in the subtalar joint at the moment of initial contact. If the heel is too far inside the projection of the leg, the foot will tend to twist into supination. This occurs in severe varus feet, in which the peroneals (especially the shortened peroneals) end up being victims of the effort in eversion required from them and for which they are not prepared (Fig. 7). When heel and leg are coaxial, a significant part of the cushioning is simply lost after the initial contact, which will end up being paid for by the upper segments in the form of overload injuries. This situation occurs in the mildest forms of varus foot. If, on the other hand, the heel is too far outward with respect to the projection of the leg, the external (passive) pronator moment that the foot will have to withstand after initial contact will be of such magnitude that the inverters will eventually be overwhelmed, giving way. The passive soft tissues, which together with the skeletal architecture are the main maintainers of the plantar vault, will become distended by the cumulative tensile damage, and the foot will eventually claudicate in a progressive pronation. The invertors (muscles), primarily the tibialis posterior, do not directly oppose to the flattening of the vault, but rather their function is to position the tarsal skeleton in such a way as to avoid joint overload positions. The tibialis posterior, in particular, rotates the leg externally, which induces a supination in the foot that causes the lax foot that had served to cushion to transform (along the second rocker) into a stiff foot, an effective propellant for the third rocker. A shock absorber can be ineffective by being excessively hard or excessively soft. When it is hard, the upper segments pay for it, and when it is soft, the lower and distal segments pay for it.

The second rocker corresponds to the period of monopodal support. The contact pattern with the ground is plantigrade, which will determine the lesional morphology of the plantar soft tissues. The stance foot during this phase is responsible for supporting the entire body weight, for which it has the most stable contact pattern. The limb must be stretched to its greatest possible length, so that the opposite foot, which is flying, does not collide with the ground. The tarsus, which started from a

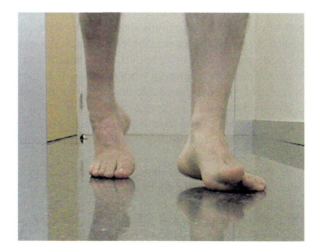

Fig. 7 If the heel is inside the axis of leg projection, the foot is twisted in supination. In this case, a patient with cavovarus feet who consulted for chronic peroneal pain and ankle instability

pronated position at the beginning of the second rocker, has to move into a supinated position, as mentioned above. The leg has to move from the talus-driven internal rotation due to pronation to an external rotation that places the head of the talus over the anterior process of the calcaneus. The passive pronation of the foot is transmitted by the talus to the leg in the form of internal rotation, and the active external rotation of the leg is transmitted to the foot in the form of supination, by means of the external rotation of the talus. The second rocker is controlled exclusively by the soleus. The calves are electrically silent during this rocker under normal conditions, so as not to produce a flexor moment in the knee, which would be undesirable because of the need to maintain as long a leg as possible. But there may be cases of relative retraction of the inactive elastic component of the calf, which could generate overloads at different levels of the foot, as long as the knee remains extended. Some authors see in these forms of equinism the evolutionary vestiges of the adaptation of the foot from a quadruped and equinized foot to a bipodal plantigrade foot, in which the heel has descended to the ground. The unanswered question is how much is equinus? Most of the population will probably barely, if at all, reach neutral ankle position when the inverted foot is brought into passive dorsiflexion and the knee remains extended. Equinism can be defined as the inability to achieve adequate heel to ground contact in static stance with the knee fully extended, without having to resort to pronation of the foot to provide additional intrinsic midtarsal dorsiflexion [16].

The function of the third rocker is to provide the necessary propulsion to allow elevation of the body center of mass. It should always be noted that here only the forefoot contacts the ground through the digit-plantar eminence and that the metatarsal is vertical to the ground. The load is passed from the external rays, protagonists during the second rocker, to the talar foot, protagonist of propulsion. The first three metatarsals are verticalized and – through three intermediate pieces, the cuneiforms – hold the navicular to the talus, so that it acts as a saddle: the "navicular stool". If the inner leg of this stool fails, the stool can tilt towards it and cause the talus to slip into adduction. If the alignment of the stool is correct, and the talus sits properly aligned on it at the third rocker, the calcaneus will behave like a wheelbarrow lifted by the triceps suralis and balanced by the other plantar flexors. But these plantar flexors, inverters or eversors, must act on a well-aligned skeleton. If proper osteoarticular alignment is not achieved, triceps and ground reaction forces can worsen skeletal malalignment when the capacity of the active and passive stabilizers is exceeded. What the foot has to do during this third rocker is to form (with the leg) a firm lever that slightly elevates the body center of mass, which advances by its moment of inertia. The transition from the second to the third rocker is a critical moment for many reasons, comparable to the moment when the pole vaulter drives his pole into the ground.

It involves a large concentric, acceleration, and power flow activity at the ankle joint. It also involves the application of a net force on the ground greater than body weight, as occurred after initial contact. With regard to the clinical applications of the mechanical study of gait, injuries that occur in this transition exhibit characteristics of both rockers, as will be seen later, which can make their identification and the establishment of the pathogenesis in a particular case difficult. On the other hand, not a few patients present disorders that produce undesirable effects during the second rocker and simultaneously others that do so during the third. External rotational forces can overcome rotational frictional forces, allowing many subjects to make a true external rotation of the foot on the ground during the third rocker. The final third of this rocker is no longer propulsive but prepares the limb for swing. The plantar flexors are activated sequentially but cease to act as the opposing limb is loaded. The third rocker requires adequate passive dorsiflexion of the toes. When the first radius loses the ability to dorsiflex while supporting body weight (functional hallux limitus), the foot can no longer rocker on the first metatarsophalangeal joint, but does so on the interphalangeal joint of the big toe, forcing the foot to supinate, with the consequent overloading of the distal end of the most lateral rays. This model explains the frequent association between functional hallux limitus and neuropathic pain of the third interdigital space, eventually leading to the development of a neuroma.

4   Gait Study

Gait analysis is the systematic study of human gait using the eyes and brain of experienced observers, supplemented by tools to measure body movements, body mechanics, and muscle activity [17]. In people with walking problems, gait analysis can be used to make a diagnosis and plan appropriate treatment.

Gait analysis can be approached from two points of view: qualitative and quantitative. In the first case, essential for any clinician, the aim is to describe the movement of the different body segments during gait based on visual inspection. It is necessary to have a sufficiently large open space for the subject to reach his normal cadence, something complicated in most of our (small) offices. The use of video recordings is very convenient, not only because of the possibility of repeating the inspection as many times as necessary but also because the human eye is incapable of recording beyond the equivalent of about 12–14 frames per second. The key to qualitative gait analysis lies in following a systematic, personal approach for each observer, so that the events seen in each of the body segments and in each of the planes of space are described in an orderly fashion, keeping in mind the five attributes of normal gait [18, 19]. A good visual gait analysis should be the beginning of any examination of a patient who consults us for a foot or ankle problem.

Biomechanical gait analysis is based on the quantification of the movement of body segments (kinematics), the forces produced as a consequence of the movement (kinetics), and complementary parameters such as muscle electrical activity and energy consumption [14, 20]. Lord Kelvin said that when one succeeded in converting a problem into a number, it ceased to be a problem [3]. Quantitative analysis requires the use of expensive equipment and highly specialized medical, engineering, and technical personnel. Its fundamental clinical application is the study of gait in infantile cerebral palsy, both to plan the appropriate treatment and to assess its results from a mechanical point of view [8]. Prosthetic fitting in amputees, the assessment of joint replacements, and the study of other neuro-orthopedic injuries are clinical fields in which quantitative gait analysis has, and will have important applications [21].

In one of the gait quantification systems (Vicon, Oxford Metrics), kinematic recording is based on stereophotogrammetry, a procedure by which the position of a series of markers in space is determined in real time. Once the position and orientation of two cameras in space with respect to a given theoretical center of coordinates are known, the pairs of coordinates (2D) with which each camera records a point (marker) can be integrated to determine the 3D coordinates of that point with respect to the Cartesian system. In this case the markers are passive, reflecting the infrared light emitted by the cameras themselves via a stroboscopic flash, and are fixed at specific anatomical locations on the subject to define the body segments pelvis, thigh, leg, and foot [18]. When using the standard Vicon Conventional Gait Model (CGM) program for the generation of kinematic and/or kinetic registration plots (Helen Hayes marker set), each body segment is actually a plane and is defined by three points, except in the case of the foot, which is an actual segment defined by only two points (which prevents inversion-eversion from being assessed) [22].

The kinetic recording of ground reaction forces is carried out with force platforms (AMTI) [6]. These record the components of the GRF vector in the three axes of space (vertical, transverse, and longitudinal). A computer system integrates the kinematic data with the ground reaction force vector (GRF) and by a calculation procedure known as inverse dynamics it deduces the internal forces necessary to generate the recorded movement [17]. To do this, it is also necessary to provide the computer with some anthropometric parameters of the subject, such as weight, height, ankle and knee width, etc., with which it can estimate the theoretical joint centers and inertial properties of each body segment. This whole study, which can nowadays be carried out in a few minutes thanks to data capture and processing systems, was developed by Braune and Fischer and presented in their book *Der Gang des Menschen* at the end of the nineteenth century, and it took them 9 years (1895–1904) to complete: three-dimensional mechanical gait analysis [4].

Finally, dynamic electromyography provides insight into the phasic electrical activity of a muscle (needle electrodes) or muscle group (surface electrodes). It cannot record the muscle force generated; it only detects whether there is electrical activity or not [3]. By knowing the joint kinematics, it can be determined whether the muscle is working in concentric or eccentric action. Much of the muscle activity in general during gait is braking, in eccentric action, with the corresponding absorption of power. The fifth attribute of normal gait refers precisely to the conservation of energy, through its transfer from one body segment to another, and to the transformation of kinetic energy to potential and vice versa of the center of mass. The kinetic component is maximum in the periods of double support and minimum in those of monopodal support, occurring inversely with the potential component. The processing of the data obtained allows the elaboration of graphs that represent the angular movement, the moments, and the generation or absorption of power (product of the other two curves) in each joint and in each of the three planes of space (Fig. 8).

Fig. 8 Patient with post-polio sequelae. The right lower limb is the least affected but presents a rigid equinus of the ankle that has produced a recurvatum of the knee by the "ankle-flexion-knee-extension" mechanism. The position of the tibia would correspond to an early stage of the second rocker (early period of intermediate stance), but the body center of mass is markedly advanced. Note the anterior pelvic tilt; this is usually due to hip flexor retraction, but in this case, it is due to gluteus maximus weakness

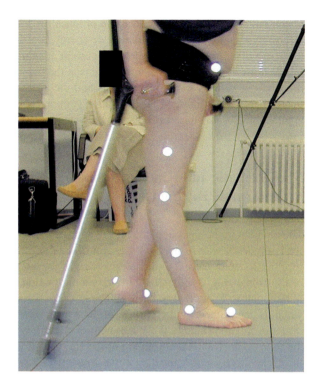

Gait is a learned process [10]. It is one of the most difficult movement patterns to acquire but, once learned, it is performed almost subconsciously [11]. Each individual's gait is so peculiar that we can identify someone without seeing them, just by the sound of their footsteps [3]. (Kirtley) We each have a peculiar way of walking, precisely because gait is a learned process. However, if we graphically represent the movement of each joint (kinematics) or the forces involved in that movement (kinetics), we can consider that there are patterns of normality, similar curves among healthy individuals, which are altered in pathological conditions.

The quantification of any natural phenomenon is an essential achievement to be able to study it from a scientific point of view. The current technological development offers different motion capture systems, thanks to which we can quantify and graphically represent what happens in each of the major joints during gait. Since the progression takes place in the sagittal plane, it is in this plane that the largest amplitude joint movements are recorded, both in the hip and in the knee and ankle. On the other hand, we also have devices that record the ground reaction forces in the three planes of space. We know from Newton's third law that the same forces will be acting along our lower extremities in magnitude and direction but in the opposite direction: the recording, in real time, of joint movements and ground reaction forces allows, by the inverse dynamics method and knowing the inertial parameters of the various body segments (mass and its distribution), the location of the joint centers of rotation and the disposition of the muscles with respect to the joints, to determine which motor actions were necessary to produce the recorded movement. Dynamic electromyography and the estimation of energy consumption, mainly through the exchange of O_2 and CO_2, complete the current quantitative analysis of human gait, whose most important clinical applications at the beginning of this millennium are the study of various forms of paralysis and the adaptation of orthoprosthetic elements, but its potential field of application is impressive with much more profitable applications such as the world of video games.

5 Kinematic and Kinetic Recordings of the Hip, Knee, and Ankle During Gait

The hip joint in the sagittal plane makes initial contact in flexion (Fig. 9). This flexion is about 40° with respect to the anatomical axis of the pelvis, which is equivalent to about 30° with respect to the vertical axis of the laboratory, since the anterior tilt of the pelvic ring is about 10°. Its maximum flexion is reached shortly after the initial contact. From that point it will progressively extend until it reaches a peak which is determined by the tension of the soft tissues ventral to the instantaneous center of rotation (mainly the Y ligament of Bertin), which occurs at about 50% of the total cycle. The total amplitude of the arc of motion is about 40°. At the end of the cycle, shortly before the next initial contact, it must be flexed, for which it relies on the action of the psoas and the inertial properties of the distal segments of the limb, since their combined mass is considerable. On the coronal plane, its kinetic behavior is very important; during the stance phase, the body weight generates an adductor moment which tends to lower the opposite hemipelvis. The abductors as a whole, captained by the gluteus medius, must generate an important action, initially eccentric, to oppose with a shorter moment arm, the weight of the passenger segment (HAT segment: head, arms, trunk) and that of the opposite motor segment, which have a greater moment arm with respect to the instantaneous center of rotation of the hip in support [6]. On the transverse plane, the rotation of the pelvis

Fig. 9 Kinematics of the hip joint in the sagittal plane

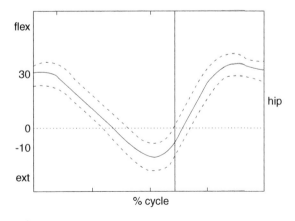

determines the movement of the hip. Initial contact is made with the ipsilateral hemipelvis maximally forward (hip external rotation) and during stance is lagging behind the contralateral hemipelvis (hip internal rotation). The internal moment generation requirements of the hip joint in the transverse plane explain the predominance of the external rotator musculature over the internal rotators. Internal rotation is largely passive, generated by an external moment due to the inertia of the opposite limb, while external rotation, which must occur during swing, is active [3].

The kinematic registration curve of the knee in the sagittal plane reproduces a double hump silhouette, with the first one having a smaller amplitude (Fig. 10). There is a first flexion peak that occurs during stance, the purpose of which is to cushion the impact of the initial contact. The first flexion peak may be absent in healthy subjects, sometimes because they perform the stance with the knee in recurvatum ("recurvatum gait") and sometimes because they walk at low speed, which decreases the damping needs. The upward ramp of damping flexion is controlled by the quadriceps in eccentric action, except for the anterior rectus, which would undesirably flex the hip during this period. After the flexion peak, which reaches approximately 15°, knee extension occurs during intermediate stance, the mission of which is to lengthen the effective length of the stance limb to facilitate the clearance of the opposing limb which is in swing. During this extension peak, the quadriceps remains inactive, a fact that can be seen on dynamic electromyography. Knee extension during intermediate stance is controlled by the soleus. Although in classical anatomy it is said that a muscle acts on the joints it crosses, the soleus is the only portion of the triceps suralis that does not cross the knee. The explanation lies in the fact that, during stance, the limb works in a closed kinetic chain (the fixed point of the muscles is the distal one). The inertia of the HAT or passenger segment due to the progression of the body center of mass, together with the brake to the anterograde rotation that the tibia would tend to perform on the ankle (for which the monoarticular portion of the triceps suralis is responsible) during the intermediate stance period, generates a net extensor moment in the knee. It is not desirable for the knee to hyperextend. In this position, the joint geometry forces locking (locking position or maximum stability) which is achieved and maintained passively by the screwing in of the femur and is very useful during static standing but requires an active

Fig. 10 Knee joint kinematics in the sagittal plane

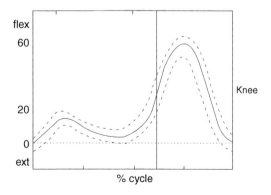

mechanism, the action of the popliteus muscle/tendon, for unlocking. If during walking we were to require an additional muscular action to unlock the knee, it would be energetically more costly and less efficient. The second flexion peak, or swing flexion, is greater than the first (around 60°), and its mission is to enable the ipsilateral limb to clear by shortening its effective length. By clearance, we mean the establishment of sufficient space between the limb and the ground to avoid contact between the two during swing. The upward slope of this second hump is greater, indicating a higher swing speed in flexion. The final extension of the knee is largely due to the inertia of the leg-foot segments, under the thigh segment being braked by the gluteus maximus. But as a matter of timing (speed), the inertial action must be completed by the action of the quadriceps; otherwise, simply with the participation of the inertial extensor moment, the knee would not reach an adequate extension at the initial contact, and the step would be shorter (which would also decrease the efficiency of gait). To modulate that active extension produced by the quadriceps as a whole (including the rectus anterior), hamstring involvement is necessary, so that just prior to initial contact, both knee flexors and extensors are active.

From a kinematic point of view in the sagittal plane, the ankle joint is represented by a more complex curve than those of the hip and knee, with two peaks of plantar flexion and two peaks of dorsiflexion (Fig. 11). The initial contact is made with the heel, the ankle joint being in neutral position. Immediately there is a passive plantar flexion of low amplitude (about 5°) as the tibia rotates forward almost as much as the sole of the foot descends. The period between initial contact and contact of the forefoot with the ground corresponds to the first rocker. During this interval, the anterograde rotation of the tibia takes the heel as its fulcrum, which is why it is also known as the heel rocker. In the kinematic recording graph, the first rocker is represented by the descending portion of a "scoop," whose peak of plantar flexion is reached at 10% of the cycle according to most authors, although it probably represents a somewhat shorter duration. Once the forefoot contacts the ground, the anterograde rotation of the tibia ceases to occur on the heel and takes as its fulcrum the geometric center of the talar trochlea. The direction of rotation is

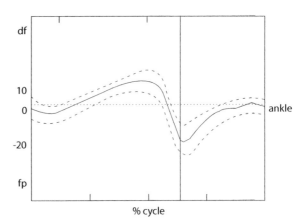

Fig. 11 Kinematics of the ankle joint in the sagittal plane

inverted towards (passive) dorsal flexion. The slope of the curve is greater in the first part of the dorsiflexion to reduce later. The second rocker, or ankle rocker, lasts until the heel comes off the ground, which is about 30% of the cycle. This is the intermediate stance period and is characterized by the plantigrade nature of the contact of the foot with the ground. From 30% of the cycle until a little over 60% at the end of the stance phase, the contact of the foot with the ground is made exclusively on the forefoot; this period corresponds to the third rocker or forefoot rocker. The continuous anterograde rotation of the tibia will then take place taking as fulcrum the metatarsophalangeal break point, which is actually a parabolic line. In the kinematic record, the first peak of dorsiflexion is reached, which is around 10–15 degrees according to different researchers [1, 3, 6]. Then, at high speed (steep slope), plantar flexion is performed at the ankle until a second maximum peak of about 10–20° is reached; the total amplitude of the ankle flexion-extension arch in the sagittal plane during normal gait is approximately 30–35°. Interestingly, most American studies attribute, of the total ankle flexion-extension motion, a greater amplitude to plantar flexion than to dorsal flexion from neutral [6], whereas our records consistently show (coinciding, e.g., with Korean studies) a predominance of dorsal over plantar flexion [16]. During the swing phase, the ankle must contribute to foot clearance by returning to dorsiflexion, although it is the functional shortening of the limb, provided by the knee, that is the most important component in avoiding toe-off during flight. The critical moment of foot-ground clearance occurs when both feet are adjacent; at that instant the separation between the foot and the ground is about 10–15 mm, which gives an idea of how easy it would be to stumble when one of the clearing mechanisms fails. In some healthy individuals, the second peak of dorsiflexion is missing; the clearance provided by the knee is sufficient, and they do not require additional ankle dorsiflexion to avoid toe strike with the ground during swing. If we study the generation of internal plantar flexor moments (assigning the + sign to plantar flexion) at the ankle during the cycle, we will see an initial negative dipper (the active muscle action would oppose plantar flexion; it would be dorsiflexive), followed by a progressive, and therefore positive, plantar flexion action. The plantar flexor moment reaches its peak in the propulsive phase, just before the pre-swing, which is determined by the support of the opposite limb, and then drops sharply and remains practically nil during the swing. From the kinetic point of view in the sagittal plane, the control of the landing of the sole of the forefoot during the first rocker is performed by the dorsiflexors as a whole, captained by the tibialis anterior and modulated by the common extensor digitorum and the third peroneus when present. Failure of these muscles, primarily the tibialis anterior, will shorten (or even obliterate) the first rocker, and an audible slap is often produced when the forefoot contacts the ground in an uncontrolled manner. L5 root lesions typically result in this phenomenon, which clinically may be evidenced by the inability to heel walk. If the tibialis anterior is functioning, but the common extensor and peroneus tertius are not, the foot will contact the ground in inversion, so the prepositioning of the foot for initial contact will be inadequate and will promote instability. The protagonism of the second rocker is carried by the soleus that, in eccentric action, stops the inertial advance of the tibia and extends the knee during the intermediate support. Plantar flexion of the ankle during stance (closed kinetic chain) is associated with knee extension, known as the "ankle plantarflexion-knee extension couple." [6, 8] In its pathological form, equinization of the foot is compensated by a recurvatum of the knee (Fig. 12). The soleus is the only portion of the triceps suralis active during intermediate stance (second rocker). If the gastrocnemius muscles were also activated during this period, undesirable knee flexion would occur. Well into the third rocker, the soleus is joined by the gastrocnemius. In concentric action, they will produce a plantar flexion whose mechanical objective is to raise the body's center of mass (provide potential energy) and then release it in the next free fall, the next step. *Human gait is a succession of potentially catastrophic free fall situations.* During most of the cycle, muscular activity is directed towards the control or braking (eccentric action) of this succession of free falls. Only during the propulsive phase, there is a net generation of power (power +) at the level of the ankle, which involves acceleration. When a child swings, he gives himself momentum by rising on the ropes in the upward leg of his swing, in order to initiate the next swing from a greater height, which will subsequently give him more kinetic energy, more speed. In the inverted pendulum model, the generation of potential energy at the end of the support is also obtained by the elevation of the

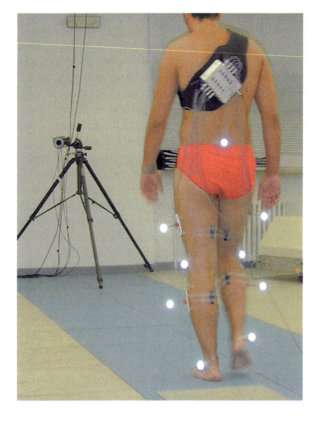

Fig. 12 Patient under study with surface EMG recording equipment (Motion Lab.) and reflective markers. In the foreground, one of the force platforms (AMTI) can be seen and in the background one of the cameras with infrared light stroboscopic flash

center of masses. It is the potential energy that will be transformed into kinetic energy at the end of the next swing and must be absorbed after the initial contact and so on and so forth.

6   Practical Applications

In recent years, we have made progress in the indications and treatment of foot and ankle disorders thanks to a better understanding of the underlying mechanical problem. The human body is capable of compensating to unsuspected limits for a constitutional ("factory-fitted") mechanical problem. Sometimes compensations hide or make it very difficult to detect or diagnose a problem [16]. Diagnosis in our specialty is a science, but it is also an art in order to know which part of the problem is due to the primary problem and which part is due to compensation. For example, a valgus flatfoot that is evident on a visual gait analysis in consultation may be completely "normal" on weightbearing x-rays if the patient still keeps his compensatory mechanisms active and functional ("the minute of glory of a weight-bearing x-ray") [23]. Even if there is no obvious abduction on the x-ray, it does exist in real life, so it would be a mistake to plan potential surgery on the x-ray and not on the patient's gait pattern in consultation. The knowledge of the "sagittal plane" has made us change the concepts of conservative and surgical treatment of disorders affecting the Achilles-calcaneal-plantar system and its understanding of its pathogenesis [24]. The knowledge of the pathomechanics of amputations has greatly improved the functional prognosis of diabetic foot and orthopedic aids [20, 21].

Industry has developed a multitude of its products in an attempt to complement the attributes of human gait. Rocker-soled shoes are an example of this and allow for a considerable decrease in the mechanical requirements of patients who have a problem in the transition between the first and third rockers of gait (e.g., hallux rigidus, ankle osteoarthritis) [25]. The world of artificial prostheses for amputees is an example of integration between mechanical knowledge, gait analysis, and bioengineering and industrial development.

7   Resources

Resources for the study of gait are currently available on the internet at sites such as http://www.clinicalgaitanalysis.com/, run by Kirtley, which is a fantastic gateway to this exciting world. The ESMAC (European Society for Movement Analysis in Adults and Children) has its website at https://esmac.org/, the ISB (International Society of Biomechanics) at https://isbweb.org/, and the International Foot and Ankle Biomechanics Community at http://www.i-fab.org/.

8 Conclusions

Throughout this work, in its different chapters, you will find continuous references to the mechanics of the foot and ankle and also to the correlation between visual gait analysis and diagnoses and treatment indications. It is essential to understand why things happen in order to know what to do with them, in health and in disease. The knowledge of foot and ankle mechanics and human gait analysis will allow us to have a comprehensive view of our specialty and put us in a privileged position to understand what happens to a patient, explain the why and how of their problem, and offer an appropriate orthopedic or surgical solution based on the mechanical resolution of their problem. We know from our experience that the restoration of an adequate mechanical environment with conservative or surgical treatment usually provides a good and lasting result.

References

1. Levine D, Richards J, Whittle MW. Whittle's gait analysis. 5th ed. Edinburgh: Churchill Livingstone; 2012.
2. Vera P, et al. Biomecánica de la Marcha Humana Normal y Patológica. Valencia: Publicaciones del Instituto de Biomecánica de; 1999.
3. Kirtley C. Clinical gait analysis: theory and practice. Edinburgh: Churchill Livingstone; 2005.
4. Fischer O. Der Gang des Menschen. Wentworth Press; 2018.
5. Inman VT, Ralston H, Todd F. Human walking. Edwin Mellen Press Ltd; Williams&Wilkins, Baltimore MD; 1981.
6. Perry J, Burnfield JM. Gait analysis: normal and pathological function. Thorofare: Slack Inc; 2010.
7. Rose J, Gamble J. Human walking. Philadelphia: Lippincott Williams & Wilkins; 2006.
8. Gage JR. Gait analysis in cerebral palsy. New York: (McKeith Press) Oxford Blackwell Sci. Pub. Cambridge University Press; 1991.
9. Gage JR, Schwartz MH, Koop SE, Novacheck TF. The identification and treatment of gait problems in cerebral palsy. London: Mac Keith Press; 2009.
10. Viladot VA. Estudio de la marcha humana. In: Lecciones Básicas de Biomecánica del Aparato Locomotor. Barcelona: Springer-Verlag Ibérica; 2001.
11. Winter DA. The biomechanics and motor control of human gait: normal, elderly and pathological. 2nd ed. Waterloo: Waterloo Biomechanics; 1991.
12. Hollander K, Zech A, Rahlf AL, Orendurff MS, Stebbins J, Heidt C. The relationship between static and dynamic foot posture and running biomechanics: a systematic review and meta-analysis. Gait Posture. 2019;72:109–22.
13. Balius X, Turró C, et al. Marcha humana vs. marcha atlética. Rev Med Cir Pie. 1995;IX(1):27–36.
14. Medved V. Measurement of human locomotion. Boca Ratón: CRC Press; 2001.
15. Sarrafian SK. Anatomy of the foot and ankle: descriptive, topographic, functional. 2nd ed. Philadelphia: JB Lippincott Company; 1993.
16. Maceira E. Análisis cinemático y cinético de la marcha humana. Rev Pie Tobillo. 2003;17(1):29–37.
17. Robertson GE. Introduction to biomechanics for human motion analysis. Waterloo: Waterloo Biomechanics; 1997.

18. Siebel A, et al. Gait Analysis Course (ESMAC). Stiftung Orthopaedische Klinik. Heidelberg: Univ; 1999.
19. Linskell JR, Gibb S, et al. The Dundee Gait Lab: Gait Analysis Course (ESMAC). Dundee: Tayside Orthopaedic Rehabilitation Technology Centre. Ninewells Hospital; 2000.
20. Winter DA, Patla AE. Signal processing and linear systems for the movement sciences. Waterloo: Waterloo Biomechanics; 1997.
21. Green C, Plyler D, Masadeh S, Bibbo C. Reconstructive amputations of the foot. Clin Podiatr Med Surg. 2021;38(1):17–29.
22. Wren TAL, Tucker CA, Rethlefsen SA, Gorton GE 3rd, Õunpuu S. Clinical efficacy of instrumented gait analysis: systematic review 2020 update. Gait Posture. 2020;80:274–9.
23. Sutter R, Pfirrmann CW, Espinosa N, Buck FM. Three-dimensional hindfoot alignment measurements based on biplanar radiographs: comparison with standard radiographic measurements. Skelet Radiol. 2013;42(4):493–80, 274–9.
24. Amis J. The split second effect: the mechanism of how equinus can damage the human foot and ankle. Front Surg. 2016;3:38. https://doi.org/10.3389/fsurg.2016.00038.
25. Taniguchi M, Tateuchi H, Takeoka T, Ichihashi N. Kinematic and kinetic characteristics of Masai Barefoot Technology footwear. Gait Posture. 2012;35(4):567–72.

Imaging in Ankle and Foot

Nicolas Zilleruelo V.

1 Introduction

The ankle and foot have a special place in musculoskeletal imaging. Due to their complex anatomy and complex clinical diagnosis, it is necessary to understand in an adequate way the use of the different imaging techniques as well as a close clinical-radiological correlation to reach an accurate diagnosis and thus provide the best treatment to each patient.

The imaging evaluation of ankle and foot pathology has led to the writing of many books on the subject. In this chapter I will try summarize the main utilities of the different imaging techniques in order to help clinicians decide when to order each image and thus achieve the greatest utility of the studies for the benefit of their patients.

2 Radiography

The initial evaluation of many musculoskeletal injuries of the ankle and foot is through plain radiographs. These are performed through variations in the absorption of ionizing radiation by the different tissues of the body, highlighting its good spatial resolution between soft tissue and bone.

Normally two projections of a body part are taken, conventionally in the antero-posterior (AP) and lateral planes. Due to the complex anatomy of the ankle and foot, this is often modified, depending on clinical suspicion. For example, in the ankle,

N. Zilleruelo V. (✉)
Musculoskeletal Radiologist, Clinica Alemana de Santiago, Santiago, Chile
e-mail: nzilleruelo@alemana.cl

© The Author(s), under exclusive license to Springer Nature
Switzerland AG 2022
E. Wagner Hitschfeld, P. Wagner Hitschfeld (eds.), *Foot and Ankle Disorders*,
https://doi.org/10.1007/978-3-030-95738-4_2

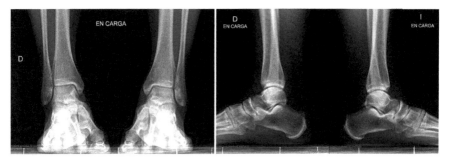

Fig. 1 Comparative ankle weight-bearing radiographs in AP and lateral projections

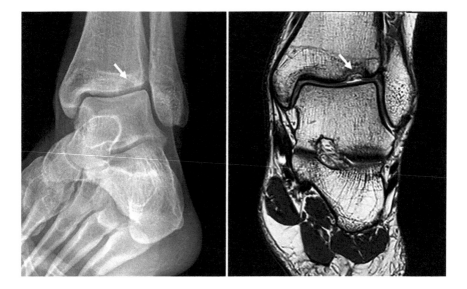

Fig. 2 Plain X-ray and MRI in T2 sequence showing an unstable osteochondral lesion of the tibial plateau (white arrow)

the use of loaded projections can make a difference in the assessment of joint spaces, revealing subtle but important changes in alignment (Fig. 1).

A modified AP projection with 15 to 20 degrees of internal rotation, the mortise projection, has demonstrated great utility, providing unobstructed evaluation of the talar dome and tibial plafond, allowing evaluation of lesions that may be hidden in standard AP projections, and is used routinely by many clinicians (Fig. 2).

In the foot, due to the overlap and orientation of the tarsal bones, oblique images can provide valuable complementary views but do not replace the standard in radiologic evaluation [1, 2].

In the foot, the use of loaded projections can also represent a great difference in the diagnosis of traumatic pathologies, for example, in Lisfranc complex injuries, where the greater amplitude of the articular space and the associated small bone fragments can be demonstrated in a comparative manner [3] (Fig. 3).

Fig. 3 Weight-bearing radiograph of feet demonstrating subtle loss of congruence of the medial aspect of the base of the second metatarsal to the medial aspect of the medial cuneiform (white arrow), typical of a ligamentary lesion of the Lisfranc complex

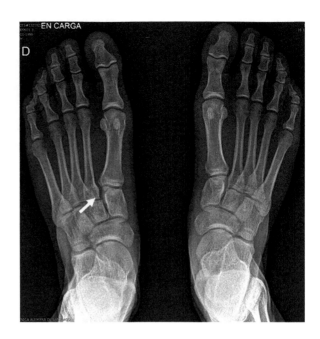

One of the main advantages of radiographic studies today is that they are widely available and relatively inexpensive. The diagnosis of bone lesions on plain radiographs is particularly useful in the acute traumatic area, although they also play a role in the evaluation of chronic ankle or foot pain. On the other hand, the demonstration of joint effusion or soft tissue enlargement becomes relevant to follow up the study of radiologically occult lesions (Fig. 4).

A relative disadvantage is that the acquisition of plain radiographs involves the use of ionizing radiation, and although the dose to the extremity is minimal, the potential dangers of radiation should not be ignored. Another disadvantage is that it fails to differentiate the various soft tissues from each other, due to the narrow range of attenuation values between them.

3 Additional Projections

Stress projection: These can be active or passive, demonstrating indirect evidence of ligamentous injury, resulting in widening of the joint space.

Gravity stress view projections: It is used in patients in which the diagnostic suspicion of medial ligament injuries is high or in which bone and ligament injuries coexist, in a patient where the projections with usual load or stress cannot be performed due to excessive pain or there is any suspicion that these were not performed in an adequate manner. The patient must only withstand the force of gravity, often enough to demonstrate some degree of altered alignment [4–6] (Fig. 5).

Fluoroscopic techniques are typically used in orthopedics to guide orthopedic and surgical fracture reduction procedures. This modality uses an X-ray source

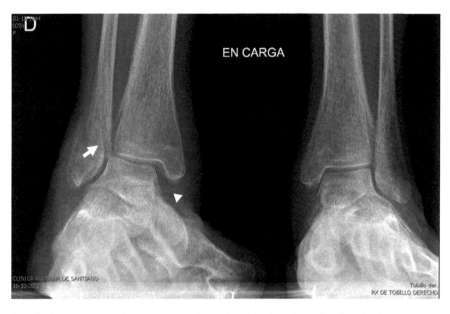

Fig. 4 Comparative weight-bearing radiograph of both ankles. Dysfunctional osteopenia. Displaced oblique fracture of the right fibula (white arrow). Displaced marginal fracture of the right medial malleolus (white arrow head). Asymmetry of the medial clear space (tibiotalar), highlighting a deltoid lesion

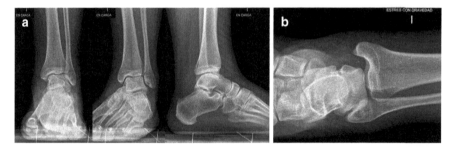

Fig. 5 (**a**) Weight-bearing ankle radiographs in AP, mortise, and lateral projections of the ankle showing a good relationship of the articular surface. (**b**) Same ankle under a gravity stress view, showing an abnormally increased medial clear space of the tibiotalar joint. Small interposed bony fragment is appreciated

but produces dynamic images in real time and allows dynamic evaluation of the joint.

Tomosynthesis is a conventional radiographic technique modified to acquire numerous low-dose images of specific bodies in a selected axis at different focal depths. The radiation dose is higher than conventional radiography but lower than computed tomography (CT). It plays a role in the possibility of evaluating occult bone lesions in any area where the anatomy is complex, such as the ankle and foot [7] (Fig. 6).

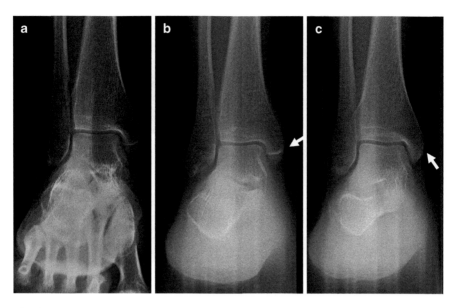

Fig. 6 Tomosynthesis of the ankle. (**a**) Ankle image in mortise projection. (**b** and **c**) Selected images of the tomosynthesis of the ankle where it is possible to differentiate structures in different planes in each image. As an example the cortices of the posterior colliculus of the medial malleolus in image **b** and the posterior colliculus of the medial malleolus in image **c** can be seen without any overlap

Ankle and foot radiographs should always be requested for the acute traumatic study as an initial study and should be attempted with weight bearing if tolerated by the patient. In the non-traumatic environment, it is very useful in the initial evaluation of chronic ankle and foot pain where different pathologies such as osteochondral lesions of the talus, bone coalitions, bone tumors, evaluation of the plantar arch, bone changes secondary to overload, and enthesopathic changes, among others, could be evaluated (Fig. 7).

4 Ultrasound (US)

Ultrasound plays a key role in the diagnosis and management of musculoskeletal pathology at the ankle and foot level. A high-frequency transducer is necessary, ideally greater than 14 MHz allowing for greater spatial resolution but limiting its depth penetration. Most of the structures to be evaluated in these areas are relatively superficial so US is an extremely useful tool in the hands of a competent operator.

Compared to other modalities, US offers the unique advantage of real-time passive and active dynamic evaluation of soft tissue, especially tendons and ligaments. It is a relatively fast, high-resolution examination that can be focused on the exact site of clinical symptoms and does not involve the use of ionizing radiation [8].

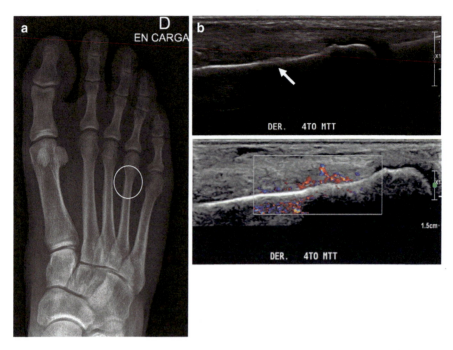

Fig. 7 (**a**) PA radiograph of the right foot. Discrete periosteal reaction of the distal diaphyseal region of the fourth metatarsal on its medial aspect (white circle). (**b**) Ultrasound of the right foot of the same patient showing the periosteal reaction (white arrow) with hypoechogenic area surrounding it secondary to edema and increased vascularization in color Doppler mode, typical of an overload (stress) fracture

As an example, dynamic ultrasound can elucidate peroneal subluxation not evident on static imaging [9] (Fig. 8).

It is also possible to perform maneuvers where stress is generated in ligaments in a specific and dynamic way for an adequate characterization of them, evaluating their continuity, thickness, reparative phenomena, and regional sequelae calcifications in a practical and simple way (Fig. 9).

The evaluation of the bone is not complete with US, but the evaluation of periosteal alterations in stress fractures can be key for the early diagnosis of these, even prior to their visualization in plain radiography or computed tomography (Fig. 7).

Power Doppler evaluation is a valuable tool mainly used in the evaluation of the vascularization of the synovium of the joints to determine active inflammation of them. It can also be used in tendons to evaluate neovascularization and also in the evaluation of the type of vascularization of a regional soft tissue lesion (Fig. 10).

Because of the superficial location of the tendons of the ankle and foot, US is an ideal modality to evaluate these structures. It also plays an important role in the

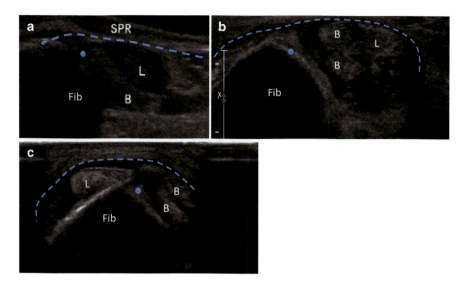

Fig. 8 (**a**) Ankle ultrasound of the long (L) and short (**b**) peroneal tendons at the site of the superior peroneal retinaculum (SPR, blue dashed line). (**a**) Shows properly positioned peroneal tendons adjacent to the fibula (Fib) and under the SPR. (**b**) Shows longitudinal rupture of the peroneus brevis and disinsertion of the SPR from the fibula. In (**c**) (same patient), dislocation of the peroneus longus over the fibula and under the disinserted SPR occurs with ankle flexion. The regional meniscus (blue circle) does not present displacement

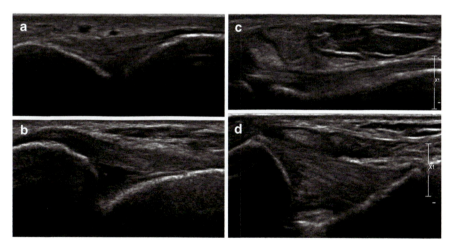

Fig. 9 Ultrasound of the ankle with ultrasound pattern of the main ankle ligaments. (**a**) Anterior inferior tibiofibular ligament of the syndesmosis. (**b**) Anterior talofibular ligament. (**c**) Fibulocalcaneal ligament, under the peroneal tendons. (**d**) Deep component of the medial deltoid ligament complex

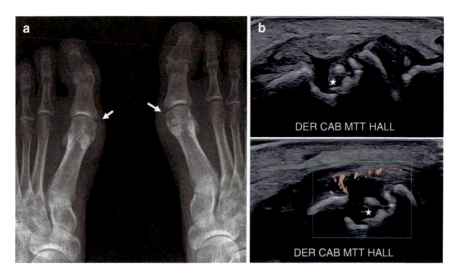

Fig. 10 Patient with rheumatoid arthritis. (**a**) AP foot radiography suggestive of erosions (white arrows) in the medial aspect of the F1 bases of both hallux and in the medial region of the first metatarsal heads, with increased volume of the soft tissues. (**b**) Ultrasound of the medial aspect of the head of the right first metatarsal, showing bone erosion and synovitis, with increased vascularization in power Doppler mode

Fig. 11 Morton's neuroma of the third intermetatarsal space of the left foot, with clearly defined continuity with the regional interdigital nerve (white arrow)

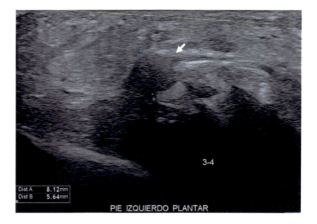

evaluation of small neurovascular bundles at the level of the ankle and foot, achieving targeted evaluations of, for example, interdigital nerves for Morton's neuromas, plantar plate lesions, and small superficial ligaments. Due to its high spatial resolution, it is able to evaluate small structures with similar resolution compared to MRI (Fig. 11).

US is also widely used as a guide for musculoskeletal procedures, allowing excellent visualization of the needle throughout the procedure (Fig. 12).

The main limitation of US is that it is an operator-dependent technique. Its results are dependent on the operator's degree of knowledge of the pathology and experience in the technique. Additionally, US has a series of specific artifacts that can

Fig. 12 Fine needle infiltration of the right ankle joint through the anterolateral recess, highlighting the adequate distance between the needle and the neurovascular bundle (white star)

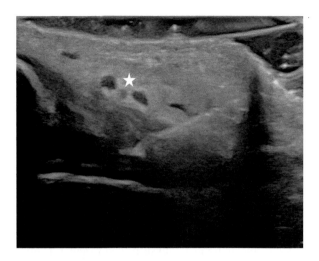

Fig. 13 Panoramic view of the Achilles tendon under ultrasound

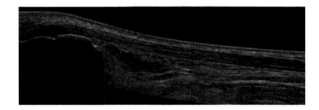

influence the quality of the image, the most frequent is anisotropy, which is when the normal tendon loses its hyperechoic fibrillar characteristic just because of the modification of the obliquity of the sound beam. This finding is easily recognized by a competent operator.

Also, the US gives us the possibility to perform panoramic images of long tendons such as the Achilles tendon or lesions that are larger than the length of the transducer, giving a continuous evaluation of the lesion, being very useful to give an adequate vision to the relevant finding for the medical referent (Fig. 13).

US elastography is an add-on that can be performed only on equipment with special software and is based on morphological changes to indicate underlying pathology. It provides a measure of tissue stiffness by gentle manual compression, for example, as part of the evaluation of Achilles tendinopathy [10].

In summary, ultrasound is a very useful tool at the level of the ankle and foot in the hands of a competent operator. Due to the superficial location of the tendons and most ligaments of the ankle and foot, US is an ideal initial modality to evaluate these structures, as well as the small regional neurovascular bundles. Its dynamic evaluation advantage is key in the diagnosis of many tendon and ligament pathologies, making a big difference when compared to all other static techniques.

5 Computed Tomography (CT)

Computed tomography is accomplished by multiple parallel images through an X-ray array and multiple detectors that move circumferentially around a patient as the patient passes through the CT scanner.

The high spatial resolution of CT makes it an ideal modality for evaluating bone and soft tissue calcifications.

As image volumes are acquired, they can be reconstructed in different planes, usually axial, coronal, and sagittal, with associated 3D reconstruction, useful for better evaluation of the overall findings and for future surgical planning if necessary. If one wishes to make any changes regarding the obliquity of the planes, this can be done thanks to the volumes acquired with isotropic voxels, which means that all sides have the same dimension, with uniform resolution in all directions (Fig. 14).

Intravenous iodinated contrast can be used to evaluate peripheral vascularization, for example, in trauma with suspected vascular involvement or for better characterization of a soft tissue tumor.

A great advantage of CT is that the acquisition process takes only a few seconds and is well tolerated by most patients. In the preoperative planning of fractures, particularly complex intra-articular fractures, CT offers a more detailed assessment of the fracture, degree of complexity, and articular bodies than other imaging modalities (Fig. 15).

As a disadvantage, CT involves the use of ionizing radiation in higher doses than conventional radiography. Multiple techniques have been developed to reduce the dose without compromising the diagnostic capacity of the study.

CT presents a limited evaluation of the soft tissues without being able to easily delimit the normal soft tissues from the adjacent abnormal ones. It is also not a study that is performed in a conventional way with load, which is why many times the study is complemented with conventional radiographs with load to evaluate bone or joint alignments.

When we face metallic materials such as osteosynthesis or prosthesis materials, a beam hardening artifact is generated that limits the study. Multiple teams have

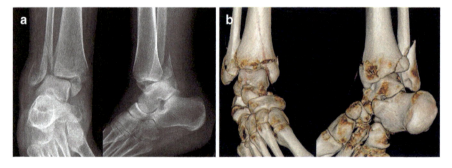

Fig. 14 AP and lateral ankle radiographs (**a**) together with computed tomography (CT) VRT bone reconstructions (**b**) of a trimalleolar ankle fracture

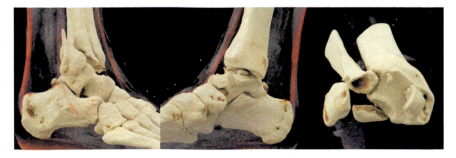

Fig. 15 Computed tomography with VRT cinematic rendering reconstructions of a trimalleolar ankle fracture

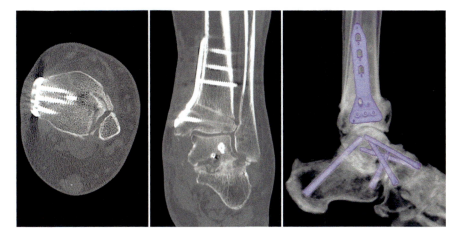

Fig. 16 Computed tomography with optimized protocol for osteosynthesis materials, highlighting the lower amount of beam artifacts in the axial and coronal images of this patient and the high quality of visualization in VRT reconstructions of the osteosynthesis materials

developed techniques and software that manage to reduce these artifacts in a remarkable way for the evaluation of pathology in relation to these metallic components [11] (Fig. 16).

Also, some equipment has the ability to acquire images with dual-energy techniques, where there are two X-ray tubes of different kilovoltage (Kv) that acquire the information simultaneously, obtaining a set of data that, by comparing the behavior of tissues with different attenuation values in the two acquisitions, can differentiate between different types of deposited crystals, for example, to differentiate the deposit of uric acid from calcium pyrophosphate deposit [12] (Fig. 17).

CT with dual energy also has the potential for the evaluation of traumatic trabecular bone lesions with the recognition of medullary bone edema, being more sensitive in the recognition of lesions not visible in a usual CT.

In recent years, technological evolution has led to smaller CT scan designs, allowing the modification of equipment that can image loaded ankles and feet

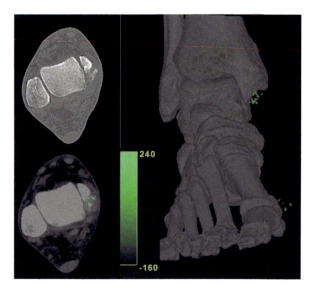

Fig. 17 Dual-energy computed tomography of a patient with gout, where it is possible to identify and calculate the load of urate crystals deposited (green dots) in the soft tissues adjacent to the medial malleolus and the medial region of the hallux

(weight-bearing CT scans). This modality better demonstrates the true orientation of the bones and joints during axial loading of the patient. It is especially useful in investigating the alignment of multiple regional pathologies such as adult-acquired flatfoot deformity, various ankle impingements, and hallux valgus, among others. In clinical practice it is increasingly used as orthopedic surgeons strive for better outcomes in the treatment of ankle and foot disorders [13].

In summary, CT is very useful for the characterization of complex fractures, with the ability to perform 3D reconstructions for surgical planning. It also has better sensitivity to small fractures than conventional radiography. Its acquisition is fast, and currently there is easy access in most institutions. Special equipment and software have been developed to eliminate metallic artifacts, reduce ionizing radiation doses, and study crystal differentiation.

6   SPECT-CT (Single Photon Emission Computed Tomography-Computed Tomography)

SPECT is based on the detection of gamma rays emitted by a radiopharmaceutical usually technetium 99 (radiotracer) injected into the patient's bloodstream, accumulating and marking the regions of greater bone turnover due to greater vascularization and osteoblastic presence. This associated to its combination with a high-resolution CT generates hybrid fused images, reflecting functional information associated to an adequate anatomical localization of the lesions [14, 15].

The use of SPECT-CT on the foot and ankle is an emerging modality, and its benefit is increasingly recognized in the localization of degenerative foci and

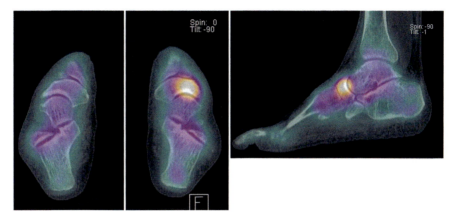

Fig. 18 SPEC-CT of the ankle with increased radiotracer uptake in the left navicular secondary to regional degenerative lesions

also in infections. Historically, the contribution of bone scintigraphy to the diagnosis of diseases of the ankle and foot has been restricted by limited resolution and low specificity. However, fused hybrid SPECT-CT imaging has significantly improved the diagnostic value in this anatomical region. Current applications of SPECT-CT in ankle and foot pathology often include patients with chronic pain symptoms that are not sufficiently explained by clinical findings and conventional imaging. These include localization of active sites of osteoarthritis, coalitions, osteoid osteomas, occult stress fractures, tendonitis, plantar fasciitis, and impingement syndromes. Assessment of response to therapy after surgical interventions such as evaluation of arthrodesis is a promising application of this technique (Fig. 18).

The main disadvantage is that both ionizing radiation and the use of radiopharmaceuticals that emit gamma rays that are distributed throughout the body are used. They also require instrumentation and image reconstruction methods that differ from those used in other medical imaging modalities.

7 Magnetic Resonance Imaging (MRI)

Magnetic resonance imaging has revolutionized musculoskeletal imaging, offering excellent spatial and contrast resolution in both superficial and deep structures. The MRI image is produced by the effect of a strong homogeneous magnetic field on the hydrogen nuclei of the different tissues of the body, achieving their differentiation. MRI does not use ionizing radiation.

Part of the complexity of MRI is centered on the wide variety of sequences available, being indispensable to have clear and directed protocols for the evaluation of the main pathologies of the study area.

MRI sequences can be simplified into three main groups. T1-weighted sequences show hyperintense fat (high signal) and hypointense fluid signal (low signal). This is a particularly useful sequence for evaluation of anatomy. T2-weighted sequences are sensitive to fluids showing them hyperintense. Fat is also hyperintense on T2. The fat signal can be suppressed (Fat Sat) and thus increase the visibility of fluids and bone or soft tissue edema. Another alternative of fat saturation is achieved through another sequence acquisition process, which is the STIR sequence (short tau inversion recovery), a sequence that has a very important characteristic in the evaluation of bone edema, since it is less sensitive to the inhomogeneities of the magnetic field.

Proton density (PD) sequences are intermediate sequences, optimized for the evaluation of hyaline cartilage; they are also sensitive to fluids, often combined with fat suppression.

MRI provides excellent spatial and contrast resolution of the major structures of the ankle and foot. MRI is widely used in the evaluation of bone, tendon, and ligament pathology, as well as detailed evaluation of cartilage and joints. Multiple new sequences have been developed as well as multiple software that have increased the diagnostic capacity of MRI [16] (Fig. 19).

Although MRI is very sensitive, it is not always specific, and the findings of the study must be interpreted in the context of the patient's clinical condition. As an example, it is common to find bone marrow signal alterations in sports patients, which are mistaken for bone edema in areas where the patient does not report regional symptoms [17]. There are also alterations of the bone marrow signal in active children under 15 years of age, which are confused with bone edema being manifestations of marrow reconversion, without pathological significance and asymptomatic [18]. Another example is ankle impingement, where images can help to better define the etiology of the clinical problem, and in other opportunities, incidental findings that are not clinically relevant are visualized. It is also very easy to

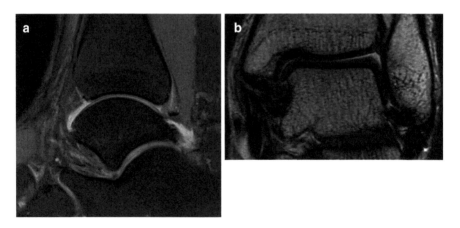

Fig. 19 3 Tesla MRI of the ankle in PD Fat Sat (**a**) and T2 (**b**) sequences with visualization of the cartilages with high contrast definition in the tibiotalar joint

determine the existence of bone edema, but it is difficult to differentiate the etiology with images alone (Fig. 20).

MRI has the disadvantage of being a study that is not fast; it requires at least 30 minutes to achieve the necessary sequences. It requires adequate equipment with a high Tesla and special coils for the ankle and foot. Due to the strong magnetic field, many pacemakers are contraindicated for use because they become misconfigured or lose battery charges. Currently most of the new pacemakers come with systems compatible with MRI use, which is done under the approval and supervision of your treating cardiologist.

Fig. 20 Anterolateral ankle impingement. MRI axial T2-weighted (**a**) and sagittal PD Fat Sat (**b**) sections. It is visualized a thickening of the anterior talofibular ligament, associated with mild tibiotalar joint effusion in anterolateral recess of the ankle where a regional meniscoid lesion is observed (white arrow)

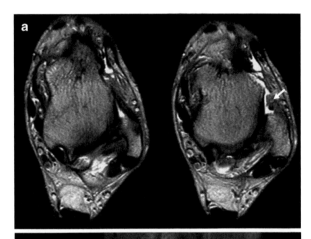

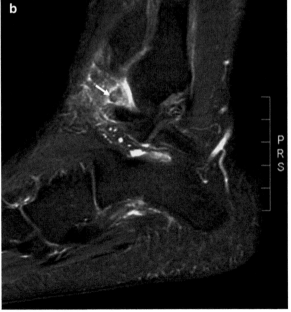

Many times, claustrophobic patients are not able to perform these studies. Low magnetic field resonators have been developed that are better tolerated by claustrophobic patients but in which the spatial and contrast resolution is suboptimal for the diagnosis of multiple key structures in the foot and ankle joints.

When osteosynthesis or prosthetic materials are present, the study should be performed in a resonator with a lower magnetic field and use sequences with certain special technical modifications to reduce the degree of magnetic susceptibility artifacts that occur, improving diagnostic sensitivity.

MR arthrography (arthro MRI) is usually performed with intraarticular (direct) contrast injection, with the benefit of joint distension with better appreciation of the intraarticular structures. However, it has potential risks as it is an invasive procedure such as the potential risk of infection. Its intention is to achieve a better characterization of ligament pathologies, impingement syndromes, chondral lesions, and synovial pathologies [19]. But with the advances of 3 Tesla resonators and special coils for these joints, they are not as widely used today.

Studies directed to articular cartilage can be performed for the characterization of acute and chronic lesions, as well as to evaluate them over time, recognizing the differentiation of hyaline cartilage from reparative fibrocartilage and the evaluation of operated chondral lesions. Sequences have been developed to evaluate the biochemical alterations of cartilage, such as the structural evaluation of collagen in lesions (T2 map) or the evaluation of the proteoglycan matrix (dGEMRIC), among others, findings that precede the arthroscopically visible lesions [20].

MRI is the technique of choice for the global evaluation of superficial and deep soft tissues, with a great information of the bone marrow signal and a very good evaluation of the intraarticular structures. Its acquisition takes quite a long time, and it is not as accessible as the rest of the images, especially the fact that resonators with a high tessellation (1.5 to 3 Tesla) with special coils for the joints are needed to achieve high-quality images in order to reach the diagnosis with greater precision (Fig. 21).

In summary, knowing the different imaging techniques and their variants is fundamental for the evaluation of the multiple pathologies of the ankle and foot, and at the same time, it is essential that they are performed in an adequate and orderly manner, ensuring that they have the minimum quality for the diagnosis. Especially dynamic techniques such as US should be performed by radiologists trained in the area because it is necessary to know the pathology and look for it in a targeted manner, passively and dynamically, achieving accurate diagnoses and in turn a better final treatment for each patient.

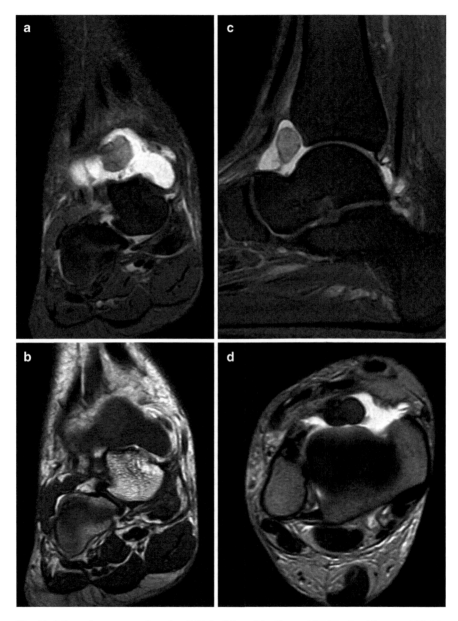

Fig. 21 Magnetic resonance imaging (MRI) of the ankle. Coronal PD Fat Sat (**a**) coronal T1 (**b**), sagittal PD Fat Sat (**c**), and axial T2 (**d**). There is a tibiotalar joint effusion where an intra-articular nodular image is observed with low signal in T2, corresponding to a focal villonodular synovitis

References

1. Clark TW, Janzen DL, Ho K, Grunfeld A, Connell DG. Detection of radiographically occult ankle fractures following acute trauma: positive predictive value of an ankle effusion. Am J Roentgenol. 1995;164:1185e9.
2. Fonseca LLD, et al. Reproducibility of the Lauge-Hansen, Danis-weber, and AO classifications for ankle fractures. Rev Bras Ortop. 2018;53:101–6.
3. Kennelly H, Klaassen K, Heitman D, Youngberg R, Platt SR. Utility of weight-bearing radiographs compared to computed tomography scan for the diagnosis of subtle Lisfranc injuries in the emergency setting. Emerg Med Australas. 2019;31:741–4.
4. Gill JB, Risko T, Raducan V, Grimes JS, Schutt RC Jr. Comparison of manual and gravity stress radiographs for the evaluation of supination-external rotation fibular fractures. J Bone Joint Surg Am. 2007;89(5):994–9.
5. Michelson JD, Varner KE, Checcone M. Diagnosing deltoid injury in ankle fractures: the gravity stress view. Clin Orthop Rel Res. 2001;387:178–82.
6. Schock HJ, Pinzur M, Manion L, Stover M. The use of gravity or manual-stress radiographs in the assessment of supination-external rotation fractures of the ankle. J Bone Joint Surg Br. 2007;89(8):1055–9.
7. Dobbins JT 3rd. Tomosynthesis imaging: at a translational crossroads. Med Phys. 2009;36:1956e67.
8. Bianchi S, Martinoli C, Gaignot C, De Gautard R, Meyer JM. Ultrasound of the ankle: anatomy of the tendons, bursae, and ligaments. Semin Musculoskelet Radiol. 2005;9:243–59.
9. Neustadter J, Raikin SM, Nazarian LN. Dynamic sonographic evaluation of peroneal tendon subluxation. AJR Am J Roentgenol. 2004;183:985–8.
10. Ooi CC, Schneider ME, Malliaras P, Chadwick M, Connell DA. Diagnostic performance of axial-strain sonoelastography in confirming clinically diagnosed Achilles tendinopathy: comparison with B-mode ultrasound and color Doppler imaging. Ultrasound Med Biol. 2015;41(1):15–25.
11. Olsen RV, Munk PL, Lee MJ, et al. Metal artifact reduction sequence: early clinical applications. Radiographics. 2000;20:699e712.
12. Desai MA, Peterson JJ, Garner HW, et al. Clinical utility of dual-energy CT for evaluation of tophaceous gout. Radiographics. 2011;31:1365–75; discussion 1376–1367.
13. Barg A, Bailey T, Richter M, Netto CDC, Lintz F, Burssens A, Phisitkul P, Hanrahan CJ, Saltzman CL. Weightbearing Computed Tomography of the Foot and Ankle: Emerging technology topical review. Foot & Ankle International. 2018;39(3):376–86.
14. Pagenstert GI, Barg A, Leumann AG, Tasch H. Mu¨ ller-brand J, Hintermann B, et al. SPECT-CT imaging in degenerative joint disease of the foot and ankle. J Bone Joint Surg Br. 2009;91(9):1191–6.
15. Knupp M, Pagenstert GI, Barg A, Bolliger L, Easley ME, Hintermann B. SPECT-CT compared with conventional imaging modalities for the assessment of the varus and valgus malaligned hindfoot. J Orthop Res. 2009;27(11):1461–6.
16. Rosenberg ZS, Beltran J, Bencardino JT. From the RSNA refresher courses. Radiological Society of North America. MR imaging of the ankle and foot. Radiographics. 2000;20(Suppl):153–79.
17. Lohman M, Kivisaari A, Vehmas T, Kallio P, Malmivaara A, Kivisaari L. MRI abnormalities of foot and ankle in asymptomatic, physically active individuals. Skelet Radiol. 2001;30:61–6.
18. Shabshin N, Schweitzer ME, Morrison WB, Carrino JA, Keller MS, Grissom LE. High-signal T2 changes of the bone marrow of the foot and ankle in children: red marrow or traumatic changes? Pediatr Radiol. 2006;36:670–6.
19. Cerezal L, Abascal F, Garcia-Valtuille R, et al. Ankle MR arthrography: how, why, when. Radiol Clin N Am. 2005;43(4):693–707.
20. Li X, Majumdar S. Quantitative MRI of articular cartilage and its clinical applications. J Magn Reson Imaging. 2013;38:991e1008.

Open vs Minimally Invasive Surgery: Advantages and Disadvantages

Mariano De Prado, Manuel Cuervas-Mons, and Virginia De Prado

1 Introduction

Minimally invasive techniques are becoming increasingly popular in modern orthopedic surgery. Their aim is to solve or minimize some of the problems encountered with open surgery, decreasing possible complications and speeding up the post-surgical recovery process. Decades ago, arthroscopy represented the spearhead, and subsequently different minimally invasive surgeries were developed, which today encompass a heterogeneous group of surgical techniques applicable to upper limb, lower limb, and spine surgery. These techniques are a point of reference towards which there is a tendency to converge and are currently the most widely used in numerous pathologies.

Percutaneous foot surgery, also known as minimally invasive surgery or MIS (minimal invasive surgery), is a surgical method that allows us to perform interventions on the foot through minimal incisions, without direct exposure of the surgical plane and under fluoroscopic control (Fig. 1), which results in a reduction of injuries to the surrounding tissues. In order to be able to offer our patients the most appropriate treatment in each case, it is necessary to know the differences and similarities between percutaneous and open surgery.

M. De Prado (✉)
Service of Orthopedic Surgery and Traumatology, Hospital Quironsalud Murcia,
Murcia, Spain

M. Cuervas-Mons
Orthopedic Surgery and Traumatology Service, Hospital General Universitario Greogrio
Marañon, Madrid, Madrid, Spain

V. De Prado
Podiatry Service, Hospital Quironsalud Murcia, Murcia, Spain

E. Wagner Hitschfeld, P. Wagner Hitschfeld (eds.), *Foot and Ankle Disorders*,
https://doi.org/10.1007/978-3-030-95738-4_3

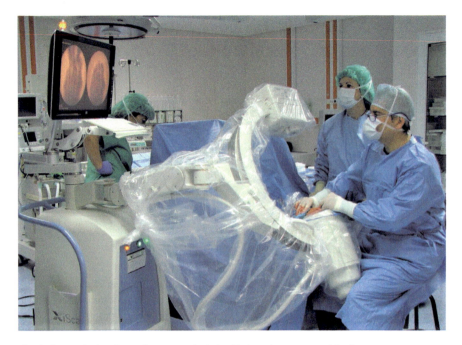

Fig. 1 Image during the performance of minimally invasive surgery of the foot

Fig. 2 Approach routes
for hallux valgus with open
surgery

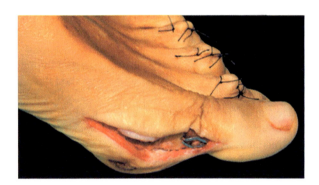

2   Fundamentals

Surgical treatment of foot deformities aims to achieve a painless and biomechanically functional foot. If we want to correct all the pathological elements of the disease, sometimes it will be necessary to perform multiple surgical gestures.

Using the postulates of open surgery, this translates into wide approach routes (Fig. 2); however, minimally invasive surgery allows us to perform the same acts, in a precise manner, through small incisions (Fig. 3).

The surgical indications are the same regardless of the surgical technique to be used, but in order to be able to perform minimally invasive surgical procedures, it is essential to have specific instruments. Surgical instruments used in open surgery

Fig. 3 Approach routes for hallux valgus with percutaneous surgery

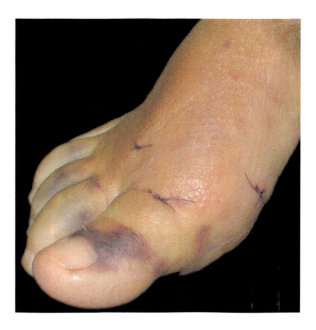

should not be adapted, as this could favor the appearance of associated complications.

We can divide the necessary material for percutaneous foot surgery into three sections: basic, motorized, and radiological control instruments.

2.1 Basic Instruments

The basic instruments include the scalpel, scrapers, and elevators (Fig. 4). Beaver 64 and Beaver 64MIS scalpels are used, allowing us to make minimal incisions (generally less than 5 mm) with a direct cut to access the desired surgical field. The scrapers and elevators, with different widths and shapes, allow us to detach and extract the bony debris through the incisions made.

In addition to these basic instruments, we must have surgical material such as needle holders and scissors, necessary for suturing surgical wounds, and hemostatic mosquito forceps, useful for resolving possible intraoperative incidences such as excessive bleeding or breakage of drills.

2.2 Motorized Instruments

Motorized instruments include the motor, a handpiece, and a complete set of drills (Fig. 5).

Fig. 4 Basic instruments

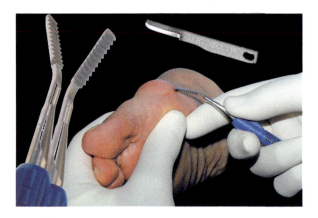

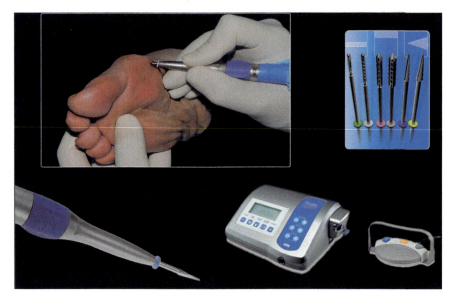

Fig. 5 Motorized instrumentation

There is a wide variety of motors that can be used in percutaneous foot surgery, both electric and compressed air, with common characteristics. The motor must have a central unit with a speed control knob to achieve the desired revolutions per minute for each surgical procedure. If we use speeds higher than 10,000 revolutions per minute, injuries and bone necrosis may occur. The ideal speed to be able to work will be the minimum speed that allows us to perform the desired gesture without blocking the drills in the bone, which can also be avoided by making slight back-and-forth movements in the direction of the cut we want to make. On the other hand, the lower the speed, the greater the control and tactile sensation of the desired surgical gesture, without performing osteotomies or bone resections greater than desired. The ideal speed for this type of surgery will be between 1000 and 8000 revolutions per minute, since it gives us a better control of the cut and at the same time a precision in the surgical gestures, all this without producing thermal injuries.

The handpiece must have a small size (similar to a pencil) in order to be handled with ease and precision. The handpiece is attached to the burs, and rotary movements are performed, not allowing circular movements of the burr or oscillating movements of the saws. The handpiece must be sterilized in order to be used freely in the surgical field.

The complete set of drills includes different drills of various shapes and lengths, in order to perform different surgical procedures (osteotomy, exostectomy-bunionectomy, wedge extraction, etc.). The most commonly used are as follows:

A. Lateral cutting drills. They are used to perform osteotomies on the metatarsals or phalanges, as well as to reduce minor bone exostoses.
B. Fine shaving drills. They are used to remove bone from the most important exostoses. They cause minimal trauma to the soft tissues; they are also used to mark the size of bone wedges as they are cone-shaped and can also be used as lateral cutting drills.
C. Coarse reaming drills. They produce a great lifting of the bone and are used, above all, to extract hallux valgus exostoses because they are very voluminous and have a powerful articular capsule that protects the rest of the soft parts from being injured, since this drill is very aggressive.

2.3   Radiological Control Instruments

It is necessary to control the exact point where osteotomies or surgical procedures on the bone are performed. For this purpose, conventional X-ray systems, such as image intensifiers, or systems such as fluoroscopes can be used. The fluoroscope is not equipped with a traditional intensifier but with an X-ray cassette that requires less radiation for its operation than traditional intensifiers, and, in addition, its design presents a mini-arch that can be rotated 360° in the three planes (Fig. 6), giving great versatility and functionality to the surgical act.

3   Relevant Anatomy

Knowing the relationships between the different anatomical structures is of vital importance for a successful surgical treatment. The objective of surgery is to correct the deformities causing the pathology while avoiding iatrogenic injuries during the intervention. Preoperative planning is necessary to know the different anatomical structures at risk (vessels, nerves, tendons, etc.) in order to choose a specific approach and protect the structures involved. In open surgery, we can visualize and protect these structures during the intervention, but in percutaneous foot surgery,

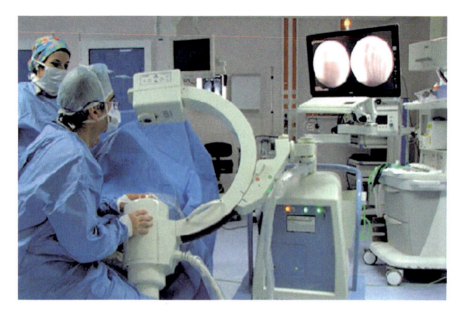

Fig. 6 Radiological control instruments

our intraoperative guide is fluoroscopy, where these structures are not visualized, in addition to losing the three-dimensional vision by relying on 2D images.

For this reason, in percutaneous surgery, it is of vital importance that the surgeon accustomed to open surgery undergoes a period of adaptation before starting the practice of MIS surgery, developing a new anatomical perspective, as we had to do when we started with arthroscopy, getting used to planning the skin incision, the angle of incidence on the surface to be treated (approach angle), and the distance from the incision to the point of surgical action (approach path), since we work with instruments that we introduce into the skin far away from the performance of the surgical gesture. We must also adapt to the use of motorized cutting instruments with burs, which are performed with a rotary movement, quite different from that described by the cutting saws with an oscillating movement. Finally, we must also adapt to the loss of the three-dimensional perception of the anatomical structures that we perceive in open surgery and that we must intuit in MIS, both in the normal anatomy and in the anatomical alterations produced by the pathology to be treated.

3.1 Incision

The skin incision should be made at an anatomical point that does not produce iatrogenic lesions, taking into account the anatomy to avoid vascular, nerve, ligamentous, tendon, etc. structures. Incisions should be made following Langer's skin lines, with 90° incidence of the scalpel (Fig. 7), regardless of the posterior direction

Fig. 7 Correct incision incidence

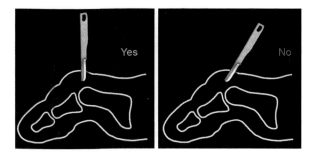

towards the surgical site. Incisions should not be made in areas of pressure with the footwear, since this would favor the appearance of hypertrophic or keloid scars and post-surgical pain at this point. The size should be small but large enough to be able to introduce the surgical instruments freely and allow the exit of the bone detritus. If an excessively small incision is made and the edges are injured, it can favor the appearance of a hypertrophic scar, perilesional calcifications due to accumulation of bone detritus, or maintenance of prolonged post-surgical inflammatory signs.

3.2 Approach Angle

The direction from the incision to the point of surgical action must allow the surgeon's hand to be free on the outside of the skin, with total freedom of movement for the use of the surgical instruments. The angle of approach from the incision should not be perpendicular to the articular surfaces (Fig. 8) on which we are going to act, except in arthrodesis, in order to avoid cartilage injury, and if, for example, we must remove an exostosis, we must bring the motorized instruments parallel to the bone surface to be removed.

3.3 Approach Path

The incision is placed at a specific distance from the point of surgical action, long enough so that the instruments (motorized or dragging) are covered by the skin and soft tissues over the whole of their cutting surface, so as not to injure the skin during their action.

The path from the incision to the surgical point of action must be unique and not multiple, one incision for each surgical procedure. No vascular, nervous, or tendon structures should be found in the path. If necessary, an extension of the trajectory can be made from the point of entry into the skin to the operative area, with a maximum angle of 60°, performing a detachment from the pivot point (skin incision) to the operative area (Fig. 9). The extension should be performed with a

Fig. 8 Incision location

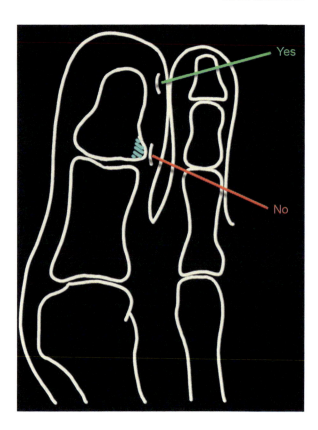

Fig. 9 Approach path

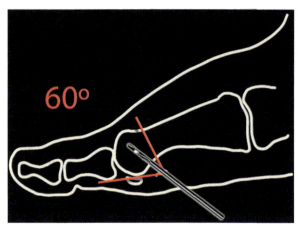

scalpel if we are within an anatomical safety zone or with blunt instruments (rasp, periosteal elevator, etc.) if there are anatomical structures in the trajectory that can be injured.

The approach path should favor, by its direction and width, the exit of bone debris after skin pressure on the surgical site.

Once the intervention is completed, the bone and blood debris are removed from the approach path, the skin incision is closed, and a light compressive bandage is applied, thus promoting subcutaneous healing. The objective is to achieve a restitutio ad integrum, provided that the subcutaneous structures have been respected.

4 Differences Between Open and Minimally Invasive Surgery

Open and minimally invasive surgery is a set of techniques with the same objective: to achieve a painless and biomechanically functional foot. The surgical indications do not vary, the main difference being in their planning and execution.

4.1 Preoperative Planning

It is necessary to have specific instruments. Under no circumstances should percutaneous techniques be performed by adapting instruments (motorized or not) similar to those specifically designed for this technique, since major complications can arise if the appropriate instrument is not used.

Similarly, radiological control is necessary during the intervention. The control allows us to see the exact position of the surgical instruments before performing the gestures, as well as the result of the same. This control avoids the logical complications that could occur as a consequence of the lack of direct vision of the surgical field.

4.2 Intraoperative Preparation

4.2.1 Anesthesia

The type of anesthesia is different in the two groups of surgical techniques. In open surgery, an anesthetic block of the sciatic nerve at the popliteal level is performed in most patients, while percutaneous surgery is performed with a peripheral block of the ankle "in sock" (Fig. 10). The type of anesthesia will condition discharge, with outpatient surgery being performed with early discharge with percutaneous surgery, since the patient has no blockage of the extrinsic musculature of the foot and can walk at the end of the intervention without the risk of falling.

4.2.2 Preparation of the Surgical Field

The correct preparation of the patient and the sterility measures of the surgical field are identical in both techniques (Fig. 11).

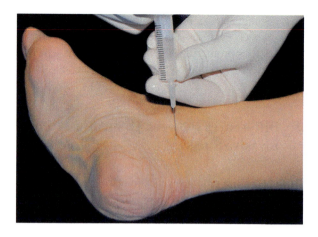

Fig. 10 Loco-regional anesthesia in percutaneous surgery

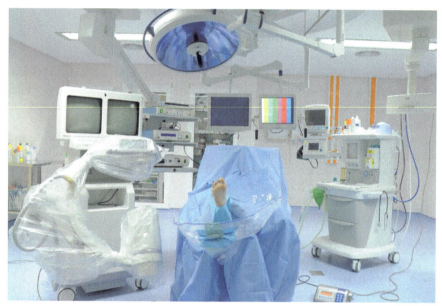

Fig. 11 Image of the prepared surgical field

One of the main differences with open surgery is that minimally invasive techniques are performed without an ischemia cuff. Intraoperative bleeding does not affect the surgery, since it is performed without direct vision and, on the other hand, blood circulation has a cooling effect on the increase in temperature produced by the motorized cutting instruments. In the same way, the bleeding favors the cleaning of the bony debris by dragging it from the surgical site to the skin entrance.

4.3   Types of Surgical Techniques

Although the surgical indications are identical in open and percutaneous surgery, not all foot surgery techniques can be performed by minimally invasive or percutaneous surgery.

The indications are precise and must be adhered to in order to obtain good results. Percutaneous surgery is a method in the surgeon's hands, not an end in itself. The techniques we practice through minimal incisions are divided into three sections: soft tissue surgery, bone surgery (osteotomies, exostectomies), and arthrodesis.

4.3.1   Soft Tissue Surgery

The indications for this type of surgery are limited. There are techniques frequently performed in foot surgery that cannot be performed, such as tendon transpositions, tendon or muscle suturing and repair, or certain tendon lengthening procedures.

On the other hand, capsulotomies and tenotomies, especially of the flexor (Fig. 12) and extensor tendons, either as a single procedure or as a procedure associated with other surgeries, are perfectly feasible by minimal incision surgery, with great efficiency and minimal aggression. Percutaneous plantar fasciotomy (Fig. 13) will be an excellent indication in the treatment of fasciitis and heel spurs.

Fig. 12 Tenotomy of the flexor tendons

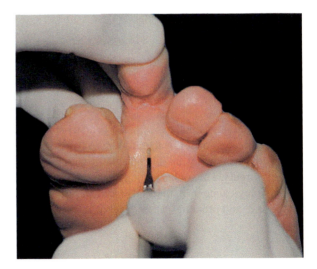

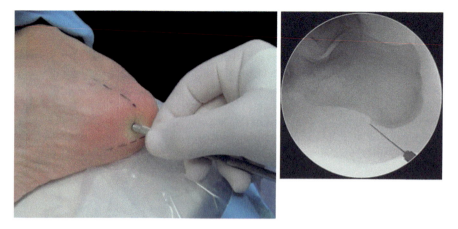

Fig. 13 Percutaneous plantar fasciotomy

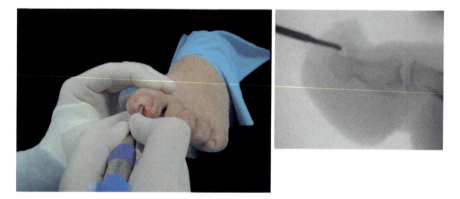

Fig. 14 Subungual exostosectomy

4.3.2 Bone Surgery

The elimination of small exostoses, especially subungual (Fig. 14), was the origin of this type of technique. It is therefore not surprising that the performance of osteotomies and exostectomy are the indications with the greatest scope of action in percutaneous surgery. The sophistication that has been reached with motorized instruments and radiological control allows us today to perform all types of osteotomies (distal, diaphyseal, and proximal) at the level of the metatarsals (Fig. 15) and phalanges.

Fig. 15 DMMO distal
metatarsal osteotomy

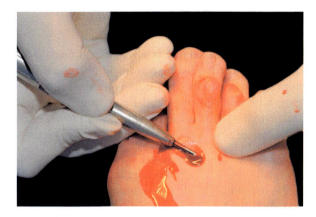

Fig. 16 Percutaneous
ankle arthrodesis

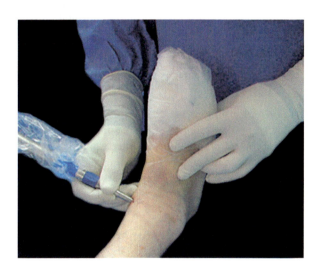

4.3.3 Arthrodesis

Although the indications are limited, articular arthrodesis can be performed (Fig. 16) by removing the articular cartilage with motorized drills, thus promoting fusion of the articular bony ends.

4.4   Advantages and Disadvantages

Percutaneous foot surgery is a very useful method for the treatment of most foot deformities, but it must be performed by experienced surgeons. With these techniques very satisfactory results are obtained, equivalent to those of traditional surgery, with minimal surgical damage, which allows a rapid incorporation of the patient to his social and working life, and a lower incidence of complications.

The main advantages of minimally invasive surgery over open surgery are:

- Surgery under loco-regional anesthesia and without the need for ischemia.
- Smaller incisions: less damage to soft tissues and improved esthetic factors.
- No use of osteosynthesis material.
- Less soft tissue trauma: reduction of postoperative pain.
- Reduction of surgical time: reduction of waiting list.
- Outpatient surgery: reduction of hospital costs and reduction of hospital infections.
- It can allow less complex revision surgery in certain cases.

The main disadvantages of minimally invasive surgery compared to open surgery are:

- Longer learning curve.
- Lack of precise control of the position and shortening of the osteotomies.
- Less control of osteotomy stabilization.
- Difficulty in the control of bleeding and localization of deep structures.
- Difficulty in spatial perception: loss of depth sensation.

5   Surgery for the Beginner in MIS

There are currently more than 200 techniques described for the treatment of forefoot pathology, but none of them alone is capable of solving all the deformities present. Therefore, nowadays, it does not seem correct to speak of a specific technique but of the specific combination for each case of different surgical gestures that can give a definitive and effective solution to the specific deformities of the patient to be treated.

There are five levels of difficulty according to the surgical techniques that we can perform in minimally invasive surgery, ranging from level 1, which expresses the minimum difficulty, to the maximum level 5. Similarly, we classify the surgeon's level of experience in four grades (beginner, initiated, advanced, and expert). It is important to start the learning curve with surgical techniques of level I or II and to increase the indications to other pathologies as the surgeon's experience in minimally invasive surgery progresses.

In the first level of experience, beginners, level I surgery should be performed, such as digital deformities or tailor's bunion, quintus varus. In the next level of experience, beginners, level II and III surgeries can be performed, reserving level IV surgeries for an advanced level of experience and level V surgeries only for experts.

5.1   Difficulty Pathology

   I. Tailor's bunion, digital deformities
  II. Achilles tendinopathy, calcaneoplasty
 III. Metatarsalgia, mild-moderate hallux valgus.
 IV. Severe hallux valgus, calcaneal osteotomy, subtalar arthrodesis
  V. Salvage surgery

5.2   Percutaneous Surgical Technique Recommended for Beginners

In our opinion, the most recommended surgical technique for the beginning of the learning curve is the treatment of the quintus varus or tailor's bunion, based on the lower complexity with respect to other techniques and on the good surgical results we obtain with this technique.

5.3   Surgical Planning

- Patient in supine decubitus with the foot outside the limit of the operating table.
- Anesthetic block at ankle level. For this technique it is not necessary to block the saphenous nerve or the deep peroneal nerve.
- Without ischemia cuff.
- Instruments for minimally invasive foot surgery.
- Basic instrumentation (Beaver-type scalpel, rasps).
- Motorized instrumentation (motor and drills).
- Radiological control instruments (fluoroscopic system).

5.4   Surgical Technique

5.4.1   Exostectomy

A 5 mm skin incision is performed, located in front of the external condyle of the fifth metatarsal. The skin is incised perpendicularly, and immediately we move towards the capsule, which is crossed towards the metatarsophalangeal joint of the

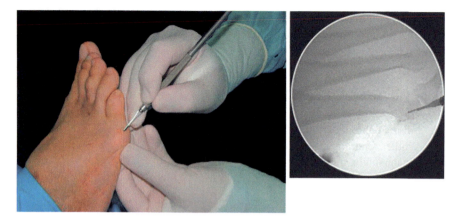

Fig. 17 Tailor's bunion approach

Fig. 18 Dorsolateral
exostectomy

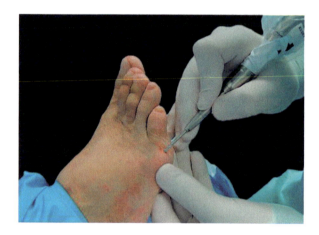

fifth toe (Fig. 17). With a dorsal and plantar movement, the entire capsule is detached
from its superior and external aspect of the lateral condyle of the fifth metatarsal,
creating a space between it and the bone where it can be "worked"; a rasp is introduced to check the space created between the condyle and the capsule, which will
protect the soft tissue from injury. The small triangular reamer is introduced, and,
with a slow speed of 2000–6000 rpm and a dorsal and plantar oscillating motion, the
dorsal and lateral exostosis is removed exactly to the desired level, which will be
checked under fluoroscopic control (Fig. 18). This process is interrupted on two or
three occasions, pressing the capsule on the head of the fifth metatarsal in the direction of the skin incision, to remove the bone paste produced, as well as to introduce
the scraper, in order to remove the fine bony debris and those adhering to the deep
side of the capsule (Fig. 19). With the repetition of these gestures, a complete exostectomy and adequate cleaning is achieved.

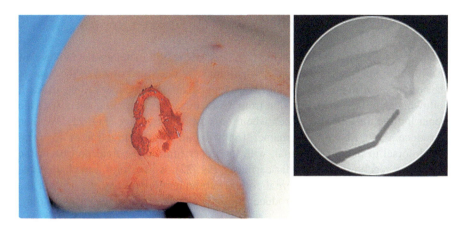

Fig. 19 Removal of the bony detritus of the exostosis

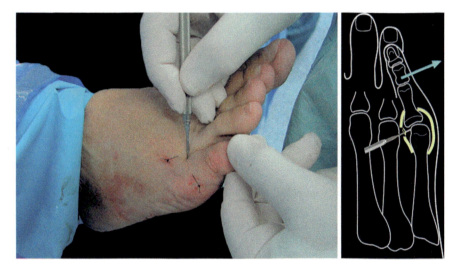

Fig. 20 Metatarsophalangeal capsulotomy

5.5 *Metatarsophalangeal Capsulotomy*

A new 5 mm incision is made at the level of the dorsal and lateral aspect of the metatarsophalangeal joint of the fifth toe (Fig. 20). Through the incision, the scalpel is introduced inside the joint, turning it 90° and leaving the cut surface facing later-ally, the finger is taken with the left hand, and a valgus movement is performed, thus tightening the medial capsule, which is incised over its entire surface, a gesture that the surgeon can appreciate perfectly by noticing how the resistance gives way in the valgus movement of the fifth finger.

5.6   Distal Metatarsal Osteotomy

A new 5 mm incision is made behind the head of the fifth metatarsal at the level of the 4th–fifth intermetatarsal space, which must be deepened down to the bone at the neck of the fifth metatarsal (Fig. 21); a long Shannon 44 reamer is then inserted, following an oblique 45° direction from distal dorsal to proximal plantar, with the upper limit at the end of the neck when it reaches the cartilage (Fig. 21). We then introduce a long Shannon 44 reamer, following an oblique direction of 45° from distal dorsal to plantar proximal, with the upper limit at the final portion of the neck upon reaching the articular cartilage (Fig. 22); we perform a medial wedge osteotomy, respecting the external cortex; subsequently, pressing the head of the fifth metatarsal medially, we produce an osteoclasty that completes the osteotomy.

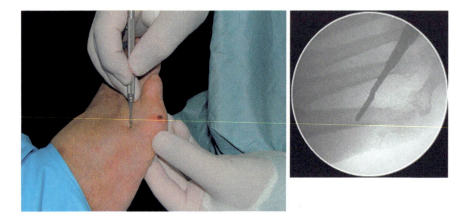

Fig. 21 Approach for distal metatarsal osteotomy

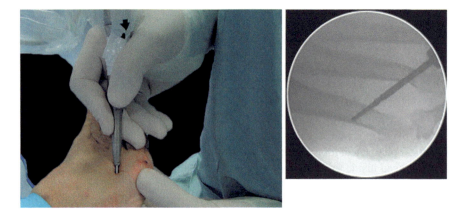

Fig. 22 Distal metatarsal osteotomy

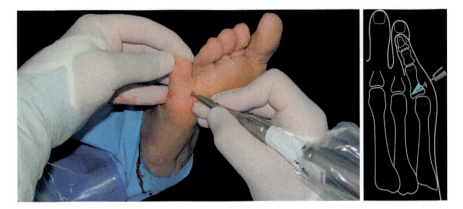

Fig. 23 Osteotomy of the base of the proximal phalanx of the fifth toe

5.7 Osteotomy of the Base of the Proximal Phalanx of the Fifth Toe

An incision is made with the Beaver blade on the plantar skin immediately behind the digitoplantar skin fold, at the mid-height of the fifth toe; a rasp is introduced and slid from the base of the phalanx through the lateral periosteum of the phalanx, displacing it; the short Shannon 44 reamer (Fig. 23) is inserted and rests on the lateral aspect of the base of the proximal phalanx, thus performing an osteotomy, which may be total or incomplete wedge osteotomy, according to the indication considered appropriate.

5.7.1 Bandaging

Post-surgical dressing plays a vitally important part in the treatment to maintain the correction obtained, since osteosynthesis is not performed. A slightly compressive bandage is applied, maintaining a moderate hypercorrection in order to close the osteotomies performed (Fig. 24).

A check-up is performed after 7 days for removal of the stitches. Subsequently, a simpler dressing is applied, the technique of which is explained to the patient so that he/she can change it daily after the toilet. The bandage consists of the placement of some plasters that maintain the correction and a metatarsal strap with a self-adhesive elastic bandage (Fig. 25). This bandage should be maintained 24 hours a day for 3 or 4 weeks after surgery, and the patient should walk with a post-surgical shoe with a rigid sole, to help maintain the stability of the osteosynthesis.

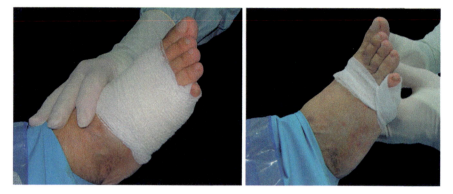

Fig. 24 Post-surgical dressing

Fig. 25 Bandage after the
first revision

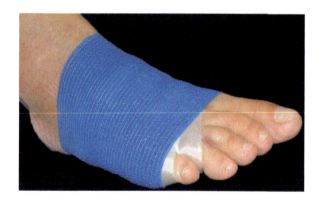

6   Complications

The poor results obtained by minimally invasive foot surgery in its beginnings,
30 years ago, were the consequence of a combination of incorrect indication, use of
nonspecific instruments, and lack of technical preparation. The rate of complications can be significantly reduced by attending specific training courses that allow
us to become accustomed to the use of the new instruments, as well as to clarify the
surgical indications.

6.1   Soft Tissues

6.1.1   Cutaneous

It is possible to find inflammation, edema, and superficial infection as a consequence of laceration or burn of the soft parts (Fig. 26). These complications are
linked to the learning curve, produced by the inadequate and repeated use of drills

Fig. 26 Burn after percutaneous surgery

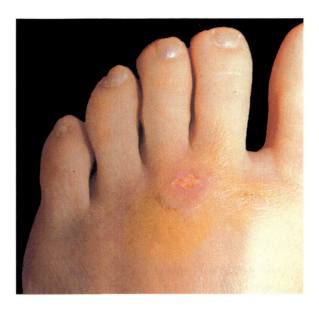

and other cutting instruments or extraction of bone detritus (rasps). They are generally caused by using the cutting drills with a speed higher than 10,000 RPM or by the pressure exerted by the drill on the skin when changing the direction of the motor during the performance of an osteotomy or exostectomy.

Occasionally, inflammation and slight exudate production can occur through the approach route, which can be mistaken for an infectious condition. This condition is caused by insufficient elimination of bone debris (detritus) produced during surgery by the action of the drills and sometimes appears as minimal bone chips through the incision after a few days.

6.1.2 Tendinous

Tendon injuries are exceptional. Contrary to what it may seem, it is not easy to section a tendon with the action of a drill, since, to section it, it is necessary for the cutting drill to be in direct contact with the tendon and to act on it while it is in contact with the bone or in the position of maximum tension.

6.1.3 Neurovascular

No vascular lesions have been described (Fig. 27) that produce ischemia of the structures distal to the surgical site, and iatrogenic neurological lesions are exceptional if we respect the access routes described for each of the different surgical techniques.

Fig. 27 Bleeding after
percutaneous surgery

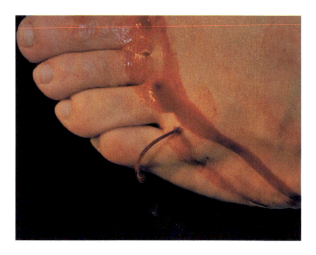

Dysesthesias may appear in up to 12% of patients, caused by inflammation or contusion of the tissues surrounding the peripheral nerves. They disappear within 2 or 3 months, persisting in time in only 0.5% of cases.

6.1.4   Edema

Persistent edema in the forefoot, especially in those cases operated of osteotomies of the lesser metatarsals, is frequent. It can be considered part of the normal evolution of this type of technique, being present up to 3 or 4 months after surgery. In some patients it requires symptomatic treatment.

6.1.5   Joint Stiffness

Joint stiffness is a relatively frequent complication, both in open surgery and in minimally invasive surgery.

In hallux valgus surgery, a limitation of 20% of the global mobility of the metatarsophalangeal joint can occur in between 1.5% and 6.8% of patients. This complication can be minimized by complete removal of bone debris, control of the action of the drills, and early mobilization of the joint (usually at 3 weeks, when there is sufficient fibrous callus to prevent displacement of the osteotomies).

In metatarsalgia surgery, joint stiffness, in the case of distal lateral metatarsal osteotomies, is exceptional, being absent or without clinical repercussions in most series, unlike in open Weil-type techniques where joint stiffness is the main complication.

6.1.6   Others

Deep infection and deep vein thrombosis occur exceptionally in minimally invasive foot surgery, with an incidence of less than 0.8% and 1.8%, respectively.

6.2   Bone

6.2.1   Secondary Displacement of Osteotomies

In osteotomies of the first radius, there is a possibility of displacement due to the absence of osteosynthesis material (Fig. 28). Technical errors in the direction of

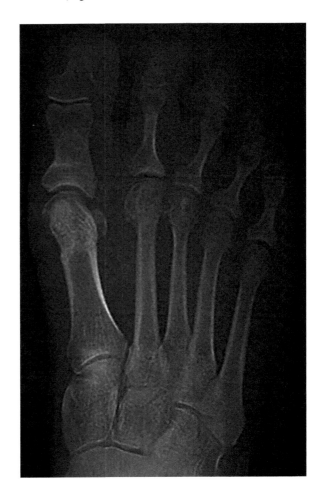

Fig. 28 Displacement after osteotomy of the first metatarsal

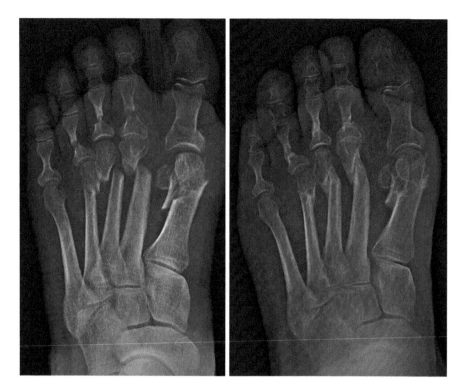

Fig. 29 Displaced DMMO and subsequent adequate consolidation

osteotomy tracing are the main cause of these secondary displacements, and early treatment should be performed. Modification of the dressing or repositioning to the correct position and the use of a percutaneous Kirchner wire synthesis may be sufficient to resolve it. If displacement is detected late after vicious consolidation of the osteotomy, surgical treatment will be necessary.

In distal lateral metatarsal osteotomies, the presence of displacement between the ends of the osteotomies, even when significant, should not be considered a complication, since it is the intended effect after surgery (Fig. 29). After these osteotomies have been performed, immediate loading is authorized so that the free metatarsal head can find its ideal functional position by receiving the weight of the body during walking. It is important to avoid dorsal rotation movements of the metatarsal head, for which it is recommended that during walking, in the first postoperative month, the use of a stiff-soled shoe without a heel, which allows loading along the sole of the foot and avoids dorsal flexion of the metatarsophalangeal joints, is recommended.

6.2.2 Healing Disorders

Delays in healing of the osteotomies of the first metatarsal are frequent, reaching consolidation after 6 months. They are well tolerated despite persistent inflammation (Fig. 30).

Fig. 30 Delayed consolidation after multiple osteotomies

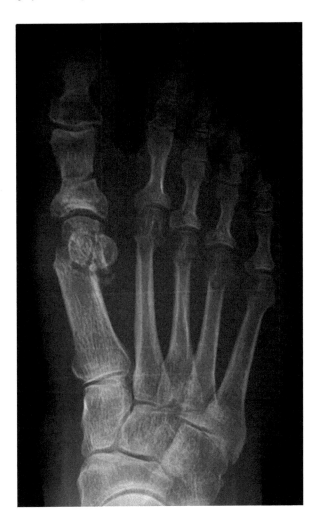

The healing time of lateral metatarsal osteotomies is very variable, ranging from 6 weeks to more than 12 months in some cases, most of which are asymptomatic. Due to the time of evolution, the presence of pseudarthrosis should not be considered until 18 months of evolution.

Pseudarthrosis and avascular necrosis of the metatarsal head are exceptional and without any clinical repercussions in most published cases.

7   Summary

The time when the complications of minimally invasive foot surgery seriously conditioned the results obtained is over. These techniques occupy an important place in our therapeutic arsenal, but not all interventions performed on the foot can or should be performed by minimally invasive techniques. Their indications are very precise, and it is necessary to adhere to them if good results are to be obtained, since minimally invasive surgery is just another method in the surgeon's hands and not an end in itself and will be reserved for surgeons with experience in both traditional and minimally invasive surgery.

To get started in these techniques, a sometimes slow and laborious learning curve will be necessary, in which we must follow a process of adaptation to the loss of direct and three-dimensional vision of the surgical field, as well as perfecting our anatomical knowledge, not only of the access route but also of the path that the instruments used follow to the place of the designed surgical gesture.

In conclusion, we can say that minimally invasive foot surgery is a surgical method that allows us to perform some interventions through minimal incisions, which in order to be performed, with respect to the anatomy, percentage of complications, and precision equivalent to open surgery, these four conditions will be necessary:

1. To limit the use of minimally invasive techniques to their indications.
2. To have an exact knowledge of the anatomical relationships of the foot, in order to be able to use adequate approach routes free of risk of injuring anatomical structures that must be respected, without producing iatrogenic lesions.
3. To have the specific instruments and to use them in the appropriate manner. Under no circumstances should these techniques be performed by adapting instruments, motorized or not, more or less similar to those designed for this surgery.
4. Use a radiological control method during the intervention not only to check the result but also to control its development under radiological vision. In this way we will avoid the complications derived from the lack of direct vision of the surgical field.

Suggested Readings

1. Addante JB. The metatarsal osteotomy, as a surgical approach to the elimination of plantar keratosis. J Foot Surg. 1969;8:3.
2. Bauer T, De Lavigne C, Biau D, De Prado M, Isham S, Laffenêtre O. GRECMIP: percutaneous hallux valgus surgery: a prospective multicenter study of 189 cases. Orthop Clin North Am. 2009;40:505–14.
3. Bauer T, Biau D, Lortat-Jacob A, Hardy P. Percutaneous hallux valgus correction using the Reverdin-Isham osteotomy. Orthop Traumatol Surg Res. 2010;96(4):407–16.
4. Bösch P, Markowski H, Rannicher V. Technik und erste Ergebnisse der subkutanen distalen Metatarsale-I-Osteotomie. Orthop Prax. 1990;26:51–6.
5. De Prado M. Minimally invasive foot surgery: a paradigma shift. In: Maffulli N, Easley M, editors. Minimally invasive surgery of the foot and ankle. Springer: London; 2011. p. 3–11.
6. De Prado M. Complications in minimally invasive foot surgery. FuB and Sprunggelenk. 2013;11:83–94.
7. De Prado M, Cuervas-Mons M, De Prado V, Golanó P, Vaquero J. Does the minimally invasive complete plantar fasciotomy result in deformity of the Plantar arch? A prospective study. Foot Ankle Surg. 2020;26(3):347–53.

8. De Prado M, Ripoll PL, Golanó P. Minimally invasive foot surgery. Barcelona: AYH; 2009.
9. De Prado M, Ripoll PL, Golanó P. Cirugía percutánea del pie. Barcelona: Elsevier (masson); 2003.
10. De Prado M, Ripoll PL, Vaquero J, Golanó P. Tratamiento quirúrgico percutáneo del Hallux Valgus mediante osteotomías múltiples. Rev Ortop Traumatol. 2003;47:406–16.
11. Dhukaram V, Chapman AP, Upadhyay PK. Minimally invasive forefoot surgery: a cadaveric study. Foot Ankle Int. 2012;33(12):1139–44.
12. García-Fernández D, Larrainzar-Garijo R, Llanos-Alcázar LF. Estudio comparativo de la osteotomía de Weil abierta: ¿es necesaria siempre la fijación? Rev Ortop Traumatol. 2006;50:292–7.
13. Giannini S, Ceccarelli R, Bevoni R, Vannini F. Hallux valgus surgery: the minimally InvasiveBunion Correction (SERI). Tech Foot Ankle Surg. 2003;2(1):11–20.
14. Henry J, Besse JL, Fessy MH. Distal osteotomy of the lateral metatarsals: a series of 72 cases comparing the Weil osteotomy and the DMMO percutaneous osteotomy. Orthop Traumatol Surg Res. 2011;97(6 Suppl):S57–65.
15. Isham S. The Reverdin-Isham procedure for the correction of hallux abductus valgus. A distal metatarsal osteotomy procedure. Clin Podiatr Med Surg. 1991;8:81–94.
16. Maffulli N. Minimally invasive surgery in orthopedic surgery. Orthop Clin North Am. 2009;4(40):491.
17. Magnan B, Pezze L, Rossi N, Bartolozzi P. Percutaneous distal metatarsal osteotomy for correction of hallux valgus. J Bone Joint Surg. 2005;87-A:1191–9.
18. Stiglitz Y, Cazeau C. Minimally invasive surgery and percutaneous surgery of the hindfoot and midfoot. Eur J Orthop Surg Traumatol. 2018;28(5):839–47.

Tumors of the Foot and Ankle

Eduardo Botello and Tomas Zamora

1 Introduction

Musculoskeletal tumors in the foot and ankle region are relatively uncommon entities, and they represent up to 5–8% of all musculoskeletal tumors [1, 2]. Moreover, sarcomas, malignant neoplasms of mesenchymal origin, arise in this region in only 2% of all sarcoma cases [3]. This being said, the implications of an error in diagnosis of a neoplasm in the foot and ankle can be frequent and can lead to significant morbidity and severe consequences in case of a malignant tumor [4], emphasizing the importance for any specialist involved to be familiar with the evaluation and diagnosis of musculoskeletal tumors in this area.

This chapter will focus on the main clinical aspects of bone and soft tissue tumors of the foot and ankle, including clinical presentation, imaging, and initial management. Common subtypes and relevant histologies will also be described.

2 Epidemiology

As previously stated, tumors of the foot and ankle are considered to be relatively infrequent. A retrospective analysis from a tumor institute in Germany described a 5.5% incidence from a total of 7487 musculoskeletal tumors treated in almost 20 years [2]. Almost two-thirds were bone tumors, and 18% were malignant tumors of bone and soft tissue. The most common benign bone tumors were simple bone cysts, enchondroma, osteochondromas, aneurysmal bone cysts, and intraosseous

E. Botello (✉) · T. Zamora
Orthopaedic Oncology and Lower Limb Reconstructive Surgery, Orthopaedic Surgery Department, Pontificia Universidad Católica de Chile, Santiago, Chile
e-mail: ebotello@med.puc.cl; tzamora@med.puc.cl

© The Author(s), under exclusive license to Springer Nature Switzerland AG 2022
E. Wagner Hitschfeld, P. Wagner Hitschfeld (eds.), *Foot and Ankle Disorders*,
https://doi.org/10.1007/978-3-030-95738-4_4

71

lipomas. From the malignant bone tumors (8%), 46% were chondrosarcomas. The most frequent benign soft tissue tumors treated in this cohort were hemangioma, followed by tenosynovial giant cell tumor (or pigmented villonodular synovitis), superficial fibromatosis, neurinoma, and schwannoma. Moreover, the most common malignant soft tissue tumors were synovial sarcoma and myxofibrosarcoma.

Similarly, a North-American series reported a 5.7% rate of tumors in the foot and ankle [5]. The most common bone tumors were giant cell tumor of bone, osteosarcoma, and chondrosarcoma, while frequent soft tissue tumors were tenosynovial giant cell tumor, hemangioma, and synovial sarcoma.

3 Anatomy

The foot and ankle anatomy is unique, given the proximity of different bone and soft tissue structures such as tendons, muscle, ligaments, nerves, and vessels. Similarly, the lack of well-defined fascial planes and complex bony anatomy can make a surgical resection complying with oncological principles and preservation of the extremity challenging.

Given the size of bony structures, especially in the foot, tumors can erode cortices relatively early during their progression, reaching the soft tissues around them. In the same way, soft tissue tumors can be diagnosed at a smaller size, compared to other anatomic sites such as the pelvis, where tumors can be extremely large before being noticed. Similarly, they can penetrate bone cortices easily, leading to more extensive surgical resections when margins are a critical consideration.

On the other hand, the distal tibia's subcutaneous location can make soft tissue coverage difficult in case of an extraosseous extension of a malignant bone tumor. Finally, the arterial supply to the distal lower extremity is given by the anterior and posterior tibial arteries, which communicate extensively through distal anastomosis around the foot, ensuring adequate blood supply in most cases. In the same way, neurological structures should be preserved when possible, especially the medial and lateral plantar divisions of the tibial nerve, which gives the sensorial innervation of the plantar weight-bearing surface of the foot.

4 Clinical Presentation

Tumors around the foot and ankle can appear at any age and are overall similarly distributed within males and females, but variations may arise depending on specific histologies.

As with musculoskeletal neoplasms in other locations, pain and a palpable lump are the most common presentations of tumors in the foot and ankle [6, 7]. Symptoms such as night or non-mechanical pain should be considered as a red flag for further investigations, as well as inflammation or swelling during examination. A soft tissue mass with a rapid increase in size, a painful lump, recurrence after a previous excision, or a size over 5 cm should prompt urgent referral to a specialized center to rule out a malignancy [8]. Given the proximity of structures in this anatomic area and the technical difficulties of a malignant neoplasm re-excision, advance imaging should be considered early in sizeable lesions. In other words, the classic 5 cm rule could underestimate the need for cross-sectional imaging in this anatomic area.

Changes in the skin color should be considered with attention, given that melanoma is not an infrequent diagnosis around the foot. Moreover, a detailed physical examination can give clues to the tumor extension, especially if a motor or sensorial deficit is present. Soft tissue tumors should also be assessed in depth, tenderness, pulsatility, and transillumination, which may be useful to suggest cystic lesions.

History of previous cancer, therapies (e.g., radiation), and risk factors (smoking) should be obtained in all patients with a bone or soft tissue lesion. Acral metastases are uncommon but should be among the differential diagnosis (mainly pulmonary and renal carcinoma).

5   Imaging

All patients with a bone or soft tissue tumor and an uncertain diagnosis or a red flag in the clinical presentation should be referred for radiographs (anteroposterior, lateral, and oblique). Plain X-rays have at least moderate evidence to support its use in evaluating all bone tumors of unknown origin. Similarly, in soft tissue tumors, they can add information like the presence of phleboliths (in hemangiomas), calcifications, or cortical erosion of the underlying bone [9]. Signs of a more aggressive lesion or malignancy include periosteal reaction, cortical erosion/breach, ill-defined margins, and signs of a soft tissue mass and should prompt further investigations. On the other hand, well-defined lesions with a sclerotic margin, without a periosteal reaction, cortical disruption, or a soft tissue mass, orientate to a more chronic and less aggressive process, usually benign.

Ultrasonography can be helpful in small and superficial soft tissue tumors by distinguishing between benign lesions such as vascular malformations, lipomas or simple cysts, and other lesions with a more solid component that warrant further investigations. On the other hand, deep and larger than 5 cm tumors should be assessed directly with cross-sectional imaging, as ultrasound could fail to discriminate in these lesions [9, 10].

Computed tomography (CT) scan and magnetic resonance imaging (MRI) are the imaging of choice when it comes to a better assessment of bone and soft tissue structures. CT provides an adequate assessment of bone involvement and cortical disruption, as well as calcifications within the lesion that could orientate to a more chronic process. MRI with gadolinium is the image of choice for soft tissue lesions and to determine bone marrow changes within the bone and other processes such as a stress fracture or osteomyelitis. MRI can also help to assess the extent of the lesion in both bone and soft tissue tumors and give details about its relationship with the surrounding tissues, being the imaging modality of choice for surgical planning.

In case that a malignant lesion is suspected, further imaging is used to assess the presence of metastatic disease. In bone sarcomas, a CT of the chest is used to rule out a pulmonary compromise, as well as a whole-body bone scan with a radiotracer (most commonly technetium-99) to assess for other skeletal lesions. In soft tissue sarcomas, a CT of the abdomen and pelvis should be included. Similarly, a whole-body MR or an 18-fluorine fluorodeoxyglucose (18F-FDG) positron emission tomography (PET)/CT is useful for this purpose, with increased sensitivity, especially for axial metastatic disease [11, 12].

6 Biopsy

Obtaining a sample for histopathology is of crucial relevance in the diagnostic process of musculoskeletal tumors around the foot and ankle as well as for other locations. This being said, the biopsy should be performed at least in communication with the referral center, as it has been reported a higher biopsy related complication rate when biopsies are performed in non-specialized centers [13].

Imaging is of particular importance when planning for a biopsy. Cross-sectional imaging should help decide the biopsy tract and the lesion area that will be sampled to avoid purely cystic or necrotic areas.

More important than the type of biopsy performed is that it complies with classic oncologic principles such as: it should be minimally invasive; should be performed by or in consultation with the surgeon/team that will perform the definitive management; should not contaminate other compartments; should be in line with the definitive/planned incision; should be representative of the lesion being biopsied; and should achieve adequate hemostasis. According to local practice and preference, after all this is reviewed, a decision whether a percutaneous or an open biopsy should be performed. Percutaneous biopsy techniques with a core needle biopsy can be performed in most tumors and are easily guided through ultrasound (soft tissue) or CT (bone). They have shown to be accurate, with most studies reporting more than 90% accuracy for bone and soft tissue tumors [14, 15], and have become the initial approach in most scenarios. On the other hand, even though fine-needle aspiration biopsy techniques have a role in general oncology and they are used in some centers for musculoskeletal tumors, we discourage their use given the high variability and lack of accuracy in some circumstances [16]. Open incisional biopsy remains a valid and commonly used technique; however, it should be reserved after a previous non-diagnostic or discordant biopsy or in young patients where a general anesthetic will be needed anyway. In the same way, an excisional biopsy is usually reserved for small tumors that can be easily excised with low risks and complying with oncological principles.

7   Principles of Treatment

General management depends on the type of tumor and its grade. For clearly benign lesions, including stage 1 latent bone lesions according to the Enneking staging system, close observation is generally the rule if the patient remains asymptomatic. Patients with benign but symptomatic lesions or active/aggressive benign bone tumors that could progress with significant morbidity are generally managed surgically with either intralesional or marginal excision depending on the type of tumor, its grade, and anatomic location, among others. On the other hand, wide resection is generally reserved for malignant tumors; however, it can also be the technique of choice in some benign aggressive lesions such as a giant cell tumor of bone with extensive bone destruction and soft tissue mass. In the foot, a radical excision usually includes some sort of amputation, given that metatarsals are the only distinct compartmental boundaries.

If limb salvage is not possible with safe margins in a high-grade malignant tumor, amputation should be considered. Most below the knee amputations can give more than acceptable function in association with adequate rehabilitation and access to prosthesis if needed.

8   Common Types of Tumors

8.1   Giant Cell Tumor (GCT) of Bone

GCT of bone is an intermediate, locally aggressive bone tumor characterized for the presence of classic multinucleated giant cells from which the tumor derives its name, distributed in a stroma of ovoid mononuclear cells, which are the true neoplastic origin. It can metastasize in its benign form and has a malignant counterpart, which is clinical and histologically different.

GCT of bone has a peak incidence in the third and fourth decade, and it is rare in children with an open physis. Even though it has been described in practically every bone of the skeleton, it is more frequent in the metaphyseal-epiphyseal region of long bones, especially around the knee in the distal femur. From all cases of GCT of bone, lesions in the foot and ankle had been reported to be up to 5% of cases, more frequently in the talus, distal tibia, and calcaneus [17–19].

Most GCT of bone present as a lytic lesion with geographic margins that can be expansile and are located eccentrically within the bone (Fig. 1). In the foot and ankle region, these lesions tend to appear more aggressive on imaging, with a more ill-defined margin, cortical disruption, and even soft tissue mass. On MRI, it has a low signal on T1 sequences and a high signal on fluid sensitive sequences such as T2, with avid enhancement on contrast-enhanced sequences.

Treatment for contained lesions (Campanacci I and II) [20] usually consists in curettage and bone grafting or cement. Given the aggressive pattern and high

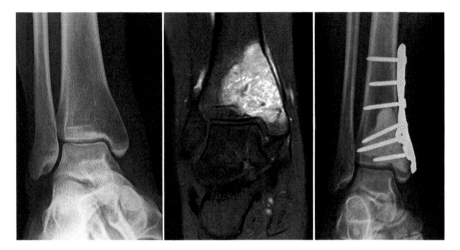

Fig. 1 35-year-old female with a bone tumor in her right ankle. (Left) AP X-ray and (center) coronal STIR reconstruction, revealing a lytic lesion in the distal epiphysis and metaphysis of the tibia. Biopsy showed a giant cell tumor of bone. (Right) AP X-ray after curettage with adjuvant treatment, plus cement filling and plate fixation with good results

recurrence risks classically described for GCT of bone, the use of some adjuvant treatment is recommended. In the foot and ankle, lesions tend to act even more aggressively with a higher recurrence rate than for other anatomic areas, with up to 30–52% of recurrence rate [17, 21]. For this reason, wide excision with resection and reconstruction and even amputation has to be considered in more advanced lesions with extensive bone destruction. On the other hand, medical treatment with neoadjuvant denosumab protocols has been used extensively in the last decade, especially in cases with a soft tissue compromise.

8.2 Chondroblastoma

Chondroblastoma is a rare and benign bone tumor of chondroid origin that typically arises in the epiphysis of long bones, especially tibia, femur, and humerus, but up to 13% of cases can involve the foot, specially tarsal bones [22, 23]. Its peak incidence is during the second decade; however, it has been described at all ages, with a 2–3:1 male preponderance.

Most cases present with severe pain and limitation of movement. The radiographic appearance is of a lytic lesion with well-defined margins. In MRI the presence of intense perilesional edema is frequent. It is most commonly found in the posterior facet of the calcaneus and the posterior body of the talus close to the tibiotalar joint [24] and can be associated with cystic features and even a secondary aneurysmal bone cyst (ABC) component.

Treatment in latent or active lesions usually consists of curettage and bone grafting or cement filling with an adjuvant treatment such as phenol or cryotherapy. Recurrence has ranged from 10% to 15% [23, 25], without a clear relationship with its location or the presence of a secondary ABC [23].

8.3   Aneurysmal Bone Cyst (ABC)

ABC was initially considered to be a reactive phenomenon; however, the identification of the constant involvement of the USP6 fusion oncogene led to a better understanding of this neoplastic, benign, but locally aggressive lesion [26]. ABC is usually observed in the metaphysis of long bones, more frequently around the knee. This being said, the foot and ankle involvement is considered infrequent, with reports stating 2–9% of ABCs located in this region [24, 27, 28]. Secondary ABC arises together with other bone tumors such as GCT of bone, chondroblastoma, osteoblastoma, or fibrous dysplasia.

Most patients with ABC are young, with a peak incidence in the second decade. Radiographic appearance includes an eccentric, expansile lytic lesion with cortical thinning, located in the metaphysis of bone. MRI shows the classic fluid-fluid levels, representing blood-filled compartments, and a CT scan is especially useful to define the extent of the lesion and cortical compromise as for other lesions. When a secondary component is present, the MRI will demonstrate an additional solid component representing the primary tumor, especially in gadolinium-enhanced sequences.

As with most benign lesions, management generally includes curettage with or without bone grafting or cement augmentation. Reported recurrence rates have been described as up to 20%, with most of them being during the first 2 years from the initial surgical treatment [28]. Lesions with extensive bone loss are treated with wide resection and reconstruction depending on the location. Other techniques, such as embolization, radiofrequency ablation, or minimally invasive methods, have also been described [24, 29].

8.4   Enchondroma

Enchondromas are one of the most common benign forms of cartilaginous neoplasms. They represent approximately 3% of all bone tumors and up to 15% of benign bone tumors. This being said, the foot will host up to 6% of all enchondromas, especially in the proximal phalanx [30].

Enchondromas are usually solitary tumors found incidentally, and therefore, their true incidence is likely to be higher than reported. Most of them are asymptomatic and are found at any age but usually from 15–40 years. Enchondromas appear as central and metaphyseal lesions, with a well-delimitated border and central mineralization. Calcifications can range in size from small punctuate to larger rings. MRI will show a cartilaginous neoplasm signal pattern with low signal intensity on T1 sequences and high signal intensity on T2-weighted sequences.

Various radiographic and clinical features can help differentiate a benign enchondroma from a more aggressive /malignant tumor; however, this remains a diagnostic challenge, even for experienced specialists [31]. Painful and larger lesions, extensive cortical compromise, and a large soft tissue mass should alert for the possibility of malignant transformation; however, this is rare for isolated lesions.

As with most benign latent lesions, enchondromas that are asymptomatic can be treated non-operatively with observation alone. Single lesions with a characteristic radiographic appearance do not need to undergo a biopsy. Indications for surgical treatment in an enchondroma are continuous symptoms, enlargement, or radiographic changes during follow-up to rule out a low-grade malignant variant, impending fracture, or an actual fracture of the host bone. If surgical treatment is decided, curettage and bone grafting or cement augmentation is usually the treatment of choice, with a low rate of recurrence if done adequately and with the addition of some form of adjuvant therapy.

Several syndromes have been described in patients with multiple enchondromas, with recent classifications based on spinal involvement and genetic inheritance. The two most frequently described syndromes are Ollier disease and Maffucci syndrome, both non-hereditary and without spinal involvement.

8.5   Osteochondroma

Osteochondromas are the most frequently biopsied bone tumors. It is usually located in the metaphysis of long bones, especially around the knee, during the second decade of life [32]. The foot and ankle region are relatively uncommon locations; however, they usually cause significant symptoms that require treatment in contrast to other anatomic areas.

Osteochondromas are usually diagnosed incidentally if they are small. However, in the distal tibia, osteochondromas can cause deformity and significant symptoms (Fig. 2). X-rays are the primary imaging modality, observing an osseous protuberance arising from the bone that can be pedunculated or sessile but has medullary and cortical continuity (Fig. 2). If there is a symptomatic or atypical lesion, MRI can accurately characterize the lesion and its cartilage cap, with a high sensitivity and specificity for malignant transformation, especially if the cap measures more than 2 cm [33].

Treatment usually consists in resection through the base of the lesion in case of significant symptoms [34], with adequate results. Multiple hereditary exostosis (MHE) is a rare autosomal dominant inherited syndrome in which patients have multiple enchondromas with a higher risk of malignant transformation (up to 5%).

Fig. 2 Coronal MRI
reconstruction and oblique
X-ray of the ankle from an
18-year-old male, with a
distal tibia
osteochondroma. A lateral
osseous protuberance is
observed in the distal tibia,
with slight fibular
deformity

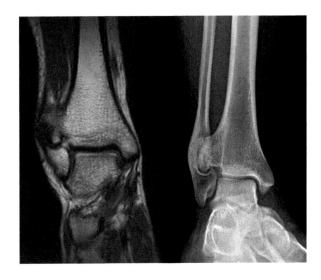

8.6   Subungual Exostosis

A subungual exostosis is a benign, painful osteocartilaginous surface lesion of the distal phalanx, mostly located in the great toe (80%); however, it can occur in any toe or finger, producing nail deformation.

X-rays show an osseous proliferation attached to the distal phalanx's side or dorsum without cortical or medullary continuity (unlike classic osteochondroma). Initially, these lesions were thought to be reactive; however, clonal cytogenetic findings in recent years have confirmed a proper neoplastic process. As with most benign lesions, marginal resection is usually adequate and curative.

8.7   Unicameral Bone Cyst (UBC)

UBCs are benign cystic lesions that are commonly seen in young patients. Their most frequent location is in the metaphysis of long bones (femur or humerus); however, the calcaneus is also a common site (sixth in frequency), and it is the most frequent location in the foot and ankle region.

Most of these lesions are found incidentally and are located in the anterolateral aspect of the calcaneus. On plain X-rays, they are observed as lytic lesions with well-defined margins and mild cortical thinning. MRI shows no solid component.

Most asymptomatic calcaneal UBC tends to be treated non-operatively, with observation alone. Levy et al. [35] showed that only a small percentage (1%) had spontaneous regression with observation, and for that reason, most symptomatic large cysts, or those with a high risk for a pathological fracture, are treated with some sort of intervention. Corticosteroid injection has shown radiographic healing in 66% of patients, while open curettage and grafting have been considered the traditional treatment with the best outcome described. Minimally invasive cannulated screws decompression and limited curettage have also been shown to be a valid technique for smaller lesions, especially in children [35].

8.8   Intraosseous Lipoma

Intraosseous lipomas are usually considered to be rare entities and are most commonly located in long bones or the calcaneus in the Ward's triangle, just inferior to the angle of Gissane [24, 36, 37].

It is unclear whether intraosseous lipoma has a predilection for a specific age or gender; however, some studies have reported a predilection for males and adult life. Most patients are symptomatic, with pain being the most frequent symptom, followed by swelling or tenderness. On plain X-rays, they appear as a lytic cystic lesion with well-defined sclerotic margins and calcifications within the margins. MRI confirms the suspected lesion with an intense signal in T1- and T2-weighted sequences, identical to subcutaneous fat.

Non-symptomatic lesions can be treated with observation, as some of them can undergo spontaneous regression. Symptomatic and large lesions are usually treated with open curettage and grafting, to prevent a pathological fracture. Lesions extending the full breadth of the calcaneus laterally to medially in the coronal plane and at least 30% of the length anteroposteriorly are considered to be of critical size and warrant surgical treatment to prevent fractures [38]. Recurrence rates are very low.

8.9   Tenosynovial Giant Cell Tumor

Tenosynovial giant cell tumors are a group of lesions that arise from the synovium of joints, bursae, or tendon sheaths that can be intra- or extra-articular and are classified by its clinical and biological behavior in localized (previously called giant cell tumor of the tendon sheath) or diffuse type (previously called pigmented villonodular synovitis). In time, cytogenetic studies have confirmed its neoplastic nature and common pathology, with a structural change involving the translocation of the CSF1 gene, causing the synthesis of a large amount of CSF1 protein [39].

The localized form of tenosynovial giant cell tumor is more frequent around the hand; however, another common location is the ankle associated with many of the tendon sheaths. They can occur at any age but are more frequent in adult life with a slight female preponderance. They present as a firm nodule, usually painless, that can grow in time and cause symptoms when compressed by footwear. Surgical resection usually gives a good outcome with a low recurrence risk if treated adequately.

The diffuse form of tenosynovial giant cell tumor usually presents in younger patients than its localized counterpart. The most commonly involved joints are the knee and ankle, but the midfoot is also a frequently involved region [3]. Patients present with pain, tenderness, swelling, and a limited range of motion. X-rays can show signs of a soft tissue mass, with bone erosions and secondary degenerative joint disease. MRI is the imaging modality of choice, showing the classic blooming artifact on gradient echo sequences and low signal on T1- and T2-weighted sequences due to hemosiderin deposits. Macroscopically, the synovium appears brown, and there can be a multinodular appearance. Surgical resection is usually the treatment of choice, with arthroscopic modalities having satisfactory outcomes in limited disease but usually needing an open radical synovectomy in diffuse and extensive lesions [40].

Recurrence can be common in diffuse forms (up to 40%) [41] but can be initially controlled by surgical re-excision. Radiation has been used as an adjuvant therapy. Molecular targeted therapy represents a new option for managing patients with recurrent or inoperable disease and has shown promising results [42].

8.10 Plantar Fibromatosis

Plantar fibromatosis or Ledderhose disease is a benign fibroblastic proliferation involving the plantar aponeurosis and is one of the most common soft tissue tumors of the foot. It is more common in younger patients and can be painful with multiple nodules in the medial and central band of the plantar aponeurosis, with a significant proportion of patients presenting with bilateral disease (one-third).

It has been associated with Dupuytren's contractures and Peyronie's disease, as well as with other systemic diseases (such as epilepsy, diabetes mellitus, and cigarette smoking), although these last ones have not been widely validated.

Asymptomatic and small lesions can be managed with observation alone; however, symptomatic lesions might require surgical excision with partial or complete resection of the plantar fascia. Direct and marginal excision of nodules has been associated with an elevated recurrence risk [43, 44]; therefore, a more extensive resection is usually needed with even a complete plantar fasciectomy indicated in cases of recurrent disease. Other therapies, such as corticoid injections, extracorporeal shock wave therapy, and radiation therapy, have been used with variable success.

8.11 Ganglion

Ganglions are one of the most common soft tissue masses in the foot and ankle region [3] and are considered to be a cystic degeneration more than a proper neoplastic condition. They appear as a firm superficial nodule that can cause symptoms depending on their location. On clinical examination, the trans-illumination test can confirm its purely cystic nature, and aspiration will reveal a gel-like fluid content, confirming the diagnosis. Surgical excision is recommended in large symptomatic lesions, and special care should be taken to remove the entire capsule and the stalk of the tumor to avoid recurrent disease.

8.12   Lipoma

Lipoma is the most common mesenchymal soft tissue tumor and is composed of mature adipocytes. It commonly arises in the foot's dorsum and is usually a painless subcutaneous mass but can cause symptoms when compressed by footwear. Clinical examination usually reveals a superficial, small, and mobile mass. Ultrasound (in small, superficial lesions) and MRI can be diagnostic, demonstrating a homogenous lesion with an isointense signal to subcutaneous fat in all pulse sequences. Thick septations, deep location, and contrast enhancement should raise suspicion for a more atypical lesion [45].

Marginal excision is indicated in symptomatic lesions and is usually a curative treatment with a low recurrence rate.

8.13   Soft Tissue Sarcoma

Soft tissue sarcomas are relatively uncommon, with fewer than 10% arising in the foot and ankle [46]. Synovial sarcoma has been described as the most frequent histology in many case series [46–48], followed by myxofibrosarcoma, clear cell sarcoma, epithelioid sarcoma, and leiomyosarcoma.

Synovial sarcoma has a variable presentation but usually presents as a soft tissue lump, which may or may not be painful, and is usually long-standing before starting to grow significantly (Fig. 3). It can occur at any age and is equally distributed

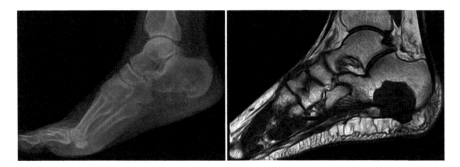

Fig. 3 Lateral X-ray (Left) and sagittal T1 MRI reconstruction (right) from a 67-year-old male's left foot, who presented with a hind foot bone and soft tissue tumor. Percutaneous biopsy resulted in a synovial sarcoma

Fig. 4 Same previous case. Surgical specimen after wide excision. Pathology report revealed a high-grade synovial sarcoma with clear margins in bone and soft tissue

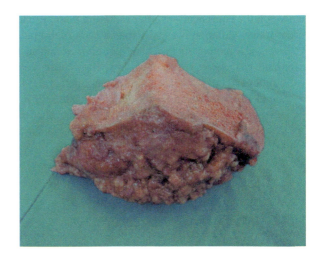

Fig. 5 Same previous case. Lateral X-ray of the left foot after wide excision and reconstruction with a femoral head allograft, with good results after 10 years

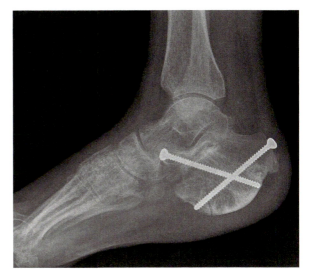

among males and females; however, most cases occur in adolescents or young adults. Synovial sarcomas are among the soft tissue sarcomas considered to have a relative predilection for lymphatic spread (compared to others).

Wide resection with limb salvage has become the treatment of choice for soft tissue sarcoma of the extremities, even distally, without compromising oncologic outcomes such as recurrence or survival [47] (Figs. 4 and 5). This has been achieved on the foot and ankle region with a combination of adjuvant therapies such as radiation therapy in selected cases and advances in plastic technique reconstruction with free flap coverage. Radiation therapy has been used with caution in the distal extremities, given the high rate of potential soft tissue complications. This being said, the difficulties in achieving an adequate margin in this anatomic location might outweigh the complications after radiation therapy, and therefore, postoperative or preoperative radiation is usually indicated in high-grade tumors of significant size.

Overall, sarcomas of the distal extremities appear to have better survival than sarcomas elsewhere. Cribb et al. [48] showed an overall mortality rate for distal extremities sarcoma of 14%, while Zeytoonjian et al. [46] showed an overall mortality rate of 10% for foot and ankle sarcoma, against 26% for all sarcomas. This might be explained by the relatively earlier presentation of these patients, given that foot masses usually become symptomatic before tumors located elsewhere.

8.14 Bone Sarcoma

8.14.1 Osteosarcoma

Osteosarcoma (OS) is the most frequent primary bone malignancy, and it has a bimodal occurrence with a peak incidence in the second decade. On the contrary, osteosarcoma of the foot is very rare, with less than 1% of all osteosarcoma arising in this location [49], and it is only slightly less uncommon in the distal tibia or fibula.

Radiographic appearance of a high-grade OS includes a lytic or sclerotic lesion with an osseous matrix, ill-defined margins, and varying amounts of periosteal reaction, including sunburst patterns or Codman's triangle. On the other hand, low-grade lesions might not show such a distinctive appearance. Because of the low grade of suspicion for malignant bone sarcoma, delays in the treatment of osteosarcomas of the foot and ankle region are often high.

Multi-agent chemotherapy and wide surgical excision are the mainstays of treatment for these lesions, but the details of medical or surgical treatment are beyond the scope of this review (Fig. 6).

8.14.2 Chondrosarcoma

Chondrosarcomas are (with Ewing's sarcoma) the most frequent primary bone sarcoma in the foot and ankle [50], but only 5% of these tumors occur in this region, being the calcaneus the most common location. Chondrosarcomas characterize for a peak incidence in middle age to older adults and are usually slow-growing malignancies.

Differentiation of a benign cartilaginous neoplasm from a chondrosarcoma remains a diagnostic challenge, even for experienced specialists [31]. Various radiographic and clinical features can help orientate the diagnostic process, including the patient's age, pain during clinical examination, size of the lesion, cortical compromise, soft tissue mass, and increased metabolic activity on bone scan or 18F-FDG PET/CT.

The recommended treatment is wide resection for all high-grade chondrosarcoma. Low-grade chondrosarcoma or atypical cartilaginous tumor could be treated

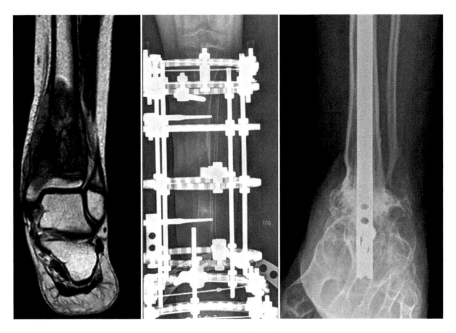

Fig. 6 7-year-old female patient with a left distal tibia high-grade conventional osteosarcoma. (Left) Coronal T1 MRI reconstruction after neoadjuvant systemic chemotherapy. AP X-ray (center) showing a bone transport technique as a reconstruction method after finishing her adjuvant chemotherapy. (Right) Two years post-op AP X-ray, with a stable ankle arthrodesis and an intramedullary nail

with an aggressive curettage, plus adjuvant treatment and cement augmentation with adequate recurrence rates and oncological outcomes [51, 52].

8.15   Ewing Sarcoma

Ewing sarcoma is a small round cell sarcoma showing a FET-ETS fusion gene derived mostly from a translocation between the chromosomes 11 and 22 – t(11;22)(q24;q12). It is more frequently located in the long bones, chest wall, and spine; however, the foot and ankle region's bones can be affected in up to 5% of cases. The calcaneus, talus, and metatarsal are the most commonly involved bones [50].

Classic radiographic appearance shows an ill-defined lesion with a permeated or moth-eaten pattern of bone destruction. Soft tissue mass is usually present.

As with osteosarcoma, multi-agent chemotherapy and local ablation are the treatment of choice. Surgical resection and radiation therapy are both forms of local control, with surgical resection being the preferred one when surgery provides acceptable morbidity and patient's tolerance [53].

8.16   Metastatic Disease

Metastatic disease in the distal extremities is less frequent than in the proximal appendicular or axial skeleton. Evans et al. [7] reported that only 0.5% of all osseous metastases, from an extensive database including more than 2500 metastatic patients, involved the foot. As described in other series for acrometastases [54], bronchogenic cancer was the most common primary disease (27% of cases), while the rest were secondary to other malignancies, including breast, prostate, kidney, and others.

Treatment for a symptomatic lesion should consider different factors such as the histology of the primary lesion, expected survival, patient's expectations and functionality, and response to other nonsurgical therapies. This being said, most patients can be managed locally with radiation therapy and marginal excision with or without internal fixation and cementation in case of persistent symptoms or impending fracture. Patients with oligometastatic disease and a primary histology that is nonresponsive to other therapies (such as renal or thyroid cancer) should be considered for wide resection to avoid local progression and surgical failure.

9   Summary

Foot and ankle tumors are rare. Although most of the time they are benign, they should not be underestimated, keeping in mind the basic oncological concepts of initial management and referral to specialized centers in the case of malignant lesions or locally aggressive behavior. Given this region's unique anatomy, where the soft tissue coverage is poor, the different pathologies' treatments can be complicated with difficult reconstructions and a higher percentage of complications.

References

1. Bos GD, Esther RJ, Woll TS. Foot tumors: diagnosis and treatment. Vol. 10, The Journal of the American Academy of Orthopaedic Surgeons. 2002. p. 259–70.
2. Toepfer A, Harrasser N, Recker M, Lenze U, Pohlig F, Gerdesmeyer L, et al. Distribution patterns of foot and ankle tumors: A university tumor institute experience. BMC Cancer. 2018;18(1).
3. Khan Z, Hussain S, Carter SR. Tumours of the foot and ankle. Vol. 25, Foot. 2015. p. 164–72.
4. Davis AM, Kandel RA, Wunder JS, Unger R, Meer J, O'Sullivan B, et al. The impact of residual disease on local recurrence in patients treated by initial unplanned resection for soft tissue sarcoma of the extremity. J Surg Oncol. 1997;66(2):81–7.
5. Chou LB, Ho YY, Malawer MM. Tumors of the foot and ankle: Experience with 153 cases. Foot Ankle Int. 2009;30(9):836–41.
6. George A, Grimer R. Early symptoms of bone and soft tissue sarcomas: could they be diagnosed earlier? Ann R Coll Surg Engl. 2012;94:261.
7. Evans S, Ramasamy A, Jeys L, Grimer R. Delayed diagnosis in metastatic lesions of the foot. Ann R Coll Surg Engl. 2014;96:536.

8. Grimer RJ, Briggs TWR. Earlier diagnosis of bone and soft-tissue tumors. J Bone Joint Surg Br. 2010;92:1489.

9. Miller BJ. Use of Imaging Prior to Referral to a Musculoskeletal Oncologist. Vol. 27, Journal of the American Academy of Orthopaedic Surgeons. 2019. p. E1001–8.

10. Nagano S, Yahiro Y, Yokouchi M, Setoguchi T, Ishidou Y, Sasaki H, et al. Doppler ultrasound for diagnosis of soft tissue sarcoma: Efficacy of ultrasound-based screening score. Radiol Oncol. 2015;49(2):135–40.

11. Harrison DJ, Parisi MT, Shulkin BL. The Role of 18F-FDG-PET/CT in Pediatric Sarcoma. Vol. 47, Seminars in Nuclear Medicine. 2017. p. 229–41.

12. Wu Q, Yang R, Zhou F, Hu Y. Comparison of whole-body MRI and skeletal scintigraphy for detection of bone metastatic tumors: A meta-analysis. Vol. 22, Surgical Oncology. 2013. p. 261–6.

13. Mankin HJ, Mankin CJ, Simon MA. The hazards of the biopsy, revisited: For the members of the musculoskeletal tumor society. J Bone Jt Surg - Ser A. 1996;78(5):656–63.

14. De Marchi A, Brach Del Prever EM, Linari A, Pozza S, Verga L, Albertini U, et al. Accuracy of core-needle biopsy after contrast-enhanced ultrasound in soft-tissue tumours. Eur Radiol. 2010;20(11):2740–8.

15. Shin HJ, Amaral JG, Armstrong D, Chait PG, Temple MJ, John P, et al. Image-guided percutaneous biopsy of musculoskeletal lesions in children. Pediatr Radiol. 2007;37(4):362–9.

16. Ogilvie CM, Torbert JT, Finstein JL, Fox EJ, Lackman RD. Clinical utility of percutaneous biopsies of musculoskeletal tumors. Clin Orthop Relat Res. 2006 Sep;450:95-100.

17. Biscaglia R, Bacchini P, Bertoni F. Giant cell tumor of the bones of the hand and foot. Cancer. 2000;88(9):2022–32.

18. About the Foot and Ankle. Vol. 56, Radiologic Clinics of North America. 2018. p. 917–34.

19. Osman W, Jerbi M, Ben Abdelkrim S, Maaref K, Ben Maitigue M, Ben Ayèche ML. Giant cell tumor of the lower end of tibia. Curettage and cement reconstruction. Foot Ankle Surg. 2015;21(1):e16–20.

20. Campanacci M, Baldini N, Boriani S, Sudanese A. Giant-cell tumor of bone. J Bone Jt Surg - Ser A. 1987;69(1):106–14.

21. Rajani R, Schaefer L, Scarborough MT, Gibbs CP. Giant Cell Tumors of the Foot and Ankle Bones: High Recurrence Rates After Surgical Treatment. J Foot Ankle Surg. 2015;54(6):1141–5.

22. Fink BR, Temple HT, Chiricosta FM, Mizel MS, Murphey MD. Chondroblastoma of the foot. Foot Ankle Int. 1997;18(4):236–42.

23. Angelini A, Arguedas F, Varela A, Ruggieri P. Chondroblastoma of the Foot: 40 Cases From a Single Institution. J Foot Ankle Surg. 2018;57(6):1105–9.

24. Reda B. Cystic bone tumors of the foot and ankle. Vol. 117, Journal of Surgical Oncology. 2018. p. 1786–98.

25. Ramappa AJ, Lee FYI, Tang P, Carlson JR, Gebhardt MC, Mankin HJ. Chondroblastoma of bone. J Bone Jt Surg - Ser A. 2000;82(8):1140–5.

26. Oliveira AM, Chou MM. USP6-induced neoplasms: The biologic spectrum of aneurysmal bone cyst and nodular fasciitis. Hum Pathol. 2014;45(1):1–11.

27. Park HY, Yang SK, Sheppard WL, Hegde V, Zoller SD, Nelson SD, et al. Current management of aneurysmal bone cysts. Vol. 9, Current Reviews in Musculoskeletal Medicine. 2016. p. 435–44.

28. Chowdhry M, Chandrasekar CR, Mohammed R, Grimer RJ. Curettage of aneurysmal bone cysts of the feet. Foot Ankle Int. 2010;31(2):131–5.

29. Rhee Y, Lee JD, Shin KH, Lee HC, Huh KB, Lim SK. Oncogenic osteomalacia associated with mesenchymal tumour detected by indium-111 octreotide scintigraphy. Clin Endocrinol (Oxf). 2001 Apr;54(4):551–4.

30. Chun KA, Stephanie S, Choi JY, Nam JH, Suh JS. Enchondroma of the Foot. J Foot Ankle Surg. 2015;54(5):836–9.

31. Zamora T, Urrutia J, Schweitzer D, Amenabar PP, Botello E. Do Orthopaedic Oncologists Agree on the Diagnosis and Treatment of Cartilage Tumors of the Appendicular Skeleton? Clin Orthop Relat Res. 2017;475(9):2176–86.

32. Kitsoulis P, Galani V, Stefanaki K, Paraskevas G, Karatzias G, Agnantis NJ, et al. Osteochondromas: Review of the clinical, radiological and pathological features. Vol. 22, In Vivo. 2008. p. 633–46.

33. Bernard SA, Murphey MD, Flemming DJ, Kransdorf MJ. Improved differentiation of benign osteochondromas from secondary chondrosarcomas with standardized measurement of cartilage cap at CT and MR imaging. Radiology. 2010;255(3):857–65.
34. Schulze S C, Valenzuela G G, Zamora H T. Manejo expectante de osteocondroma solitario interóseo de la tibia distal: reporte de un caso y revisión de la literatura. Rev Chil Ortop y Traumatol. 2018;59(03):100–4.
35. Levy DM, Gross CE, Garras DN. Treatment of Unicameral Bone Cysts of the Calcaneus: A Systematic Review. Vol. 54, Journal of Foot and Ankle Surgery. 2015. p. 652–6.
36. Aumar DK, Dadjo YBA, Chagar B. Intraosseous Lipoma of the Calcaneus: Report of a Case and Review of the Literature. J Foot Ankle Surg. 2013;52(3):360–3.
37. Chow LTC, Lee KC. Intraosseous lipoma: A clinicopathologic study of nine cases. Am J Surg Pathol. 1992;16(4):401–10.
38. Narang S, Gangopadhyay M. Calcaneal intraosseous lipoma: A case report and review of the literature. J Foot Ankle Surg. 2011;50(2):216–20.
39. Gouin F, Noailles T. Localized and diffuse forms of tenosynovial giant cell tumor (formerly giant cell tumor of the tendon sheath and pigmented villonodular synovitis). Vol. 103, Orthopaedics and Traumatology: Surgery and Research. 2017. p. S91–7.
40. Noailles T, Brulefert K, Briand S, Longis PM, Andrieu K, Chalopin A, et al. Giant cell tumor of tendon sheath: Open surgery or arthroscopic synovectomy? A systematic review of the literature. Vol. 103, Orthopaedics and Traumatology: Surgery and Research. 2017. p. 809–14.
41. Mastboom MJL, Palmerini E, Verspoor FGM, Rueten-Budde AJ, Stacchiotti S, Staals EL, et al. Surgical outcomes of patients with diffuse-type tenosynovial giant-cell tumours: an international, retrospective, cohort study. Lancet Oncol. 2019;20(6):877–86.
42. Staals EL, Ferrari S, Donati DM, Palmerini E. Diffuse-type tenosynovial giant cell tumour: Current treatment concepts and future perspectives. Vol. 63, European Journal of Cancer. 2016. p. 34–40.
43. Carroll P, Henshaw RM, Garwood C, Raspovic K, Kumar D. Plantar Fibromatosis: Pathophysiology, Surgical and Nonsurgical Therapies: An Evidence-Based Review. Vol. 11, Foot and Ankle Specialist. 2018. p. 168–76.
44. Aluisio F V., Mair SD, Hall RL. Plantar fibromatosis: treatment of primary and recurrent lesions and factors associated with recurrence. Foot Ankle Int. 1996 Nov;17(11):672-8.
45. Knebel C, Neumann J, Schwaiger BJ, Karampinos DC, Pfeiffer D, Specht K, et al. Differentiating atypical lipomatous tumors from lipomas with magnetic resonance imaging: A comparison with MDM2 gene amplification status. BMC Cancer. 2019;19(1).
46. Zeytoonjian T, Mankin HJ, Gebhardt MC, Hornicek FJ. Distal lower extremity sarcomas: Frequency of occurrence and patient survival rate. Foot Ankle Int. 2004;25(5):325–30.
47. Branford-White H, Giele H, Critchley P, Cogswell L, Gibbons CLM, Dean BJF, et al. Management and outcome of acral soft-tissue sarcomas. Bone Jt J. 2018;100B(11):1518–23.
48. Cribb GL, Loo SCS, Dickinson I. Limb salvage for soft-tissue sarcomas of the foot and ankle. J Bone Jt Surg - Ser B. 2010;92(3):424–9.
49. Blscaglia R, Gasbarrini A, Böhling T, Bacchini P, Bertoni F, Picci P. Osteosarcoma of the bones of the foot-an easily misdiagnosed malignant tumor. Mayo Clin Proc. 1998;73(9):842–7.
50. Mascard E, Gaspar N, Brugières L, Glorion C, Pannier S, Gomez-Brouchet A. Malignant tumours of the foot and ankle. EFORT Open Rev. 2017;2(5):261–71.
51. Verdegaal SHM, Brouwers HFG, Van Zwet EW, Hogendoorn PCW, Taminiau AHM. Low-grade chondrosarcoma of long bones treated with intralesional curettage followed by application of phenol, ethanol, and bone-grafting. J Bone Jt Surg - Ser A. 2012;94(13):1201–7.
52. Schreuder HWB, Pruszczynski M, Veth RPH, Lemmens JAM. Treatment of benign and low-grade malignant intramedullary chondroid tumours with curettage and cryosurgery. Eur J Surg Oncol. 1998;24(2):120–6.
53. DuBois SG, Krailo MD, Gebhardt MC, Donaldson SS, Marcus KJ, Dormans J, et al. Comparative evaluation of local control strategies in localized Ewing sarcoma of bone: A report from the Children's Oncology Group. Cancer. 2015;121(3):467–75.
54. Chung TS. Metastatic malignancy to the bones of the hand. J Surg Oncol. 1983;24(2):99–102.

Care and Management of Surgical Wounds, Wounds Dehiscence, and Scars

Leonardo Parada and Günther Mangelsdorff

1 Introduction

Although the skin is not the key issue in foot and ankle surgery, wound healing has a fundamental role for a successful outcome.

A wound that does not close properly can lead to severe problems with bone and/or osteosynthesis hardware exposure, leading to known consequences such as infections, delayed consolidation, and the need for reoperations, among others.

A defective scar, from either a functional or an aesthetic point of view, could be a nightmare for the surgeon. Even though the main problem may be resolved, a scar that is annoying for the patient could be related to multiple consultations and discrepancies with the result obtained.

Bearing these points in mind, it is essential to take serious precautions and manage surgical wounds with care, trying to procure the most effective results in the context of global treatments.

Anatomical considerations and the considerable mobility exerted at the ankle level make the management of wounds in this body segment even more challenging. A separate topic corresponds to traumatic wounds that add even more significant difficulties and usually require a plastic surgery specialist's assistance to achieve a suitable improvement.

L. Parada (✉)
Department of Plastic Surgery and Burns, Hospital del Trabajador, Santiago, Chile

Department of Plastic Surgery, Clínica Las Condes, Santiago, Chile
e-mail: lparada@hts.cl

G. Mangelsdorff
Department of Plastic Surgery and Burns, Hospital del Trabajador, Santiago, Chile

Department of Plastic Surgery, Clínica Santa Maria, Santiago, Chile
e-mail: gmangelsdorff@hts.cl

© The Author(s), under exclusive license to Springer Nature Switzerland AG 2022
E. Wagner Hitschfeld, P. Wagner Hitschfeld (eds.), *Foot and Ankle Disorders*,
https://doi.org/10.1007/978-3-030-95738-4_5

89

In this chapter, we will review practical recommendations to adequately treat surgical wounds performed during foot and ankle surgery, both in elective and trauma surgery, as well as advices to follow when complications such as dehiscences and pathological scars occur.

2   Relevant Anatomy

The lower limbs, especially the foot and ankle, are functionally very relevant and highly demanded areas for developing the human standing characteristic. By being upright, they support all body weight, generally for long periods, and, furthermore, are responsible for producing our displacements.

Despite this, it could be stated that the ankle and the foot are relatively unprotected areas highly exposed to trauma. The skin on the distal third of the leg and around the ankle is thin, with a little subcutaneous tissue layer; moreover, essential structures like bones and tendons are poorly covered and can be easily exposed in trauma.

Conversely, the glabrous skin of the sole possesses completely different characteristics, being thick and firm, designed to resist weight. Unfortunately, its characteristics are unique, and there are no similar structures that could replace it.

2.1   Irrigation

As in all the functioning of the human body and each surgical intervention, the blood supply is central for a favorable result.

The foot and ankle are supplied by arteries dependent on three main axes, the anterior tibial, posterior tibial, and peroneal arteries, each of which feeds specific segments interconnected by vessels of a smaller caliber.

To better understand how a body segment is irrigated, it is essential to keep in mind the concept of angiosome described by Ian Taylor [1]. An angiosome corresponds to a three-dimensional anatomical unit of tissue supplied by a source artery. In his experimental study, Taylor maps the whole body describing 40 territories or angiosomes, of which 6 correspond to the foot and ankle. These angiosomes are unrigid structures intercommunicated between adjacent angiosomes through a network of so-called shock vessels. Specifically, at the ankle and foot level, six angiosomes are described (Fig. 1).

- The posterior tibial artery originates three angiosomes that supply the medial ankle and the sole through the calcaneal branch (heel), the medial plantar artery (arch of the foot), and the lateral plantar artery (lateral midfoot and forefoot).
- The peroneal artery is the source of two angiosomes that supply the anterolateral ankle and the lateral hindfoot, thanks to the anterior perforating branch (superior anterolateral ankle) and the calcaneal branch (plantar heel).

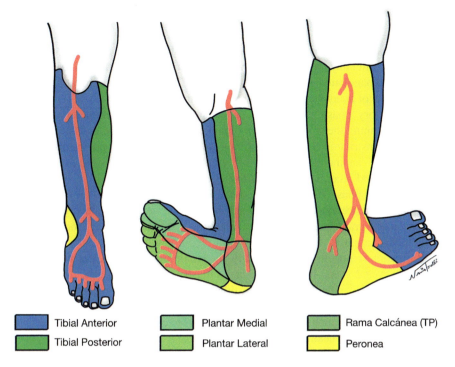

Tibial Anterior   Plantar Medial   Rama Calcánea (TP)

Tibial Posterior   Plantar Lateral   Peronea

Fig. 1 A schematic representation of the angiosomes at the level of foot and ankle

- An angiosome that supplies the anterior ankle depends on the anterior tibial artery and then like the dorsal artery of the foot that feeds the entire foot dorsum [2].

Knowing these angiosomes allows for the correct planning of the location of the surgical incisions. The usual designs consider these angiosomes, reducing the risk of complications. In the case of traumatized feet or with chronic pathologies, such as diabetic foot [3], that can alter the vasculature, an easy-to-use tool is mapping these arteries with a portable Doppler pencil, noting alterations to the normal anatomy and allowing adjustment of surgical plans [2].

3   Wound Healing Process

To understand how to manage a wound, it is a prerequisite to have notions about the normal healing process and the factors that can alter it.

Every time a wound occurs, our body triggers a series of processes that lead to tissue repair and scar formation. This process has been divided into stages that help understand it better, yet these stages are intertwined in a dynamic process [4, 5].

3.1   Phases of Wound Healing Process

- Hemostasis: While it is not considered a stage in the healing process, it is the first to happen after any injury. Initially, vasoconstriction occurs, and the intrinsic and extrinsic coagulation pathways are triggered. This process culminating in the production of a clot acts as a bridge to the inflammatory phase.
- Inflammatory phase: Immediately after the injury, an inflammatory process begins cleaning the wound of microorganisms and foreign bodies. After the initial vasoconstriction occurs vasodilation, an increase in the blood vessels permeability, and an increased arrival of lymphocytes and macrophages releasing cytokines and other biologically active agents.
- Proliferative phase: From the second day and approximately until the third week, fibroblasts represent the predominant cells in the wound, producing collagen deposits, granulatory tissue formation, angiogenesis, and finally epithelialization.
- Maturation/remodeling phase: Finally, the repair process can be extended for up to 1 or even 2 years. Initially, the scar is mostly composed of type III collagen, achieving approximately 20% of healthy skin strength. This collagen predominantly changes to type I through remodeling, reaching 80% of the original strength after 2–3 months. Later the scar begins to contract and never reaches the initial strength of healthy tissue.

3.2   Factors Affecting Wound Healing

From a practical point of view, understanding the factors that can alter the wound healing process is more important than understanding the physiological process of wound repairs. Keeping these factors in mind is essential to avoid problems later.

- Oxygen: The cellular growth proper to the healing process is dependent on oxygen, and adequate arterial oxygen pressure and tissue perfusion are fundamental factors for tissue repair.
- Age: Age, by itself, affects healing. At an older age, the stages described previously begin late, occur more slowly, and generally do not obtain the same results as at younger ages.
- Nutrition: Healing requires an increased production of cells and their products, so a state of malnutrition will negatively affect the entire process. On the other hand, poor nutrition due to excess has also shown an increase in complications such as infections and dehiscences.

Ideally, a patient who will undergo elective surgery should arrive in good nutritional condition at the surgery. In trauma cases, the nutritional status should be evaluated, and the necessary corrections and supplements should be adjusted early.

- Tobacco: The deleterious effects of tobacco are multifactorial. Nicotine is a vaso-constrictor that decreases cell proliferation; carbon monoxide decreases oxygen transport capacity; and tobacco also increases platelet aggregation and blood viscosity. These and other facts explain why a single cigarette generates cutaneous vasoconstriction for about 90 minutes.

The recommendation for elective surgeries is to stop smoking at least 4 weeks before and 4 weeks after surgery.

- Infection: Infection prolongs the inflammatory phase, interfering with later phases, especially collagen deposition, epithelialization, and contraction. In addition, the granulatory tissue growing under local infection is of lower quality, therefore being more abundant, edematous, hemorrhagic, and fragile, not allowing an adequate closure of the wounds.
- In chronic wounds, attention should be paid to biofilm, although it does not imply an active infection, alters, and inhibits wounds healing. Actions must be taken to eliminate it.
- Radiation: Apart from the beneficial effects sought with radiotherapy, it also causes deleterious effects on the tissues, altering the DNA, and reduces the irrigation, the deposit of collagens, and the tensile strength obtained. Unfortunately, irradiated skin is chronically damaged, forever affecting the wound healing processes.
- Chronic diseases: A series of chronic diseases alter the overall state of health and wound healing. The classic example is diabetes mellitus, but others such as obesity, COPD, cancer, liver and kidney failure, connective tissue diseases, and venous and arterial failure, among others, are involved in alterations to the healing process and should be compensated as much as possible prior to any elective surgery.

4   Elective Surgical Wounds

As previously mentioned, the anatomical characteristics at the foot and ankle require the correct management of surgical incisions to achieve the best result.

4.1   Location of Incisions

The approach to be used will remain a fundamental matter for the orthopedic surgeon, who will consider anatomical factors, such as irrigation of the area and the need for adequate access to the element to be intervened.

When deciding on these approaches, it is crucial always to be concerned about the possible complications in the future and the soft tissue deficit existing at the time or that could develop in the expected evolution of the wound, paying particular attention to signs of skin suffering. In these cases, being aware of the situation and the options to reconstruct later will always guide a fair decision-making process.

In complex cases, it is always advisable to discuss the case with the plastic surgery team if, in the future, the patient requires their assistance to reconstruct a skin coverage deficit.

4.2   *Incisions*

In general, the incision should be the smallest to achieve adequate exposure, limiting the scars' extension. However, it is inadvisable to save on the incision extension at the cost of having poor access and hindering subsequent repair and results.

The skin must be handled with care avoiding unnecessary traumatization, handling the skin with grasps pressing the dermis, and leaving the epidermis free is a way to protect it, especially with delicate skin like those of aged people. Using hooks to catch the skin, instead of grasps, is also an excellent alternative.

The use of skin retractors is recommended to avoid damage to the soft tissues. These could be self-retaining retractors or individual elastic retractors (Lone Star™ Cooper Surgical™/CooperSurgical Inc., USA), which, given their versatility, can be adjusted to any size and wound position.

The incision closure is presumably the most critical surgeon-dependent aspect to achieve the best possible scar, this means making it as unnoticeable as possible, not depressed, not raised, and similar in color to the surrounding skin [6]. With this, the core objective is to close in layers and avoid, whenever possible, a closure only in a single cutaneous plane. When facing deep planes, dead spaces are closed, avoiding scar depression and reducing skin tension. Ideally, before placing the last suture line over the skin, the wound margins should be seen practically closed, leaving minimal tension on this layer (Fig. 2).

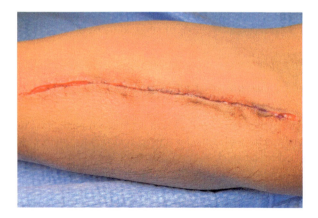

Fig. 2 Skin suture: before performing the last suture plane, for example, with a running subcuticular suture, the wound edges have to be almost completely opposite without tension

4.3 Suture Materials

Absorbable suture materials are preferably used to target muscles, fascia, and subcutaneous tissues. Our preferred material is polydioxanone (PDS™, Ethicon Inc., Somerville, NJ, USA), a strand of easy maneuverability that, being monofilament, reduces trauma to tissues and risk of infection. Also, its durability profile allows maintaining extended support while healing occurs.

A valid and high-quality alternative corresponds to polyglactin (Vicryl™, Ethicon), probably the most used suture for deep planes. In very thin patients and incisions over areas with scarce subcutaneous tissue between the skin and the bone, it can be especially useful, since by being more flexible, it would be less noticeable by patients. The use of a colorless strand prevents it from showing through the skin.

For superficial layers, a continuous subdermal suture is recommended, avoiding the excessive accumulation of knots, with 3–0 or 4–0 material depending on the patient's wound location and characteristics.

Finally, for the last plane, non-absorbable materials should be used that causes the least possible inflammatory reaction. Nylon (Ethilon™, Ethicon) is usually the first alternative, and in general, a 4–0 size should be adequate. However, in less demanding areas such as the foot dorsum, smaller diameter sutures could be used. On the contrary, in greater demand areas such as the sole or closed with a certain degree of tension, larger sutures should be used. An alternative is polypropylene (Prolene™, Ethicon), which advantage is having a higher tensile strength, being useful when approaching tissues with some tension degree.

4.4 Suturing Technique

Before closing any wound, hemostasis should be appropriately checked in order to stop any active bleeding. It is ideal to coagulate promptly only at the bleeding sites and not aimlessly reducing the tissues' irrigation, with the risks that it entails in terms of infections and dehiscences.

For deep layers, inverted stitches are used in which the needle enters and exits through a deep plane, leaving the knots inwards, which reduce the chances of extrusion or even being felt by the patient, especially at the ankle in the case of very thin patients. The steps to perform an inverted suture are demonstrated in Fig. 3. When there is greater tension or risk of infection, it is advisable to use simple interrupted stitches. Once the tension has been decreased, a continuous suture could be used with the advantage of reducing time and resulting in fewer knots.

There are different options for suturing skin, always remembering that wound edges must be everted. The first corresponds to the simple interrupted stitches whose advantage lies in its ease of execution, ability to adapt the tissues' margins, and

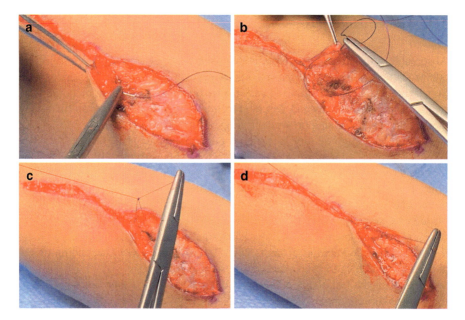

Fig. 3 Inverted stitches are used to suture deep planes. (**a**) The needle penetrates from a deep plane; (**b**) at the opposite edge, it enters from a superficial plane to a deep one; (**c**) edges are approaching; (**d**) the knot is hidden inward

speed. An excellent option is to perform an intradermal suture in wounds well faced in their deep layers, which generates a more aesthetic linear scar. It could be done with absorbable material avoiding the need to remove stitches or with a non-absorbable suture, in which case it can be removed deferred. It is important regarding long incisions, to leave intermediate exits of the strand, in order to be able to remove it easily.

In the case of wounds closed at higher tension, it is ideal to use a stitch that provides greater firmness and a coapted surface. In this case, vertical or horizontal mattress points are the alternative of choice.

In the situation where one of the edges of the wound has borderline irrigation, it is advisable to use a less ischemic technique, such as Gillies' stitches in which the suture enters and exits the surface on only one side and passes through the other edge only by dermis (as in an intradermal suture). This same point is recommended to close flap wounds.

Regarding surgical staples, no evidence shows the superiority of one method over another [7–9] except for faster with stapling [10] and a trend towards better aesthetics with suturing [11]. In our practice, the use of staples is unusual, and we recommend always using them after correctly closing deep planes and removing them promptly, no later than 10 days, to avoid excess marks on the skin.

4.5   Wound Dressing

Once the suture is finished, the skin must be protected. The ideal dressing generates an environment with controlled humidity, which prevents desiccation and reduces edema, with an easy application and removal, painless, and inexpensive.

In simple wounds that do not have a higher risk of complication, our recommendation is to apply a skin protector and then cover with paper tape (Micropore™ 3 M, Ltd., USA), applying at least four tape layers.

In the case of bruised or traumatized skin, it is important to use a product for advanced wound management. At this point, the most used primary dressing is a *tulle gras*, applied to the wound and covered with a secondary dressing. The telfa has similar characteristics.

For highly exudative wounds, alginate or foam is the most suitable alternative.

In general, wound dressings should be changed every 3 to 5 days, depending on the product used. When healthy skin has been noticed, it can continue using paper tape.

Regarding the right time to wet a wound, we recommend not doing it for the first 48 to 72 hours, and then, for example, if using paper tape, it is possible to wet it with extreme caution in order to completely dry it later. Other dressings require keeping it dry until removal.

Other essential precautions are respecting rest, keeping the leg up, and evaluating the use of compression bandages [12], all measures that reduce edema and its negative consequences.

In the same way, it is crucial to maintain adequate glycemic and nutritional management and suspend the use of tobacco.

4.6   Incisional Negative Pressure Wound Therapy

Negative pressure wound therapy (NPWT) since its introduction in 1997 [13] has been a significant contribution to wound management. Traditionally it has been used in open wounds, being widely accepted as a bridging or even definitive therapy.

Its applications have gradually expanded, including its use in closed surgical wounds, known as incisional negative pressure wound therapy (iNPWT) described by Gomoll et al. in 2006 [14] precisely in patients undergoing ankle and foot surgery.

iNPWT refers to the application over closed wounds, acting as a dressing that transmits pressure on the suture line.

The advantages it provides are fundamentally an improvement in the microcirculation of the wound, a decrease in tension on the wound edges, a decrease in edema, and a more effective obliteration of dead spaces [15].

Its use is increasingly popular, thanks to a decrease in dehiscences and wounds infections [16–19]. Our group demonstrated a decrease in complications in the donor area of the anterolateral thigh flap, allowing large defects to be closed with minimal consequences [15]; however, systematic reviews have not been able to strongly demonstrate a global utility of this therapy nor its clear cost-effectiveness [20, 21].

We recommend the use of iNPWT in any high-risk injury:

- Closed with a certain degree of tension.
- Performed on traumatized tissues.
- Patients with risk factors for dehiscence (obese and smokers, among others).
- Presence of significant edema.
- Arthroplasty, considering that the consequences of a wound infection are so dire that any preventive measures seem reasonable.

Its application is straightforward. There are ready-to-use devices such as the VAC Prevena™ (KCI, San Antonio, Texas, USA). If this type of device is not available, it can be easily made with the material of a standard NPWT. Once the wound is closed, both sides of the lesion are covered with a transparent dressing, leaving only the suture line uncovered, and over this, the standard NPWT foam is placed covering the sutured area and then is connected to the suction motor (Fig. 4). In general, a pressure of −125 mm Hg continuously is the most suitable.

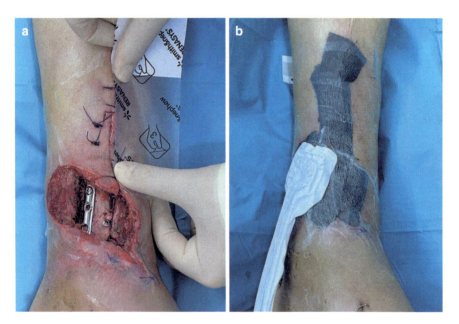

Fig. 4 An incisional negative pressure wound therapy (NPWT) can be assembled using a traditional one. (**a**) Start protecting the edges of the wound with a transparent dressing, (**b**) cover with foam over protected areas. In this case, a traditional NPWT is used to cover an open wound and an incisional segment over a closed one

Its removal is recommended between 5 and 7 days later, being earlier in the case of doubts about infection or other complications. A second cycle can then be applied if the wound is not yet completely closed or if there are reasonable doubts of subsequent favorable evolution. If the wound is seen to be in good condition, it will be possible to continue with the usual care.

4.7 Suture Removal

A frequent question for patients, and surgeons, is when to remove sutures.

The first thing to point out is that there is no standard recipe applicable to every case, but rather, it will be customized according to the characteristics of the injury, the quality of the tissues, and the technique used.

In general, at the ankle, they should remain in place for 10 to 14 days for young patients and up to 21 days for older patients or in case of high-risk wounds (fracture cases, limb with more edema, greater risk of dehiscence). On the dorsum, they could be removed between 7 and 10 days. On the contrary, those located on the sole should be removed deferred, especially if the patient has the authorization to support. In these circumstances we recommend not to do so, before 21 days.

A suture that remains on the wound for a long time will leave more imprints, especially marking each site where the suture passes through the skin. If a useful, aesthetically result is sought, the sutures should be removed early; however, it should never be done before ensuring that the wound will not become dehiscent. A good alternative is to make partial removals, which reduce the areas where there could be marks of the suture material in the scar but maintains adequate support. After removal, reinforce the wound with paper tape or adhesive skin suture (Steri-Strip™, 3 M).

4.8 Wound and Scar Care Management

Once the wound is closed and the stitches have been removed, it is still essential to continue with the scar's management in order to obtain the best possible result.

In this sense, there are three significant actions to develop:

- Adequate moistening, keeping the scar moisturized properly, promotes better healing and a better aesthetic result. Simply use any moisturizer to achieve this effect, to be used two to three times a day.
- Compression: It has been shown that a scar's compression improves their quality and prevents the appearance of complications such as hypertrophic scars. In case of a normal scar, it is enough to cover it with a few layers of paper tape [22, 23] that needs to be changed each 3 to 4 days.

- Of better quality is the use of the silicone sheet, which, due to its characteristics, has been demonstrated as an excellent tool for the improvement of the quality of scars [6]. It has the advantage of being self-adhesive and transparent.
- In both cases, we recommend its use for 2 to 3 months after surgery.
- Sun protection: One key point when looking for the least noticeable scar possible is to protect it adequately from the sun. During all wound healing process, the skin is much more vulnerable to the sun's damaging effects and may become hyperpigmented. We recommend the daily use of sunscreen, ideally SPF 50, reapplying to the scar, at least three times a day and ideally every 2–3 hours if are extensively exposed to the sun.

In the circumstance of presenting a pathological scar, this care should be reinforced, which will be reviewed later in this chapter.

5 Traumatic Wounds

A particular situation occurs with injuries originating after trauma. Open fractures, ulcers, and degloving are common in this body segment. Any soft tissue injury could complicate the orthopedic surgeons work and could be a risk factor for future complications.

In general terms, the treatment is similar and follows the same rules previously presented, with some necessary adaptations to remember:

- They should undergo surgical debridement, removing all necrotic tissue. If there are tissues with borderline vitality, it is appropriate to keep it until the following intervention.
- The ideal surgical incision could be located over injured areas and therefore not available, needing to adjust in an individual approach.
- Avoid using braided sutures.
- Perform advanced wound care that protects and allows damaged skin to recover.

5.1 I Cannot Close the Wound

Unfortunately, a wholly unpleasant and not uncommon circumstance occurs when the surgeon has finished performing the central actions of the surgery and proceeds to close the wound, which is not possible or has to do it with extreme tension or with injured tissues.

Faced with this situation, we recommend three actions:

- Try closing the wound with few single total stitches, separated and away from the edges. Doing this makes possible to approximate the wound margins generously or even close it completely, avoiding future surgeries. An example is presented in Fig. 5.

- If there are not enough tissues to close, the ideal method is to try to cope the tissues as much as possible and not leave them in a relaxed position, as they will quickly retract and will be unavailable for future closures leaving a larger defect and requiring the use of other reconstructive techniques.
- Ultimately, we recommend using NPWT or iNPWT, which helps to improve the condition of the tissues, and in a future intervention, try a definitive closure or request the plastic surgeon's assistance for this.

In the case of having a soft tissue deficit and especially if it involves exposure of noble structures or any hardware, the limb's reconstruction should be performed as early as possible [24]. Management in conjunction with the plastic surgeon is an excellent alternative. If this is not possible, the NPWT gives a time window to schedule the reconstruction.

A practical recommendation is always to take pictures of the injury to discuss the case with the plastic surgeon and have reconstructive options planned for the next intervention.

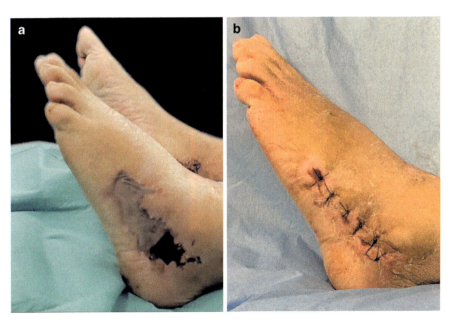

Fig. 5 (**a**) Due to an accident, the patient develops an eschar on the lateral aspect of the foot. (**b**) After resection, it is closed advancing skin flaps on both sides of the wound that are sutured in a single plane with simple interrupted stitches. If a complete closure is not achieved, at least the skin edges are approximated, preventing their retraction

6 Wound Dehiscence

6.1 Definition and Classification

Wound dehiscence corresponds to the partial or total disruption or opening of a previously closed wound. A complication, with an incidence in the foot and ankle surgery difficult to estimate, both due to a lack of consensus in defining dehiscence and because of communications that use slightly broader expressions such as *problems of the wound*. Considering these factors, reports show an overall incidence of 4–6% [25], between 8.6% and 16.5% in fractures [18] up to values as high as 28% in ankle arthroplasty [26].

To standardize concepts in 2018, the World Union of Wound Healing Societies generates a consensus that defines dehiscence as the separation of the margins of a closed surgical incision that involves the skin with or without exposure or protrusion of underlying tissue, organs, or implants. It can occur at single or multiple regions or involve the entire length of the incision and one or all tissue layers [27]. In the same consensus, they adapt the Sandy Grading System for Surgical Wound Dehiscence Classification [28], generating a new classification that allows an efficient systematization and the treatment options suggested, which graduates surgical wound dehiscences into four levels according to the depth of affected tissues:

- Grade 1: Epidermis only.
- Grade 2: Exposed subcutaneous tissue.
- Grade 3: Exposed subcutaneous tissue and fascia.
- Grade 4: With exposure of organs, viscera, bones, or implants.
- A: In addition to each of these degrees, add the presence or absence of signs and symptoms of wound infection.

6.2 Risk Factors

There are several risk factors for the occurrence of operative wound dehiscence. These factors can be:

- Related to the patient and modifiable: Obesity considering that the higher the BMI, the greater the risk, malnutrition, especially protein deficit, anemia, diabetes mellitus, smoking, and alcohol consumption.
- Related to the patient and difficulty or non-modifiable: Age over 65 years, emergency surgery, and other comorbidities such as cancer, liver failure, kidney failure, use of steroids, and prior irradiation.
- Intraoperative: Prolonged duration of surgery, perioperative hypothermia, inadequate closure technique, non-obliteration of dead spaces, tension closure, and wide dissections.
- Postoperative: Wound infection, premature removal of sutures, edema, failure to rest, and other complications such as hematomas and seromas.

Managing these risk factors is essential to avoid complications. Optimizing the patient's global state prior to elective surgery, especially by stopping tobacco consumption 1 month prior, making nutritional corrections, and maintaining controlled comorbidities are unavoidable actions.

Similarly, after surgery, adequate care must be provided, generating a good follow-up plan, especially in patients undergoing outpatient surgeries, reinforcing the importance of complying with indications such as rest and wound care.

6.3 Treatment

If despite taking all possible safeguards a dehiscence occurs, which unfortunately is not unusual in ankle and foot surgery, an adequate treatment can help resolve it successfully.

Its management will depend on the extension and mainly on the depth of this and the presence or not of wound infection.

We will systematize its management in the following aspects:

6.3.1 Prevention

Already stated in the risk factors section, we cannot fail to reinforce these measures, which are by far the most important.

In addition to stopping tobacco consumption, optimizing nutritional status, and compensating for any chronic disease, there are some specific actions to be carried out by the medical team:

- Closure technique appropriate to the type of surgery and patient's characteristic. It is important to remember the closure by layers and avoid prolonged surgeries [29].
- Wound dressings: keep the wound closed, with dressings that maintain a controlled moist environment. In the case of traumatic wounds, they should also allow adequate recovery of the epidermis.
- Do not remove the dressing in the first 48 to 72 hours, at which time a re-epidermization should have already occurred, thus reducing the risk of wound infection.
- Use of iNPWT: its use on closed wounds is gradually gaining more acceptance; the cause has been shown to reduce the risk of infection and complications, like dehiscences. Its use is recommended in wounds or patients at high risk for dehiscence [18] [16].
- Prevention of edema: during the postoperative period through compression bandages [7] and the limb's elevation.
- Rest/immobilization: reinforcing the previous point, it is necessary to maintain rest and eventually use immobilizers to avoid excessive movements subjecting the wound to excessive stress.

6.3.2 Infection

In the case of wounds with local signs of infection, limited to the wound, the main treatment tool corresponds to advanced dressings adapted to each wound's needs. The use of topical antimicrobial and antibiotic dressings for a limited period should also be added [27].

In the case of systemic signs of infection or local signs that extend beyond the wound's limits, systemic antibiotic therapy is indicated.

Antibiotic therapy should be adjusted to the local epidemiological reality and, if possible, guided by cultures, ideally of tissues, since those with superficial exudate usually show cutaneous flora and do not represent accurately soft tissue infection status.

6.3.3 Superficial Dehiscence

Superficial dehiscences, grades 1 and 2, that is, that exposes even the subcutaneous tissue, can be effectively treated with advanced dressings.

In most cases, products will be used to control the exudate and debride while there are detritus and then continue with another dressing type that allows better granulatory tissue growth.

In early dehiscence, generally linked to an inadequate closure technique, a primary delayed closure can be performed, as in totally clean wounds without other associated complications. In all other circumstances, which covers most cases, a closure by secondary intention is chosen.

6.3.4 Deep Dehiscence

For dehiscences of grades 3 and 4, that is, with exposure of fascia and other elements such as viscera, bones, and implants, in addition to what is exposed for those more superficial parts, management is usually more aggressive and involves surgeries. Surgical toilets will be performed, removing all the devitalized tissue present. The ideal situation in these circumstances is, when the wound is clean and without other complications, to try a new closure by re-advancing the skin flaps and applying iNPWT.

In wounds that cannot be closed, an attempt should be made to advance the flaps and approximate the tissues as much as possible to avoid their retraction. In a second intervention, they can be re-advanced again and eventually achieve closure.

We strongly recommend using NPWT as bridging therapy in these circumstances, especially in dehiscences of great extension and with abundant exudate. If bone or tendons are exposed, hydrophilic foam, VAC Whitefoam™ Dressing (KCI, San Antonio, Texas, USA), should be used to prevent drying out (Fig. 6).

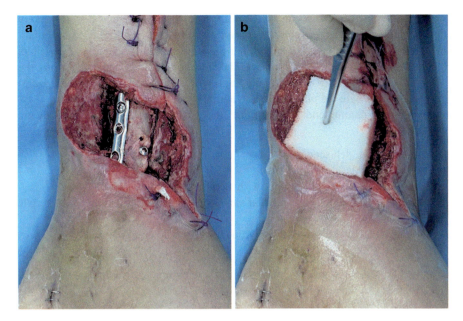

Fig. 6 (**a**) A traumatic injury with exposure of bone and osteosynthesis hardware is appreciated. (**b**) If it is not possible to close the wound, to avoid desiccation of the bone, a hydrophilic foam (VAC Whitefoam™) is used together with a traditional VAC

In the case of contaminated wounds, between any toilets, it is advisable to use NPWT with irrigation (VAC VERAFLO™ Therapy, KCI), which will help to clean the wound and promote the development of granulatory tissue [30].

Finally, in these cases, it is possible to continue treating with wound dressings or NPWT until a closure by second intention is achieved or when local conditions allow performing a closure by the third intention. If there are no tissues available to close the wound after extensive dehiscence, it will be necessary to work together with the plastic surgeon who will eventually require the use of grafts or flaps for definitive treatment [31].

7   When to Consult the Plastic Surgeon

By far, most of the wounds can be managed entirely and successfully by any orthopedic surgeon, being quite unlikely to need a reconstructive specialist for their management. Nonetheless, this may be necessary, especially in foot and ankle injuries due to the anatomical characteristics and frequently high-energy trauma.

A wound that does not close and has tendon, bone, or implants exposure can be a disaster if it is not promptly well managed.

Although the orthopedist can successfully execute the first steps, it is very likely that they will require a reconstructive plastic surgeon's support for the correct treatment. In these cases, we recommend that the consultation be as early as possible. Depending on the characteristics of each hospital, it can be immediately during the surgery. If this is not possible, a photograph will always be an excellent bridge to discuss the case with the plastic surgeon and plan actions to follow.

We highly recommended consulting the plastic surgeon in the following circumstances:

- Wide and deep dehiscences.
- Infected wounds.
- Traumatized surrounding tissues with signs of poor irrigation.
- Wounds with tendon, neurovascular structures, bone, or osteosynthesis materials exposure.
- Patients with a clear history of previous hypertrophic or keloid scars.

Working together to plan a reconstructive option, basically, grafts or flaps will give the best result for patients, minimizing the occurrence of significant complications such as osteomyelitis and its consequences.

8 Pathological Scar

Despite all care taken to manage wounds, some scars do not evolve favorably. Beyond a bad aesthetic result, which can generate high psychosocial stress in the patient, some scars transform into a new pathology, specifically hypertrophic and keloid scars.

8.1 Hypertrophic and Keloid Scars

One of the most feared problems is when a scar evolves into a hypertrophic one or, worse yet, to a keloid. Both carry a series of problems not only from an aesthetic point of view, but they can also be symptomatic.

Traditionally, both types of scars have been considered as distinct entities characterized by generating an excessive amount of scar. Hypertrophic scars are limited to the original margins of the wound, unlike keloids that grow beyond the limits of the initial wound; they also possess a genetic factor involved and can be symptomatic, mainly due to the pain and itching and, unfortunately, of very complex treatment. An example of a scar with both a hypertrophic segment and also a keloid part could be appreciated in Fig. 7.

In recent years, however, there is a tendency to consider both types of scars as a continuum on the same spectrum, in which the initial state would correspond to the

Fig. 7 A lateral foot surgical incision develops an excessive pathological scar of both types. (**a**) A hypertrophic scar respecting the original scar boundaries. (**b**) A keloid growing outside the borders of the original scar

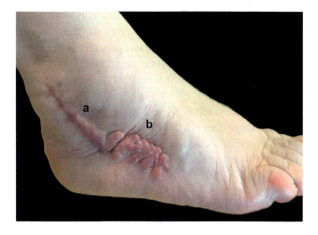

hypertrophic scar and its most severe level to the keloid [32]. All this is based on physiopathological appraisals and histological findings.

Although there is still no complete understanding of these conditions, there are related factors, mainly the tension over the wound. Indeed, those sutured under tension or in areas of great mobility where the tissues are exposed to forces have a greater risk of progressing to hypertrophy in different degrees.

The treatment of these pathologies has several modalities. None of them are 100% effective. Among these, we can mention the infiltration with corticosteroids infiltration compression, use of silicone sheets, cryotherapy, and laser, among others, to reach the most effective keloid treatment that corresponds to the resection followed by radiotherapy. All of these generally have discrete results, with high recurrence rates, with radiotherapy being the most successful alternative in avoiding keloid recurrence, with success rates close to 90%.

8.2   Prevention

For the ankle and foot specialist, perhaps the most relevant action is prevention and, if one develops, its prompt referral to plastic surgery for definitive management. The prevention actions will be grouped into two areas: patient with no history and patient with a previous history.

8.2.1   Patient with No Previous History of Pathological Scars

This situation could occur in any patient and any scar; however, some risk factors such as wounds closed at high tension, in highly traumatized tissues, or with a slow healing process should make us suspect the appearance of problematic scars. In these cases, we recommend being very strict in the care of scars, with the elements already exposed, namely, adequate lubrication of the skin and the fundamental compression of the scar with paper tape or silicone sheet [33].

If the problem is already established and a hypertrophic or keloid scar begins developing, the ideal step is to address it promptly, so it is essential to warn the patient to consult immediately if they notice that the scar begins to grow abnormally.

If a scar is evidently hypertrophic, it should be immediately compressed, ideally with a silicone sheet. After this, we believe the best course of action would be referring the patient to a specialist, generally plastic surgeons or dermatologists, to establish the appropriate treatment and perform a follow-up.

8.2.2 Patient with a Personal History of Hypertrophic/Keloid Scars

Although the ankle and foot are not among the most common areas of the body for the development of this type of scar, if a patient has already developed them elsewhere, especially a keloid previous history, they are at high risk of producing another keloid if they suffer any additional skin injuries.

For patients with hypertrophic scars, we recommend closing the wound, handling the tissues with care, avoiding over-trauma, achieving a tension-free closure, and immediately starting compression with a silicone sheet. If in the healing process it begins to hypertrophy, promptly refer to a plastic surgeon.

In terms of patients with keloids, extreme precautions must be taken. Even if it sounds like a truism, the first action is to warn the patient about the risk of developing a new keloid, owing to the way they cicatrize and mostly independent of the suture technique used.

At the time of surgery, we recommended using sutures that react as little as possible and that generate the minimum inflammatory effect on the wound. In this sense, an excellent option is to use nylon to close deep planes, although it is nonabsorbable, since it avoids producing a reaction with tissues. It could be colorless for more superficial planes. For the final closure of the skin, ideally perform intradermal sutures avoiding multiple passes of the needle through the epidermis and dermis, as would occur with simple stitches or staples, since in each of these points a wound is produced with the risk of evolving into a keloid. Again, it is important to compress the wound initially with paper tape and, after removing the sutures, start using silicone.

All of the above can be accompanied by even more aggressive actions like infiltration of corticosteroids, generally triamcinolone, into the wound at the time of closure or the early use of tapes impregnated with corticosteroids [34] to avoid the appearance of a keloid; however, we recommend that under these circumstances refer the patient previously to the plastic surgeon, for a joint treatment planning. Once again, teamwork can deliver the best solutions for the patient.

9 Summary

The human being's ability to stand lies mainly on the foot and ankle, so on a daily basis, this body segment is overstressed and vulnerable to trauma. However, its anatomical characteristics leave it relatively unprotected. The skin at the ankle is very thin and bones and tendons can be easily exposed in any high-energy trauma or also in case of complications from elective surgery. Thus, correctly managing skin injuries is a skill to be developed by the foot and ankle surgeon.

The treatment of these wounds requires careful handling of the skin, making sutures by layers and posteriorly with adequate wound healing dressings, in which the use of negative pressure wound therapy plays an increasingly relevant role. The early recognition of complications such as dehiscences is essential to treat them successfully.

In the case of complex wounds and skin coverage deficits, working together with the plastic surgeon is essential.

If, despite everything, the patient develops hypertrophic or keloid scars, nowadays, there are a series of treatments that allow them to be treated with good results.

References

1. Taylor GI, Palmer JH. The vascular territories (angiosomes) of the body: experimental study and clinical applications. Br J Plast Surg. 1987;40:113–41.
2. Attinger CE, Evans KK, Bulan E, Blume P, Cooper P. Angiosomes of the foot and ankle and clinical implications for limb salvage: reconstruction. Incisions, and Revascularization: Plast Reconstr Surg. 2006;117:261S–93S.
3. Clemens MW, Attinger CE. Angiosomes and wound care in the diabetic foot. Foot Ankle Clin. 2010;15:439–64.
4. Broughton G, Rohrich RJ. Wounds and scars. Sel Read Plast Surg. 2005;10
5. Kaufman MG, Louis MR, Qiu SS, Buchanan EP. Wound healing. In: Fundam. Top. En Plast. Surg. 1st ed. New York: Thieme, Stuttgart; 2018. p. 13–30.
6. Lee Peng G, Kerolus JL. Management of Surgical Scars. Facial Plast Surg Clin N Am. 2019;27:513–7.
7. Biancari F, Tiozzo V. Staples versus sutures for closing leg wounds after vein graft harvesting for coronary artery bypass surgery. Cochrane Database Syst Rev. 2010;(5):CD008057.
8. Iavazzo C, Gkegkes ID, Vouloumanou EK, Mamais I, Peppas G, Falagas ME. Sutures versus staples for the management of surgical wounds: a meta-analysis of randomized controlled trials. Am Surg. 2011;77:1206–21.
9. Krishnan RJ, Crawford EJ, Syed I, Kim P, Rampersaud YR, Martin J. Is the risk of infection lower with sutures than with Staples for skin closure after Orthopaedic surgery? A Meta-analysis of randomized trials. Clin Orthop. 2019;477:922–37.
10. Krishnan R, MacNeil SD, Malvankar-Mehta MS. Comparing sutures versus staples for skin closure after orthopaedic surgery: systematic review and meta-analysis. BMJ Open. 2016;6:e009257.

11. Cochetti G, Abraha I, Randolph J, Montedori A, Boni A, Arezzo A, Mazza E, Rossi De Vermandois JA, Cirocchi R, Mearini E. Surgical wound closure by staples or sutures?: systematic review. Medicine (Baltimore). 2020;99:e20573.
12. Winge R, Bayer L, Gottlieb H, Ryge C. Compression therapy after ankle fracture surgery: a systematic review. Eur J Trauma Emerg Surg. 2017;43:451–9.
13. Argenta LC, Morykwas MJ. Vacuum-assisted closure: a new method for wound control and treatment: clinical experience. Ann Plast Surg. 1997;38:563–76. discussion 577
14. Gomoll AH, Lin A, Harris MB. Incisional vacuum-assisted closure therapy. J Orthop Trauma. 2006;20:705–9.
15. Mangelsdorff G, Cuevas P, Rodriguez J, Pereira N, Ramirez E, Yañez R. Reduced anterolateral thigh flap donor-site morbidity using incisional negative pressure therapy. J Reconstr Microsurg. 2019;35:229–34.
16. Agarwal A. Management of closed incisions using negative-pressure wound therapy in orthopedic surgery. Plast Reconstr Surg. 2019;143:21S–6S.
17. Nam D, Sershon RA, Levine BR, Della Valle CJ. The use of closed incision negative-pressure wound therapy in orthopaedic surgery. J Am Acad Orthop Surg. 2018;26:295–302.
18. Stannard JP, Volgas DA, McGwin G, Stewart RL, Obremskey W, Moore T, Anglen JO. Incisional negative pressure wound therapy after high-risk lower extremity fractures. J Orthop Trauma. 2012;26:37–42.
19. Wang C, Zhang Y, Qu H. Negative pressure wound therapy for closed incisions in orthopedic trauma surgery: a metaanalysis. J Orthop Surg. 2019;14(1):427.
20. Norman G, Goh EL, Dumville JC, Shi C, Liu Z, Chiverton L, Stankiewicz M, Reid A. Negative pressure wound therapy for surgical wounds healing by primary closure. Cochrane Database Syst Rev. 2020;5(5):CD009261.
21. Iheozor-Ejiofor Z, Newton K, Dumville JC, Costa ML, Norman G, Bruce J. Negative pressure wound therapy for open traumatic wounds. Cochrane Database Syst Rev. 2018;7(7):CD012522.
22. Atkinson J-AM, McKenna KT, Barnett AG, McGrath DJ, Rudd M. A randomized, controlled trial to determine the efficacy of paper tape in preventing hypertrophic scar formation in surgical incisions that traverse Langer??S skin tension lines. Plast Reconstr Surg. 2005;116:1648–56.
23. Gold MH, McGuire M, Mustoe TA, Pusic A, Sachdev M, Waibel J, Murcia C, International Advisory Panel on Scar Management. Updated international clinical recommendations on scar management: part 2--algorithms for scar prevention and treatment. Dermatol Surg Off Publ Am Soc Dermatol Surg Al. 2014;40:825–31.
24. Soltanian H, Garcia RM, Hollenbeck ST. Current concepts in lower extremity reconstruction. Plast Reconstr Surg. 2015;136:815e–29.
25. Lehtonen E, Patel H, Phillips S, Correia Pinto M, Naranje S, Shah A. Staple versus suture closure for ankle fracture fixation: retrospective chart review for safety and outcomes. Foot. 2018;37:71–6.
26. Whalen JL, Spelsberg SC, Murray P. Wound breakdown after Total ankle arthroplasty. Foot Ankle Int. 2010;31:301–5.
27. World Union of Wound Healing Societies. World Union of Wound Healing Societies (WUWHS) consensus document. Surgical wound dehiscence: improving prevention and outcomes. 2018;
28. Sandy-Hodgetts K. Clinical innovation: the Sandy grading system for surgical wound dehiscence classification — a new taxonomy. Wounds Int. 2017;2017(8):6–11.
29. Gowd AK, Bohl DD, Hamid KS, Lee S, Holmes GB, Lin J. Longer operative time is independently associated with surgical site infection and wound dehiscence following open reduction and internal fixation of the ankle. Foot Ankle Spec. 2020;13:104–11.
30. Kim PJ, Attinger CE, Constantine T, et al. Negative pressure wound therapy with instillation: international consensus guidelines update. Int Wound J. 2020;17:174–86.
31. Ieropoli G, Villafañe JH, Zompi SC, Morozzo U, D'Ambrosi R, Usuelli FG, Berjano P. Successful treatment of infected wound dehiscence after minimally invasive locking-plate

osteosynthesis of tibial pilon and calcaneal fractures by plate preservation, surgical debridement and antibiotics. Foot. 2017;33:44–7.

32. Köse O, Waseem A. Keloids and hypertrophic scars: are they two different sides of the same coin? Dermatol Surg. 2008;34:336–46.

33. Del Toro D, Dedhia R, Tollefson TT. Advances in scar management: prevention and management of hypertrophic scars and keloids. Curr Opin Otolaryngol Head Neck Surg. 2016;24:322–9.

34. Ogawa R, Akaishi S, Kuribayashi S, Miyashita T. Keloids and hypertrophic scars can now be cured completely: recent Progress in our understanding of the pathogenesis of keloids and hypertrophic scars and the Most promising current therapeutic strategy. J Nippon Med Sch Nippon Ika Daigaku Zasshi. 2016;83:46–53.

Part II
Pediatric Orthopaedics and Traumatology

Biomechanics, Assessment, and Management Principles for Pediatric Foot Deformities

Vincent S. Mosca

We, as orthopedic surgeons, were obviously drawn to our profession by a desire to help relieve musculoskeletal pain and related dysfunction using surgical techniques. However, techniques change. Principles are forever. For such a complex anatomic site as the child's foot with its 26 bones and at least 19 major articulations and almost innumerable congenital and developmental deformities and malformations, one must, therefore, study principles. A principle is a basic generalization that is accepted as true and can be used as a basis for reasoning or conduct.

The following principles were personally conceived, developed, organized, explained, presented, and finally published in 2014 in my book, *Principles and Management of Pediatric Foot and Ankle Deformities and Malformations* [1]. I am pleased to share with you some of my excerpted principles in condensed form in this book. Note that the number of the principle in this chapter does not necessarily match the number of the principle in my book because all of them are not included here.

1 Biomechanics

Biomechanics Principle #1
"The foot is not a joint!" In all congenital and developmental deformities and most malformations of the child's foot, there are at least two segmental deformities that are often in rotationally opposite directions from each other, "as if the foot was wrung out." Before one can surgically treat the pain and disability associated with

V. S. Mosca (✉)
Orthopedics, University of Washington School of Medicine, Seattle, WA, USA

Pediatric Orthopedic Surgeon, Seattle Children's Hospital, Seattle, WA, USA
e-mail: vincent.mosca@seattlechildrens.org

© The Author(s), under exclusive license to Springer Nature Switzerland AG 2022
E. Wagner Hitschfeld, P. Wagner Hitschfeld (eds.), *Foot and Ankle Disorders*,
https://doi.org/10.1007/978-3-030-95738-4_6

115

foot deformities and malformations, each segmental deformity and malformation must be identified, characterized, and understood so a plan can be created to individually, yet concurrently, manage each one.

Biomechanics Principle #2

Before treating deformities and malformations of the child's foot, whether non-operatively or operatively, a thorough and working knowledge of the normal anatomy of the child's foot and ankle is required.

Biomechanics Principle #3

The average foot shape of a child is different than the average foot shape of an adult. And the range of normal foot shapes in a child is different than the range of normal foot shapes in an adult, though with significant overlap between age groups. For example, many or most babies are flatfooted, a shape less commonly seen in adults. Many babies have metatarsus adductus, a shape rarely seen in adults.

Biomechanics Principle #4

Age-related anatomic variations in the shape of the foot and the natural history of each one must be appreciated. In most cases, anatomic variations in the shape of the child's foot change spontaneously to adult norms through normal growth and development.

For example, most babies are flatfooted, whereas about 25% of adults are flatfooted. Approximately 1 in 100 babies has metatarsus adductus, almost none receive treatment, and very few adults have that foot shape. Knowledge of anatomic variations and their natural history should prevent unnecessary and potentially harmful interventions.

Biomechanics Principle #5

One must understand subtalar joint positions and motions in a manner that supersedes the confusing and inconsistent terminology in the literature. The static deformity positions of the subtalar joint can appropriately be described using the terminology used for other joints, i.e., varus (the calcaneus angles inwards in relation to the talus) and valgus (the calcaneus angles outwards in relation to the talus). Hindfoot varus is the static position of the subtalar joint found in cavovarus feet and clubfeet. Hindfoot valgus is the static position of the subtalar joint seen in flatfeet, skewfeet, and vertical tali. Some healthcare professionals use the term "pronated" when referring to a foot with hindfoot valgus. I disagree. Forearms pronate and supinate. There is a lot more going on in foot deformities with a valgus hindfoot than can be captured with the simplistic and specific term "pronated."

The motions that result in those static positions should, in my opinion, be described using terms that recognize the unique and complex features of the subtalar joint. The subtalar joint differs from all other joints in the body in several ways: it is not a hinge joint or a ball-and-socket joint; its axis is not in the sagittal, coronal, or transverse plane; and it is a compound joint (several bones articulate) rather than a diarthrodial joint (two bones articulate). The subtalar joint complex is comprised of three bones (possibly four, if one includes the cuboid), several important ligaments, and multiple joint capsules that function together as a unit. Almost 200 years ago, Scarpa saw similarities between the hip joint and the subtalar joint complex. He coined the term "acetabulum pedis," referring to a cuplike structure made up of the proximal articular surface of the navicular, the spring ligament, and the facets of the anterior end of the calcaneus. He compared the femoral head to the talar head and the pelvic acetabulum to his so-called acetabulum pedis. I believe that the unique term "inversion" best captures the three-dimensional motions of the acetabulum pedis around the head of the talus that result in the static position termed "varus." The acetabulum pedis plantar flexes (down), internally rotates (in), *and* supinates. Simply stated, inversion is a "down and in" movement of the acetabulum pedis around the talus. Conversely, "eversion" motion results in the static position termed "valgus." It is a combination of dorsiflexion (up), external rotation (out), *and* pronation of the acetabulum pedis around the talar head. Simply stated, eversion is an "up and out" movement of the acetabulum pedis around the talus.

Biomechanics Principle #6
A thorough and working knowledge of the biomechanics of the foot and of the subtalar joint complex in particular are mandatory for assessment and management of foot deformities in children. The functions of the foot include provision of a stable, but supple, platform that helps it accommodate to the changing terrain below and propel the body in space. And the subtalar joint is the machinery used by the foot to adapt to the ground during the early stance phase of gait and then convert to a rigid lever during push-off.

The foot acts as the most efficient and effective lever for the generation of power during push-off when the subtalar joint is inverted/locked and the foot is pointing directly forward, i.e., perpendicular to the transverse axis of the knee joint. This is the concept of lever arm function. Lever arm dysfunction can result from shortening the lever arm and/or weakening the triceps surae. The lever arm is shortened when the foot is externally rotated in relationship to the sagittal plane of the knee. This can be due to an everted/unlocked subtalar joint and/or external tibial torsion. The force coupling (force x distance to the center of the axis of motion, i.e., length of the lever arm) can be further diminished by weakness of the triceps surae. This can occur if the triceps surae is inappropriately lengthened and, thereby, weakened.

Biomechanics Principle #7
In the normal foot, the overall shape is determined by the shapes and interrelationships of the bones, coupled with the strength and flexibility of the ligaments. Muscles maintain balance, accommodate the foot to uneven terrain, protect the ligaments from unusual stresses, and propel the body forward.

Biomechanics Principle #8
Don't use the term "pronated" as a substitute for the term "flatfoot." There's very little pronation in a flatfoot, yet many healthcare professionals refer to a flatfoot as a pronated foot. It's true that pronation is one of the components of eversion of the subtalar joint, but the dorsiflexion and external rotation components are far more significant deformities. And the forefoot in a flatfoot is supinated! If it were not supinated, but instead followed the subtalar joint into eversion/"pronation," it might be appropriate to use the term pronated. In that situation, however, the lateral forefoot would be elevated off the ground, a deformity that almost never exists except in some cases of congenital subtalar synostosis.

Another misnomer for flatfoot that is often used when discussing adult flatfoot is "dorsolateral peritalar subluxation." It is true that eversion of the subtalar joint results in dorsal and lateral alignment of the navicular in relation to the head of the talus, i.e., peritalar. But there is no subluxation of any component part of the subtalar joint complex with even severe eversion. Subluxation is defined as incomplete or partial dislocation of a joint, i.e., only partial contact between articular surfaces that normally have full contact. Think of Scarpa's analogy of the hip and the acetabulum pedis. Congenital and developmental hip subluxations occur, and these are characterized by partial contact (incongruity) of the articular surfaces due to translation of the femoral head from the center of the acetabulum. There is no analogy for that pathology in the foot. Severe eversion, which might be called dorsolateral peritalar *positioning*, is a rotational malalignment of the subtalar joint. It is perhaps analogous to severe abduction or adduction of the hip without translational loss of contact of the articular surfaces, i.e., without subluxation.

The term flatfoot has historical precedence and, though not specific, is associated with a good visual for most people.

Cavus is defined as plantar flexion of the forefoot on the hindfoot. It does not mean "high arch," although that's the resultant effect. There may be plantar flexion of the medial column, the lateral column, or the entire forefoot on the hindfoot. Coincidentally, the subtalar joint can be inverted, everted, or in neutral alignment. And the ankle can be plantar flexed, dorsiflexed, or in neutral alignment. When describing a cavus foot, it is best to describe all of its features. Some examples are cavovarus, equinocavovarus, calcaneocavus, and transtarsal cavus. I've seen congenital and iatrogenic calcaneo-abducto-cavo-valgus.

Biomechanics Principle #9
The foot deformity may be the primary problem or the result of the primary problem, i.e., a neuromuscular disorder. Differentiation is important. A cavovarus foot deformity is the result of a neuromuscular disorder until proven otherwise. This is important to remember because a treatable neuromuscular disorder, such as a tethered spinal cord or spinal tumor, is not necessarily readily apparent when a child presents with a cavovarus foot deformity. However, it should be diagnosed and treated before the foot deformity is treated. Further permanent neuromuscular deterioration should be arrested as soon as possible. Flatfoot is most often either a normal anatomic variant or the primary problem. Examples of the latter include flexible flatfoot with short Achilles tendon, tarsal coalition, congenital vertical talus, and skewfoot. Flatfoot can also be associated with neuromuscular disorders, such as cerebral palsy, but these underlying disorders are usually apparent.

2   Clinical Assessment

Assessment Principle #1
A complete and detailed clinical and radiographic assessment of the child's foot is required before treatment is instituted.

Assessment Principle #2

Clinical evaluation of the child's foot begins with a clinical evaluation of the child. Although the foot deformity or malformation is the reason for the requested evaluation by you, children with these conditions often have underlying neuromuscular, genetic, or chromosome disorders as well as other deformities and/or malformations of the lower extremities and spine. These must be recognized and factored into the decision-making process to ensure that the most appropriate of the possible non-operative and operative interventions are chosen.

Assessment Principle #3

Congenital and developmental deformities should be differentiated. Congenital deformities are rarely progressive in their natural history, yet rarely regressive. Tendons and joint capsules are usually co-contracted. For example, in a clubfoot (congenital talipes equinocavovarus) in an older child that does not correct with non-operative management, posterior ankle capsulotomy is often required in addition to Achilles tendon lengthening.

Developmental deformities, by definition, are progressive in their natural history, though the rate of progression is variable. Contracture of tendons precedes contracture of joint capsules. In a developmental equinocavovarus foot deformity in an older child, an Achilles tendon lengthening is usually enough to correct the equinus deformity.

Assessment Principle #4

Static and progressive deformities should be differentiated, and the rate of progression established, if possible. As stated in *Assessment Principle #3*, most congenital foot deformities are static, rather than progressive, in nature. Muscle imbalance is the underlying problem in many acquired foot deformities. The muscle imbalance can be static, as in children with myelomeningocele, lipomeningocele, and post-infectious poliomyelitis, or it can be progressive, as in children with Charcot-Marie-Tooth disease, muscular dystrophy, spinal cord tumors, tethered cord, and diastematomyelia. Whether the muscle imbalance is static or progressive, the deformity is likely to progress. Unfortunately, the rate of progression is rarely predictable for either static or progressive muscle imbalances. Progression and increased time to treatment will increase the complexity of reconstruction.

Assessment Principle #5

It is often more challenging to ascertain the history of pain and/or dysfunction that is related to the foot deformity in a child than in an adult, but it's worth the effort. Reasons for children to be poor historians include that they are too young, "too adolescent," intellectually challenged, and neurologically impaired. The importance of an accurate assessment of the pain and dysfunction is that there are many clinically and radiographically apparent normal anatomic variations of the child's foot. If the pain location, severity, and temporal and activity-related patterns do not match the known pain pattern of an identified deformity/condition, the two might not be related.

Assessment Principle #6

Assessment of pain must be specific – where, when, what level/severity, and what associations. There are many anatomic variations of the foot, including a host of accessory ossicles, which could be the source of pain or merely incidental findings. It is easy, for example, to ascribe reported foot pain to a tarsal coalition or an accessory navicular that is identified on an x-ray. However, since most anatomic variations including tarsal coalitions and accessory naviculars don't hurt, it is important to know the exact site(s) of pain, as well as the activities that insight and relieve the pain. Severity of the pain should be quantified. Visual analog pain scales have been shown to be reliable in even very young children. The pain location, pattern, and severity must all match those of the presumed diagnosis. Chronic pain in a non-physiologic distribution that occurs continuously during all waking hours and is reported to be of an exaggerated severity suggests chronic regional pain syndrome, aka reflex sympathetic dystrophy, reflex neurovascular dystrophy, and pain amplification syndrome.

Assessment Principle #7
If pain is a complaint, ask the child to point to the exact location(s). By having the child identify the point(s) of maximal tenderness, you can start your physical examination away from that site(s) and learn about the surrounding area(s) before creating pain that might limit the rest of the examination. You can also quickly determine if your working diagnosis (based on the history) is valid even before you touch the foot.

Assessment Principle #8
Physical evaluation of the child's foot begins with a physical evaluation of the child. This includes a careful examination of the hips and spine in a newborn. Visual gait analysis, torsional profile analysis, and angular alignment assessment are used for older children and adolescents. Visual gait analysis is carried out by watching the child walk, run, toe walk, heel walk, squat and stand, and hop on each foot. These observations are used to evaluate symmetry, strength, coordination, and comfort. The child's torsional profile must be ascertained with the child prone on an examination table.

Assessment Principle #9
The foot must be clinically assessed in weight-bearing, not just on the exam table. Do this first to learn about the true deformities and functions/dysfunctions of the foot. The foot deformity will look very different when weight-bearing and non-weight-bearing. A flatfoot looks better than it truly is when it is not bearing weight. And a cavovarus foot looks worse than it truly is when non-weight-bearing. Pain and/or disability are usually, if not always, experienced when weight-bearing. Observation of the weight-bearing foot helps understand the pattern of pain and disability.

Assessment Principle #10
Assessment of each of the segmental deformities of the foot and ankle is imperative before planning treatment, as a plan needs to be established to correct each one.
   The segments are:

1. Forefoot – pronated or supinated; plantar flexed (equinus) or dorsiflexed.

   (a) Recall that alignment (and deformity) is defined as the relationship between a more distal anatomic part and the next more proximal anatomic part. Therefore, pronation or supination refers to the alignment of the forefoot in relation to the midfoot/hindfoot, not the tibia/leg. This has been a source of confusion for many who believe the forefoot in a flatfoot is neutrally aligned (in relation to the tibia) when, in fact, it is supinated – in relation to the mid/hindfoot.

2. Midfoot – abducted or adducted.
3. Hindfoot – varus/inverted or valgus/everted.
4. Ankle – varus or valgus; plantar flexed (equinus) or dorsiflexed (calcaneus).

Assessment Principle #11

Each segment of the foot should be evaluated for shape/deformity, flexibility, and skin integrity. Documentation should be specific. Accurate assessment of the shape of each segment of the foot is the first step.

For a cavovarus foot deformity, the segmental deformities are pronation of the forefoot, adduction of the midfoot, varus of the hindfoot, and possibly equinus of the ankle. Equally important is the flexibility of each segment. The first segment to lose flexibility is the forefoot. Loss of flexibility of the hindfoot, which is assessed by the Coleman block test, eventually follows.

Skin integrity should be assessed, as it can identify unsafe foot pressures. This is especially important in children with insensate skin. In the cavovarus foot, exaggerated pressures are seen at the base of the fifth metatarsal and under the first and fifth metatarsal heads.

The segmental deformities of a flatfoot include supination of the forefoot, abduction or straight alignment of the midfoot, valgus of the hindfoot, and equinus of the ankle. Equally important is the flexibility of each segment. Flexibility of the hindfoot is assessed in a different manner than that used for a cavovarus foot. There is not a reliable "reverse" Coleman block test. Instead, toe standing and the Jack toe raise test are utilized to assess hindfoot flexibility.

Evidence of exaggerated skin pressures in a flatfoot are identified under the medial midfoot. The skin in this area is rarely stressed except when a flatfoot is associated with contracture of the gastrocnemius or the entire triceps surae (Achilles tendon).

Assessment Principle #12

The accurate assessment of subtalar motion is an inexact science, but you can better at it by practicing. There are no studies documenting the accuracy of assessment of subtalar motion. It is particularly challenging in very small feet and fat feet.

The best way to improve your skills for assessing subtalar joint motion is to practice in the OR during a foot deformity correction operation while observing your technique and the resultant motions of the subtalar joint under mini fluoroscopy.

Assessment Principle #13

There may also be a deformity in the ankle joint. An ankle joint deformity may coexist with a foot deformity or it may be an isolated deformity. It must be differentiated.

The ankle joint is in valgus orientation to the anatomic axis of the tibia in all newborns. In otherwise normal children, the distal fibula and lateral distal tibia grow relatively faster than the medial distal tibia until about age 3–4 years at which point the ankle joint/tibial plafond becomes perpendicular to the tibia. It maintains that anatomic alignment through skeletal maturity.

That spontaneous change from physiologic neonatal ankle valgus to neutral alignment does not occur in children with myelomeningocele, lipomeningocele, early onset poliomyelitis, other early onset flaccid paralytic conditions, and approximately 66% of limbs with a clubfoot. The clinical assessment of ankle joint alignment and the differentiation from subtalar joint alignment are helpful in older children, particularly in those with the stated underlying conditions. In spastic conditions, such as cerebral palsy, normal spontaneous correction of neonatal ankle valgus to neutral occurs.

The frontal plane angle between the ankle joint and a line connecting the distal tips of the medial and lateral malleoli is 15 degrees. Therefore, with a valgus ankle joint deformity of approximately 15 degrees, the line connecting the distal tips of the medial and lateral malleoli is in a transverse plane that is perpendicular to the tibia. When the ankle joint has assumed its adult alignment perpendicular with the tibia, the distal tip of the lateral malleolus is closer to the floor and further from the knee than the medial malleolus. This assessment of the relative heights of the malleoli is helpful in the clinical determination of frontal plane ankle alignment. It is particularly helpful in the clinical determination of the site of hindfoot valgus deformity, which can exist in the ankle joint, the subtalar joint, or in both joints.

The ankle joint can also have a procurvatum or recurvatum deformity. These are almost always acquired deformities. A flat-top deformity of the talus can occur following both non-operative and operative treatment of clubfoot deformity and result in a true or "functional" procurvatum deformity of the ankle. Iatrogenic posterior distal tibial physeal arrest following clubfoot surgery can cause a true procurvatum deformity.

Assessment Principle #14

The Achilles tendon or gastrocnemius muscle may be contracted. The presence of a gastrocnemius or an Achilles tendon contracture must be identified and differentiated from each other.

Many foot deformities do not cause pain or functional disability unless they are accompanied by a contracture of the heel cord (the gastrocnemius alone or the entire triceps surae/Achilles tendon). The ankle joint should have at least 10° of dorsiflexion with the knee extended and the subtalar joint in neutral alignment. The Silfverskiold test should be used to determine if there is a contracture of the heel cord and, if so, whether the contracture is of the gastrocnemius alone or the Achilles tendon. This will ensure that the proper tendon is lengthened if surgery is indicated, thereby avoiding under- or overlengthening. The Silfverskiold test must be mastered.

The cavus foot presents a different challenge to the assessment of a possible heel cord contracture. Cavus means plantar flexion of the forefoot on the hindfoot, i.e., equinus of the forefoot. Therefore, assessment of ankle equinus can only be performed by isolating the hindfoot. The forefoot should be obscured from your vision with your hand so that only the hindfoot can be seen.

Assessment Principle #15

A detailed examination of strength, sensation, reflexes, and vascularity is required. This is particularly true for the cavovarus foot but is important for all foot deformities. Don't rely on EMG findings or on someone else to do it.

Assessment Principle #16

Signs and symptoms must match the presumed pathology, so ensure that you have enough clinical information before focusing on a radiographic finding.

There are many common anatomic foot variations, such as tarsal coalitions and accessory naviculars, that do not cause pain or functional disability in most affected individuals. Therefore, it's important to ensure that the signs and symptoms match those associated with the radiographic finding. If they don't, the two are unrelated, and a more thorough investigation is required.

3   Radiographic And Other Imaging Assessment

Assessment Principle #17

All standard initial/screening radiographs for assessment of foot deformities should be obtained in weight-bearing, or simulated weight-bearing if the former is not possible because of young age or inability to stand.

This is the radiographic version of *Assessment Principle #9*. The appropriate clinical assessment of foot deformities is performed in weight-bearing. Radiographs must, therefore, be obtained in weight-bearing to correlate the anatomic alignment of the bones and joints with the outward appearance of the foot. Specialized views, such as oblique views, can be taken non-weight-bearing because they are used to identify anatomic abnormalities other than bone and joint alignment. The standard radiographic views for assessing foot deformities are *standing* AP, lateral, and (medial or standard) oblique. Additional views include lateral oblique, Harris axial, and Saltzman views.

Assessment Principle #18

The foot-CORA method should be used pre-, intra-, and postoperatively for the most objective evaluation of foot deformities and malformations.

There are several radiographic features of the foot bones in children that make it unreliable or impossible to apply the CORA method, as used in the long bones of the extremities, to the assessment of pediatric foot deformities. These features justify a unique CORA method for assessment of pediatric foot deformities.

The basis of the "foot-CORA" method is the assessment of the relationship between the axis of the talus and the axis of the first metatarsal in the transverse (AP) and sagittal (lateral) planes. Unlike the ossification centers of the bones of the midfoot, those of the metatarsals, talus, and calcaneus are present at birth and reliably represent the shapes of the incompletely ossified bones. The first metatarsal is a proxy for the calcaneopedal unit (CPU), which is the term for all the bones of the foot except the talus. The major deformities of subtalar varus/inversion and valgus/

eversion exist between the CPU and the talus. The foot-CORA method readily identifies and defines those deformities by an intersection of those axis lines in the head of the talus in the AP plane. The lines are adducted in varus/inversion deformities and abducted in valgus/eversion deformities.

There may also be static deformities in the shapes of the small bones within the CPU. Based on the acknowledged challenges of assessing them directly, the foot-CORA method assessment of the relationship between the axis of the talus and that of the first metatarsal accurately identifies those as well, by proxy.

The CORA in a long bone is the site of deformity and the ideal site for deformity correction by means of an osteotomy. The foot-CORA for varus and valgus hindfoot deformities, that is in the talar head, is the site of deformity but never the site for deformity correction. Instead, soft tissue procedures and/or osteotomies of the peritalar structures are performed to align the axes of the talus and the first MT at the foot-CORA. The talus-first metatarsal angle can be used to quantify the degree of inversion and eversion deformities before and after correction.

The center of the medial cuneiform (within the CPU) is the foot-CORA for the two most common midfoot deformities, cavus and metatarsus adductus. Like the CORA in long bones, the medial cuneiform is the site of deformity and the ideal site for deformity correction for these deformities.

Assessment Principle #19
There will be a projectional artifact on the lateral radiograph of a foot with a varus or valgus hindfoot deformity and an adduction or abduction midfoot deformity. Therefore, order specifically positioned views.

When a foot is C-shaped due to inversion or eversion of the hindfoot and adduction or abduction of the midfoot, the lateral x-ray creates an unusual appearance of the hindfoot. The reason is that an x-ray beam cannot simultaneously pass perpendicular to the forefoot and the hindfoot when there is a curve in the plane of the beam. Therefore, order specifically positioned views to see each segment in a true lateral projection. The radiology technicians can easily visualize the forefoot and will generally aim the x-ray beam perpendicular to the metatarsals. That creates a rotational projectional artifact of the hindfoot in varus/inversion and valgus/eversion hindfoot deformities and in adduction and abduction midfoot deformities. Recall that one component of inversion is internal rotation of the subtalar joint/acetabulum pedis in relation to the talus/ankle and that one component of eversion is external rotation of the subtalar joint/acetabulum pedis in relation to the talus/ankle.

Finally, be aware that the best way to assess proper hindfoot positioning for a lateral radiograph is to note the relationship between the distal fibula and tibia. The posterior cortex of the distal fibula metaphysis and the posterior ossification margin of the distal tibial epiphysis are colinear in a true lateral x-ray of the hindfoot/ankle. It is unreliable to use the shape of the dome of the talus to determine a true lateral projection, because the ossification of the dome is not particularly dome-shaped in young children. Furthermore, there are many instances in which the dome had been crushed, devascularized, or otherwise injured, thereby flattening its dome shape.

And, as has just been discussed, flattening of the dome can be a projectional artifact. Therefore, use the distal fibula to tibia relationships to determine if the projection is a true lateral of the hindfoot/ankle.

Assessment Principle #20

Don't forget about ankle radiographs.

Ankle radiographs (*standing* AP, lateral, mortis) are not a standard part of every assessment of a foot deformity or malformation but should be ordered if clinically indicated. See *Assessment Principle #13*.

Assessment Principle #21

CT scan in all three orthogonal planes and with 3D reconstruction is the best imaging modality for more detailed assessment of complex foot deformities and malformations. It is the definitive imaging study for the diagnosis and management of tarsal coalitions.

For most deformities and malformations, plain radiographs provide enough information to corroborate the physical examination findings. CT scans show the shapes of bones and the alignment of joints in three dimensions, the exact information needed to assess the more complex deformities and malformations, particularly those that have been operated on previously. MRI scans are best for the assessment of soft tissue pathology, which is not the intent of structural assessment. The exorbitant cost of an MRI (even in comparison with a CT scan) makes it fiscally irresponsible to obtain this study without careful consideration of the indications and the information desired, considerations that apply to all imaging studies. CT scans use ionizing radiation but at a distance far from the most radiation sensitive parts of the body.

Importantly, the CT scan is the *definitive imaging study* for the diagnosis and management of talocalcaneal tarsal coalitions, because the published criteria for choosing the appropriate treatment modality are based on CT scan findings. Fibrocartilaginous as well as osseous coalitions can be easily identified on CT scans.

Assessment Principle #22

MRI is rarely helpful for assessment of pediatric foot deformities and malformations. Radiographs and CT scans are most helpful for these indications.

MRI scans are useful in assessing soft tissue abnormalities, such as infections and soft tissue tumors. The exorbitant cost of an MRI of the foot might be justified in the assessment of a complex deformity or malformation in a very young child who has minimal ossification of the tarsal bones.

4   Management

Management Principle #1

The decision (to operate) is more important than the incision (i.e., the surgical technique). And the decision to operate on a foot deformity or malformation is based on

(1) the known natural history of the condition, (2) the symptomatic and/or functional responses to non-operative treatment (where appropriate), and (3) the reported risks and complications of surgery. A "well-executed" operation for the right indication is far better for the patient than the "most skillfully executed operation in the history of surgery" for the wrong indication. The best surgeon is not necessarily the most skillful, but the one who knows when to operate. Of course, it's nice to make the best decisions and be technically excellent. We all strive for that combination of knowledge and skills.

Management Principle #2

A less than ideal surgical outcome can be due to a poor technique, a poor technician, or both.

This principle assumes that the patient satisfies reasonable indications for the technique in question. A surgical or non-surgical (e.g., Ponseti) technique is developed and, hopefully, tested by the originator before it is presented to the medical community. There is perhaps no technique that is so simple or foolproof that mere knowledge of the concept allows another surgeon to perform the procedure as well as the originator. And for some/many techniques, attention to all the fine details of the procedure is critical for success. Failure to perform the procedure as described by the originator might result in a good outcome, but a poor outcome cannot automatically be attributed to the technique. It can only, perhaps, be considered a poor technique if other surgeons skillfully follow the fine details of the procedure (as published and without modifications) and fail to achieve outcomes comparable to the originator. Before abandoning or modifying a procedure that has been shown by others to be effective, make sure to perform it as described by the originator. Personal observation of, or tutoring by, an expert might be required, depending on the complexity and uniqueness of the technique.

Management Principle #3

You can't un-operate on anyone. Foot deformities and malformations are never lethal. Non-operative treatment might prolong the temporary pain and disability but might eliminate both, thereby avoiding the reported risks and complications of surgery.

Management Principle #4

The (surgical) treatment could be worse than the condition itself.

No operation is without potential risks and complications that are unacceptable if the natural history of the condition or the response to non-operative treatment provides favorable outcomes with little to no long-term disability. Non-operative treatment corrects a high percentage of many congenital deformities (clubfoot and metatarsus adductus) and/or resolves pain and functional disability in a high percentage of certain other conditions (tarsal coalition, juvenile hallux valgus, and accessory navicular). Natural history trumps all treatment modalities. Many anatomic variations correct spontaneously through normal growth and development (flexible flatfoot, metatarsus adductus, and position calcaneovalgus) or persist without resulting in pain or functional disability (flexible flatfoot, metatarsus adductus, skewfoot).

Management Principle #5

Modalities that *correct structural* deformities: (1) natural history, (2) physical stretching, (3) serial casting, and (4) surgery.

Surgery is the final common pathway for foot deformities that do not correct spontaneously or respond fully to non-operative treatment. Surgical techniques include soft tissue releases and/or plications, osteotomies, and, rarely, arthrodeses. Tendon transfers do not correct structural deformities.

As a corollary, natural history is the only modality that results in permanent deformity correction. There is a risk of deformity recurrence following all treatment modalities.

A commonly held belief by some healthcare professionals and most grandparents is that special "orthopedic shoes" and orthotics correct foot deformities in children. There is no scientific evidence to support that belief. The myth has been perpetuated because those devices have been credited with the deformity correction that has, in fact, occurred as a result of the natural history of the condition.

Management Principle #6

Modalities that *correct dynamic* deformities: (1) focal injection of tone-reducing medication into muscles (such as BOTOX) and (2) muscle-balancing tendon surgery.

Tendon lengthening/weakening, shortening, and transfer techniques are more permanent solutions to muscle imbalance, but they are not entirely reliable, predictable, or definitive. The main problem with a dynamic deformity is that it is the result of the problem (an underlying neuromuscular disorder) and not the primary problem. After tendon surgery, the child still has the underlying nerve or muscle disorder. Therefore, recurrence of deformity and overcorrection are real possibilities.

Management Principle #7

Modalities that *maintain* deformity correction: (1) focal injection of tone-reducing medication into muscles, (2) physical stretching, (3) special shoes/braces, (4) orthotics, and (5) balanced muscles.

Surgically balanced muscles can maintain deformity correction, but achieving balance is an art and may not be achievable. Maintaining muscle balance is particularly challenging in progressive neuromuscular disorders.

Management Principle #8

Treatment (non-operative and/or operative) is indicated for:

1. Congenital deformities and malformations that are known, or expected, to cause pain and/or functional disability unless corrected.

   (a) These include congenital clubfoot, congenital vertical talus, rigid metatarsus adductus, rigid skewfoot, polydactyly, and macrodactyly. They are treated well before they become symptomatic.

2. Developmental deformities that are creating pain and/or functional disability.

    (a) These include cavovarus foot, flexible flatfoot with short Achilles tendon, idiopathic equinus, tarsal coalition, accessory navicular, spastic and paralytic foot deformities, and iatrogenic deformities.

For both pain and functional disability, the treatment is disease-specific and can be non-operative and/or operative.

Management Principle #9
Surgical treatment is indicated for:

1. Congenital deformities and malformations that do not, or cannot, correct with non-operative treatment and are known to cause pain and/or functional disability unless corrected.

    (a) These include congenital clubfoot and vertical talus that do not respond to non-operative (Ponseti and reverse Ponseti) management, macrodactyly, longitudinal epiphyseal bracket of the first metatarsal, and polydactyly.

2. Progressive cavovarus foot deformities that are associated with pain and/or functional disability.
3. Other developmental, persistent, and recurrent deformities that do not adequately respond to prolonged attempts at non-operative treatment designed to relieve pain and/or diminish or relieve functional disability that are related to the deformity.

    (a) These include skewfoot, recurrent and overcorrected congenital clubfoot and vertical talus, idiopathic equinus, flexible flatfoot with short Achilles tendon, tarsal coalition, accessory navicular, juvenile hallux valgus, and spastic and paralytic foot deformities.

Management Principle #10
Provide clear, accurate, and reasonable expectations to the patient and family of the short- and long-term outcomes of non-operative and operative management.

Foot deformities and malformations are rarely "cured", i.e., made normal. But long-term comfort and function can be anticipated for many or most of them. For deformities that are due to neuromuscular disorders, the foot deformity is the result of the problem and not the primary problem. Recurrence of deformity and the need for future treatment can be anticipated in many of these cases. Normal growth and development of a foot with a primary deformity can have an anticipated or unanticipated effect on the long-term outcome of the intervention. Share your predictions about future comfort and function and about the need for future treatment with the patient and family. That way there should be few surprises down the line.

Management Principle #11
A surgical plan for each of the segmental deformities and muscle imbalances needs to be established before proceeding with surgery.

This means creating a list of the multiple related and unrelated procedures that are to be performed either during a single operative session or sequentially in cases of staged procedures. Some deformities are not evident until others are corrected. This needs to be anticipated before the start of the operation, based on one's knowledge and understanding of deformities, with a surgical plan ready for each additional deformity that might be identified intraoperatively. Be prepared, rather than surprised.

Management Principle #12

Correct deformity at the site of the deformity, unless the only option is arthrodesis of the subtalar joint.

That means:

1. Perform a calcaneal lengthening osteotomy (CLO) rather than posterior calcaneal medial displacement osteotomy (PCDO) for valgus/eversion deformity of the hindfoot. The former procedure (CLO) corrects all components of subtalar joint eversion at the site of deformity, whereas the latter procedure (PCDO) creates a compensatory deformity to "correct" valgus alignment of the hindfoot.
2. Perform a plantar-medial soft tissue release (PMR) of the subtalar joint rather than posterior calcaneal lateral displacement osteotomy (PCDO) for varus/inversion deformity of the hindfoot. The former procedure (PMR) corrects all components of subtalar joint inversion at the site of deformity, whereas the latter procedure (PCDO) creates a compensatory deformity to "correct" varus alignment of the hindfoot.
3. Perform a medial cuneiform opening wedge osteotomy rather than first metatarsal osteotomy for cavus deformity (plantar flexion deformity of the first ray). The foot-CORA for cavus is in the medial cuneiform.
4. Perform a medial cuneiform opening wedge osteotomy and cuboid closing wedge osteotomy rather than metatarsal osteotomies or tarsometatarsal capsulotomies for metatarsus adductus. The foot-CORA for metatarsus adductus is in the medial cuneiform.

Management Principle #13

Preserve joint motion (particularly subtalar joint motion) in the feet of children and adolescents by utilizing soft tissue releases/plications and osteotomies instead of arthrodeses.

Arthrodesis of the subtalar joint results in debilitating stress transfer to adjacent joints, particularly the ankle joint, leading to premature degenerative arthritis. Arthrodesis also has a detrimental effect on future growth and development of the foot. The subtalar joint is the shock absorber of the foot and, in fact, the entire lower extremity. Preserve its function at all costs.

Management Principle #14

Use biologic, rather than technologic, interventions, i.e., rearrange and/or reshape anatomic parts rather than replace or interfere with them.

The overall reported short-term complication rate of subtalar arthroereisis with synthetic implants is 3.5–30%, with more recent reports of 3.5–11%. However, the actual rates are much higher if one includes the inappropriate implantation of these devices into normal physiologic flexible flatfeet, a practice employed by some healthcare providers. Complications can be categorized as surgeon error, biomaterials problems, biologic problems, and inappropriate implantations. Long-term outcome studies have not been reported. Pain after insertion of these implants may be greater than the pain that predated their implantation. This is particularly concerning if none preexisted, as when they are implanted in normal, physiologic flexible flatfeet.

Management Principle #15
Correct deformities and balance muscle forces.

1. Deformity correction will not correct muscle imbalance.

   Deformity correction without muscle balancing can result in recurrent deformity. If muscle imbalance created the deformity, as is usually the case in cavovarus foot deformities, persistence of the muscle imbalance will recreate the deformity, despite adequate initial deformity correction.

2. Tendon transfers will not correct structural deformities.

   Muscle balancing without deformity correction will create a balanced deformity. That's not the goal.

Management Principle #16
The calcaneocuboid joint is the most distal site at which the lateral column of the foot can be shortened or lengthened to realign the talonavicular joint/acetabulum pedis in a foot with a varus/inverted or a valgus/everted hindfoot deformity. The body of the cuboid is too far distal.

Management Principle #17
The medial cuneiform is the foot-CORA for cavus and for metatarsus adductus. Osteotomies in the medial cuneiform can and should be used to correct forefoot pronation and supination, midfoot adduction and abduction, as well as combinations of those deformities.

When treating pronation (plantar flexion of the first ray) and supination (dorsiflexion of the first ray) deformities of the forefoot, it is important to recognize the alignment of the midfoot, i.e., adduction or abduction. Knowledge of this second plane alignment can help determine whether an opening or closing wedge osteotomy should be used. Opening wedge osteotomies of the medial cuneiform to dorsiflex or plantar flex the first ray inadvertently create mild abduction of the midfoot, whereas closing wedge osteotomies inadvertently create mild adduction of the midfoot. This can be used to your advantage or detriment. For the supination forefoot deformity in a skewfoot, a plantar-based closing wedge osteotomy will pronate the forefoot but increase the midfoot adduction. The better choice is a dorsomedially based opening wedge osteotomy that will pronate the forefoot and abduct the adducted forefoot.

Management Principle #18

The iliac crest is the ideal bone graft source for foot deformity correction surgery in children and adolescents. Allograft has advantages over autograft.

Management Principle #19

Principles of tendon transfers:

1. Move the right tendon to the right location at the right tension.
2. Tendon transfers will not correct structural deformities.
3. Tendon transfers are based on existing and anticipated patterns of muscle imbalance.
4. Tendon transfers are much more challenging with joint preserving reconstruction.

Management Principle #20

Correct deformities in a complex multi-segmental foot/ankle deformity in the proper order.

1. Cavovarus – forefoot before hindfoot.
2. Equinocavovarus – cavovarus before equinus.
3. Planovalgus – hindfoot before forefoot.
4. Equinoplanovalgus – planovalgus concurrent with equinus.
5. Planovalgus or cavovarus deformity with real or apparent ipsilateral tibial torsion – foot deformity before tibial deformity.
6. Coincident subtalar joint and ankle joint valgus – ankle before foot.

Management Principle #21

Order of events during complex foot reconstruction surgery:

1. Expose and prepare everything before completing anything.
2. Perform and stabilize deformity corrections.
3. As you proceed, close incisions that will no longer be accessed.
4. Set proper tension on tendon lengthenings/plications/transfers.
5. Close final incisions.

Reference

1. Mosca VS. Principles and management of pediatric foot and ankle deformities and malformations. Philadelphia: Wolters Kluwer/Lippincott Williams & Wilkins; 2014.

Clubfoot

Dalia Sepúlveda Arriagada and Nicolas Valdivia Rojo

Summary Clubfoot or congenital talipes equinovarus is the most common congenital deformity affecting the lower extremities. It can occur in approximately 50% bilaterally and is more frequent in males.

Despite its frequency, its etiology is not completely clear. What is recognized is that there is a group of genes that jointly influence the appearance of this deformity.

The gold standard for treatment of idiopathic clubfoot is the Ponseti technique, which presents studies with long follow-up and which confirms it as a safe, low cost, reproducible technique with very good results.

1 Introduction

Clubfoot or talipes equinovarus is one of the most common pediatric orthopedic disorders. It affects approximately 1 per 1000 live newborns [1]. In the world about 174,000 children are born with this pathology, and of these, approximately 90% are born in developing countries [2]. It is currently the leading cause of disability in these countries and carries a heavy social stigma if left untreated.

About 80% of patients with clubfoot present in isolation, the remainder being associated with chromosomal or genetic abnormalities, neurological disorders,

D. Sepúlveda Arriagada (✉)
Private Practice, COTI Chile, Santiago, Chile
e-mail: dsa@cotichile.org

N. Valdivia Rojo
Servicio de Salud Bio bio, Concepción, Chile

Hospital Base Los Angeles, Concepción, Chile

Sanatorio Alemán, Concepción, Chile

© The Author(s), under exclusive license to Springer Nature   133
Switzerland AG 2022
E. Wagner Hitschfeld, P. Wagner Hitschfeld (eds.), *Foot and Ankle Disorders*,
https://doi.org/10.1007/978-3-030-95738-4_7

arthrogryposis, myelomeningocele, or muscular dystrophies. A family history of clubfoot is found in only about 25% of cases [3].

Approximately 50% affect both feet, and in the case of being unilateral, it slightly more frequently affects the right lower extremity [4]. The Polynesian race has the record of having an affection seven to eight times greater than the rest of the world population.

Its etiology is not very clear, but apparently genetic inheritance and maternal smoking are the factors that recur most frequently in clubfoot without associated pathologies or syndromes.

In the last 20 years, the treatment of clubfoot has changed radically, taking a conservative line less and less surgical. In the past, wide posteromedial releases became very common (generating greater scarring, stiffness, and painful arthrosis in the long term); nowadays, they are in frank withdrawal, to the point of being considered contraindicated in the management of children with clubfoot.

Currently the gold standard for the treatment of clubfoot is the Ponseti method; it is a very minimally invasive method that consists of serial manipulation of the foot using modeling casts that progressively correct the deformity and culminate with percutaneous tenotomy of the Achilles tendon (95% of the cases). The correction must be maintained with the use of an orthosis designed by Dr. Ponseti and must be worn until at least 4 years of age. This method has gained more and more followers due to its good long-term results and the low rate of complications [5].

The objective of this chapter is to understand the specific characteristics of clubfoot and the pillars for its diagnosis, its causes, and specific treatment, as well as to show some other types of clubfoot.

2 Diagnosis

In order to make an accurate diagnosis of clubfoot, one must initially recognize what deformities are present. Its diagnosis is clinical, and no additional examination is required. Radiographic study has proven not to be necessary because it does not change the form of treatment according to Ponseti's method.

Classically, clubfoot is described as a set of deformities recognized by the old mnemonic CAVE, midfoot cavus, forefoot adductus, varus, and hindfoot equinus. For this to occur, it is accepted that there is an anomalous position of the tarsal bones (described below) (Figs. 1, 2, 3, 4, and 6).

In addition to these characteristics, we can find a foot generally smaller than the contralateral foot (in unilateral cases), a thinner calf due to the presence of shorter gastrocnemius (occupying only 1/3 of the calf length), and hypodevelopment of the lateral compartment of the leg.

Histological and imaging studies with 3D magnetic resonance imaging show less muscle volume throughout the calf, increased subcutaneous adipose tissue, smaller tibia and fibula, abnormal tendon insertions, shortened ligamentous structures, and

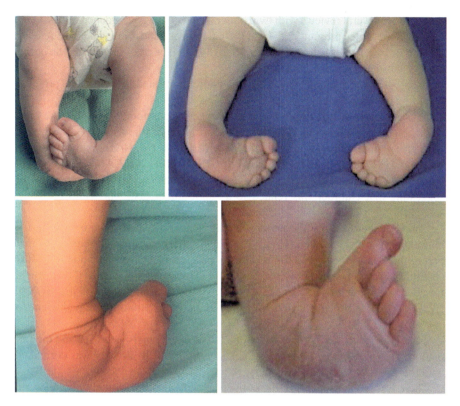

Figs. 1, 2, 3, and 4 Four examples of clubfoot patients

smaller diameter, with abundant fibrous tissue (medial and posterior areas of the foot); this includes shortening of the tendons: posterior tibial, Achilles, deltoid, and calcaneal navicular plantar ligament. Finally, hypoplasia or vascular alterations in the calf territory such as absence of posterior tibial artery [6–9].

3 Etiology

The etiology of clubfoot is well studied, but its origin is not completely clear (assuming that we are talking about the most prevalent orthopedic deformity in pediatrics). A precise origin is not yet known for the group of patients with idiopathic clubfoot which corresponds to 80% of the cases. Researchers have proposed several theories (lack of intrauterine mobility, neurological, vascular, alterations in the connective system and genetic), histological and structural alterations that affect the whole leg and not only the foot are described in several publications [10], so the genetic theory of those genes responsible for the development of the lower limbs is the one that is currently being studied.

There are several reviews with twin patients, where the concordance rate is 2.9%, while monozygotes present 32.5% [11]. On the other hand, having a direct relative (sibling or parent) with clubfoot has a 10 to 20% higher risk of suffering the deformity versus the general population.

In recent years, anatomical and genetic studies have made considerable progress regarding the origin of this pathology [11].

Genetics plays a crucial role in the appearance of clubfoot; however, there is no single gene involved or predominant in the presence of this deformity. There is a wide group of genes involved in clubfoot such as HOXD13, NAT2 (associated with smoking), PITX1, TBX4, HOXC13, UTX, CHD1, RIPPLY2, CAND2, andWNT7. In addition, it is highlighted that there are two regions on chromosomes 3 and 13 suggesting that clubfoot was related to a single major gene but with multigenic susceptibility [12, 13].

The HOX gene family (homeobox family genes) plays an essential role in the morphogenesis process of embryonic development. It determines the correct formation of the axial skeleton and limbs. Several publications have found a genetic susceptibility locus where the presence of clubfoot is associated with the HOX domain. Based on the emerging evidence, we can assume that disruption of the HOXA, HOXC, and HOXD gene clusters may play a role in the etiology and pathogenesis of clubfoot.

The CASP gene family plays an essential role in apoptosis, necrosis, and inflammation. This family was studied by Heck's group, since its activity was correlated with the development of the members.

There is a group of genes of the collagen family also associated with the origin of clubfoot. Recent studies [14] comparing a healthy population versus a population with idiopathic clubfoot show an overexpression of COL1A1 (including mutations of COL1A1), which would correlate even more with the presence of clubfoot.

Mutations of the GLI3 gene would also be involved in the appearance of idiopathic clubfoot. It is noteworthy that this group of genes interacts with HOXD13 with the GLI3 promoter. This was proven by observing that GLI3 mRNA levels and the levels of its expression protein were elevated in rat models of clubfoot.

This would mean that HOXD13 is a transcription factor of GLI3. Its low levels (HOXD13) could lead to elevated levels of GLI3 expression during limb formation which would play an important role in the occurrence of clubfoot.

The role of the T-box gene family would play important roles in embryogenesis and morphogenesis. There are only associations of mutations of these genes with the appearance of clubfoot.

The transcription factors PITX1-TBX4 are responsible for early limb development. There are numerous reports about mutations at this level where less muscle development and the classic phenotype of clubfoot are observed in both rats and humans [15]. Studies by Gurnett, Alvarado, and Dobbs show that there is a close relationship of this pathway with the development of clubfoot and even with the presence of congenital vertical talus.

The family of genes in charge of encoding the troponin and tropomyosin proteins, responsible for muscle contraction, would also be involved in the presence of clubfoot, which clinically would be responsible for the shortening and poor development of the musculature around the calf. This group of genes could also be responsible in cases of syndromic clubfoot associated with distal arthrogryposis. Variations in genes at this level (MYH3, TPM2, TNNT3, TNNI2, and MYH8) would result in muscle contractures at this level. It is unclear which specific alterations would lead to the development of distal arthrogryposis or clubfoot.

The presence of hypoplasia or muscle atrophy around the calf which is maintained over time [16], which is also replaced by fat, has been demonstrated in some MRI studies. On the other hand, studies rule out the presence of histological alterations that suggest a neuromuscular origin of this pathology [17]. This would lead to think of a genetic origin mainly oriented to this group of genes as the ones responsible for clubfoot.

As we can see, there are multiple gene families involved in the etiopathogenesis of VEP. It is clear that external stimuli (tobacco or others) could influence the abnormal expression of these genes, so the multifactorial theory is the one that is currently most supported, and it would not be only one responsible for the presence of this disease.

4   Functional Anatomy

The detailed analysis of the multidirectional movements in the multiple joints of the normal foot, which we know and call the functional anatomy of the foot, is the fundamental pillar of the principle of the correction of the clubfoot with the conservative method technique of Dr. Ignacio Ponseti; he was the one who used the normal kinematics proper and exclusive to the joints surrounding the talus to simultaneously reduce the many deformities of the clubfoot.

5   Normal Anatomy

The subtalar joint complex is one of the most complex and difficult to explain joints in the entire human skeleton. It plays a fundamental role in the adaptation of reaction forces to the ground during lower extremity rotation and gait, as well as in the adaptation of a movable foot to surfaces inclined to the ground plane.

The talus has three articular facets, posterior, medial, and anterior, and two functional components.

- Talocalcaneal joint is housed in the posterior articular facet, which is oblique in the coronal plane and saddle-shaped in the sagittal plane.
- Talocalcaneonavicular joint or "acetabulum pedis" sits on the anterior and medial facets (Fig. 5).
- Interosseous talocalcaneal ligament constitutes the center of rotation of the subtalar joint consisting of two bands: "acetabulum pedis" and Interosseous ligament.

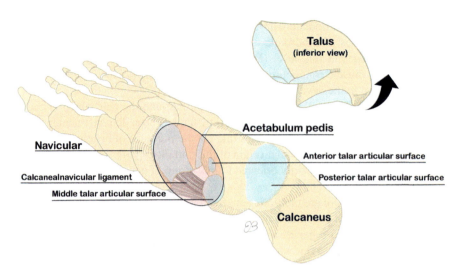

Fig. 5 Anatomy diagram of the acetabulum pedis (talocalcaneonavicular joint). Drawing by Dr. Estefanía Birrer

6   Subtalar Kinematics

Functionally, all the bones of the foot move as a unit around the talus. There is very little intertarsal motion [18] (Inman 1976).

The foot normally moves around the two functional entities of the subtalar joint, the talar calcaneal joint and the "acetabulum pedis" (talocalcaneonavicular), with the interosseous ligament as the center of rotation.

On the other hand, the subtalar axis is not fixed but a dynamic axis that allows displacement and sliding around the limiting or restraining mechanism of the interosseous ligaments, as determined by Inman, Husen, and Van Langelann [19–21].

The motion achieved by the subtalar joint in this oblique plane is supination and pronation. Supination consists of the kinematically coupled movements of adduction, inversion, and plantar flexion, and pronation consists of the kinematically coupled movements of abduction, eversion, and dorsiflexion.

Correction of the rearfoot and midfoot can be fully achieved by abduction of the forefoot. Pressure thus applied on the first metatarsal lever can "motorize" the motion of the calcaneus pedis, thus demonstrating that abduction and eversion are "kinematically coupled."

7   Kinematic Coupling

It is common for orthopedic surgeons to analyze joint movements in reference to standard body planes: coronal, sagittal, and axial. Thus, we have adduction/abduction, inversion/eversion, and plantar flexion/dorsiflexion of the foot.

But when a joint is in the oblique plane, as is the case with the subtalar joint, all these movements are inextricably linked to each other, or "kinematically coupled." Therefore, calcaneal abduction cannot occur without simultaneous eversion and extension. The Ponseti technique allows correction by simultaneously producing the movements in the oblique plane, using abduction as the motor [21–28].

With this explanation of the functional anatomy of the foot, it is possible to understand why abduction of the foot alone simultaneously leads to abduction of the calcaneus and why the entire block pedis during Ponseti manipulation, including the calcaneus, moves or follows in conjunction around the talus.

The Ponseti technique, as we can see, is both simple and profoundly complex. The forefoot is abducted around the talus, which must be kept in the shroud and held in that reduction position by pressure on its head and counterpressure on the widest part of the tibial malleolus, thus obtaining simultaneous abduction, eversion, and extension (dorsiflexion) of the foot with heel valgus.

The normal maximum reduction of the talus in the tibioperoneal mortise of an infant provides full range of motion of the subtalar joint, also reducing the scaphoid at the head of the talus and obtaining full eversion and pronation with dorsiflexion of the calcaneus which simultaneously corrects heel varus.

The clubfoot is not adequately corrected until full abduction is obtained, and calcaneal extension or dorsiflexion occurs primarily during extreme abduction. An infant's foot normally abducts 70°–80°, and the single correction of the clubfoot to a neutral or functional position is not sufficient to achieve all kinematically coupled movements, for this reason recurrence is inevitable [29].

Based on this same mechanism of the kinematic coupling of the tarsal bones, it is also possible to understand the error of the Kite technique [29–32] and other similar treatments, which attempt to correct the foot sequentially, dividing or separating the combined movements into their component parts. Fixing the calcaneus when displacing the forefoot does nothing but block its normal kinematically coupled movement, and then we have to accept that the pseudo correction of the badly manipulated foot only obeys to an iatrogenic deformation of the tarsal bones; for example, blocking the abduction of the calcaneus causes an iatrogenic deformation of the midtarsal bones and joints creating the "bean-shaped or bunioned foot."

8   Classification

The clubfoot can be classified in different ways:

- According to its origin or association to other diseases or syndromes: idiopathic, complex, and syndromic.
- Severity classification: Pirani (currently most used), Dimeglio.

The most currently used classification is that of Pirani, which has a greater interobserver similarity than Dimeglio's classification, and some publications state that both age and the Pirani score at the beginning of treatment could even suggest the number of casts to be used. The important point is that the higher the Pirani score, the longer the treatment (higher number of casts) and the higher the risk of recurrence.

9   Pirani Score (Fig. 6)

10   Treatment

The treatment of congenital clubfoot with Ponseti's method is one of the treatments with the longest follow-up in the world of pediatric orthopedics; in fact, its first publications date back to 1996; however, the method was only adopted and accepted by orthopedic doctors in the world in the last two decades. Since the beginning of the twenty-first century, the news has spread both in the scientific field of specialists and in the social networks of parents with children treated with the bloodless method of Dr. Ignacio Ponseti [20, 33–35].

The excellent functional results of the feet treated with the method slowly convinced parents and orthopedic surgeons of its superiority over any of the surgical techniques in vogue in the last half of the twentieth century, techniques that never came close to the near 100% success achieved with Dr. Ignacio Ponseti's method and technique (Evans, Crawford, Turco).

It is recommended that parents start treatment after the first 2 to 3 weeks of the child's life, once the mother, child, and family unit becomes stable and once they have been informed and explained in great detail the strict route already mapped out for the successful correction of their child's feet.

The method of reduction, to a normal position and appearance, consists first of a very specific and efficient technique of manipulations that return the calcaneal foot (block pedis) to its normal location below the subtalar joint. The advantage and multidirectional kinematic capacity of the subtalar joint (explained in the functional anatomy section) is used to this effect, which progressively allows all components of the clubfoot deformity to be corrected simultaneously.

11   Description of the Two-Handed Manipulation Technique

This is the classic form recommended by Dr. Ponseti whereby the soft tissues of the medial aspect of the foot that are firm and thickened and which cause the retraction and adduction deformity of the forefoot are stretched or elongated (etiology).

The procedure room in which the procedure will be performed should maintain as comfortable an environment as possible, both for the child and accompanying person and for the operators of the treating medical team. The orthopedist or

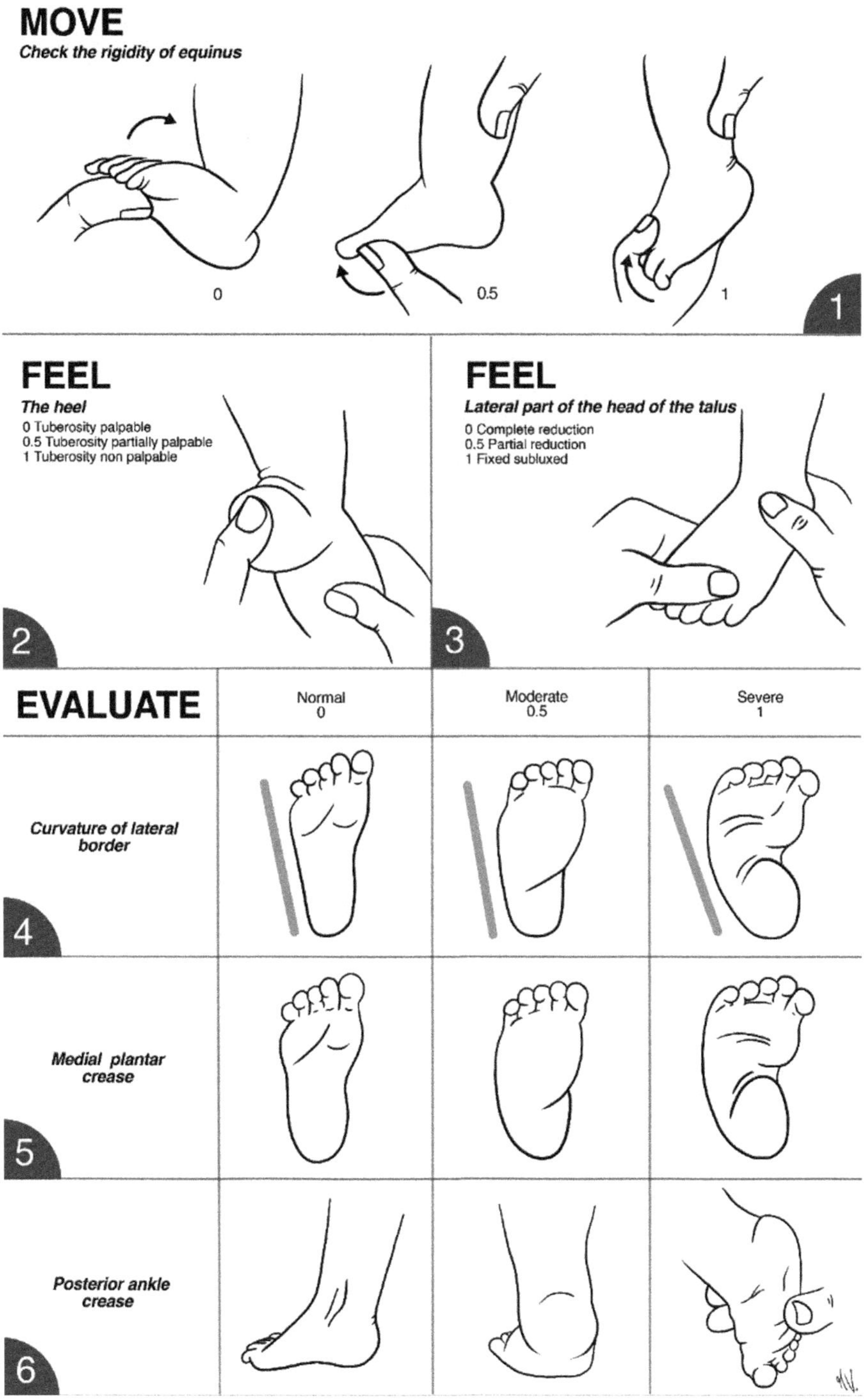

Fig. 6 Pirani Score

operator can be seated or standing and positions himself on the side of the foot to be manipulated; his assistant should not interfere in this positioning and should be positioned on the opposite side to the operator who will perform the manipulations; the assistant's task is fundamental, because he must neutralize the limb to be corrected by firmly holding the knee and only the tip of the toes. The operator then first looks, touches, and then looks for the bony prominences of the tibial (medial) and peroneal (lateral) malleoli as a reference, as well as the prominence of the head of the talus which is located immediately below the lateral or peroneal malleolus just below the anterior ankle interline [36].

The operator supports the tip of the thumb of the hand opposite to the foot that is treating on the lateral prominence of the head of the talus, at the same time that with the index and/or middle fingers of the same hand takes and makes counterpressure on the widest and posterior aspect of the tibial malleolus lodging, controlling and stabilizing completely the talus inside the tibioperoneal mortise.

The opposite hand (hand on the same side as the foot being corrected) grasps with the middle and index fingers the medial and plantar aspect of the midfoot and forefoot up to the scaphoid and with the thumb of the same hand embraces the dorsum covering up to the level of the toes and metatarsals. Next, combine a firm but delicate traction maneuver and then move the foot in supination and abduction seeking to align the midfoot and forefoot with the rearfoot (Fig. 7); this maneuver is held and repeated for a few seconds until the child tolerates it; ideally the child should not cry (Figs. 8, 9, and 10).

A frequent error during this manipulation and application of the Ponseti technique is pronating the forefoot, which worsens the cavus and keeps the calcaneus in varus. Other errors during the application of the technique include pressure on the calcaneocuboid joint instead of the heel head, also known as the Kite error, which blocks calcaneal abduction and prevents correction of heel varus and foot adduction and may even damage the Lisfranc joint (be careful and respect the area of the thumb that presses on the small head of the talus in infants starting treatment); it can also be observed that by seeking abduction of the foot without properly containing the head of the talus in the mortise, a posterior translation of the peroneal malleolus

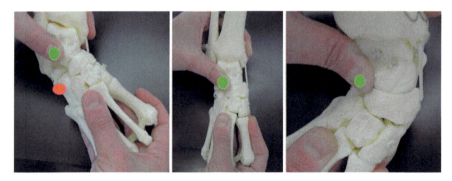

Fig. 7 Kinematic of the subtalar joint. Midfoot and forefoot move around green dot. Recreation of the Ponseti method motion

Fig. 8 Manipulation with
two hands, holding the
forefoot as described in
Fig. 7. Foot position after
casting

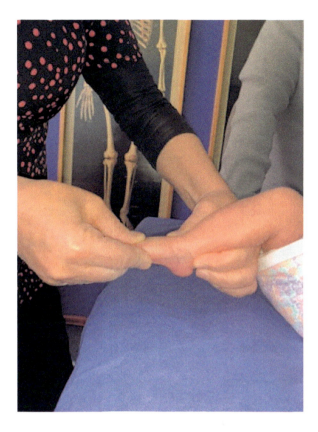

is produced by rotating the talus and opening the syndesmosis, while the calcaneus will fail to correct itself and will remain in varus. On the other hand, if the operator asserts the calcaneus during the manipulation, which tends to correct the foot and does not allow it to follow the movement spontaneously offered by the subtalar joint, he will also be blocking the correction of the varus to valgus instead of improving it.

Finally, you should not apply forces against plantar flexion with fulcrum in the ankle without first having corrected the abduction and varus of the calcaneus; some less experienced operators believe that this could correct the equinus; however, this bad manipulation leads to a rocker deformity by stress and breakage of the Lisfranc joint. This same bad anti-equinus force can compromise the future congruence of the talus in the mortise causing a flat talus by compromise of its ossification nucleus very moldable and sensitive at that stage of the child's life, and that is thus compressed between the anterior zone of the mortise and the calcaneus [29].

On average, after five sessions with progressive serial casts containing the abduction obtained after manipulation with the Ponseti technique, the foot should reach the next stage of treatment consisting of a transcutaneous tenotomy of the tricipital tendon or Achilles tendon (Figs. 11 and 12).

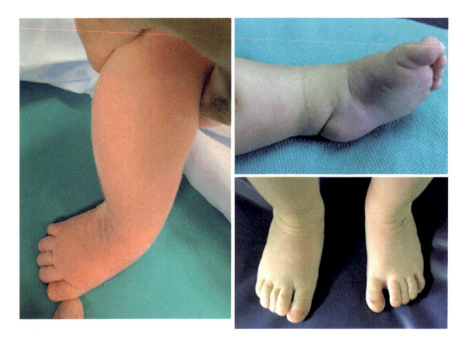

Figs. 9 and 10 Another case before and after casting

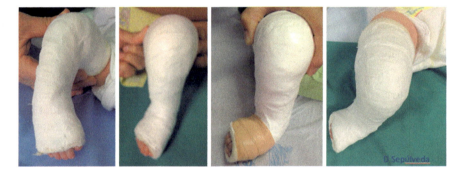

Fig. 11 Correct 15–25 degrees of abduction in each cast. Before tenotomy, abduction external rotation should be 60–70 degrees with valgus heel and 90° of ankle dorsiflexion

12   Description of One-Handed Manipulation

In this one-handed technique, the operator faces the child and rests the index finger of the hand opposite to the foot to be treated on the head of the talus and embraces the foot with the thumb on the plantar and medial aspect at the level of the scaphoid; applying with this one-handed gripper, a slight traction is made while bringing the rest of the foot in supination and abduction, thus achieving the same as with the

Fig. 12 Final cast, after
Achilles tenotomy

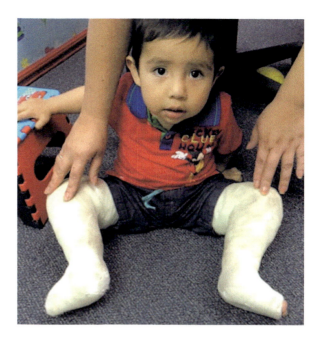

two-handed technique. If the assistant does not exercise good firm control of the leg
during this maneuver, with only one hand, the same effect of external rotation of the
tibioperoneal mortise can be generated instead of stretching the medial and plantar
soft tissues of the foot, with the same risk of producing a posterior displacement of
the peroneal malleolus. It is advisable to be used in very young children who offer
less resistance, and a single hand can do the maneuver as if turning a key in a lock
to achieve the task (Fig. 13).

13 Casting

13.1 Materials

It is necessary to have cotton for the protection of the patient's skin, which should
ideally be hypoallergenic soft and come prepared in bandages of width and length
appropriate to the size of the foot we are going to treat. Traditional plaster bandages
(plaster of Paris) are needed of 5, 7.5, and 10 cm wide according to the size of the
foot, leg, and thigh. Other necessary items are scissors plaster spreaders and forceps
to open and remove casts of appropriate size to the dimensions of the child under
treatment (Fig. 14).

Warm water is needed as well that does not offer burns risk.

Fig. 13 One-handed
manipulation technique

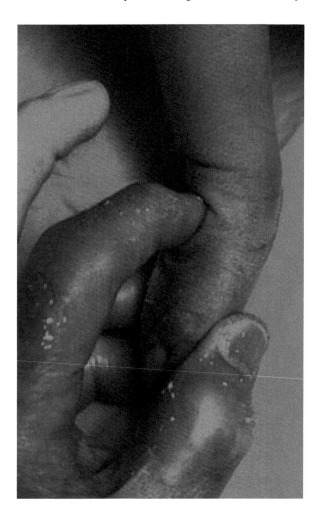

14   Procedure

On a healthy, clean, and dry skin, place the protective material you have at your disposal, which should cover the entire limb leaving it long in excess both in the toes and thigh.

Add a small piece of padding around the heel, malleoli, popliteal fosa and fibular head.

Being the cast operators in the positions indicated in the previous paragraph, ideally with the patient calm, you must begin to roll the cast from the tip of the toes, covering them and moving proximally after giving about three cast revolutions in

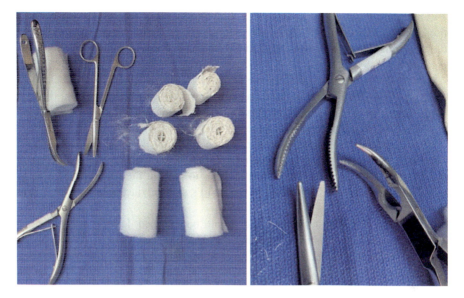

Fig. 14 Casting and cast removal materials

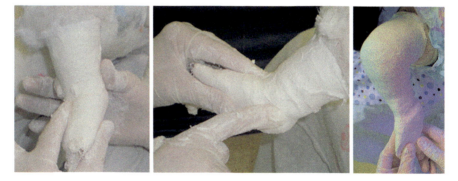

Fig. 15 Cast molding around the talar head, forefoot, and medial malleolus

each section of the limb until the tibial tuberosity, taking care to remove excess air and water with a dragging maneuver in each cast revolution.

The operator applies the cast at this time, neatly demarcating the areas and points of anchorage of the cast to the ankle and foot – forefoot, heel, anterior ankle, and malleoli – maintaining the reduction of the talus and giving the degree of correction corresponding to the degree of correction achieved at the time of this procedure and immobilization (Ponseti 1,2,3, 4,....) (Fig. 15).

The forefoot should be molded until obtaining in a lateral view a triangular section and perfectly flat finish dorsal and plantar; the leg should also be molded to the tibia as straight as possible, avoiding that it adopts a curved shape as a banana by its anterior face (frequent error).

Wait a few minutes maintaining the reduction position achieved until the plaster dries out. Continue casting in the same way above the knee until reaching the root of the thigh. At this stage, do not forget to remove the air at each turn, mold the popliteal fosa, and leave the knee flexed at 90°.

It is customary that some operators, when finishing the boot below the knee, make cuts of 1.5 cm, radial and perpendicular to the circular section of the cast at the level of the proximal tibia. This is in order to prevent the formation of a waist that could compress and/or embed in the child's skin producing compression and even a wound.

At the end of the cast, the toes end should be trimmed, leaving only the third phalanx uncovered, keeping the plantar support a little longer, so that the toes are restricted to perform plantar flexion (Figs. 16 and 17).

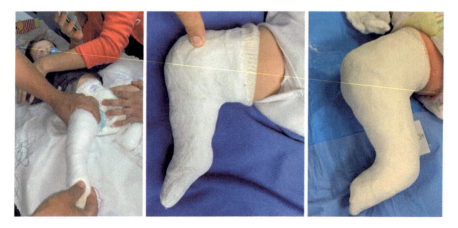

Fig. 16 Photos of casting procedure at different stages

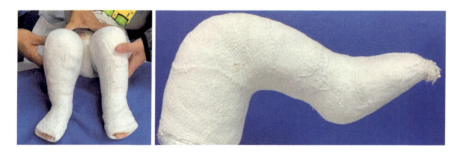

Fig. 17 Ponseti cast in position 3, with details of the plaster finish

15   Percutaneous Tenotomy of the Achilles Tendon

Immediately after corrective casts, it is time to decide on percutaneous or transcutaneous tenotomy; for this purpose, it is required that all components of the deformity are already corrected (achieve a minimum of 60° of foot abduction, complete correction of the cavus and a hindfoot ideally in valgus or neutral) (except for the equinus). A dorsiflexion of less than 20 degrees is an indication for Achilles lenghtening (surgery needed in 95–99% of cases).

Percutaneous tenotomy of the Achilles tendon is a quick and simple procedure, which can be performed under local anesthesia in a procedure box with sterile technique or in the ward under general anesthesia or sedation (this varies between different health centers).

The patient should be positioned so that the operator feels comfortable and safe in the procedure to be performed, which will certainly be different if this procedure is done under local or general anesthesia. With the foot in maximun dorsiflexion, insert a scalpel N°11 or an ophthalmologic straight scalpel 2 cm proximal to its insertion in the calcaneus along the medial border of the Achilles tendon. Then proceed to rotate the blade laterally and transect the tendon completely. A sudden loss of resistance reflecting the complete section of the tendon will be felt and heard, and an increase in dorsiflexion of at least 10 to 20° will be observed (Fig. 18).

After the tenotomy, apply the post-tenotomy cast. This cast is placed in 60°–70° of foot abduction and maximum ankle dorsiflexion (minimum 20°). The cast, always with the knee included, should remain in place for 3–4 weeks.

16   Abductor Orthosis

The use of the abductor orthosis is intended to maintain the correction of the affected foot(s). It has no corrective function. There are several models and designs of brace in the market (Mitchell, Dobbs, handmade, etc.); the important thing is that it complies with certain characteristics included in Dr. Ponseti's design.

The ideal brace is one that is as anatomical as possible, made of soft materials that do not injure the skin, durable, easy to install, as comfortable as possible, ideally with adjustable degrees of abduction, with a resistant bar, hopefully telescopic, and affordable. The length of the bar should be equivalent to the distance of the midpoint between shoulders (adjustable and rigid models are available). The position of the brace boots should ideally have 10° to 15° of dorsiflexion. In the case of unilateral clubfoot, it should be positioned in 60° of abduction in the affected foot and 35–40° in the healthy foot (Figs. 19 and 20).

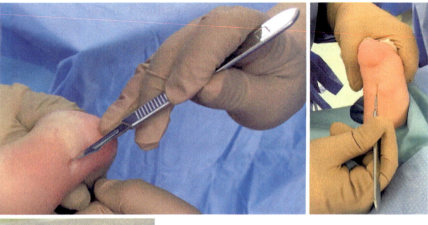

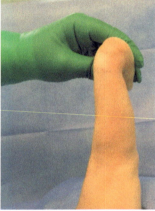

Fig. 18 Photos showing different ways of performing the Achilles tenotomy with n°11 blade. Posterior view post-tenotomy showing heel in valgus and dorsiflexion greater than 20°

Fig. 19 Ponseti bar

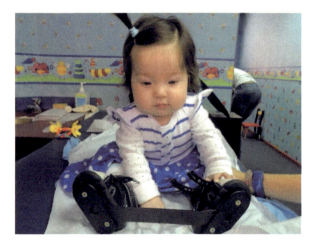

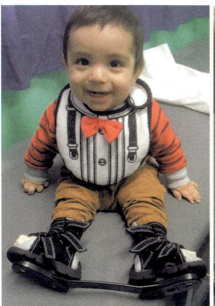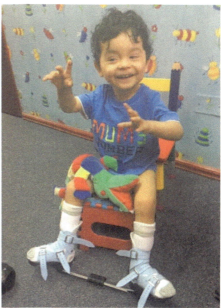

Fig. 20 Ponseti bar examples

The brace use starts immediately after the last cast.

The first 3 to 4 months of splint use should be 23 hours/day, and then the number of hours should be reduced according to various factors (age, motor development, reliability of use, number of casts needed before the tenotomy, etc.), until reaching 12–14 hours/day (at this stage rather during nights and naps) at least until 4 years of age.

17 Recurrences

A recurrence is defined as the appearance of any of the previously corrected club-foot deformities. It is initially characterized by loss of dorsiflexion of the foot due to increased tension of the gastrosoleus complex which leads to plantar flexion of the calcaneus, which progresses to hindfoot varus, forefoot adduction and finally cavus.

The severity of the relapse depends directly on the time of evolution. In some occasions only loss of dorsiflexion will be evident. In others, all the deformities present in clubfoot can reappear.

It should be remembered that the relapses are an evolutionary process, where gastrosoleus complex shortening is present. This shortening worsens with the longitudinal bone growth which in turn ncreases the ankle plantar flexion (Fig. 21).

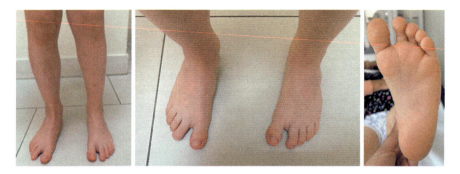

Fig. 21 Late relapse in patient with previously treated clubfoot. Note the subtle adductus in the left foot

It is a mistake to consider that the clubfoot is a "foot deformity," but it is a sign of a disease that affects the entire limb.

The early identification of a relapse will allow simpler and less invasive treatments.

Recurrences can be found from 11 to 48% of corrected feet [37, 38]. In spite of a correct management and an adequate adherence to the brace use, the appearance of recurrences is quite frequent.

The main reasons for recurrence are incomplete correction of the foot (not complying with the principles of the Ponseti method), poor adherence to the brace use, and failures in the strict follow-up of these patients. Poor adherence to bracing is directly correlated with the educational and socioeconomic level of the parents.

As is well known, the Ponseti method is often promoted as a conservative and minimally invasive method, but even the staunchest proponents of the method acknowledge that at least one surgical procedure should be performed: Achilles tenotomy (95%), tibialis anterior tendon transfer (15–40%), and even a second Achilles tenotomy [39].

When evaluating a patient with a recurrence, it is extremely important to assess the correct use of the abduction splint and its adherence. Understanding the family environment and evaluating the various difficulties (economic, logistical, religious, etc.) or any other variable that could hinder the correct use of the orthosis should be identified and discussed with the parents patient.

Correct bracing is a critical step. The orthosis should be the right one, with an adequate fit, and the parents themselves should demonstrate how to install it in order to correct key points of its use.

A foot with recurrence is approached in exactly the same way as an uncorrected foot, that is, it begins with the installation of molding casts and correcting each of the deformities present in the foot, achieving an abduction of 60°. Once achieved, the dorsiflexion of the foot is evaluated. If 15 or more degrees of dorsiflexion are achieved, the bracing protocol is initiated; if this is not achieved, Achilles lengthening tenotomy should be performed. It is recommended to perform the classic technique of single tenotomy in children under 3 years of age, or triple tenotomy in older patients.

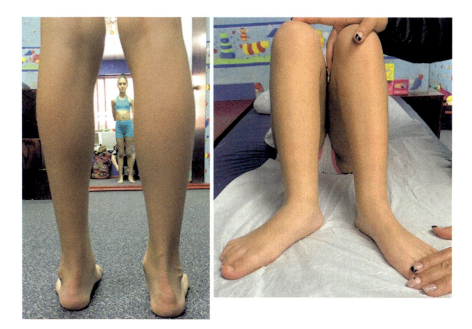

Fig. 22 Corrected feet and long-term follow-up

After the age of 4 years, the splint can be discontinued since recurrences are uncommon (5–10% of cases). If a contracted Achilles tendon is observed achieving 10° of ankle dorsiflexion, 1 more year of brace use is recommended. In addition, daily Achilles stretching exercises are prescribed (Fig. 22).

The indication to perform an anterior tibial tendon transfer is very specific. It should be performed only in children older than 4 years of age who present a dynamic supination. Those patients have to have all other deformities corrected. It should be kept in mind that this procedure is not useful to correct any deformity but only helps to maintain the correction of the deformity together with the splint.

18 Complex Clubfoot

We speak of complex clubfoot when we have an idiopathic clubfoot, and that due to a bad manipulation of the foot and/or incorrectly installed casts generated changes in the structure of the affected foot.

It is described as a foot that characteristically has a midfoot flexion (a midfoot plantar crease is evident) and a shortened hallux in hyperextension. The foot may be swollen and even have trophic changes in the skin if it was recently casted (Fig. 23).

Its management depends on the general condition of the foot. If the foot presents skin lesions, edema, or erythema and is currently being treated with casts, it is

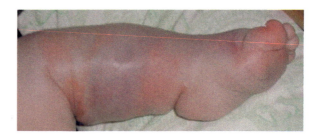

recommended to suspend the installation of casts. It is advisable to wait 3–4 weeks (or even longer if necessary) until the foot is in optimal condition to reinstall a cast.

The technique of manipulation and correction of a complex clubfoot consists of placing one thumb under the head of the first metatarsal and the other under the head of the fifth metatarsal, pushing the forefoot in dorsiflexion, and the index and middle fingers push the heel in the opposite direction, sliding the talus into the ankle and thus avoiding flattening it. To prevent the foot from slipping into the cast (these feet are very short and difficult to manipulate), it is recommended that the cast have 100 to 120° of knee flexion.

Once the plantar crease (secondary to midfoot flexion) is corrected, with the rearfoot in neutral, achieve 30° of forefoot abduction and 0° of ankle dorsiflexion. It is at this point that the Achilles tendon tenotomy is performed. The abduction splint should not go beyond 35° of abduction since the forefoot can commonly present a lateral crease suggestive of hypercorrection of the forefoot. The protocol of splinting in the complex foot has no other differences compared to the idiopathic clubfoot.

19   Syndromic Clubfoot

Syndromic clubfoot, as the name implies, is a clubfoot associated with another pathology, whether neuromuscular, neurological, or genetic syndrome. In recent years, Ponseti's method has been extrapolated to be used in other pathologies such as spinal dysraphism and arthrogryposis, but there is still no consensus on when this method can be applied.

References

1. Dobbs MB, Gurnett CA. Update on clubfoot: etiology and treatment. Clin Orthopaed relat res. 2009;467(5):1146–53. https://doi.org/10.1007/s11999-009-0734-9.
2. Owen RM, Capper B, Lavy C. Clubfoot treatment in 2015: a global perspective. BMJ Glob Health. 2018;3(4):e000852. https://doi.org/10.1136/bmjgh-2018-000852. PMID: 30233830; PMCID: PMC6135438.

3. Gurnett CA, Boehm S, Connolly A, Reimschisel T, Dobbs MB. Impact of congenital talipes equinovarus etiology on treatment outcomes. Dev Med Child Neurol. 2008;50(7):498–502. https://doi.org/10.1111/j.1469-8749.2008.03016.x. PMID: 18611198.

4. Miedzybrodzka Z. Congenital talipes equinovarus (clubfoot): a disorder of the foot but not the hand. J Anat. 2003;202(1):37–42. https://doi.org/10.1046/j.1469-7580.2003.00147.x. PMID: 12587918; PMCID: PMC1571059.

5. Laaveg SJ, Ponseti IV. Long-term results of treatment of congenital club foot. J Bone Joint Surg Am. 1980;62(1):23–31. PMID: 7351412.

6. Duce SL, D'Alessandro M, Du Y, Jagpal B, Gilbert FJ, Crichton L, Barker S, Collinson JM, Miedzybrodzka Z. 3D MRI analysis of the lower legs of treated idiopathic congenital talipes equinovarus (clubfoot). PLoS One. 2013;8(1):e54100. https://doi.org/10.1371/journal.pone.0054100. Epub 2013 Jan 30. PMID: 23382871; PMCID: PMC3559654.

7. Ippolito E, De Maio F, Mancini F, Bellini D, Orefice A. Leg muscle atrophy in idiopathic congenital clubfoot: is it primitive or acquired? J Child Orthop. 2009;3(3):171–8. https://doi.org/10.1007/s11832-009-0179-4. Epub 2009 May 6. PMID: 19418086; PMCID: PMC2686819.

8. Merrill LJ, Gurnett CA, Siegel M, Sonavane S, Dobbs MB. Vascular abnormalities correlate with decreased soft tissue volumes in idiopathic clubfoot. Clin Orthop Relat Res. 2011;469(5):1442–9. https://doi.org/10.1007/s11999-010-1657-1. Epub 2010 Nov 2. PMID: 21042891; PMCID: PMC3069258.

9. Dobbs MB, Gordon JE, Schoenecker PL. Absent posterior tibial artery associated with idiopathic clubfoot. A report of two cases. J Bone Joint Surg Am. 2004;86(3):599–602. https://doi.org/10.2106/00004623-200403000-00022. PMID: 14996890.

10. Dobbs MB, Walton T, Gordon JE, Schoenecker PL, Gurnett CA. Flexor digitorum accessorius longus muscle is associated with familial idiopathic clubfoot. J Pediatr Orthop. 2005;25(3):357–9. https://doi.org/10.1097/01.bpo.0000152908.08422.95. PMID: 15832155.

11. Pavone V, Chisari E, Vescio A, Lucenti L, Sessa G, Testa G. The etiology of idiopathic congenital talipes equinovarus: a systematic review. J Orthop Surg Res. 2018;13(1):206. https://doi.org/10.1186/s13018-018-0913-z. PMID: 30134936; PMCID: PMC6104023.

12. Gurnett CA, Alaee F, Kruse LM, Desruisseau DM, Hecht JT, Wise CA, Bowcock AM, Dobbs MB. Asymmetric lower-limb malformations in individuals with homeobox PITX1 gene mutation. Am J Hum Genet. 2008;83(5):616–22. https://doi.org/10.1016/j.ajhg.2008.10.004. Epub 2008 Oct 23. PMID: 18950742; PMCID: PMC2668044.

13. Alvarado DM, Buchan JG, Frick SL, Herzenberg JE, Dobbs MB, Gurnett CA. Copy number analysis of 413 isolated talipes equinovarus patients suggests role for transcriptional regulators of early limb development. Eur J Hum Genet. 2013;21(4):373–80. https://doi.org/10.1038/ejhg.2012.177. Epub 2012 Aug 15. PMID: 22892537; PMCID: PMC3598331.

14. Zhao XL, Wang YJ, Wu YL, Han WH. Role of COL9A1 genetic polymorphisms in development of congenital talipes equinovarus in a Chinese population. Genet Mol Res. 2016;3:15(4). https://doi.org/10.4238/gmr15048773. PMID: 27819742.

15. Alvarado DM, McCall K, Aferol H, Silva MJ, Garbow JR, Spees WM, Patel T, Siegel M, Dobbs MB, Gurnett CA. Pitx1 haploinsufficiency causes clubfoot in humans and a clubfoot-like phenotype in mice. Hum Mol Genet. 2011;20(20):3943–52. https://doi.org/10.1093/hmg/ddr313. Epub 2011 Jul 20. PMID: 21775501; PMCID: PMC3177645.

16. Ippolito E, De Maio F, Mancini F, Bellini D, Orefice A. Leg muscle atrophy in idiopathic congenital clubfoot: is it primitive or acquired? J Child Orthop. 2009;3(3):171–8. https://doi.org/10.1007/s11832-009-0179-4. Epub 2009 May 6. PMID: 19418086; PMCID: PMC2686819.

17. Herceg MB, Weiner DS, Agamanolis DP, Hawk D. Histologic and histochemical analysis of muscle specimens in idiopathic talipes equinovarus. J Pediatr Orthop. 2006;26(1):91–3. https://doi.org/10.1097/01.bpo.0000188994.90931.e8. PMID: 16439910.

18. Inman VT. The joints of the ankle. Williams & Wilkins; 1976.

19. Ponseti IV. Congenital clubfoot. Fundamentals of treatment. Oxford: Oxford Medical Publications; 1996.
20. Ponseti IV, Smoley EN. Congenital club foot: the results of treatment. Bone Joint Surg. 1963;45-A:261–27.Plaster cast treatment of clubfoot.
21. van Langelaan EJ. A kinematical analysis of the tarsal joints. An X-ray photogrammetric study. Acta Orthop Scand Suppl. 1983;204:1–269. PMID: 6582753.
22. The Ponseti method of manipulation and casting Morcuende 1994. J Pediatr Orthop Part B. 1994;3:161–7.
23. Close JR, Inman VT, Poor PM, Todd FN. The function of the subtalar joint. Clin Orthop Relat Res. 1967;50:159–79. PMID: 6029014.
24. Huson A. Functional anatomy of the foot. In: Jahs JH, editor. Disorders of the foot and ankle, vol. 1. 2nd ed. Philadelphia: Saunders; 1991.
25. Kapandji IA. The Physiology of the joints. 2nd ed. Churchill Livingstone.
26. Ponseti IV. Congenital clubfoot. Fundamentals of treatment. Oxford, New York: Oxford University Press; 1996.
27. Sarrafian SK. Biomechanics of the subtalar joint complex. Clin Orthop Relat Res. 1993;290:17–26. PMID: 8472445.
28. Sarrafian SK. Functional anatomy of the foot and ankle. 2nd ed. J.B.Lippincott Company.
29. Ponseti IV. Common errors in the treatment of congenital clubfoot. Int Orthop. 1997;21(2):137–41. https://doi.org/10.1007/s002640050137. PMID: 9195271; PMCID: PMC3616653.
30. Kite JH. The clubfoot. New York London: Grune & Stratton; 1964.
31. Kite JH. Nonoperative treatment of congenital clubfoot. Clin Orthop. 1972;
32. Manter JT. Movements of the Subtalar and transverse Tarsal Joints. The Anatomical Record. 1941;80(4)
33. Ponseti IV, Campos J. The classic: observations on pathogenesis and treatment of congenital clubfoot. 1972. Clin Orthop Relat Res. 2009;467(5):1124–32. https://doi.org/10.1007/s11999-009-0721-1. Epub 2009 Feb 14. PMID: 19219518; PMCID: PMC2664437.
34. Miller NH, Carry PM, Mark BJ, Engelman GH, Georgopoulos G, Graham S, Dobbs MB. Does strict adherence to the ponseti method improve isolated clubfoot treatment outcomes? a two-institution review. Clin Orthop Relat Res. 2016;474(1):237–43. https://doi.org/10.1007/s11999-015-4559-4. Epub 2015 Sep 22. PMID: 26394639; PMCID: PMC4686485.
35. Arana Hernández EI, Cuevas De Alba C. Método de Ponseti en el tratamiento del pie equino varo: técnica de enyesado y tenotomía percutánea del tendón de Aquiles. Orthotips. 2015;11(4)
36. Morcuende JA, Abbasi D, Dolan LA, Ponseti IV. Results of an accelerated Ponseti protocol for clubfoot. J Pediatr Orthop. 2005;25(5):623–6. https://doi.org/10.1097/01.bpo.0000162015.44865.5e. PMID: 16199943.
37. Ponseti IV. Common errors in the treatment of congenital clubfoot. Int Orthop. 1997;21(2):137–41. https://doi.org/10.1007/s002640050137. PMID: 9195271; PMCID: PMC3616653.
38. Morcuende JA, Dolan LA, Dietz FR, Ponseti IV. Radical reduction in the rate of extensive corrective surgery for clubfoot using the ponseti method. Pediatrics. 2004;113:376. https://doi.org/10.1542/peds.113.2.376.
39. Eidelman M, Kotlarsky P, Herzenberg JE. Treatment of relapsed, residual and neglected clubfoot: adjunctive surgery. J Child Orthop. 2019;13(3):293–303. https://doi.org/10.1302/1863-2548.13.190079.

Pediatric Metatarsus Adductus and Cavovarus Foot

Maryse Bouchard

1 Metatarsus Adductus

1.1 Introduction

Metatarsus adductus is the most common congenital foot deformity [1]. It consists of medial angulation of the forefoot relative to the hindfoot. The longitudinal medial arch is present, and the hindfoot alignment is neutral to valgus [1] (Fig. 1). The true incidence remains unknown with reports from 0.1% to 12% [2–4]. Associations with twin births [3] and hip dysplasia [5] have been reported, although the latter has been refuted in more recent studies [6, 7].

1.2 Etiology

The etiology of metatarsus adductus is unknown. Given the deformity often resolves spontaneously, intra-uterine positioning is suspected as a possible cause [3, 8, 9]. Other theories include anomalous morphology of the medial cuneiform [10] and muscle imbalance of the tibialis anterior, tibialis posterior, or abductor hallucis [5, 11–13].

M. Bouchard (✉)
The Hospital for Sick Children, Division of Orthopaedic Surgery, University of Toronto, Toronto, ON, Canada
e-mail: Maryse.bouchard@sickkids.ca

© The Author(s), under exclusive license to Springer Nature Switzerland AG 2022
E. Wagner Hitschfeld, P. Wagner Hitschfeld (eds.), *Foot and Ankle Disorders*,
https://doi.org/10.1007/978-3-030-95738-4_8

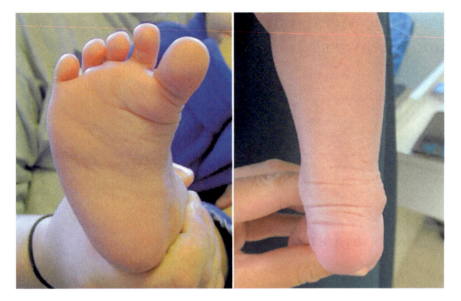

Fig. 1 Plantar and posterior photographs of an infant with right metatarsus adductus deformity. The foot has a curved convex lateral border and neutral hindfoot alignment. (From the private collection of Maryse Bouchard, MD)

1.3 Anatomy

The foot with metatarsus adductus presents with a medially deviated forefoot relative to the hindfoot creating a convex curved lateral border. There is full ankle and subtalar motion, and hindfoot is in neutral to slight valgus [14].

On anteroposterior (AP) radiographs of the foot, there is often a trapezoidal shape to the medial cuneiform [15]. Instead of a square bone with its distal and proximal articular surfaces being parallel to one another, the distal articular surface is angulated medially resulting in a varus alignment of the first metatarsal (Fig. 2) [10]. There may also be milder adductus through the lesser metatarsals. The hindfoot alignment is normal on AP and lateral foot radiographs [14].

1.4 Diagnosis

Metatarsus adductus is a clinical diagnosis based on the shape of the foot. Radiographs are not necessary for diagnosis. Radiographs are indicated in the case of significant residual deformity and pain in the older child or adolescent and if surgical intervention is being considered [1].

The majority of metatarsus adductus deformities in children resolved spontaneously by age 3–4 years [8, 16]. In a prospective natural history study by Rushforth

Fig. 2 AP radiograph of an older child's foot with metatarsus adductus. Note the medially deviated distal articular surface (red line) contributing to the adducted alignment of the first metatarsal. Normally, the distal and proximal articular surfaces are parallel to one another (yellow dashed and solid lines, respectively). (From the private collection of Maryse Bouchard, MD)

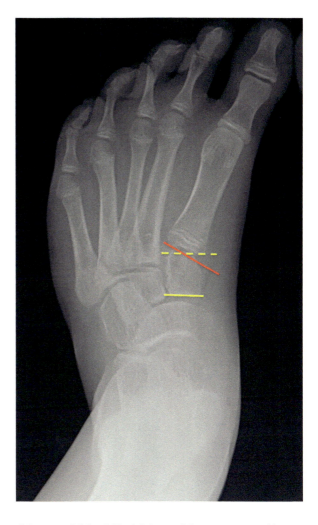

et al. with mean follow-up of 7 years, 86% of 83 children with metatarsus adductus (130 feet) received no treatment and developed normal foot shapes. Ten percent had persistent moderate deformities but were asymptomatic, and 4% of feet were deformed and stiff [8]. In a cohort of 335 children with flexible metatarsus adductus studied by Ponseti and Becker, 88% of feet improved by age 4 years, with only 12% requiring corrective casting. No poor long-term results or functional disabilities in patients with mild or moderate residual deformity have been reported [8, 16, 17].

There are two commonly used classifications for metatarsus adductus [18–20]. One classification is based on severity and is determined by the heel bisector when examining the foot's plantar surface anatomy (Fig. 3) [20]. The other is based on flexibility of the foot deformity [18]. Metatarsus adductus is defined as flexible if the forefoot can be passively abducted beyond the midline heel bisector rendering the lateral border concave (Fig. 4) [14]. A partly flexible foot can be abducted only

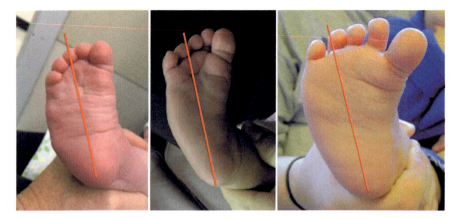

Fig. 3 The heel bisector method. Severity is determined by how medial a line bisecting the heel ends in the toes distally. The closer the line ends to the fifth ray, the more severe the deformity. Red lines denote the heel bisector. (From the private collection of Maryse Bouchard, MD)

Fig. 4 Clinical photos demonstrating a foot with flexible metatarsus adductus. Using the calcaneal cuboid joint as the fulcrum, the foot is abducted. Note the curved lateral border is now corrected denoting a flexible foot (yellow lines). (From the private collection of Maryse Bouchard, MD)

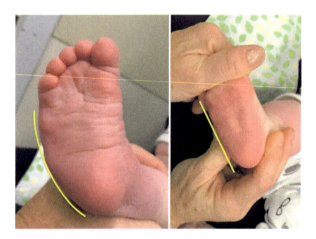

to the midline, with the lateral border only correcting to straight. An inflexible, or rigid, foot is one that cannot be abducted to the midline, and the lateral border remains convex [14].

1.5   Non-operative Management

Given the high rate of spontaneous resolution of metatarsus adductus [15–17, 21], observation is recommended for children under the age of 1 year, especially when the deformity is flexible [22]. Although passive stretching exercises are commonly performed, there is no evidence of their efficacy [4, 16]. In a study of 94 newborns with metatarsus adductus who were randomized to a parental stretching program or observation, there was no significant difference in resolution or rate of correction [23].

Other non-operative modalities for management for metatarsus adductus include orthoses, corrective shoes, and corrective casts. The efficacy of shoes and orthoses in correcting metatarsus adductus has never been clearly demonstrated, and some authors believe excessive manipulation into valgus can create harm to the foot causing an iatrogenic skewfoot deformity [4, 16, 24]. A recent systematic review demonstrated no evidence for treatment of flexible metatarsus adductus and only limited evidence for partly flexible feet with no supportive high-level studies [22].

Multiple studies have shown efficacy of manipulation and serial casting for the correction of partly flexible and rigid deformities and recommend initiation under the age of 1 year [16, 18, 24, 25]. No upper age limit has been reported, and there is no clear indication to initiate treatment before the age of 6 months [1]. The technique for manipulation and casting is important to avoid excessive valgus of the hindfoot. Ponseti and Becker originally describe a technique with long-leg casts where the fulcrum of the manipulation is on the lateral border of the foot at the cuboid [16]. An abduction moment is applied at the medial aspect of first metatarsal head while maintaining the hindfoot in neutral [16]. Orthoses and shoes are often used after correction to decrease the risk of recurrence. Recurrence ranges between 8% and 37% [2, 18, 26].

Katz et al. published on the use of short-leg casts for correction of partly flexible and rigid deformities and reported similar correction and recurrence rates to studies using long-leg casts [25]. Herzenberg et al. prospectively randomized 27 infants with residual metatarsus adductus deformity aged 3–9 months to treatment with either serial plaster casts or a triplanar-hinged orthoses. There was no difference in outcomes or rate of correction; however, parental compliance was critical for success with the orthosis [27].

1.6   Surgical Management

Although surgery is rarely indicated for metatarsus adductus in children, many operative procedures have been recommended for resistant deformities [1].

Described soft tissue procedures include release of the abductor hallucis and medial midfoot capsulotomies [12, 13]. When capsulotomies were combined with intermetatarsal ligament releases, there was a 41% long-term complication rate with skin sloughing, avascular necrosis of the middle and lateral cuneiforms, prominence of the first metatarsal-tarsal joint, and early degenerative changes [28]. Hallux valgus has been reported after abductor hallucis release [12]. For children between 1 and 3 years old with rigid deformities rendering who recur after casting and bracing and have persistent problems with shoe wear and skin breakdown, this author has performed mini-open distal abductor hallucis recessions followed by use of straight last shoes for 6 months. Anecdotally, this small improvement in flexibility of the first ray resolved symptoms, and no hallux valgus has occurred in short- to medium-term follow-up.

If an older child experiences ongoing pain and disability from residual metatarsus adductus deformity, surgery may be indicated after failure of non-operative interventions such as insoles and shoe modification. On standing radiographs of the foot, skewfoot deformity should be ruled out. Corrective osteotomies are ideally performed at the apex of deformity. In metatarsus adductus, the site is typically the misshapen trapezoidal medial cuneiform [14]. This author's preferred technique is therefore a medial opening wedge osteotomy of this bone. In more severe or rigid deformities, additional closing wedge osteotomy of the cuboid or base of second, third, or fourth metatarsals may be required [29–32] (Fig. 5). It is important to recognize the high risk of resulting shortening due to osteotomies of the first

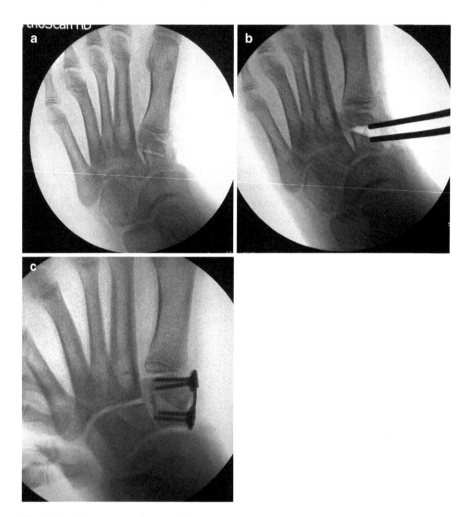

Fig. 5 Medial opening wedge medial cuneiform osteotomy for correction of residual metatarsus adductus in the older child. (**a**) Direction of the osteotomy aiming to wards the second tarsometatarsal joint. (**b**) Distraction of the osteotomy to achieve correction of the adducted first ray. (**c**) Placement of tricortical allograft. Internal fixation can be added if there is insufficient press-fit of the graft. (From the private collection of Maryse Bouchard, MD)

metatarsal. Shortening from nonunion or physeal injury is reported in 5–30% of patients [33]. Recently, good results have been reported with percutaneous lesser metatarsal osteotomies and first tarsometatarsal joint capsule release in children with a mean age of 5.7 years and mean follow-up of 55 months [34].

2   Cavovarus Foot

2.1   Introduction

The cavovarus foot is challenging to treat. The concurrent deformities in the fore, mid-, and hindfoot are typically coupled with muscle imbalance and joint contractures. Successful correction relies on determining the underlying diagnosis and the application of deformity-based principles to select the appropriate surgical procedures.

2.2   Etiology

Cavovarus foot deformity is rare in children under 3 years. Incidence in adults is 10–20% [35–38]. In up to two-thirds of patients, the underlying etiology is secondary to a spinal cord or neuromuscular disorder, with Charcot-Marie-Tooth (CMT) disease, a hereditary sensorimotor neuropathy (HSMN), being one of the most common causes [36, 37, 39]. CMT rarely presents in children under age 10 years and is causative in approximately half of adults with a neuromuscular cavovarus foot [37, 40]. Other common pathologies include tethered cord, myelodysplasia, and post-traumatic injuries [37, 39, 41]. Poor prognosis is associated with early age of onset. The subtle, flexible cavovarus foot may be a normal variant, but a neuromuscular etiology in all cavovarus feet must be considered and ruled out [36]. Table 1 includes a comprehensive list of differential diagnoses.

Establishing the etiology is important to understand the natural history of the deformity and risk of recurrence. Some conditions are static (cerebral palsy (CP), post-traumatic injury), while others are progressive (HSMN and tethered cord) [37, 39, 42]. However, typically bilateral, cavovarus deformities can be unilateral in hemiplegic CP, poliomyelitis, peripheral nerve lesions or tumors, or after compartment syndrome or trauma [37, 39, 41, 42].

2.3   Anatomy

Muscle imbalance in the cavovarus foot causes deformities of the fore-, mid-, and hindfoot and if left untreated can progress to rigid deformities.

Table 1 Differential diagnosis for cavovarus foot deformity

Brain	Cerebral palsy
	Friedrich's ataxia
	Tumor
	Spinocerebellar degeneration
Spine	Tumor
	Spinal dysraphism (tethered cord, myelomeningocele, diastematomyelia)
	Spinal muscular atrophy
	Poliomyelitis
Peripheral nervous system	Hereditary sensorimotor neuropathy (Charcot-Marie-Tooth)
	Traumatic or neoplastic nerve lesions
Muscle and tendon	Leg compartment syndrome
	Residual clubfoot deformity
	Muscular dystrophy
Bone	Tarsal coalition
	Post-traumatic (fracture malunion)

Weakness of the foot intrinsics leads to shortening of the plantar fascia and the short flexors of the toes, thereby increasing the height of the medial arch [39]. Plantarflexion of the first ray, also described as pronation of the forefoot, is further accentuated by the relative over-pull of peroneus longus versus the tibialis anterior [14]. Flexibility of the plantarflexed first ray is assessed manually by elevating the first metatarsal head. If the arch can be completely flattened, the forefoot pronation is flexible, and the hindfoot will remain aligned in valgus [43].

In stance, the weight through a normal-shaped foot is evenly distributed as a tripod between the first and fifth metatarsal heads and the heel. When there is excessive plantarflexion of the first ray, the foot rolls onto the lateral border and the heel is forced into varus alignment to keep all three points on the ground [44]. The flexibility of the hindfoot varus is assessed with the Coleman block test [45]. This author performs a modified version of the Coleman block test as described by Mosca where only the fourth and fifth metatarsal heads are placed on a 2.5 cm block [14]. With the first ray in its plantarflexed position, the heel will correct to its normal valgus if the hindfoot deformity is flexible [39, 44, 46] (Fig. 6). If the hindfoot varus is rigid, the heel remains in varus or only partially corrects to neutral. Relative weakness of tibialis anterior versus the tibialis posterior and peroneus longus further contributes to hindfoot varus [44].

Dynamic supination occurs when there is over-pull of tibialis anterior compared to peroneus brevis. This can be appreciated in gait or with active dorsiflexion of the ankle on seated exam [44, 47]. A fixed supination in stance phase and at rest occurs with a rigid hindfoot varus deformity or when there is excessive over-pull of tibialis posterior over the peroneals [47]. When the hindfoot is in varus, the Achilles tendon exacerbates the supination deformity acting as a secondary inverter [37, 44].

Fig. 6 Photograph demonstrating the modified Coleman block test showing correction of hindfoot varus to valgus. This is therefore a flexible hindfoot deformity. (From the private collection of Maryse Bouchard, MD)

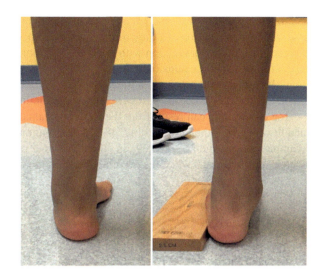

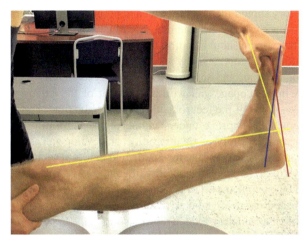

Fig. 7 When examining for equinus, be sure to evaluate the hindfoot relative to the tibia. If severe cavus is present, this can confuse the examiner as it gives the appearance of equinus. The horizontal yellow line represents the axis of the tibia. The vertical yellow line shows the inclination of the hindfoot and the blue the inclination of the forefoot. The red line represents the plantar aspect of the foot. Relative to the tibial axis, if referencing the red line, it would suggest significant lack of dorsiflexion at the ankle. Manually covering the forefoot can help visualize the true hindfoot position. In this patient, the hindfoot is dorsiflexed (yellow lines), and therefore correction of the cavus and not Achilles lengthening is required. (From the private collection of Maryse Bouchard, MD)

Assessment for equinus contracture can be challenging in feet with severe cavus as the midfoot deformity gives the appearance that the ankle cannot dorsiflex above neutral [46]. A more accurate examination of ankle equinus can be achieved by manually covering forefoot to better visualize only the hindfoot position versus the tibial axis (Fig. 7). The Silfverskiold test must also be performed to determine if the contracture is due to the entire triceps surae complex or the gastrocnemius alone, as this will inform selection of the appropriate surgical procedure [47]. The Silfverskiold test assesses ankle dorsiflexion with the knee in flexion relaxing the gastrocnemius and with the knee in extension tensioning the gastrocnemius as it crosses the knee joint. If equinus is present when the knee is in extension, but improves or resolves when the knee is flexed, the gastrocnemius is predominantly shortened [14].

Toe deformities can result from the relative weakness of the long toe extensors and flexors versus the intrinsics [47, 48]. Most common are toe flexion contractures (hammer toes) and claw toes [39, 46, 48]. A hammer toe is flexible if it straightens with a "push-up test," when the examiner elevates the metatarsal head manually.

2.4   Diagnosis

A thorough history and physical examination, and elucidation of the underlying etiology, are imperative to inform optimal management of the cavovarus foot.

Focused history should include the onset and progression of deformity, pain, disability, problems with shoe wear, and presence of neurologic symptoms such paresthesias [43]. The surgeon should confirm the family history, birth and developmental history, past surgical history, and any antecedent trauma [39].

Foot position in stance and during gait is necessary to identify static and dynamic deformities. A high-steppage gait with recruitment of toe extensors is typical in CMT [39]. Assessment of the feet for calluses and evaluation of the patient's shoes for wear patterns will improve understanding of the deformity [36]. With longstanding cavovarus deformity, ankle instability can develop and should be tested for [43]. Passive range of motion of the for-, mid-, and hindfoot should be performed as described above to determine the flexibility of identified deformities. The spine and hips must also be examined [44].

A complete neurological exam is required including manual strength testing, sensory examination, and deep tendon reflex testing of the upper and lower extremities [29, 37, 47]. Assessment of muscle bulk is important as conditions such as CMT can present with muscle wasting of the calves and hand intrinsics [43].

Weight-bearing AP and lateral radiographs of the foot and ankle are essential to assess the cavovarus deformity [39, 42, 44]. Hindfoot alignment is best evaluated on a Saltzman view [43].

There are many angles described to assess foot deformities. This author prefers measures that identify the location of the deformity as they inform the surgical plan. Assessment of midfoot deformity on the AP and lateral views is determined by the intersection of the longitudinal axes of the first metatarsal and talus. The angle between these axes on both views is normally 0–5 degrees [36, 39] (Fig. 8a and b). The location of the intersection, as opposed to the magnitude of angle, identifies the site or apex of deformity. In a cavovarus foot, this is typically in the medial cuneiform [14]. When there is hindfoot varus, the intersection on the AP view may occur in the head of the talus [14]. On the lateral, calcaneal pitch (normal 20–30 degrees) may be decreased if equinus is present or increased if there is calcaneocavus [36, 39] (Fig. 8b). On the Saltzman view, the axis of the calcaneus to the tibia is normally in slight valgus but may be in varus in a cavovarus foot [35, 47] (Fig. 8c).

When a clinical Coleman block test is equivocal, Saltzman x-rays taken with the foot on and off the Coleman block are helpful to confirm if hindfoot alignment has improved [14, 45] (Fig. 8c).

In especially rigid deformities, tarsal coalitions and degenerative changes should be ruled out on radiographs. If suspected, or in cases of severe deformity, a CT scan can be helpful [41, 44]. Magnetic resonance imaging (MRI) of the ankle or foot is rarely indicated [4].

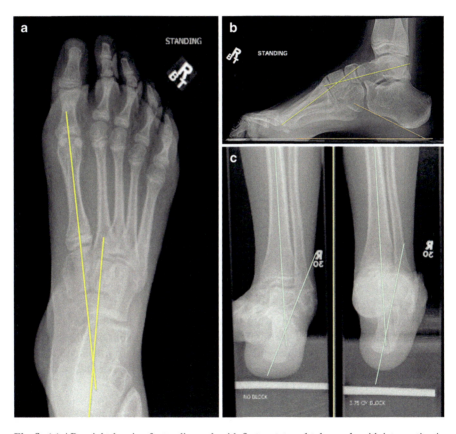

Fig. 8 (**a**) AP weight-bearing foot radiograph with first metatarsal-talar angle with intersection in the talar head demonstrating the site of hindfoot varus deformity (yellow lines). (**b**) Lateral weight-bearing foot radiograph with first metatarsal-talar angle with intersection in the medial cuneiform demonstrating the site of cavus deformity (yellow lines). The lateral calcaneal pitch is also demonstrated and in normal range (orange lines). (**c**) Saltzman view radiographs on and off a Coleman block. Note improvement of the calcaneal-tibial alignment (green lines) and foot position when positioned on the Coleman block. This confirms improvement of hindfoot varus and flexibility of the hindfoot deformity. (From the private collection of Maryse Bouchard, MD)

Acetabular dysplasia can occur in patients with CMT. A screening AP pelvis radiograph is recommended [36, 39]. Additional diagnostic investigations may include electromyography, nerve conduction studies, radiographs of the spine, and/or MRI of the brain, spine, or affected extremity [36, 39, 41]. Referral to neurology is also recommended.

2.5   Non-operative Management

For progressive cavovarus foot conditions, there is a very limited role for non-operative intervention. Physical therapy [36], orthotics [35–37], bracing, casting [48, 49], and botulinum toxin [50] have all been described without success at correcting or preventing worsening of the cavovarus deformity [39].

D'Astorg et al. published a series of 23 children (35 feet) with cavovarus feet treated with serial casting and turnbuckle bracing [49]. Bracing and casting achieved better outcomes than bracing alone. After 4.5 years, 10 feet required surgery. No patient required triple arthrodesis. This is the only study to date supportive of non-operative intervention [49].

Accommodative orthotics or gait aids may have a role in the mild non-progressive deformity [36, 37].

2.6   Surgical Management

In almost all cavovarus feet, surgical correction is recommended. Goals of surgery are to achieve a plantigrade, supple foot to alleviate pain, improve function, and prevent development of rigid deformities and degenerative changes [46]. In the child or adolescent, with rare exception, procedures should be joint and physeal sparing [35, 37, 38, 43, 46].

Surgical correction may involve a combination of soft tissue releases, tendon transfers, and osteotomies. Determining the necessary procedures will depend on the flexibility of the deformities and their location. When deformities are flexible, soft tissue procedures are typically sufficient, while rigid deformities require the addition of bony procedures [36, 39, 42].

The order in which procedures are performed is important to ensure optimal deformity correction. Performing soft tissue before bony procedures helps avoid unnecessary bony overcorrection [14]. Tendon transfers should be secured after deformity correction is achieved to avoid overly taught or lax tension [14, 37, 39, 51]. Osteotomies should be done at the site of deformity or as close to it as possible to avoid creating secondary deformities [14, 37, 51].

Consider staging procedures in severe rigid feet. Performing simultaneous soft tissues and osteotomies may not allow for full and immediate deformity correction due the tight plantarmedial skin [14, 43]. By staging the plantarmedial soft tissue releases in a first surgery then allowing the patient to walk in a short-leg cast allows for gradual stretching of the skin and soft tissues. When the second surgery for the required osteotomies and tendon transfers is performed 2–3 weeks later, there is now more flexibility in the foot and improved ability to obtain full correction [14, 43].

There are many procedures described in the literature and in textbooks. Determining the optimal treatment for individual cavovarus feet can be challenging. Each foot is different in etiology, flexibility, severity, and muscle imbalance and requires careful assessment. A one-size-fits-all approach is not adequate. This author determines the operative plan based on five questions to assess and qualify the deformities present in the cavovarus foot [43].

2.6.1 Is the Forefoot Pronation Flexible or Rigid?

First, the surgeon must assess if there is adduction of the first ray in addition to plantar flexion. Secondly, through manual testing, they must determine if the pronation is flexible or rigid.

In flexible deformities, soft tissue releases are sufficient. As described above, the weakened plantar intrinsic muscles and plantar fascia shorten elevating the arch. The abductor hallucis is typically spared in CMT and therefore can cause adduction of the first ray. If only plantarflexion is present, the plantar fascia is released. If there is adduction and plantarflexion, through a medial incision, the plantar fascia and three bellies of the abductor hallucis are released from the calcaneus, decompressing the tarsal tunnel [14, 35]. Care must be taken not to injure the lateral and medial plantar nerves [35].

To augment a relatively weak peroneus brevis and to minimize the plantarflexion moment of the peroneus longus on the first ray, the longus can be transferred to the brevis. This can be performed through a lateral approach at the midfoot or posterolaterally if performing a concurrent calcaneal osteotomy. A side-to-side tenodesis or Pulvertaft weave may be used to dock the longus tendon to the brevis [42, 43, 46].

If the forefoot pronation is rigid, a dorsiflexion osteotomy through the apex of the deformity is required in addition to the above soft tissue releases [14]. A variety of midfoot osteotomies, in isolation or in combination, have been described to correct cavus including first and lesser metatarsal osteotomies, cuboid closing wedges, and medial cuneiform dorsiflexion opening and closing wedges [52].

In most cavovarus feet, the apex of the midfoot deformity as described above is in the medial cuneiform [36, 41]. This author therefore performs a plantarmedial-based opening wedge osteotomy of the medial cuneiform to correct both the plantarflexion and adduction of the first ray [14, 43]. A tricortical triangular piece of allograft is used [14, 43], but autograft is an equal alternative [41]. As this osteotomy is under tension, fixation of the graft or bone is rarely required [14]. If unstable, a Steinman pin is usually sufficient [52].

2.6.2   Is the Hindfoot Varus Flexible or Rigid?

Flexibility of the hindfoot varus is assessed clinically and/or radiographically by the Coleman block test. If the hindfoot varus corrects to valgus, it is considered flexible and is treated by correcting the forefoot pronation that is driving the deformity as described above [14, 43].

If the hindfoot does not correct into valgus on the Coleman block, additional soft tissue releases and a lateralizing posterior calcaneal displacement osteotomy are needed [14, 43, 52]. The tibialis posterior requires lengthening or a recession [53], and release of the talonavicular joint capsule, sparing the lateral aspect, may be needed in particularly rigid feet [14, 47]. For the lateral displacement posterior calcaneal osteotomy, this author prefers a percutaneous minimally invasive technique using a cooled Shannon burr. There is little published on results in children [54]; however, the adult literature strongly supports the technique with equivalent deformity correction, less postoperative pain, swelling and wound issues, and no increased infection or neurovascular injury rates [55, 56] (Fig. 9). Alternatively, this author uses a posterolateral open approach, taking care to preserve the sural nerve and peroneal tendons [43]. To prevent unwanted lengthening or shortening of the calcaneus, the osteotomy is made in the plane of the metatarsal heads, as opposed to perpendicular to the lateral wall of the calcaneus [14].

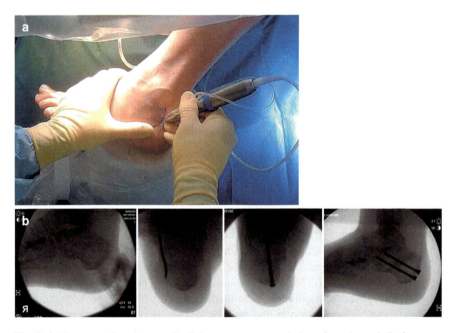

Fig. 9 (**a**) Intraoperative photograph of the percutaneous technique for calcaneal displacement osteotomy with a cooled Shannon burr. (**b**) Intraoperative radiographs demonstrating the percutaneous osteotomy of the posterior calcaneus, using a Williger to translate and final screw fixation. (From the private collection of Maryse Bouchard, MD)

Other osteotomies of the calcaneus have been described. The Dwyer osteotomy is a biplanar calcaneal osteotomy that adds a lateral closing wedge to the slide, and Malerba described a concurrent translational and rotational "Z" cut osteotomy [35, 41, 46, 47]. The Z osteotomy provides the most powerful correction but also has the highest complication rate [57].

2.6.3 Is There Dynamic or Fixed Supination of the Foot?

When there is dynamic supination resulting from relative overpower of tibialis anterior to peroneus brevis, a tendon transfer should be performed though this is not routinely needed in patients with CMT.

To correct dynamic supination, the tibialis anterior should be transferred in full or partially to the dorsolateral foot [14]. Selecting the appropriate transfer technique depends on the degree of eversion weakness and severity of deformity. This author prefers a split transfer to the lateral cuneiform when there is ≥4 out of 5 peroneal strength on manual testing [43]. If there is weak or no peroneal function (<4 out of 5), a full transfer can be performed with docking as far lateral as the cuboid if necessary for optimal muscle balance [43].

If the supination is fixed, and the eversion and dorsiflexion function are weak or absent, consider full or partial tibialis posterior tendon transfer through the interosseous membrane to the lateral cuneiform [39, 42, 48]. Consider transfer to the cuboid if there is no eversion function. It is important to include plantar fascia, abductor hallucis, and talonavicular joint capsule releases as needed, and to ensure correction of the hindfoot varus is also achieved, to avoid recurrence or persistence of deformity.

Dreher et al. report improved active balanced dorsiflexion in swing phase and maintained active plantarflexion with total split posterior tibialis tendon transfers in adults with CMT [42]. There is no literature supporting this technique routinely in children, and there is scant evidence on the minimum age to perform a tibialis posterior transfer. Turner and Cooper describe a cohort of 33 patients with equinovarus from multiple etiologies in children aged 1–25 years [58]. Overcorrection occurred predominantly in children with spastic CP and spina bifida. Age at the time of surgery was not reported. Aydin et al. report on 24 patients with post-traumatic foot drop (75%) and myelodysplasia (25%) aged 7–18 years [59]. No patient developed a flatfoot after a mean of 32 months follow-up. To avoid overcorrection, this author reserves full transfers of the tibialis posterior to children aged 8 years and older and selects split transfers when there is significant risk of muscle imbalance such as in spastic or myelodysplastic conditions [43].

2.6.4 Is There Concurrent Equinus?

In a cavovarus foot without equinus, Achilles lengthening is contraindicated as the tendon acts as the counterforce in the correction of the cavus after the plantarmedial tissues are released from the calcaneus [48]. If there is equinus based on clinical and radiographic assessment, the appropriate lengthening should be performed. If the gastrocnemius alone is tight, a recession of this muscle (Strayer) is done [35]. If there is <10 degrees of equinus with the knee extended, this author performs a recession of the gastrocnemius and soleus (Vulpius), or a percutaneous or mini-open tendoachilles release, such as the double-cut lengthening described by Mosca [14, 43]. If equinus is ≥10 degrees with the knee extended and there is little risk of overlengthening, an open z-lengthening of the tendon is preferred [43].

2.6.5 Are There Toe Deformities and Are They Flexible or Rigid?

If hammer toes are present and remain flexible as per the push-up test, percutaneous long toe flexor tenotomy performed distally, with temporary pinning as needed, is indicated [42, 43]. For a flexible first claw toe, most surgeons perform a modified Jones procedure (first interphalangeal joint fusion with EHL transfer to dorsal metatarsal neck) with good results [36, 37, 39, 46]. For flexible lesser claw toes, a variety of tendon transfers have been described including the Girdlestone-Taylor (flexor digitorum longus [FDL] to the extensor hood [36, 39] and extensor digitorum longus [EDL] to the neck of the metatarsals [39, 46, 48]) but with less predictable outcomes. Alternatively, a Hibbs transfer of the EDL to the cuboid or the peroneus tertius can be performed with percutaneous tenotomy of the distal FDL tendons [14]. If the toe deformities are rigid and symptomatic, an arthrodesis [39] or resection arthroplasty of the affected joints is necessary.

2.7   Intraarticular and Tibial Deformity

The surgeon must also assess for concurrent coronal and/or rotational deformity of the distal tibia. A supramalleolar osteotomy may be required if present [42, 44]. Similarly, the chronic lateral overloading of the foot and ankle from the rigid hindfoot varus alignment may lead to lateral ankle instability [44, 47]. If present on examination and the ankle joint is healthy, a lateral ligament repair should be considered especially if laxity persists after deformity correction [43]. The modified Brostrom, Brostrom-Gould, and repairs with allo- and autograft augment have been described for this indication [35, 41, 44]. Lateral ankle instability with concurrent degenerative ankle joint changes typically does not occur until adulthood and often requires arthrodesis or arthroplasty.

2.8   Gradual Deformity Correction

For the isolated cavovarus foot, indications for gradual deformity correction with a circular external fixator are rare and should only be employed if severe deformities cannot be corrected acutely, in patients whose feet are significantly shortened from prior surgeries, or have a poor soft tissue envelope preventing standard surgical approaches [60, 61]. In cases with concurrent equinus, an external fixator may be more useful [60, 61]. Typically under 8–10 years of age, correction by soft tissue distraction is possible. Osteotomies through the calcaneus or midfoot can be added in older children with acute or gradual correction [43]. The typical complications of external fixators remain, such as pin site infections and pain, and residual stiffness and recurrence are common [51, 60].

2.9 Arthrodesis and Midfoot Wedge Resections

Arthrodesis and large wedge resections should only be considered in the older child with severe rigid deformity [43].

Classically, severe midfoot deformity was corrected with a dorsal or dorsolateral closing wedge resection through the joints or tarsal bones. Multiple techniques have been described including the Cole, Jahss, Japas, or Akron dome [46, 51, 53]. Although powerful, the foot is left stiff and shortened [39]. Better results and lower recurrence are reported in patients over 8 years of age with non-progressive disorders [37, 39, 51].

Other described resection techniques include navicular excision and dorsolateral cuboid closing wedge as described by Mubarak and Dimeglio in a small series of patients with good results at 5 years [62]. Shariff et al. obtained good results with partial or complete excision of the base of the fifth metatarsal in adults with residual lateral overloading after cavovarus deformity correction with a triple fusion or osteotomies [47, 63].

Arthrodesis is not recommended before the age of 10–12 years [39, 64]. There is scant literature on the outcomes of arthrodesis in the pediatric foot and minimal evidence supporting its use in isolated cavovarus deformity. Specifically in adults with CMT undergoing triple arthrodesis, satisfaction ranges from excellent to good with development of adjacent joint disease in 24–77% [65–69]. Saltzman et al. reported on their 40-year follow-up of triple arthrodesis in adult patients and found 75% good and 25% fair outcomes at 25 years, whereas at 40 years, 28% had good results, 69% were fair, and 3% had poor results [65]. Aarts et al. reported 58% of adult patients at 7.5 years following triple fusion showed no signs of adjacent joint disease [66]. Generally results are better in the setting of non-progressive motor conditions and if sensation is spared [53]. It is important for the surgeon to remember that the arthrodesis alone will not correct the forefoot pronation or muscle imbalance and should be addressed separately as described above [53].

2.10 Postoperative Protocol

Most patients are placed in a short-leg cast after surgery. If only soft tissue releases were performed, weight-bearing is allowed [43]. If tendon transfers or osteotomies were required, the patient is non-weight-bearing for a minimum of 6 weeks [14, 42,

43]. If the etiology of the cavovarus foot is progressive, they are transitioned to custom articulated ankle-foot-orthosis for maintenance of deformity correction [37, 39, 43]. Monitoring and surveillance of the children throughout growth to watch for and, if needed, manage recurrence are critical. Transition to an adult surgeon should be made for ongoing care if the underlying etiology is progressive [43].

3 Summary

Spontaneous resolution of the metatarsus adductus can occur up to age 4 years, and minor residual deformity rarely leads to disability. The cavovarus foot can be challenging to manage. It requires an understanding of the etiology, concurrent deformities, and muscle imbalances to determine the optimal treatment. Recurrence in progressive deformities is common, and close follow-up is mandatory.

References

1. Mosca V, Bouchard M. Chapter 28: The foot. In: Weinstein SL, Flynn JM, editors. Lovell and Winter's pediatric orthopedics. 8th ed. Philadelphia: Lippincott Williams and Wilkins; 2020. p. 1431–4.
2. Wynne-Davies R. Family studies and the cause of congenital club foot. Talipes equinovarus, talipes calcaneo-valgus and metatarsus varus. J Bone Joint Surg Br. 1964;46:445–63.
3. Hunziker UA, Largo RH, Duc G. Neonatal metatarsus adductus, joint mobility, axis, and rotation of the lower extremity in preterm and term children 0–5 years of age. Eur J Pediatr. 1988;148:19–23.
4. Kite JH. Congenital metatarsus varus. J Bone Joint Surg Am. 1967;49:388–97.
5. Kumar SJ, MacEwen GD. The incidence of hip dysplasia with metatarsus adductus. Clin Orthop Relat Res. 1982;164:234–5.
6. Gruber MA, Lozano JA. Metatarsus varus and developmental dysplasia of the hip: is there a relationship? Orthop Trans. 1991;15:336.
7. Kollmer CE, Betz RR, Clancy M, et al. Relationship of congenital hip and foot deformities: a national Shriner's Hospital survey. Orthop Trans. 1991;15:96.
8. Rushforth GF. The natural history of hooked forefoot. J Bone Joint Surg Br. 1978;60-B:530–2.
9. Wynne-Davies R, Littlejohn A, Gormley J. Aetiology and interrelationship of some common skeletal deformities. (Talipes equinovarus and calcaneovalgus, metatarsus varus, congenital dislocation of the hip, and infantile idiopathic scoliosis). J Med Genet. 1982;19:321–8.
10. Morcuende JA, Ponseti IV. Congenital metatarsus adductus in early human fetal development: a histologic study. Clin Orthop Relat Res. 1996;333:261–6.
11. Browne RS, Paton DF. Anomalous insertion of the tibialis posterior tendon in congenital metatarsus varus. J Bone Joint Surg Br. 1979;61:74–6.
12. Asirvatham R, Stevens PM. Idiopathic forefoot-adduction deformity: medial capsulotomy and abductor hallucis lengthening for resistant and severe deformities. J Pediatr Orthop. 1997;17:496–500.
13. Mitchell GP. Abductor hallucis release in congenital metatarsus varus. Int Orthop. 1980;3(4):299–304. https://doi.org/10.1007/BF00266025. PMID: 7399770
14. Mosca VS. Principles and management of pediatric foot and ankle deformities and malformations. Philadelphia: Wolters Kluwer/Lippincott Williams & Wilkins; 2014. p. 21, 26, 32–33, 43, 45, 68–69, 145–160, 176–177, 226–235.

15. Cappello T, Mosca VS. Metatarsus adductus and skewfoot. Foot Ankle Clin. 1998;3:683–700.
16. Ponseti IV, Becker JR. Congenital metatarsus adductus: the results of treatment. J Bone Joint Surg Am. 1966;48:702.
17. Farsetti P, Weinstein SL, Ponseti IV. The long-term functional and radiographic outcomes of untreated and non-operatively treated metatarsus adductus. J Bone Joint Surg Am. 1994;76:257–65.
18. Bleck EE. Metatarsus adductus: classification and relationship to outcomes of treatment. J Pediatr Orthop. 1983;3:2–9.
19. Bleck EE. Developmental orthopaedics. III. Toddlers. Dev Med Child Neurol. 1982;24:533.
20. Smith JT, Bleck EE, Gamble JG, et al. Simple method of documenting metatarsus adductus. J Pediatr Orthop. 1991;11:679–80.
21. Ghali NN, Abberton MJ, Silk FF. The management of metatarsus adductus et supinatus. J Bone Joint Surg Br. 1984;66:376–80.
22. Williams CM, James AM, Tran T. Metatarsus adductus: development of a non-surgical treatment pathway. J Paediatr Child Health. 2013;49(9):E428–33. https://doi.org/10.1111/jpc.12219. Epub 2013 May 6. PMID: 23647850.
23. Eamsobhana P, Rojjananukulpong K, Ariyawatkul T, Chotigavanichaya C, Kaewpornsawan K. Does the parental stretching programs improve metatarsus adductus in newborns? J Orthop Surg (Hong Kong). 2017;25(1):2309499017690320. https://doi.org/10.1177/2309499017690320. PMID: 28215117.
24. Berg EE. A reappraisal of metatarsus adductus and skewfoot. J Bone Joint Surg Am. 1986;68:1185–96.
25. Katz K, David R, Soudry M. Below-knee plaster cast for the treatment of metatarsus adductus. J Pediatr Orthop. 1999;19(1):49–50. PMID: 9890286.
26. McCauley J Jr, Lusskin R, Bromley J. Recurrence in congenital metatarsus varus. J Bone Joint Surg Am. 1964;46:525–32.
27. Herzenberg JE, Burghardt RD. Resistant metatarsus adductus: prospective randomized trial of casting versus orthosis. J Orthop Sci. 2014;19(2):250–6. https://doi.org/10.1007/s00776-013-0498-7. Epub 2013 Nov 19. PMID: 24248551.
28. Stark JG, Johanson JE, Winter RB. The Heyman-Herndon tarsometatarsal capsulotomy for metatarsus adductus: results in 48 feet. J Pediatr Orthop. 1987;7:305–10.
29. McHale KA, Lenhart MK. Treatment of residual clubfoot deformity—the "bean-shaped" foot—by opening wedge medial cuneiform osteotomy and closing wedge cuboid osteotomy. Clinical review and cadaver correlations. J Pediatr Orthop. 1991;11:374–81.
30. Anderson DA, Schoenecker PL, Blair VPI. Combined lateral column shortening and medial column lengthening in the treatment of severe forefoot adductus. Orthop Trans. 1991;15:768.
31. Conklin MJ, Kling TF. Open-wedge osteotomies of the first cuneiform for metatarsus adductus. Orthop Trans. 1991;106.
32. Feng L, Sussman M. Combined medial cuneiform osteotomy and multiple metatarsal osteotomies for correction of persistent metatarsus adductus in children. J Pediatr Orthop. 2016;36(7):730–5. https://doi.org/10.1097/BPO.0000000000000559. PMID: 26057072.
33. Holden D, Siff S, Butler J, et al. Shortening of the first metatarsal as a complication of metatarsal osteotomies. J Bone Joint Surg Am. 1984;66:582–7.
34. Knörr J, Soldado F, Pham TT, Torres A, Cahuzac JP, de Gauzy JS. Percutaneous correction of persistent severe metatarsus adductus in children. J Pediatr Orthop. 2014;34(4):447–52. https://doi.org/10.1097/BPO.0000000000000122. PMID: 24276227.
35. Kim BS. Reconstruction of cavus foot: a review. Open Orthop J. 2017;11:651–9. https://doi.org/10.2174/1874325001711010651.
36. VanderHave KL, Hensinger RN, King BW. Flexible cavovarus foot in children and adolescents. Foot Ankle Clinic N Am. 2013;18(4):715–26.
37. Schwend R, Drennan J. Cavus foot deformity in children. J Am Acad Orthop Surg. 2003;11(3):201–11.
38. Dwyer FC. The present status of the problem of pes cavus. Clin Orthop. 1975;106:254–75.
39. Lee MC, Sucato DJ. Pediatric issues with cavovarus foot deformities. Foot Ankle Clin. 2008;13(2):199–219, v. https://doi.org/10.1016/j.fcl.2008.01.002.

40. Alexander IJ, Johnson KA. Assessment and management of pes cavus in Charcot-Marie-Tooth disease. Clin Orthop Relat Res. 1989;246:273–81.
41. DeVries JG, McAlister JE. Corrective osteotomies used in cavus reconstruction. Clin Podiatr Med Surg. 2015;32(3):375–87. https://doi.org/10.1016/j.cpm.2015.03.003.
42. Dreher T, Beckmann NA, Wenz W. Surgical treatment of severe cavovarus foot deformity in Charcot-Marie-Tooth disease. JBJS Essent Surg Tech. 2015;5(2):e11. https://doi.org/10.2106/JBJS.ST.N.00005.
43. Bouchard M. Assessment and Management of the Pediatric Cavovarus Foot. Instruct Course Lect. 2020;69:321–90.
44. Krause F, Seidel A. Malalignment and lateral ankle instability: causes of failure from the varus tibia to the cavovarus foot. Foot Ankle Clin. 2018;23(4):593–603. https://doi.org/10.1016/j.fcl.2018.07.005.
45. Coleman SS, Chestnut WJ. A simple test for hindfoot flexibility in the cavovarus foot. Clin Orthop Relat Res. 1977;123:60–2.
46. Barton T, Winson I. Joint sparing correction of cavovarus feet in Charcot-Marie-Tooth disease: what are the limits? Foot Ankle Clin. 2013;18(4):673–88. https://doi.org/10.1016/j.fcl.2013.08.008.
47. Kaplan JRM, Aiyer AA, Cerrato RA, Jeng CL, Campbell JT. Operative treatment of the cavovarus foot. Foot Ankle Int. 2018;39(11):1370–82.
48. Wicart P. Cavus foot, from neonates to adolescents. Orthop Traumatol Surg Res. 2012;98(7):813–28. https://doi.org/10.1016/j.otsr.2012.09.003.
49. d'Astorg H, Rampal V, Seringe R, Glorion C, Wicart P. Is non-operative management of childhood neurologic cavovarus foot effective? Orthop Traumatol Surg Res. 2016;102(8):1087–91.
50. Burns J, Scheinberg A, Ryan MM. Randomized trial of botulinum toxin to prevent pes cavus progression in pediatric Charcot-Marie-Tooth disease type 1A. Muscle Nerve. 2010;42:262–7.
51. Weiner DS, Jones K, Jonah D, Dicintio MS. Management of the rigid cavus foot in children and adolescents. Foot Ankle Clin. 2013;18(4):727–41. https://doi.org/10.1016/j.fcl.2013.08.007.
52. Mubarak SJ, Van Valin SE. Osteotomies of the foot for cavus deformities in children. J Pediatr Orthop. 2009;29:294–9.
53. Simon A-L, Seringe R, Badina A, Khouri N, Glorion C, Wicart P. Long term results of the revisited Meary closing wedge tarsectomy for the treatment of the fixed cavavarus foot in adolescent with Charcot-Marie-Tooth disease. Foot Ankle Surg. 2018;15: pii: S1268-7731(18)34087-9.
54. Uglow MG. Percutaneous pediatric foot and ankle surgery. Foot Ankle Clin. 2016;21(3):577–94. https://doi.org/10.1016/j.fcl.2016.04.005. Epub 2016 Jun 29. PMID: 27524707.
55. Mourkus H, Prem H. Double calcaneal osteotomy with minimally invasive surgery for the treatment of severe flexible flatfeet. Int Orthop. 2018;42(9):2123–9. https://doi.org/10.1007/s00264-018-3910-2. Epub 2018 Mar 26. PMID: 29582117.
56. Gutteck N, Zeh A, Wohlrab D, Delank KS. Comparative results of percutaneous calcaneal osteotomy in correction of hindfoot deformities. Foot Ankle Int. 2019;40(3):276–81. https://doi.org/10.1177/1071100718809449. Epub 2018 Nov 9. PMID: 30413133.
57. Pfeffer GB, Michalski MP, Basak T, Giaconi JC. Use of 3D prints to compare the efficacy of three different calcaneal osteotomies for the correction of heel varus. Foot Ankle Int. 2018;39(5):591–7.
58. Turner JW, Cooper RR. Anterior transfer of the tibialis posterior through the interosseous membrane. Clin Orthop Relat Res. 1972;1(2):41–9.
59. Aydin A, Topal M, Tuncer K, Canbek U, Yildiz V, Kose M. Extramembranous transfer of the tibialis posterior for the treatment of drop foot deformity in children. Arch Iran Med. 2013;16(11):647–51.
60. Grill F, Franke J. The Ilizarov distractor for the correction of relapsed or neglected clubfoot. J Bone Joint Surg Br. 1987;69:593–7.
61. Ferreira RC, Costo MT, Frizzo GG, et al. Correction of neglected clubfoot using the Ilizarov external fixator. Foot Ankle Int. 2006;27:266–73.
62. Mubarak SJ, Dimeglio A. Navicular excision and cuboid closing wedge for severe cavovarus foot deformities: a salvage procedure. J Pediatr Orthop. 2011;31:551–6.

63. Shariff R, Myerson MS, Palmanovich E. Resection of the fifth metatarsal base in the severe rigid cavovarus foot. Foot Ankle Int. 2014;35(6):558–65.
64. Penny JN. The neglected clubfoot. Tech Orthop. 2005;20(2):153–66.
65. Saltzman CL, Fehrle MJ, Cooper RR, et al. Triple arthrodesis: twenty-five and forty-four-year average follow-up of the same patients. J Bone Joint Surg Am. 1999;81-A(10):1391Y1402.
66. Aarts CAM, Heesterbeek PJC, Jaspers PEM, Stegeman M, Louwerens JWK. Does osteoarthritis of the ankle joint progress after triple arthrodesis? A midterm prospective outcome study. Foot Ankle Surg. 2016;22:265–9.
67. Wukilch DK, Bowen JR. A long-term study of triple arthrodesis for correction of pes cavovarus in Charcot-Marie-Tooth disease. J Pediatr Orthop. 1989;9:433–7.
68. Wetmore RS, Drennan JC. Long-term results of triple arthrodesis in Charcot-Marie-Tooth disease. J Bone Joint Surg Am. 1989;71:417–22.
69. Mann DC, Hsu JD. Triple arthrodesis in the treatment of fixed cavovarus deformity in adolescent patients with Charcot-Marie-Tooth disease. Foot Ankle. 1992;13(1):1–6.

Pediatric Flexible and Rigid Flatfoot

Kyle M. Natsuhara and Jacob R. Zide

1 Introduction

Children and adolescents commonly present to orthopedic providers with concerns about a flatfoot deformity. While the etiology and management of flatfeet in this population differ substantially from that in adults, there is a lack of consensus as to what constitutes a consistent definition of the deformity as well as what the optimal treatment should be. The majority of flatfoot deformities in children are flexible, painless, and functional and do not require any treatment whatsoever [1, 2].

Despite the fact that most patients with flatfeet will never develop symptoms, there still exists a widespread negative sentiment associated with the "low-arched" foot. The genesis of this is unclear, but it may stem somewhat from historic military reports. In 1944, it was reported that foot symptoms were the cause of 30–40% of US Army medical discharges. Among soldiers with foot symptoms, many had flatfeet which led to the assumption that it was the flatfoot that was the source of pain and disability [3]. This simplistic interpretation resulted in a lingering stigma still present today and may, in part, explain parental concerns for future pain, physical dysfunction, or deformity progression in children with asymptomatic flatfeet.

A small percentage of children with flexible flatfeet are symptomatic, and when this is the case, treatment is often indicated. Additionally, a subset of patients with

K. M. Natsuhara
Department of Orthopaedic Surgery, Baylor University Medical Center, Dallas, TX, USA

J. R. Zide (✉)
Department of Orthopaedic Surgery, Baylor University Medical Center, Dallas, TX, USA

Department of Orthopaedic Surgery, UT Southwestern Medical School, Dallas, TX, USA

Department of Surgery, Texas A&M Health Science Center College of Medicine, Dallas, TX, USA
e-mail: Jacob.Zide@bswhealth.org

© The Author(s), under exclusive license to Springer Nature
Switzerland AG 2022
E. Wagner Hitschfeld, P. Wagner Hitschfeld (eds.), *Foot and Ankle Disorders*,
https://doi.org/10.1007/978-3-030-95738-4_9

179

painful flatfeet have rigid deformities suggesting an underlying disorder that warrants further investigation and treatment.

2   Etiology-Pathophysiology

The challenge of creating an agreed upon definition of the pediatric flatfoot has resulted in an unusually wide range of prevalence of 0.6–77.9% found in the literature [1, 2]. Moreover, the reporting is inconsistent, and disparities related to variable sampling, different assessment measures, and age groups must be taken into account [2].

Before defining what constitutes a pathologic flatfoot, it is crucial to understand what comprises the normal development and common variations of a child's foot. Infants are born with flatfeet, and the longitudinal arch forms over the course of the first decade of life [4, 5]. In a Cochrane review, children aged 2–6 years were found to have a mean flatfoot prevalence of 46.3% [2]. In studies that investigated children ages 8–13 years old, the mean prevalence decreased to 14.2% [2]. A study by Pfeiffer et al. investigated 835 children aged 3–6 years and observed that boys and obese children were at higher risk for flatfeet than girls and normal weight children [4]. In fact, boys were twice as likely as girls to have a flatfoot deformity, and children who were obese were three times as likely as those with a healthy weight [4]. El et al. found that hypermobility, based on Beighton's assessment method, was a risk factor for pediatric flatfoot [6].

The conundrum of the pediatric flexible flatfoot is that there remains no understanding as to why some patients become symptomatic while others do not. Furthermore, when patients are symptomatic, the underlying source of pain has not been fully elucidated and is likely multifactorial. It has been postulated that increased hindfoot valgus and collapse of the longitudinal arch elevate stress within the subtalar joint which in turn provokes synovial and ligamentous irritation at the subtalar and midtarsal joints. This irritation, along with overload of the intrinsic musculature, may be one source of hindfoot pain associated with the deformity [7].

Certain clinical characteristics such as a short Achilles tendon associated with a flexible flatfoot have been correlated with symptoms and are reported to have an increased prevalence of pain and disability [1]. Some radiographic parameters also correspond to symptomatology. For example, a study of 135 pediatric patients over the age of 7 with idiopathic flexible flatfeet demonstrated that increased lateral displacement of the navicular on the AP radiograph (measured by talonavicular coverage) was found to relate to the presence of symptoms [8]. This study found that no other measurements of hindfoot alignment including longitudinal arch, lateral column length, or pronation/supination of the forefoot correlated to symptomatology [8].

In contrast to flexible flatfeet, rigid flatfeet occur at a lower prevalence but are more often symptomatic. There are multiple causes of rigid flatfeet in children and adolescents, with tarsal coalitions being the most common [1, 9]. However, in patients without an identifiable structural cause, one must consider and rule out other potential underlying pathologies including but not limited to neoplastic, neurologic, and rheumatologic etiologies [1, 9]. Peroneal and Achilles spasticity are also associated with rigid flatfoot deformities, so it is important to identify neurologic conditions such as cerebral palsy, hypoxic brain injury, Chiari malformation, syrinx, trauma, and central nervous system tumors [9, 10].

3   Anatomy

The medial longitudinal arch develops during the first decade of life along with the bones, muscles, and ligaments of the foot. Maintenance of the longitudinal arch is thought by some to rely on muscular strength and that a flexible flatfoot is the result of subclinical muscle weakness [1, 7]. Others theorize that while the surrounding musculature functions to support balance, propel the body forward, and navigate uneven terrain, the shape of the longitudinal arch is truly determined by the bone-ligament complex [1, 7]. Despite the lack of consensus on how the longitudinal arch is maintained, the biomechanical function of the bony ligamentous complex is well understood.

In early stance phase, the hindfoot complex of the flexible flatfoot is aligned in accentuated valgus with the transverse tarsal joint unlocked. As stance phase progresses, the transition to a locked transverse tarsal joint and varus hindfoot position requires increased intrinsic muscle activity to stabilize the hindfoot joints at toe off. It is thought that these demands on the intrinsic musculature may subsequently lead to foot fatigue and pain.

Contractures of the gastroc-soleus complex and peroneal tendons play an important role in flatfoot deformities. The decrease in calcaneal pitch seen in a flatfoot allows for shortening and contracture of the gastroc-soleus. In concert with the valgus alignment of the hindfoot, the shortened Achilles acts as a deforming force, driving the calcaneus further into valgus and equinus. Contractures of the peroneus brevis are associated with midfoot abduction deformity. Whether these contractures are a primary force that drive and exacerbate the deformity or a consequence of the foot position is not known.

Overt peroneal tendon spasticity as a primary cause of flatfoot deformity in the pediatric flatfoot is well described but poorly understood. It has been theorized that the peroneals are dynamically contracted due to subtalar pain and eventually become shortened [9].

Tarsal coalitions are the most common cause of a rigid flatfoot deformity. They are thought to be the product of failure of mesenchymal segmentation and are characterized by a fibrous, cartilaginous, or osseous connection between two or more tarsal bones [11, 12]. The most common coalitions are calcaneonavicular (CN) and talocalcaneal (TC). While it is thought that coalitions are present from birth in cartilaginous form, ossification of the coalition occurs between the ages of 8 and 12 years and correlates closely with the most common age range for symptomatic clinical presentation [11].

4 Diagnosis

4.1 History

Children and adolescents commonly present for evaluation secondary to parental concern regarding the cosmetic appearance of the foot or the potential for future disability rather than for pain or dysfunction. Determining whether or not the patient is symptomatic is the most important part of the interaction as it guides all further discussion with the patient and family.

The physician should inquire as to recurrent injuries, calluses, or skin irritation. Difficulties with shoe wear, walking bare foot, or walking on uneven surfaces may also provide clues regarding the underlying diagnosis. A history of frequent ankle sprains with activity is common in the setting of a coalition since the hindfoot cannot properly accommodate to the inversion and eversion stresses typically seen in sports. Additionally, adolescents with a stiff hindfoot often describe worsening of their symptoms with a corrective arch support [1, 2, 13].

When pain is present, identifying its precise location is critical in the diagnosis of flatfoot deformity. Most frequently, pain is found at the plantarmedial aspect of the midfoot as a result of the talar head pressing into the floor, but sinus tarsi pain and calcaneofibular impingement symptoms are common as well [1, 10, 13]. Occasionally, pain along the course of the posterior tibial tendon (PTT) may be present. True pathology of the PTT however is essentially a nonissue in the pediatric population except in cases of trauma or iatrogenic injury. In the setting of a tarsal coalition, pain may be localized to the coalition itself. Rigid deformities also commonly present with anterior ankle pain as a result of stress transfer from the stiff hindfoot [10, 13].

Flatfeet may be associated with rheumatologic, neoplastic, traumatic, neurologic, or connective tissue disorders so it is important to ask if there is any known patient or family history related to such conditions. Of note, night pain, swelling, warmth, and redness are all unusual in both flexible and rigid flatfoot, and the presence of these symptoms warrants investigation for other potential underlying pathology [1].

4.2 Exam

The physical examination begins with evaluation of the patient's entire lower extremity for additional sources of angular or rotational deformity that may be related to the presenting foot symptoms. Genu valgus or external tibial torsion can make a flatfoot appear exaggerated when standing [13]. Assessing the child's gait pattern especially when their attention is elsewhere, such as when they first walk into an exam room, is helpful as children often alter their gait when being observed. Asymmetry in gait or inability to perform a heel or toe walk may indicate an underlying neuromuscular disorder that requires further evaluation [10]. The patient's shoes should be examined for clues of abnormal wear due to an underlying deformity. Asymmetric medial wear of the sole of the shoe is common in patients with a flexible flatfoot, and when the Achilles tendon is tight, wear can be seen at the medial midfoot [7]. Finally, one should examine the patient for signs of ligamentous laxity and other connective tissue disorders such as Ehlers-Danlos, Marfan syndrome, or Down syndrome.

Recognition of a contracture of the gastroc-soleus complex is important since pediatric patients with a flatfoot and associated short Achilles tendon are often symptomatic [1, 2, 13]. The Silfverskiöld test is used to differentiate between an isolated gastrocnemius contracture and a contracture of the entire gastroc-soleus complex. During this examination maneuver, it is important to restrict dorsiflexion through the subtalar joint by locking it in a neutral or slightly inverted position, thus isolating sagittal motion of the talus. When less than 10 degrees of ankle dorsiflexion is obtained with the knee in both flexion and extension, the entire gastroc-soleus complex is contracted. If more than 10 degrees of ankle dorsiflexion is obtained with the knee in flexion, but dorsiflexion beyond 10 degrees is not possible with the knee in extension, the gastrocnemius alone is affected [1, 4, 13].

One of the primary goals of the diagnostic process is determining whether a flatfoot is flexible or rigid because this has a substantial impact on the treatment algorithm. There are several ways to assess for flexibility. First, a double-limb heel rise should elicit correction of the hindfoot to a varus heel position through contraction of the posterior tibialis if the deformity is flexible. Performing a heel rise without correction of the hindfoot into a varus position is suspicious for a rigid deformity. Another method to check for rigidity is to manually assess subtalar joint motion with the patient seated and the ankle in neutral dorsiflexion. Maintaining neutral dorsiflexion during this maneuver is key as it minimizes the coronal plane motion contribution from the tibiotalar joint by bringing the wider anterior portion of the talar dome into the mortise. Perhaps the simplest way to evaluate hindfoot flexibility is to observe the patient's resting foot position when seated with the feet dangling off the edge of the bed. A patient with a stiff hindfoot will often have a resting foot position that is dorsiflexed and everted compared to the other side, assuming no contralateral hindfoot stiffness (Fig. 1).

There is an approximately 50% incidence of bilateral tarsal coalitions so it is of course necessary to examine the contralateral foot [14]. Patients with TC coalitions may have a palpable eminence inferior to the medial malleolus and may also be tender to palpation in the sinus tarsi. CN coalitions may be palpable as well and are confluent with the anterior process of the calcaneus [12].

4.3 Imaging

Symptomatic patients should be assessed with standard weight-bearing ankle (anteroposterior [AP] and mortise) and foot (AP, 45° external rotation oblique, and lateral) radiographs to evaluate for signs of planovalgus alignment and assess for a coalition or other osseous abnormality. The AP foot radiograph is used to analyze talonavicular joint alignment as the navicular is laterally positioned relative to the

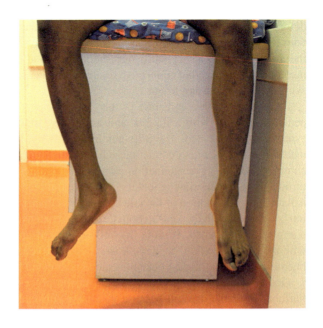

Fig. 1 Resting foot position of a patient with a rigid flatfoot on the patient's right side. The resting foot position of the rigid hindfoot (patient's right) is dorsiflexed and everted compared to the contralateral side

head of the talus in a flatfoot. This can be difficult to interpret however in the pediatric population since the navicular does not normally ossify until the age of 3–4 years, and ossification begins asymmetrically toward its lateral aspect [7]. Alternatively, the AP talus-first metatarsal angle may be used to evaluate the talonavicular joint relationship (Fig. 2), but it may be unreliable, as in the case of metatarsus adductus and skewfoot deformity [7].

On the lateral view, the lateral talus-first metatarsal angle (Meary's angle), formed by lines drawn through the mid-axis of the talus and the mid-axis of the first metatarsal, is evaluated (Fig. 3) [7, 15]. In a flatfoot deformity, there is an apex plantar break in this angle, but it is important to note that this measurement has been shown to vary off the neutral axis up to 13 degrees even in "normal" feet [15]. The lateral radiograph of a flatfoot will also reveal an equinus position of the calcaneus, measured by the calcaneal pitch (Fig. 4). The average calcaneal pitch in the pediatric population is approximately 17 degrees [15].

It is often possible to identify a CN coalition on the oblique view of the foot (Fig. 5), whereas an axial or Harris heel view of the hindfoot has traditionally been obtained to help identify a middle facet TC coalition or dysmorphic middle facet. It should be noted that literature examining the utility of the Harris view has found that it is poor for diagnostic purposes in children and adolescents [16]. Other radiographic features suggestive of a coalition may be seen on the lateral view and include talar beaking (TC and CN coalitions), a C sign (TC coalition), or an anteater sign (CN coalition).

The C sign, formed by the medial outline of the talar dome and the posteroinferior outline of the sustentaculum tali (Fig. 6), is not always present in TC coalitions and may also be seen in children with flexible flatfeet who do not have a coalition [17]. One study used computed tomography (CT) scans to verify the presence of a TC coalition and correlated them with the identification of a C sign on the lateral

Fig. 2 Standing anteroposterior (AP) foot radiograph demonstrating the AP talus-first metatarsal angle, formed by lines drawn through the mid-axis of the talus and the mid-axis of the first metatarsal

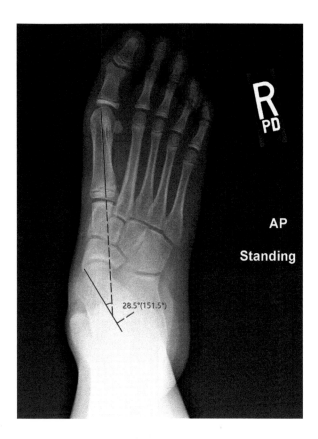

Fig. 3 Standing lateral foot radiograph demonstrating the lateral talus-first metatarsal angle (Meary's angle), formed by lines drawn through the mid-axis of the talus and the mid-axis of the first metatarsal

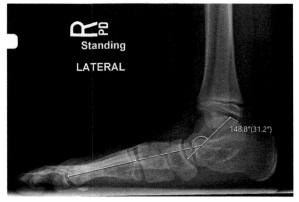

radiograph. They found that a "true C sign," defined as complete or a near complete (with a linear interruption and rarefaction of the edges), was present in only 41% of patients with a TC coalition. However, if a true C sign was present, then it was 97% specific for a TC coalition [17].

Whether or not a coalition is identified on plain radiographs, advanced imaging with CT or magnetic resonance imaging (MRI) is mandatory for the complete

Fig. 4 Standing lateral
foot radiograph
demonstrating the
calcaneal pitch, which is
the angle between the
horizontal line parallel to
the ground and the line
drawn between the plantar
prominence of the
calcaneus proximal to the
calcaneocuboid articular
surface and the plantar
aspect of the most plantar
prominence of the
calcaneal tuberosity

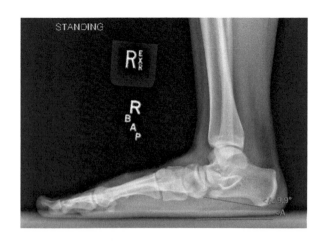

Fig. 5 Oblique foot
radiograph demonstrating a
calcaneonavicular coalition

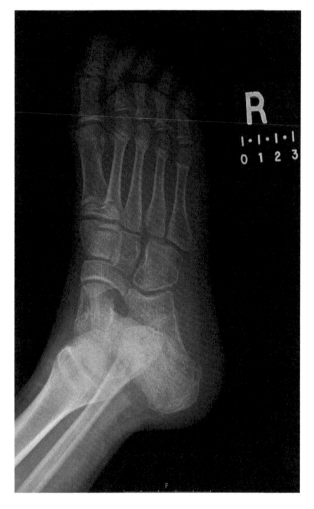

Fig. 6 The C sign (arrows) is formed by the medial outline of the talar dome and the posteroinferior outline of the sustentaculum tali

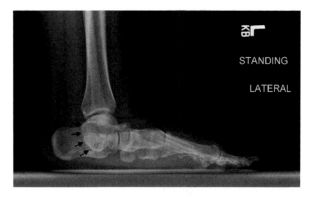

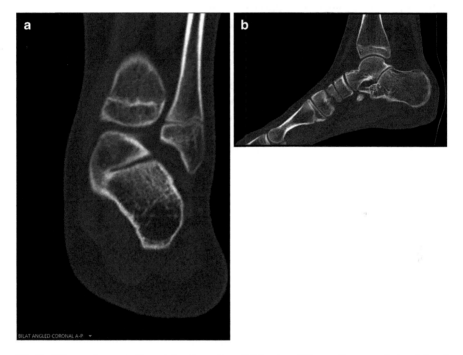

Fig. 7 CT scan demonstrating a talocalcaneal medial facet coalition on the coronal view (**a**) and associated narrowing of the posterior facet on the sagittal view (**b**)

workup of a rigid hindfoot. These studies are important to accurately evaluate the characteristics of a coalition as well as to identify the presence of a second ipsilateral coalition which occurs in 20% of cases [18]. We recommend bilateral ankle CT scans to assess for contralateral pathology and as a comparison to the unaffected side since subtle differences in the relationships of the joint surfaces may be difficult to identify. CT is especially helpful to aid surgical planning for a TC coalition as morphology of the coalition, joint space narrowing of the posterior facet, and extension of the coalition into the posterior facet are all important factors to guide treatment (Fig. 7).

If no coalition is identified on advanced imaging studies, exam findings concerning for rigidity warrant further workup with neurological consultation. Electromyography can be a useful objective tool to confirm and quantify spasticity affecting the hindfoot.

5   Conservative Treatment

The first line of treatment for pediatric flexible flatfeet is always nonsurgical. When asymptomatic, observation alone is the rule as orthoses will neither help correct alignment nor prevent future pain and dysfunction. Despite this, intervention is often requested by parents or suggested by other medical providers, and in this setting, it is essential to provide patient and parental education and reassurance.

When symptomatic, pain can often be lessened through the use of in-shoe prefabricated or custom orthoses to invert the hindfoot, offload the plantarmedial soft tissues, and decrease exaggerated muscle activity [1, 2, 13]. While most physicians find orthoses and arch supports to be a useful treatment tool, there are mixed results in the literature regarding their effectiveness and the overall quality of evidence is poor [2]. In one of the few randomized controlled studies, Whitford and Esterman showed that although orthoses improved pain and physical function, the improvement was not statistically significant compared to the control group with no treatment. They also showed there was no benefit to custom orthoses over prefabricated inserts [19]. A 2010 Cochrane Review concluded that due to the heterogeneity of the studies evaluating nonoperative management in pediatric flatfoot patients, there was no clear evidence to support that foot orthoses affect the long-term shape of the foot or decrease potential future disability [2]. However, there was limited evidence that orthoses and supportive shoes improve pain and function, although there were varying degrees of baseline symptoms in the patients included. Despite a lack of evidence, over-the-counter foot orthoses may help reduce pain and relieve activity related symptoms. They certainly seem to be a reasonable and relatively inexpensive adjunct to the initial management of flexible flatfeet [2, 13, 20].

Pain is more common in flexible flatfeet with a short Achilles tendon, so heel cord stretching should be part of the treatment plan for these patients [1, 2, 10, 13]. The patient should perform heel cord stretching with the knee extended and the subtalar joint in neutral to slightly inverted alignment as this helps to isolate motion to the tibiotalar joint and avoids dorsiflexion through the everted subtalar joint [1, 7].

When a flatfoot is rigid, the foot shape cannot be manipulated with a corrective orthotic device. In fact, adding material to the arch may actually exacerbate symptoms by increasing pressure under the head of the talus [7]. Instead, it may be worthwhile to first treat symptomatic tarsal coalitions with 4–6 weeks of immobilization with a walking boot or short leg cast. A University of California Berkeley Laboratories (UCBL) orthosis is another alternative. These rigid orthoses can be cumbersome and painful for some, but for those patients who find them comfortable, they can provide relief and may be used for long-term stabilization of the hindfoot. Nonoperative interventions as a whole are valuable in the setting of a symptomatic tarsal coalition and have shown durable pain relief in approximately 50% of patients at 1.5 year follow-up after initial presentation [21].

6 Surgical Management, Timing, and Post-op Protocol

6.1 Flexible Flatfoot

The primary indication for surgery is pain specifically related to the flatfoot that affects the patient's ability to participate in activities and failure of at least 3–6 months of nonsurgical treatment. As a result of the variability in the literature of both the definition of the flexible flatfoot and surgical results, more specific surgical indications are debatable [2, 7].

The mainstay of surgical treatment is a combination of soft tissue procedures and osteotomies for rebalancing and realigning the foot. Other bony procedures including osseous excision and arthrodesis procedures have been described for management of the deformity but are not recommended in the treatment of an otherwise uncomplicated flexible flatfoot. Excision procedures have been largely abandoned due to their destructive nature. Hindfoot arthrodesis procedures are not typically indicated in an otherwise healthy patient with a flexible flatfoot because the decrease in mobility and shock absorbing capacity of the hindfoot can increase the risk of adjacent joint degeneration, especially in children [7].

Osteotomies have the benefit of realigning the foot without sacrificing mobility. The most popular techniques are the calcaneal lengthening osteotomy (CLO) with or without a concomitant plantarflexion producing cuneiform osteotomy and the calcaneo-cuboid-cuneiform osteotomy [1, 7, 13].

Evans originally described the CLO in 1975, and it was later modified by Mosca in 1995 [22, 23]. Lateral column lengthening occurs via the use of a distraction wedge osteotomy of the anterior calcaneus between the anterior and middle facets. The location of the osteotomy positions the center of rotation near the center of the talar head rather than the medial cortex of the calcaneus, and the opening wedge trapezoid-shaped graft produces lengthening and adduction of the calcaneus. The result is correction of hindfoot valgus and restoration of talar head coverage via correction of midfoot abduction. One of Mosca's modifications to allow distraction of the osteotomy included releasing the lateral plantar fascia and abductor digiti minimi aponeurosis [23]. His study reported satisfactory clinical and radiographic outcomes in 29 of 31 patients at an average of 32 months follow-up [23]. Figure 8 demonstrates an example of this procedure.

Rathjen and Mubarak first reported the technique of combining of a medial displacement calcaneal osteotomy, an opening wedge cuboid osteotomy, and a plantar-based closing wedge osteotomy of the medial cuneiform to correct severe valgus deformity in the pediatric population [24]. This calcaneo-cuboid-cuneiform osteotomy technique is alternatively referred to as the "triple C." The medial displacement calcaneal osteotomy provides correction of heel valgus; the cuboid opening wedge lengthens the lateral column, helps to realign the talonavicular joint, and dorsiflexes

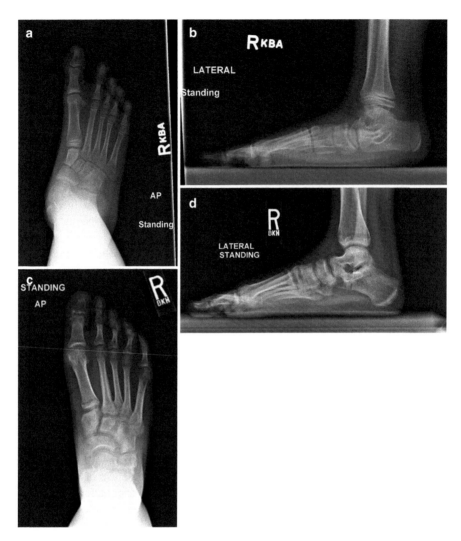

Fig. 8 Preoperative anteroposterior (**a**) and lateral (**b**) radiographs demonstrating severe flatfoot deformity. Postoperative anteroposterior (**a**) and lateral (**b**) radiographs of the same foot after calcaneal lengthening osteotomy showing correction of the deformity

the talus; and the plantarflexion medial cuneiform osteotomy introduces increased arch height and corrects forefoot supination. Rathjen and Mubarak reported "good" or "excellent" outcomes in 23 of the 24 patients included in their original study at an average of 18 months follow-up [24].

Moraleda et al. compared the modified Evans CLO and the triple C osteotomy in symptomatic pediatric patients with flexible flatfeet who had failed nonsurgical management. They found that both techniques obtained good clinical and radiographic results with an average follow-up of 2.7 years in the triple C group and 5.3 years in the CLO group. In their prospective series, the CLO provided better correction of talonavicular subluxation and of the talus-first metatarsal angle, but it was associated with a slightly increased complication rate. It should be noted that greater than 10% subluxation of the calcaneocuboid joint was included as a potential complication and was present in 51.5% feet of the CLO group [25]. Other studies have shown that calcaneocuboid subluxation after calcaneal lengthening osteotomy improves and often resolves over time, and therefore it is not clear if the subluxation noted intraoperatively has a significant clinical consequence [25, 26]. Other complications associated with the CLO procedure included nonunion, neuropraxia of the popliteal portion of the sciatic nerve, pain and stiffness of the subtalar joint, and delayed wound healing [25]. Complications with the triple C group included wound complications and delayed union [24, 25].

A variety of bony and soft tissue procedures are added to the CLO and triple C procedures to help remove deforming forces and balance the foot reconstruction. Contracture of part or all of the gastroc-soleus complex is often present and contributes to the deformity because of the increased lateral line of pull of the Achilles seen in patients with valgus heel alignment. The Silfverskiöld test should be performed intraoperatively to determine whether a contracture is present and an Achilles lengthening or gastrocnemius recession should be performed [1, 23, 24]. Z-lengthening of the peroneus brevis removes its deforming force on the midfoot and decreases resistance to lateral column distraction. Mosca also recommends recession of the abductor digiti minimi [27]. The posterior tibial tendon and spring ligament/talonavicular joint capsule will be redundant after correcting the bony alignment and should be imbricated to reset their tension and maintain deformity correction. Finally, if there is residual forefoot supination after correction of the hindfoot deformity, a plantarflexion medial cuneiform osteotomy is performed to bring the metatarsal heads into a neutral alignment and recreate the longitudinal arch of the foot through plantarflexion of the first ray [24].

A more controversial surgical option is the arthroereisis procedure which involves inserting a bioabsorbable, silicone, or titanium cone-shaped implant into the sinus tarsi. This may be performed in conjunction with other bony and soft tissue surgeries or as a stand-alone. The device functions by restricting external rotation of the subtalar joint and results in elevation the arch and improved talonavicular congruity. However, the popularity of arthroereisis has declined due to implant pain, risk of misplacement or displacement of the device, subtalar joint degeneration, and incomplete deformity correction or recurrence [1, 7, 13]. In a critical review of the literature including 76 small studies, satisfactory patient-reported outcomes were reported between 79 and 100% with improvement of most radiographic measures. However, there was a complication rate of 5–19% with an unplanned removal rate between 7 and 19% [28]. Overall, there is insufficient evidence to support its use for adolescent deformity.

6.2   Rigid Flatfoot

A rigid flatfoot may be the result of a variety of causes, some obvious and others less so. If nonoperative treatment fails to provide satisfactory relief, surgery may be considered only after an underlying source of the rigidity has been identified, as this will significantly impact surgical planning. Here we will discuss options for surgical treatment in the setting of TC or CN coalitions as well as the flatfoot with a neurogenic cause.

6.2.1 Talocalcaneal Coalition

Multiple techniques have been described for TC coalition resection along with methods to prevent regrowth by coating the resection surfaces with bone wax and/ or interposing fat graft or tendon into the defect [1, 13, 29]. Historically, subtalar or triple arthrodesis was the standard surgical treatment for a TC coalition. While arthrodesis procedures still have an important role in their management, the concern for long-term adjacent joint degeneration and functional issues associated with a rigid hindfoot led to a transition toward the goal of motion restoration and preservation in the adolescent population [29].

Results of motion sparing surgery for TC coalitions were initially mixed so studies began to focus on appropriate indications to guide the decision of joint preservation rather than sacrifice. In a widely referenced article, Wilde et al. concluded that middle facet coalitions with a cross-sectional area measuring 50% or more than that of the adjacent posterior facet were associated with poorer outcomes after coalition resection [30]. Although many still use this guideline, the use of coalition size as an indication was based on an incidental finding of the study and has largely not been validated in the literature [30–32]. Multiple studies have shown that when TC coalitions are appropriately excised, approximately 90% of patients report decreased levels of pain and significant improvement in outcome scores, even in patients with large coalitions measuring more than 50% of the surface area of the middle facet [29, 31, 32]. While there are no formal published guidelines for resection versus arthrodesis, our recommendation is that all adolescent TC coalitions indicated for surgery should be resected *unless* (1) there is narrowing of the subtalar joint space on CT scan (essentially indicating subtalar arthritis) or (2) if the coalition involves any portion of the posterior facet. If either of these two are the case, then subtalar arthrodesis is preferred.

When one does decide to proceed with resection, it is essential to take the time to excise the coalition completely in order to prevent recurrence and improve clinical outcomes. Assessing the adequacy of a TC coalition resection during surgery can be difficult. Kemppainen et al. found that use of intraoperative CT scan improved resection quality and altered surgical decision-making with 21% of their cases requiring further resection [33]. Presently, there are no studies of long-term clinical outcomes available to justify the increased cost and radiation incurred by use of intraoperative CT.

When a TC coalition is present in the setting of planovalgus deformity, it is important to discern whether the source of the pain is related to the deformity, to the coalition, or to both as correction of the foot alignment is often necessary for pain relief, whether or not the coalition is resected [34]. This differentiation of symptoms is helpful for surgical planning as well as for guiding patient and family expectations.

   Surgical treatment of a TC coalition with an associated flatfoot deformity depends on whether or not the coalition is amenable to resection. When joint preservation is possible, resection of the coalition may proceed concomitantly with the osteotomies and soft tissue procedures described in the flexible flatfoot section of the chapter. If the coalition is unresectable, subtalar arthrodesis with correction of hindfoot alignment either through the subtalar joint or via additional calcaneal osteotomy is preferred. Other bony and soft tissue procedures are included as necessary. In the specific setting of an osseous coalition, one may consider performing the flatfoot correction and leaving the bony coalition intact since it essentially represents an already fused subtalar joint.

   It has been shown that CLO fully corrects the flatfoot deformity even when a bony TC coalition is left unresected [34]. Mosca and Bevan reported on a cohort of patients with planovalgus deformity associated with TC coalitions that were treated with CLO, with or without coalition resection. Treatment was based on the patient's individual signs, symptoms, and imaging, and they showed that CLO provided good deformity correction and pain relief. Most importantly, their algorithmic approach demonstrated that treatment of the valgus deformity is just as important as the management of the coalition itself and the coalition cannot necessarily be assumed to be the primary pain generator among symptomatic patients [34].

6.2.2   Calcaneonavicular Coalition

Symptomatic CN coalitions are treated with resection and interposition after failing conservative management. Extensor digitorum brevis (EDB), fat graft interposition, and bone wax have all been described to decrease recurrence rate and provide long-term pain relief [11].

   Mubarek et al. noted that the calcaneocuboid bony prominence after interposition of the EDB can lead to shoe wear difficulties and cosmetic differences in the lateral contour of the foot [11]. They also used a cadaver model to demonstrate that when EDB muscle belly was used for interposition, it filled an average of 64% of the resected gap, which could potentially allow partial regrowth of the coalition [11]. In the same study, fat graft was found to fill 100% of the resection gap. Cosmetically, harvest of fat graft from a remote site (usually the medial calf or the gluteal fold) avoids the change in contour of the lateral hindfoot seen after harvest of the EDB muscle but requires a second surgical site and can leave a scarred soft tissue dimple at the harvest site [11].

   Masquijo et al. performed a retrospective study comparing fat graft, EDB, and bone wax interposition after CN coalition resection and found that fat graft and bone wax interposition techniques provided greater pain relief, resulted in better functional scores, and avoided more coalition reossification than the EDB technique [35]. Their study did not discuss whether or not the size of the EDB was adequate to fill the defect left by the resection.

Percutaneous and arthroscopic resection techniques have been proposed for CN coalitions in small patient cohorts with good short-term results, but long-term follow-up with regard to pain relief or recurrence has not yet been reported [20].

As with a TC coalition, flatfoot deformities may occur along with a CN coalition. The location of pain, symptomatology, and physical examination findings determine if the coalition can be treated in isolation or if correction of the deformity is necessary as well. Flatfoot correction in the setting of a CN coalition may be performed as described in the flexible flatfoot section above either concurrently or as a staged procedure [27].

6.2.3 Neurogenic Flatfoot

The neurogenic flatfoot often presents as a severe deformity with variable patterns of contracture, spasticity, and weakness. This poses a difficult challenge with concerns for recurrence, undercorrection, and overcorrection [10].

In Mosca's study describing his modified CLO technique, there were 24 flatfeet treated with an underlying neurogenic disorder (16 with a myelomeningocele and 8 with cerebral palsy). Of these, only two patients had unsatisfactory outcomes [23]. Subsequently, Ettl et al. reported on 24 children (28 feet) with cerebral palsy that were treated with CLO and organized the results based on ambulatory status [36]. Although they had good results in the ambulatory group, 44% of the nonambulatory group had relapse and unsatisfactory outcomes. Therefore, they recommended against CLO in nonambulatory children with cerebral palsy and severe planovalgus deformities [36].

Correction of deformity through the use of fusion procedures such as a triple arthrodesis may lead to a more predictable result in these patients and can provide good long-term patient satisfaction [37]. However, one must recognize and counsel patients and parents that fusions have been shown to lead to progressive adjacent joint degeneration even in the low-demand neurogenic population [37].

7 Summary

Pediatric and adolescent flatfoot deformities can be flexible or rigid and present with a variable degree of symptomatology. The flexible pediatric flatfoot is usually painless and does not require treatment other than reassurance and education. Occasionally, flexible flatfeet can be symptomatic, and a trial of generic orthoses is the preferred first-line treatment option. If the patient continues to have pain and disability after a concerted attempt at nonsurgical management, surgical correction may be indicated. This most commonly consists of a combination of soft tissue procedures and osteotomies. It is crucial for the surgeon to be diligent and confirm that the deformity is the true source of the patient's pain since conditions aside from the flatfoot can occur concurrently and may be overlooked.

Rigid flatfeet are more commonly symptomatic than their flexible counterparts. When a rigid flatfoot is identified, identification and appropriate treatment of the source of the deformity are critical. Surgery must be tailored to the specific underlying cause, and although there are some promising short-term surgical results, studies are needed to confirm long-term outcomes for this challenging pathology.

References

1. Bouchard M, Mosca VS. Flatfoot deformity in children and adolescents: surgical indications and management. J Am Acad Orthop Surg. 2014;22(10):623–32.
2. Evans AM, Rome K. A Cochrane review of the evidence for non-surgical interventions for flexible pediatric flat feet. Eur J Phys Rehabil Med. 2011;47(1):68–9.
3. Ilfeld FW. Pes planus: military significance and treatment with simple arch support. J Am Med Assoc. 1944;124(5):281–3.
4. Pfeiffer M, Kotz R, Ledl T, Hauser G, Sluga M. Prevalence of flat foot in preschool-aged children. Pediatrics. 2006;118(2):634–9.
5. Gould N, Moreland M, Trevino S, Alvarez R, Fenwick J, Bach N. Foot growth in children age one to five years. Foot Ankle. 1990;10(4):211–3.
6. El O, Akcali O, Kosay C, Kaner B, Arslan Y, Sagol E, et al. Flexible flatfoot and related factors in primary school children: a report of a screening study. Rheumatol Int. 2006;26(11):1050–3.
7. Mosca VS. Flexible flatfoot in children and adolescents. J Child Orthop. 2010;4(2):107–21.
8. Moraleda L, Mubarak SJ. Flexible flatfoot: differences in the relative alignment of each segment of the foot between symptomatic and asymptomatic patients. J Pediatr Orthop. 2011;31(4):421–8.
9. Luhmann SJ, Rich MM, Schoenecker PL. Painful idiopathic rigid flatfoot in children and adolescents. Foot Ankle Int. 2000;21(1):59–66.
10. Dare DM, Dodwell ER. Pediatric flatfoot: cause, epidemiology, assessment, and treatment. Curr Opin Pediatr. 2014;26(1):93–100.
11. Mubarak SJ, Patel PN, Upasani VV, Moor MA, Wenger DR. Calcaneonavicular coalition: treatment by excision and fat graft. J Pediatr Orthop. 2009;29(5):418–26.
12. Takakura Y, Sugimoto K, Tanaka Y, Tamai S. Symptomatic talocalcaneal coalition its clinical significance and treatment. Clin Orthop. 1991;269:249–56.
13. Ford SE, Scannell BP. Pediatric flatfoot. Foot Ankle Clin. 2017;22(3):643–56.
14. Cowell H, Elener V. Rigid painful flatfoot secondary to tarsal coalition. Clin Orthop. 1993;177:54–60.
15. Davids JR, Gibson TW, Pugh LI. Quantitative segmental analysis of weight-bearing radiographs of the foot and ankle for children: normal alignment. J Pediatr Orthop. 2005;25(6):769–76.
16. Lee M, Harcke H, Bassett G. Subtalar joint coalition in children: new observations. Radiology. 1989;172(3):635–9.
17. Moraleda L, Gantsoudes GD, Mubarak SJ. C sign: talocalcaneal coalition or flatfoot deformity? J Pediatr Orthop. 2014;34(8):814–9.
18. Clarke DM. Multiple tarsal coalitions in the same foot. J Pediatr Orthop. 1997;17(6):777–80.
19. Whitford D, Esterman A. A randomized controlled trial of two types of in-shoe orthoses in children with flexible excess pronation of the feet. Foot Ankle Int. 2007;28(6):715–23.
20. Bauer K, Mosca VS, Zionts LE. What's new in pediatric flatfoot? J Pediatr Orthop. 2016;36(8):865–9.
21. Shirley E, Gheorghe R, Neal KM. Results of nonoperative treatment for symptomatic tarsal coalitions. Cureus. 2018;10(7):e2944.

22. Evans D. Calcaneo-valgus deformity. J Bone Joint Surg Br. 1975;57(3):270–8.
23. Mosca V. Calcaneal lengthening for valgus deformity of the hindfoot. Results in children who had severe, symptomatic flatfoot and skewfoot. JBJS. 1995;77(4):500–12.
24. Rathjen K, Mubarak SJ. Calcaneal-cuboid-cuneiform osteotomy for the correction of valgus foot deformities in children. J Pediatr Orthop. 1998;18(6):775–82.
25. Moraleda L, Salcedo M, Bastrom TP, Wenger DR, Albiñana J, Mubarak SJ. Comparison of the calcaneo-cuboid-cuneiform osteotomies and the calcaneal lengthening osteotomy in the surgical treatment of symptomatic flexible flatfoot. J Pediatr Orthop. 2012;32(8):821–9.
26. Ahn JY, Lee HS, Kim CH, Yang JP, Park SS. Calcaneocuboid joint subluxation after the calcaneal lengthening procedure in children. Foot Ankle Int. 2014;35(7):677–82.
27. Mosca VS. Principles and management of pediatric foot and ankle deformities and malformations. Philadelphia: Lippincott Williams & Wilkins; 2014.
28. Metcalfe SA, Bowling FL, Reeves ND. Subtalar joint arthroereisis in the management of pediatric flexible flatfoot: a critical review of the literature. Foot Ankle Int. 2011;32(12):1127–39.
29. Gantsoudes GD, Roocroft JH, Mubarak SJ. Treatment of talocalcaneal coalitions. J Pediatr Orthop. 2012;32(3):301–7.
30. Wilde P, Torode I, Dickens D, Cole W. Resection for symptomatic talocalcaneal coalition. J Bone Joint Surg Br. 1994;76(5):797–801.
31. Khoshbin A, Law PW, Caspi L, Wright JG. Long-term functional outcomes of resected tarsal coalitions. Foot Ankle Int. 2013;34(10):1370–5.
32. Mahan ST, Spencer SA, Vezeridis PS, Kasser JR. Patient-reported outcomes of tarsal coalitions treated with surgical excision. J Pediatr Orthop. 2015;35(6):583–8.
33. Kemppainen J, Pennock AT, Roocroft JH, Bastrom TP, Mubarak SJ. The use of a portable CT scanner for the intraoperative assessment of talocalcaneal coalition resections. J Pediatr Orthop. 2014;34(5):559–64.
34. Mosca VS, Bevan WP. Talocalcaneal tarsal coalitions and the calcaneal lengthening osteotomy: the role of deformity correction. JBJS. 2012;94(17):1584–94.
35. Masquijo J, Allende V, Torres-Gomez A, Dobbs MB. Fat graft and bone wax interposition provides better functional outcomes and lower reossification rates than extensor digitorum brevis after calcaneonavicular coalition resection. J Pediatr Orthop. 2017;37(7):e427–31.
36. Ettl V, Wollmerstedt N, Kirschner S, Morrison R, Pasold E, Raab P. Calcaneal lengthening for planovalgus deformity in children with cerebral palsy. Foot Ankle Int. 2009;30(5):398–404.
37. Saltzman CL, Fehrle MJ, Cooper RR, Spencer EC, Ponseti IV. Triple arthrodesis: twenty-five and forty-four-year average follow-up of the same patients. JBJS. 1999;81(10):1391–402.

Foot Osteochondrosis

Pablo J. Echenique Díaz and Pablo Schaufele Muñoz

1 Introduction

Osteochondrosis is a focused alteration of the endochondral ossification process. It is manifested by a variety of diseases that affect growing cartilage [1].

There are two areas of specialized growth cartilage present at the ends of developing bones: the physis, responsible for longitudinal growth, and the epiphyseal cartilage (epiphyseal-articular cartilage complex), responsible for the bone end shapes. In both areas, the growing cartilage is replaced by bone through a sequential process of cell proliferation, cell hypertrophy, extracellular matrix synthesis, and matrix mineralization, where vascular invasion contributes to endochondral ossification. Through this process, a continuous addition of cartilage is achieved, which will be replaced by bone, thus allowing the individual to carry weight while growing. Both the chondrocytes of the epiphysis and those of the physis are organized in different zones. The resting zone contains chondrocytes that divide slowly and are precursors of the proliferative zone, in which cells divide rapidly forming easily identifiable columns at the physiological level, while in the epiphyseal growth zones, this column formation is less obvious, and they tend to form groups. Finally, hypertrophic chondrocytes mature and secrete a highly specialized matrix, whose function is to promote calcification of the cartilage that serves as a template for bone formation by osteoblasts. In the calcification zone, the osteoclasts reabsorb the transverse septa, allowing vascular and osteoprogenitor cell invasion into

P. J. Echenique Díaz (✉)
Universidad Austral de Chile, Valdivia, Chile

Hospital Base Valdivia, Los Ríos, Chile

P. Schaufele Muñoz
Universidad de Concepción, Concepción, Chile

Hospital Clínico Regional de Concepción Dr. Guillermo Grant Benavente, Biobío, Chile

© The Author(s), under exclusive license to Springer Nature Switzerland AG 2022
E. Wagner Hitschfeld, P. Wagner Hitschfeld (eds.), *Foot and Ankle Disorders*,
https://doi.org/10.1007/978-3-030-95738-4_10

the gaps formed by the hypertrophic chondrocytes [2, 3]. Vascular endothelial growth factor secreted by mature chondrocytes appears to be the factor responsible for vascular invasion of growth cartilage, a factor necessary for endochondral ossification. When this angiogenesis is interrupted by any mechanism, whether genetic, biochemical, or mechanical, a thickening of the growth cartilage occurs due to the persistence and expansion of the hypertrophic layer (osteochondrosis) [4].

Multiple local factors have been identified as responsible for the proliferation and differentiation of chondrocytes and subsequent ossification at the growth plate. Thus, regulation mechanisms are described through expression mediators of at least 60 specific genes [5, 6], some of them related to osteochondrosis such as ATP6V0D2 and TMSB4. In addition, gene transcription factors and molecules secreted by chondrocytes and other perichondrial cells are part of this complicated local control network. The most important are Indian Hedgehog ligating protein (IHH), parathyroid hormone-related peptide (PTHrP), and transforming growth factor beta (TGF-beta).

There are other factors that may have a role in the etiology of osteochondrosis such as inheritance, anatomical features, repetitive trauma, dietary factors, and alterations in the irrigation of epiphyseal or physiological cartilage that coincide with the period of rapid growth. This pathology has been studied in animals and humans, finding similarities in its presentation and origin.

At least two hypotheses indicate a vascular origin of this alteration. The first one is based on a study carried out in birds, which experimentally demonstrates that when the apoptosis of the vascular endothelium that covers the vascular channels of the cartilage is artificially induced, a lesion of the surrounding cartilage is initiated that ends up showing an aspect very similar to the lesion observed in mammals. Hypothetically, a focused interruption of the irrigation of the growth cartilage causes the necrosis of the chondrocytes near the metaphyseal side of the physis (where the ischemia would be greater). This can create an abnormal bone matrix plate, impervious to penetration by the capillaries of the ossification front. Such a barrier would isolate a group of hypertrophic chondrocytes on the epiphysis side thus creating a thick mass of abnormal physiological cartilage in the affected area, stopping its ossification. The second vascular theory attributes repeated microtraumas to the metaphysical blood vessels that can disrupt the irrigation of the ossification front, causing a failure to differentiate hypertrophic cartilage and leaving an abnormally thickened area of physeal cartilage as a result. This theory is based on experimental studies and evidence from animal studies.

Siffert in 1981 classified osteochondroses into three groups [7]. The first group originates in the cartilage of the articular epiphyseal complex, basically secondary to necrosis of the articular hyaline cartilage or epiphyseal nucleus (Köhler's disease of the tarsal navicular, Freiberg's disease of the second metatarsal). The second group affects the growth cartilage of the apophyses that are zones of tendon insertion, being osteochondrosis by traction (Sever's disease of the calcaneus, Iselin's disease, Sinding-Larsen-Johansson's disease of the inferior pole of the patella). Finally a third group, that classifies alterations of the spine and long bones physis (Blount's disease, Scheuermann's disease).

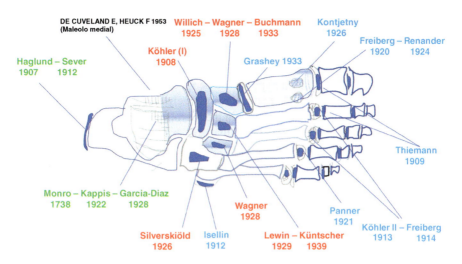

Fig. 1 Osteochondrosis of the foot bones described with author's name and date of publication. (Copyright 2020, Dr. Pablo Echenique Díaz. Used with permission from Dr. Pablo Schaufele Muñoz)

In this chapter the osteochondroses that are presented in the bones of the foot are reviewed (Fig. 1), except for the osteochondrosis and osteochondral lesions of the talus that will be the subject of another chapter of this work.

2   Diagnosis

The diagnosis of these diseases is eminently clinical, in the presence of pain in the growing foot, with its own characteristics for the different entities. In imaging studies [8], it is difficult to make a diagnosis in the early stages, with evidence of soft tissue edema and increased joint space. However, in more advanced stages, signs of necrosis are observed, with the appearance of sclerosis, irregularity of the edges of the ossification nuclei, fragmentation, deformity, and finally collapse. Later, scarring and recovery to its normal shape occur, which occurs during the remaining growth within months or years.

The radiographs in standard projections, comparative of both extremities, allow the follow-up.

Computed tomography (CT) can contribute to the differential diagnosis and quantify the three-dimensional extent of bone involvement. It allows evaluating the evolution of the fragmentation and articular free bodies and showing osteolytic images of another origin. It is also capable of defining in detail the resulting deformity.

Magnetic resonance imaging (MRI) is also useful for differential diagnosis. Usually, low-signal intensity images are observed in T1 and T2 sequences, consistent with avascular necrosis. In the early stages, the findings are variable and show the bone marrow with an isointense signal, highlighting a decreased signal area in T1-weighted images at the level of the transition zone between normal and ischemic tissue. Hyperintense images in T2 and STIR show diffuse edema, an early but unspecific finding. Therefore, there may be cases of heterogeneous images, depending on the degree of necrosis in the different areas of the affected bone. In addition, there is the sign of a double line in cancellous bone, evident in T2 sequence, with a hyperintense internal line and a hypointense peripheral line, which indicate hypervascular granulation tissue and necrosis, respectively. The addition of gadolinium would not produce signal reinforcement in the necrotic zone [9].

Nuclear medicine has been successfully used in the diagnosis of this type of disease [10], especially three-phase bone scintigraphy, with pinhole collimator-enhanced images, and tomographic images with SPECT. These tests demonstrate the lowest radiopharmaceutical uptake in necrotic bone and its recovery later in the healing stage. However, their specificity and sensitivity are surpassed by the MRI.

3 Sever's Disease

The picture of heel pain in children and adolescents was described initially by Haglund in 1907 and later characterized by Sever in 1912 as an inflammatory disease of the posterior process of the calcaneus, secondary ossification center in which the Achilles tendon is directly inserted.

This apophysitis of the calcaneus is the most frequent cause of pain in the heel in adolescents. It affects mainly to the active population of children between 6 and 13 years. The disease is intermittent and self-limited, without evidencing sequels, lasting until the physis closure. Although it has been demonstrated that it affects the quality of life of the affected ones, the parents are usually more worried than patients. Its prevalence goes between 2% and 16% of the consultations by muscular skeletal pathology in children, with bilateral presentation in 60–65% of the cases.

The apophysis grows on the posterior inferior part of the calcaneus, between 4 and 7 years in girls and between 7 and 10 years in boys. Characteristically it is developed from several nuclei of ossification that converge and fuse with the tuberosity of the calcaneus at the age of 12–13 years in girls and from 15 years in boys. The Achilles tendon is inserted in the cartilaginous surface of the most proximal portion of the apophysis, and the plantar fascia and the musculature originate in the lowest part of the apophysis [11].

The most accepted theory about the etiology of the calcaneal apophysitis is an overuse syndrome, related to chronic repeated microtraumas, by traction or impact along the calcaneal process, or through the union with the Achilles tendon. Intrinsic and extrinsic biomechanical alterations have been described in patients with Sever's disease. Intrinsic factors include increase in plantar pressure [12], greater body mass index, decreased capacity of impact absorption because of conditions like genu varum, cavus foot, flat foot and short Achilles tendon. On the other hand, extrinsic factors include, intense practice of sports with great impact such as jogging and jumping, sports on hard surfaces and the use of inadequate sports shoes. The repeated presence of these factors would take tissues to the limit, causing the appearance of injuries such as microfractures secondary to compression or traction.

The diagnosis of this disease is eminently clinical. It can affect one or both feet. The patients refer pain in the posterior plantar part of the heel, during physical activity and relieves with rest. Normally, they do not refer pain at night. Several weeks can pass before the first consultation. In the physical examination, there is absence of edema and erythema or increase in local temperature. Three diagnostic maneuvers have been validated with a high sensitivity and specificity [13]: (1) monopodal heel load (painful in 100% of cases). (2) pain on direct posterior calcaneus palpation (positive in 80% of cases), and (3) pain on simultaneous medial and lateral posterior calcaneal tuberosity compression (positive in 97% of cases).

The radiological findings in calcaneal apophysitis have been cause of controversy for decades. At the moment it is accepted that the greater radiological density of the apophysis compared with the calcaneal tuberosity is not an apophyisitis sign, but is secondary to the orientation of its trabeculae. Some trabeculae are oblique that provide resistance to the Achilles tendon traction and other perpendicular giving resistance to compression. Some authors describe fragmentation of the apophysis of the calcaneus, with the appearance of a fragment in the lowest part of the apophysis. Another interesting factor is that Sever's disease only appears in a specific period of development coinciding with the stages I to III of calcaneus ossification, described by Nicholson [14, 15]. Therefore, in patients with a suspicion of Sever's disease in a more advanced stage of ossification of the calcaneus, other etiologies must be ruled out. In MRI images it is possible to rule out other diagnoses and detect stress fractures (Fig. 2).

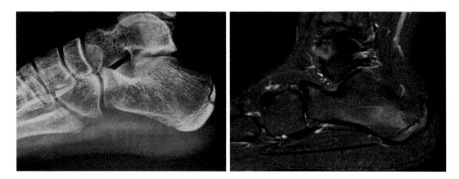

Fig. 2 Sever's disease in male patient with heel pain, fragmentation, and increase of radiological bone density is observed in posterior apophysis of the calcaneus, frequent finding in asymptomatic patients. MRI shows signs of bone edema in the posterior apophysis and in the posterior tuberosity around the physis. (Copyright 2020, Dr. Pablo Schaufele Muñoz. Used with permission from Dr. Pablo Schaufele Muñoz)

The treatment of this self-limited condition is aimed at reducing pain. The recommendation is to limit the sport activity that causes the symptoms, while the crisis lasts or until the child feels comfortable, or can change to another activity that produces less discomfort. Symptoms are intermittent and it is important to warn and educate family and sports coaches accordingly [16]. The use of sports shoes that reduce impact, viscoelastic heel pads, orthopedic insoles, therapeutic bandages in conjunction with local ice, nonsteroidal anti-inflammatory drugs, and elongation exercises for the gastro-soleus system are useful [17, 18]. In severe cases that do not respond to these measures, a walking boot or a plaster boot can be used for 2–4 weeks [19]. There are reports of the benefit of prolotherapy consisting of local injections of substances that would activate healing (good results in follow-up to 1 year in cases of Osgood Schlatter osteochondrosis) [20]. More studies of high methodological quality are needed to include this therapeutic alternative in the pediatric population with benign musculoskeletal pain refractory to treatment. The authors have an ongoing study of prolotherapy in Sever's disease (Dr Pablo Schaufele) with dextrose at 12.5% with promising results so far.

4 Köhler's Disease

Navicular osteochondrosis was described by Köhler in 1908. It has been described in children from 2 to 9 years of age. It is more common in boys than in girls (6:1), and it may present bilaterally in 20–30% of the cases. It refers to history of isolated trauma or repetitive microtraumas in 35–50% of the cases [21]. It is a self-limited condition and usually without sequelae. Köhler's disease has been associated with patients with delayed ossification of the navicular, which would increase the risk of injury due to ischemia or venous congestion in a mostly cartilaginous bone. The navicular is subject to continuous compression forces between the talus and the forefoot, that could end up in avascular necrosis. The extensive presence of blood vessels ensures the complete recovery of the bone structure.

The symptoms of Köhler's disease are gait claudication and occasionally inability to carry weight due to pain in the medial longitudinal arch of the foot. Edema, increased local temperature, and erythema may occur. Compression of the navicular and the talonavicular joint can be painful. If pain is found in the rest of the tarsal, subtalar, and talar joints, an inflammatory disease should be suspected. On the other hand, if a rigid flat foot is found, a tarsal coalition should be suspected. The laboratory tests and clinical evolution will serve to rule out cases of osteomyelitis or septic arthritis, which can also occur with pain and claudication in this area.

Two patterns of radiological presentation are described. The first is with an increase in the bone density of the navicular (sclerosis) without loss of shape. The second is characterized by thinning or flattening in the proximal-distal direction of

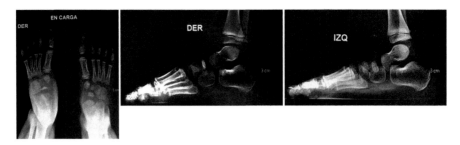

Fig. 3 Bilateral weight-bearing foot X-rays of a 4-year-old patient with Köhler's disease. Significant reduction in size and sclerosis of the navicular nucleus in the right foot (label DER) is observed. In addition, there is a slight tendency to cavus foot in the affected foot. (Copyright 2020, Dr. Pablo Echenique Díaz. Used with permission from Dr. Pablo Echenique Díaz)

the navicular (Fig. 3). In cases where the diagnosis is doubtful, the CT or MRI study can be useful, allowing the identification of arthritis, posterior tibial tendonitis, os naviculare, infection, tarsal coalition, or tumor pathology. It is recommended that radiographic control be performed for follow-up until healing, which usually takes up to a year. After 6 months to 4 years from the onset of symptoms, the radiological appearance becomes normal [22].

Treatment of Köhler's disease consists of immobilization with a short walking boot for 4–8 weeks, with unloading and use of canes if necessary. After this, the use of an insole or brace with medial arch support is recommended. In most cases, when the cast is removed, the foot is already asymptomatic [23]. Exceptional cases are described that result in degenerative changes in the talonavicular joint, which could require surgery in the long term.

5 Freiberg's Disease

Alfred Freiberg [24] reported in 1914 a series of six patients who presented a similar pattern of infarction of the second metatarsal head, with flattening and collapse of the head resulting in progressive degenerative changes.

Freiberg's disease [25] is the fourth most frequent osteochondrosis. It is described as a condition of the heads of the minor metatarsals. It involves almost exclusively the head of the second metatarsal (80%), rarely the third metatarsal (27%), and more rarely the fourth or fifth metatarsal (3%). It is usually unilateral and affects only one metatarsal. It is the only osteochondrosis that preferentially affects the female sex (5:1), between 10 and 18 years of age, the majority of cases being around 12 years of age. The disease can remain asymptomatic for a long time, being diagnosed in older patients by presenting symptoms in advanced stages.

It most frequently affects patients who present a short first metatarsal, an unfavorable biomechanical situation that results in a second metatarsal overload. In addition, the second ray is the least mobile of the forefoot, exposing it increased pressure, thus contributing to the disease. The metatarsal heads have two sources of arterial irrigation, the dorsal metatarsal arteries, originating from the dorsalis pedis artery, and the plantar metatarsal arteries, originating from the posterior tibial artery. These vessels are anastomosed in two places near the metatarsal heads in a vascular ring, forming an extensive extra-bony arterial network around them. Small branches of this network run distally and penetrate the metaphysis near the insertion of the joint capsule and ligaments. This network irrigates the distal metaphysis, the growth cartilage, the epiphyseal growth nucleus, and the subchondral bone of the epiphysis [26]. Villadot and Villadot proposed that mechanical compression and repeated trauma of the arteries that irrigate the metatarsal head can cause vessel spasm and thrombosis of these vessels, with consequent necrosis of the metatarsal head. Possible causes have also been linked to vascular anatomical variations, iatrogenic complication, diabetes mellitus, systemic lupus erythematosus, and hypercoagulability syndromes.

The diagnosis of Freiberg's disease is based on clinical history, physical examination, and radiological findings. Patients typically report intermittent pain and limited mobility of the affected metatarsophalangeal joint. In some cases, they report a history of trauma prior to the onset of symptoms. Pain increases with activity or weight-bearing and is relieved by rest. Discomfort increases when wearing high-heeled shoes or walking barefoot.

A mild limp is found secondary to pain, increased temperature and soft tissue edema. These findings are secondary to metatarsophalangeal joint synovitis. Pain can be elicited by dorsal or plantar palpation of the affected metatarsal joint.

Early stage radiological studies can only identify an increase in the space of the involved metatarsophalangeal joint and signs of edema of the periarticular soft tissues. In advanced stages, X-rays show sclerosis and flattening due to collapse of the metatarsal head. In lateral oblique projection, more information can be obtained about the extent of the metatarsal head damage. MRI is useful for the differential diagnosis in early stages, in which X-rays are normal, doubtful, or with atypical changes. It should be noted that a normal variant with bilateral flattening of the head of the second metatarsal associated with a widening of the joint space has been reported as a finding in asymptomatic patients. Differential diagnoses are stress fractures of the metatarsals, osteomyelitis of the metatarsal head, idiopathic metatarsophalangeal synovitis or capsulitis, tendonitis of extensors or flexors, injury of collateral ligaments or plantar plate of the metatarsophalangeal joint, Morton's neuroma, metatarsalgia or stress injury, juvenile idiopathic arthritis or Still's disease, and subacute inflammatory periostitis, among others.

In 1957, Smillie [27] described the first classification of Freiberg's disease, still in use (Fig. 4). In stage I, a subchondral fracture is observed in the ischemic and sclerotic epiphysis. In stage II there is an alteration of the articular surface of the epiphysis. After the cancellous bone resorption, the central part of the metatarsal head begins to collapse, leaving a bone bridge in the plantar area unharmed. Progressive bone resorption gives way to stage III, which is when the metatarsal head sinks into the metatarsal neck, keeping the neck edges intact but prominent on

Fig. 4 Diagram of Smillie's classification in five progressive stages for Freiberg's disease, useful in treatment planning. Upper row: anteroposterior metatarsal view. Lower row: lateral metatarsal view. (Copyright 2020, Dr. Pablo Schaufele Muñoz. Used with permission from Dr. Pablo Schaufele Muñoz)

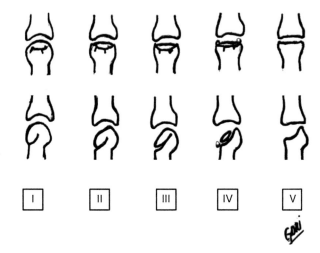

each side. In stage IV, the plantar rim collapses and a subchondral fracture occurs, creating free articular fragments. The anatomy is lost. In stage V, the final stage, osteoarthritis appears, with marked flattening and deformity of the metatarsal head with joint space narrowing.

Although there are no prospective studies to determine the effectiveness of conservative management of Freiberg's disease, most authors recommend it in Smillie stages I to III [28]. The success of the conservative treatment is related to the progression of the disease, having great importance to the early diagnosis, despite the fact that most of the symptomatic patients have radiological evidence of articular free bodies (stage IV), while most of the asymptomatic patients did not have free bodies. Immobilization, discharge, and activity restriction are the pillars of conservative treatment in the acute stage. The use of a walker boot or surgical shoe, with or without canes, is recommended for a period of 2–6 weeks, or until symptoms subside. Alternative treatments such as corticosteroid and anesthetic infiltrations, nonsteroidal anti-inflammatory analgesics, physiotherapy, and ultrasound have been described as effective in the acute phase of the disease. The patient should be advised to limit participation in sports and not to wear high-heeled shoes until the disease is completely resolved. Alternative low-impact activities such as swimming, cycling, and water aerobics are recommended for very active adolescents. To decrease the pressure on the affected metatarsal head, the use of a brace or insole is recommended to elevate and thus unload the metatarsal head. This, in combination with stretching exercises, can alleviate pain and prevent the claw deformity of the affected toe. Shoes with thick, rigid soles or rocker bottoms are also useful. It is recommended to maintain this treatment until radiological evidence of healing, which usually takes 2–3 years.

Surgical management is indicated in advanced cases (stages IV and V) and in those that do not respond to conservative management. The surgical techniques described can be divided into two groups: those that preserve the joint and those that sacrifice the joint. There is no consensus on which procedure to choose. Recent studies show that the techniques that preserve the joint would have better results (over 90% success) in relation to those that sacrifice the joint (70% success) [29], so the latter would be less recommended. The surgical complications are persistence of pain, joint stiffness, floating toe, transfer metatarsalgia, dorsiflexion weakness and painful scar.

Freiberg recommended removal of the free joint bodies. Many authors agree with this behavior, noting improvement of symptoms in most cases. Other authors also recommend a partial synovectomy. It has also been proposed to add a head decompression, performed by perforating it with a drill or Kirschner wire. This procedure should be performed preferably before significant structural changes occur showing good results [30].

According to Smillie, a devitalized bone curettage, reduction of the collapsed joint surface, and filling of the defect with autologous cancellous bone graft should be considered. This principle has been considered in recent works applying the technique of osteochondral autotransplantation and replacement with osteogenic implants [31]. In 1979, Gauthier [32] designed a dorsal closing wedge osteotomy of the metatarsal neck, as a variation of a Weil's osteotomy, including part of the necrotic zone and also resecting free bodies and osteophytes. This technique manages to dorsally rotate the intact plantar articular cartilage. Given its good results, it has become the most used technique nowadays, being used as reference to evaluate other techniques (Fig. 5). Different forms of fixation are described, from sutures, cerclages, Kirschner wires, resorbable wires, plates, and screws, all with good results and few complications [33, 34]. These osteotomies produce shortening, either by resecting a segment of the metatarsal neck or by sliding. This shortening

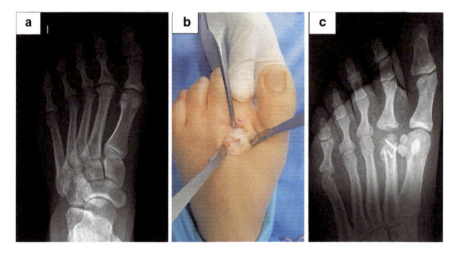

Fig. 5 (**a**) 24-year-old patient with Freiberg's disease in stage IV. (**b**) Debridement of free articular fragments and necrotic bone was performed. (**c**) Finally, a dorsal subtraction wedge osteotomy was performed, fixed with two mini fragment screws, which allows dorsal reorientation of the articular surface. (Copyright 2020, Dr. Pablo Echenique Díaz. Used with permission from Dr. Pablo Echenique Díaz)

is 2.3 mm on average, with few clinical consequences. Pedobarographic studies have shown a reduction in the pressure load on the operated metatarsal. The appearance of floating toes is reported as a complication, but the appearance of transfer metatarsalgia is not mentioned. Osteotomies without fixation have been used, but it has not proven to be the optimal approach to the problem.

Kehr [35], in 1982, described an interposition arthroplasty for Freiberg's disease. This technique is recommended if the whole joint surface is compromised. After debridement of the metatarsal head, the extensor tendon and the joint capsule are interposed in the joint. An alternative to this procedure is to perform a "U" capsulotomy which is placed over the metatarsal head, holding it in place with a pull-out suture on the sole of the foot, over a button or pad. It is also possible to carve a periosteal and adipose flap, with less morbidity and excellent results [36]. In recent years, mini-invasive arthroscopic techniques have been developed, performing the interposition of the extensor digitorum brevis for this purpose, with good results [37].

Historically, the resection of the metatarsal head was reported. This technique leads to the appearance of transfer metatarsalgia and hyperkeratosis, shortened and floating toe, hallux valgus, alteration of the metatarsal parabola, and gait alteration. It has been proposed to perform joint replacement arthroplasties [38], with total silicone prosthesis or partial prosthesis, which could work in some patients. However, in young and active patients, complications are frequent: bone resorption at the interface with the implant, loosening and fracture of the prosthesis that forces the removal of the implant, synovitis, stiffness, loss of stability, floating toe, etc. Recently it has been reported the use of synthetic joint covering implants (NEXA OsteocureTM [39], Cartiva [40]) initially designed for the treatment of hallux rigidus, with good results. Prospective, comparative studies are needed to weigh the results and draw conclusions. In joints with very severe osteoarthritis, with or without dorsal toe dislocation, another option is to perform a debridement of the metatarsal head and resection of the base of the proximal phalanx, in conjunction with syndactylization to the adjacent toe. This procedure can improve symptoms and preserves the metatarsal parabola.

6   Iselin's Disease

In 1912, Hans Iselin described a traction apophysitis at the base of the fifth metatarsal. It occurs infrequently in adolescent athletes and is more common in boys than in girls. It is a benign and self-limited condition, caused by the traction of the peroneus brevis, whose tendon is inserted into it [41]. The apophysis is located longitudinally on the lateral plantar surface at the fifth metatarsal base. Sports that involve running, jumping, or lateral pivoting movements can predispose child to develop this disease, but it must be distinguished from other pathologies of the base of the fifth metatarsal, such as acute or stress fractures, and supernumerary bones (os vesalianum). The diagnosis is clinical and radiological [42]. The symptoms are pain at the base of the fifth metatarsal, which is exacerbated with activity and subsides with rest. Palpation of the tuberosity can reproduce the pain. Increased local temperature, erythema, and edema can be found. Eversion against resistance and maximum foot inversion can also evoke the symptoms [43]. It appears normally at age 10 in girls and at age 12 in boys. A thin ossification is observed with an oblique orientation to the axis of the diaphysis, located at the lateral plantar edge of the proximal tuberosity of the fifth metatarsal. The secondary nucleus fuses with the rest of the metatarsal about 2–4 years after its appearance [44]. Treatment consists of limiting physical activity and restraining from sport. Functional bandaging and foot orthoses can decrease the traction of the peroneus brevis tendon. In refractory cases, a short walking cast boot can be used for 2–4 weeks [45]. Surgical treatment has been reported in an exceptional way, with resection of loose bone fragments and fenestrations that accelerate the fusion of the apophysis.

7   Cuneiform Osteochondrosis

An extremely rare disease, cuneiform osteochondrosis first reported in 1930 by Harbin M. and Zollinger R. [46] and later by Buchman J. [47] in 1933. It most often affects boys (80%) between 5 and 13 years of age (most often 4–6 years). Most cases correspond to the medial cuneiform [48], to a lesser extent to the middle and rarely to the lateral. It can be bilateral in half of the cases. Patients report discomfort around the medial or dorsal side of the midfoot. The pain increases with activity and is relieved with rest. It has been postulated that this disease may be underdiagnosed, given the age of the patients and the null or low intensity of the symptoms. In X-rays, a decrease in the size of the affected cuneiform is characteristic of the disease. The changes are recovered within 6–24 months. It is possible to find its association with navicular osteochondrosis. Consider differential diagnosis with lesions that may have a similar radiological appearance (Ewing's sarcoma, eosinophilic granuloma) and rule out osteomyelitis. An erroneous diagnosis can delay treatment or subject the patient to unnecessary surgery. Treatment is aimed at reducing impact, activities, and treating pain [49].

8   De Cuveland's Disease

It is an osteochondrosis of the tibial medial malleolus described in 1953 [50]. The triggers of this condition would be the sport, especially with boot-type footwear, the calcaneus valgus, and the presence of an accessory nucleus of ossification. Clinically it is characterized by pain and slight local soft tissue edema, presenting pain to palpation and with foot eversion. In the radiography, irregular ossification is evident, and many times the presence of an accessory ossification nucleus can be seen [51]. The MRI helps with diagnostic confirmation and shows malleolar fragmentation and bone edema. The treatment is symptomatic, sport rest, with improvement in 100% of the cases [52].

9 Sesamoid Osteochondrosis

The medial sesamoid is the most affected, described in 1925 by A. Renander, who published two cases. It is characterized by pain at progressive pressure and stress-related discomfort, especially with dorsiflexion of the first toe. Foot radiograph shows a fragmented bone, sclerotic and slightly enlarged or reduced. Changes are evident 6–12 months after symptoms start. MRI confirms the previous diagnosis, showing bone fragmentation and edema. The differential diagnosis is with sesamoid bone fracture, sesamoiditis, arthritic changes, and bi- or tripartite sesamoid. The treatment is based on rest and orthoses (cushioning or unloading insoles) with very good response. The few cases that do not respond are managed with walking boots or short boot casts. In rare cases, sesamoidectomy is necessary [53].

10 Osteochondrosis of the First Metatarsal Base

Described by Grashey in 1933, it occurs between the ages of 6 and 13 years [54]. It is characterized by insidious discomfort or pain and swelling over the base of the first metatarsal which interrupts physical activity. The radiography shows a fragmented, dense, and flattened epiphysis. Its treatment includes non weight bearing in a boot for 3 weeks. Its resolution takes between 4 and 6 months.

11 Osteochondrosis of the First Metatarsal Head

First described by Kontjetny and Wagner [55] in the years 1927 and 1930, respectively. Clinically it is similar to Freiberg's disease, characterized by first metatarsophalangeal joint swelling and increased local temperature. Pain at palpation and mobilization of the joint is always present. The radiographic study may initially show an increase in comparative size of the head of the affected metatarsal and a subchondral radiolucent line, to later account for signs of necrosis and lytic changes. MRI shows bone edema. The recommended treatment is non-weight-bearing, rest, and analgesia. Then, at 10–12 weeks, it is changed to partial load with a walking boot. The pain resolves completely within 6–8 months. However, there is a chance of having persistent pain, even requiring surgery. Smillie's classification for Freiberg's disease, which is also used for osteochondrosis of the third metatarsal head (Panner) and the fourth and fifth metatarsal head (Ehrlach), is useful in deciding on the indication for surgery.

12 Thiemann's Disease

It is a form of genetic multifocal osteochondrosis [56] to be considered in the differential diagnosis of juvenile arthritis. Described in 1909, it is considered an idiopathic avascular necrosis with progressive affection of the interphalangeal joints (feet and hands). It can start at 4 years old, but the usual age of onset is around 13 years old. It is characterized by a painless increase in volume in the proximal interphalangeal joint; however, it can present as a painful swelling with joint stiffness that increases with cold. The radiological image shows alterations in the epiphysis and metaphysis of the phalanxes (of the feet and hands), with widening, flattening, and the appearance of scalloped and irregular edges. Its handling is symptomatic and has a favorable evolution.

13 Summary

Osteochondroses are a group of abnormalities of the endochondral ossification process of the growing skeleton. We will review the current knowledge and most accepted theories about the etiology and treatment of those that occur in the ankle and foot. Most of these diseases are rare and produce self-limited pain and functional limitation.

References

1. Achar S, Yamanaka J. Apophysitis and osteochondrosis: common causes of pain in growing bones. Am Fam Physician. 2019;99(10):610–8.
2. McCoy AM, Toth F, Dolvik NI, Ekman S, Ellermann J, Olstad K, Ytrehus B, Carlson CS. Articular osteochondrosis: a comparison of naturally-occurring human and animal disease. Osteoarthr Cartil. 2013;21(11):1638–47.
3. Ytrehus B, Carlson CS, Ekman S. Etiology and pathogenesis of osteochondrosis. Vet Pathol. 2007;44(4):429–48. https://doi.org/10.1354/vp.44-4-429.
4. Sun MM, Beier F. Chondrocyte hypertrophy in skeletal development, growth, and disease. Birth Defects Res C Embryo Today. 2014;102(1):74–82.
5. Mirams M, Ayodele BA, Tatarczuch L, Henson FM, Pagel CN, Mackie EJ. Identification of novel osteochondrosis – associated genes. J Orthop Res. 2016;34(3):404–11.
6. Liu CF, Samsa WE, Zhou G, Lefebvre V. Transcriptional control of chondrocyte specification and differentiation. Semin Cell Dev Biol. 2017;62:34–49.

7. Siffert RS. Classification of the osteochondroses. Clin Orthop Relat Res. 1981;158:10–8.
8. West EY, Jaramillo D. Imaging of osteochondrosis. Pediatr Radiol. 2019;49(12):1610–6.
9. Enge Junior DJ, Fonseca EKUN, Castro ADAE, Baptista E, Santos DDCB, Rosemberg LA. Avascular necrosis: radiological findings and main sites of involvement – pictorial essay. Radiol Bras. 2019;52(3):187–92.
10. Danger F, Wasyliw C, Varich L. Osteochondroses. Semin Musculoskelet Radiol. 2018;22(1):118–24.
11. Arbab D, Wingenfeld C, Rath B, Lüring C, Quack V, Tingart M. Osteochondrosen des kindlichen Fußes [Osteochondrosis of the pediatric foot]. Orthopade. 2013;42(1):20–9. German.
12. Rodríguez-Sanz D, Becerro-de-Bengoa-Vallejo R, López-López D, Calvo-Lobo C, Martínez-Jiménez EM, Perez-Boal E, Losa-Iglesias ME, Palomo-López P. Slow velocity of the center of pressure and high heel pressures may increase the risk of Sever's disease: a case-control study. BMC Pediatr. 2018;18(1):357.
13. Perhamre S, Lazowska D, Papageorgiou S, Lundin F, Klässbo M, Norlin R. Sever's injury: a clinical diagnosis. J Am Podiatr Med Assoc. 2013;103(5):361–8.
14. Duong M, Nicholson A, Li S, Gilmore A, Cooperman D, Liu R. Relationship of Sever's disease with skeletal maturity and implications for radiographic findings. Pediatrics. 2018;142 (1_MeetingAbstract):278.
15. Nicholson AD, Liu RW, Sanders JO, Cooperman DR. Relationship of calcaneal and iliac apophyseal ossification to peak height velocity timing in children. J Bone Joint Surg Am. 2015;97(2):147–54.
16. James AM, Williams CM, Haines TP. Health related quality of life of children with calcaneal apophysitis: child & parent perceptions. Health Qual Life Outcomes. 2016;14:95.
17. James AM, Williams CM, Haines TP. Effectiveness of footwear and foot orthoses for calcaneal apophysitis: a 12-month factorial randomised trial. Br J Sports Med. 2016;50(20):1268–75.
18. Wiegerinck JI, Zwiers R, Sierevelt IN, van Weert HC, van Dijk CN, Struijs PA. Treatment of calcaneal apophysitis: wait and see versus orthotic device versus physical therapy: a pragmatic therapeutic randomized clinical trial. J Pediatr Orthop. 2016;36(2):152–7.
19. Ramponi DR, Baker C. Sever's disease (calcaneal apophysitis). Adv Emerg Nurs J. 2019;41(1):10–4.
20. Topol GA, Podesta LA, Reeves KD, Raya MF, Fullerton BD, Yeh HW. Hyperosmolar dextrose injection for recalcitrant Osgood-Schlatter disease. Pediatrics. 2011;128(5):e1121–8.
21. Chan JY, Young JL. Köhler disease: avascular necrosis in the child. Foot Ankle Clin. 2019;24(1):83–8.
22. Tuthill HL, Finkelstein ER, Sanchez AM, Clifford PD, Subhawong TK, Jose J. Imaging of tarsal navicular disorders: a pictorial review. Foot Ankle Spec. 2014;7(3):211–25.
23. Sferopoulos NK. Tarsal navicular osteonecrosis in children. Int J Ortho Res. 2019;2(1):1–5.
24. Freiberg A. Infraction of the second metatarsal bone a typical injury. Surg Gynecol Obstet. 1914;19:191–3.
25. Carter KR, Chambers AR, Dreyer MA. Freiberg infarction. [Updated 2020 Aug 10]. In: StatPearls [Internet]. Treasure Island: StatPearls Publishing; 2020 Jan-.
26. Petersen WJ, Lankes JM, Paulsen F, Hassenpflug J. The arterial supply of the lesser metatarsal heads: a vascular injection study in human cadavers. Foot Ankle Int. 2002;23(6):491–5.
27. Smillie IS. Freiberg's infarction. J Bone Joint Surg (Br). 1957;39:580.
28. Longworth R, Short L, Horwood A. Conservative treatment of Freiberg's infraction using foot orthoses: a tale of two prescriptions presented as a case study to open debate. The Foot (Edinb). 2019;41:59–62.
29. Schade VL. Surgical management of Freiberg's infraction: a systematic review. Foot Ankle Spec. 2015;8(6):498–519.
30. Viladot A, Sodano L, Marcellini L. Joint debridement and microfracture for treatment late-stage Freiberg-Kohler's disease: long-term follow-up study. Foot Ankle Surg. 2019;25(4):457–61.
31. Miyamoto W, Takao M, Miki S, Kawano H. Midterm clinical results of osteochondral autograft transplantation for advanced stage Freiberg disease. Int Orthop. 2016;40(5):959–64.

32. Gauthier G, Elbaz R. Freiberg's infraction: a subchondral bone fatigue fracture. A new surgical treatment. Clin Orthop Relat Res. 1979;(142):93–5.
33. Trnka HJ, Lara JS. Freiberg's infraction: surgical options. Foot Ankle Clin. 2019;24(4):669–76.
34. Balakumar B, Maripuri SN, Kotecha A, et al. The functional outcome of four-in-one technique: dorsal closing-wedge & shortening osteotomy, debridement, micro-fracture in the treatment of Freiberg's disease. MOJ Clin Med Case Rep. 2017;7(6):315–9.
35. Kehr LE. A new surgical technique for the correction of Freiberg's deformity. J Am Podiatry Assoc. 1982;72(3):130–4.
36. Abdul W, Hickey B, Perera A. Functional outcomes of local pedicle graft interpositional arthroplasty in adults with severe Freiberg's disease. Foot Ankle Int. 2018;39(11):1290–300.
37. Lui TH. Arthroscopic interpositional arthroplasty of the second metatarsophalangeal joint. Arthrosc Tech. 2016;5(6):e1333–8.
38. Miller ML, Lenet MD, Sherman M. Surgical treatment of Freiberg's infraction with the use of total joint replacement arthroplasty. J Foot Surg. 1984;23(1):35–40.
39. Kilmartin TE, Posmyk L. Synthetic cartilage implant hemiarthroplasty for second MTP joint osteoarthrosis. J Foot Ankle Surg. 2020;59(5):942–8.
40. Brandao B, Fox A, Pillai A. Comparing the efficacy of Cartiva synthetic cartilage implant hemiarthroplasty vs osteotomy for the treatment of conditions affecting the second metatarsal head. Foot (Edinb). 2019;41:30–3.
41. Forrester RA, Eyre-Brook AI, Mannan K. Iselin's disease: a systematic review. J Foot Ankle Surg. 2017;56(5):1065–9.
42. Kishan TV, Mekala A, Bonala N, Sri PB. Iselin's disease: traction apophysitis of the fifth metatarsal base, a rare cause of lateral foot pain. Med J Armed Forces India. 2016;72(3):299–301.
43. Deniz G, Kose O, Guneri B, Duygun F. Traction apophysitis of the fifth metatarsal base in a child: Iselin's disease. BMJ Case Rep. 2014;2014:bcr2014204687.
44. Ralph BG, Barrett J, Kenyhercz C, DiDomenico LA. Iselin's disease: a case presentation of nonunion and review of the differential diagnosis. J Foot Ankle Surg. 1999;38(6):409–16.
45. Sylvester JE, Hennrikus WL. Treatment outcomes of adolescents with Iselin's apophysitis. J Pediatr Orthop B. 2015;24(4):362–5.
46. Harbin M, Zollinger R. Osteochondritis of the growth centers. Surg Gynec Obstet. 1930;51:145–61.
47. Buchman J. Osteochondritis of the internal cuneiform. J Bone Joint Surg Am. 1933;15:225–32.
48. Godoy IRB, Yamada AF, Skaf A. MRI findings of intermediate cuneiform osteochondrosis as a rare cause of foot pain in a child. Radiol Case Rep. 2020;15(6):765–8.
49. Sferopoulos NK. Juvenile osteochondrosis of the cuneiform bones. Clin Res Pediatr. 2019;2(2):1–4.
50. de Cuveland E, Heuck F. Osteochondropathie eines akzessorischen Knochenkernes am Malleolus tibiae (des sog. Os subtibiale) [Osteochondropathy of accessory apophyseal ossification center on malleolus tibiae, so-called os subtibiale]. Fortschr Geb Rontgenstr. 1953;79(6):728–32. Undetermined Language.
51. Turati M, Glard Y, Griffet J, Afonso D, Courvoisier A, Bigoni M. Osteochondrosis of the medial malleolar epiphysis: a case report and review of the literature. Int J Surg Case Rep. 2017;39:176–80.
52. Farsetti P, Dragoni M, Potenza V, Caterini R. Osteochondrosis of the accessory ossification centre of the medial malleolus. J Pediatr Orthop B. 2015;24(1):28–30.
53. Bartosiak K, McCormick JJ. Avascular necrosis of the sesamoids. Foot Ankle Clin. 2019;24(1):57–67.
54. Souverijns G, Peene P, Cleeren P, Raes M, Steenwerckx A. Avascular necrosis of the epiphysis of the first metatarsal bone. Skelet Radiol. 2002;31(6):366–8.
55. Wagner A. Isolated aseptic necrosis in the epiphysis of the first metatarsal bone. Acta Radiol. 1930;os-11(1):80–7.
56. Damseh N, Stimec J, O'Brien A, Marshall C, Savarirayan R, Jawad A, Laxer R, Kannu P. Thiemann disease and familial digital arthropathy – brachydactyly: two sides of the same coin? Orphanet J Rare Dis. 2019;14(1):156.

Fibular Hemimelia: Principles and Techniques of Management

Philip K. McClure and John E. Herzenberg

1 Introduction

Fibular hemimelia (FH), also known as congenital fibular deficiency, has an annual incidence of approximately one in 50,000 live births (~75 cases per year in the United States; about 330 cases per year in Latin America and the Caribbean) [1]. The classic hallmark is a variable degree of absence of the fibula. In some cases, however, the fibula appears near normal in length and shape. The degree of fibular involvement does not necessarily predict the severity of other, arguably more important, factors.

The known manifestations of fibular hemimelia include foot deformity (equinovalgus and sometimes equinovarus), central or lateral ray deficiency, tarsal coalitions, ankle stiffness/deformity, anteromedial tibial bowing, cruciate ligament insufficiency or absence, genu valgum (often due to hypoplastic lateral femoral condyle), and leg length discrepancy. The skin at the apex of the tibial bow often has a characteristic dimple. While it is primarily a unilateral lower extremity phenomenon, upper extremity manifestations may include syndactyly, cleft hand, and ulnar hemimelia [2, 3]. Bilateral cases occur but are less common than unilateral cases. Rodriguez-Ramirez et al. [4] examined the prevalence of associated congenital osseous anomalies in patients with fibular hemimelia and found that lateral femoral condyle hypoplasia was the most common associated anomaly (93%) followed by ball-and-socket ankle joint (80%), congenital short femur (72%), tarsal coalition (51%), and forefoot ray deletion (44%) [4]. While ray deficiency has often been assumed to be limited to the lateral rays, a subset of patients have intact lateral

P. K. McClure (✉) · J. E. Herzenberg
International Center for Limb Lengthening, Rubin Institute for Advanced Orthopedics, Sinai Hospital of Baltimore, Baltimore, MD, USA
e-mail: Pmcclure@lifebridgehealth.org; jherzenb@lifebridgehealth.org; http://www.limblength.org; http://www.limblength.org

E. Wagner Hitschfeld, P. Wagner Hitschfeld (eds.), *Foot and Ankle Disorders*, https://doi.org/10.1007/978-3-030-95738-4_11

Fig. 1 Ten-month-old female with fibular hemimelia (FH) and congenital femoral deficiency (CFD). AP (**a**) and lateral (**b**) view radiographs demonstrate leg length discrepancy, anterior bowing of the tibia, and equinus position of the foot. (**c**) and (**d**) Two-year-old with FH and CFD. Mild genu valgum and ankle valgus are present on AP and lateral view long leg images. (**e**) and (**f**) Twelve-year-old with limb length discrepancy, genu valgum, and talocalcaneal coalition with resultant ball-and-socket ankle joint. (Used with permission from the Rubin Institute for Advanced Orthopedics, Sinai Hospital of Baltimore)

columns and appear to have central ray deletions [5]. Equinovalgus is much more common than equinovarus. Absence of the anterior cruciate ligament (ACL) is common and may require reconstruction, either as a preparatory surgery for lengthening or for symptomatic treatment of instability. ACL deficiency can contribute to anterior subluxation of the tibia during tibial lengthening due to the deforming force of the proximal gastrocnemius tendons that cross the knee to insert on the posterior femoral condyles.

Fibular hemimelia has a very broad phenotype, as demonstrated in Fig. 1. This spectrum should be considered carefully in the settings of family preferences, functional needs, anticipated outcomes, and available resources. It is safe to say that if a surgeon always treats fibular hemimelia using the same formulaic method, at least some of the patients are being poorly served. Not every case is reconstructible to the level of desired function, nor is amputation an appropriate automatic response to all cases. Careful assessment of the patient is required, but extensive discussion with family and caregivers is equally important for appropriate care. Prosthetic-mediated reconstruction (amputation) is widely available in the United States and has predictable outcomes in most surgeons' experience [3, 6–14]. Limb reconstruction requires more from all parties involved, including the family, the patient, the surgeon, and the therapists. Similar to traumatic reconstruction, the end outcomes remain similar in the short to medium term: true long-term outcomes are not yet available for either route of treatment [10, 13].

Ideally, the patient and family will meet with a surgeon who is experienced in both amputation and reconstruction early in the child's first year of life. While there is generally no need for early intervention (prior to 1 year of age), developing a trusting relationship is critical to optimize the care delivered. The surgeon must strive to understand the family's desires (and the realism thereof), while delivering realistic expectations and risks for both pathways. Whether reconstruction or amputation is chosen, the patient will require a long-term care relationship with a dedicated physician and medical team.

2   Classification

Classifications are an important component of any orthopedic pathology. In the effort to categorize, these systems can serve two major functions: demonstrating the spectrum of disease and directing treatment depending on classification type. In the

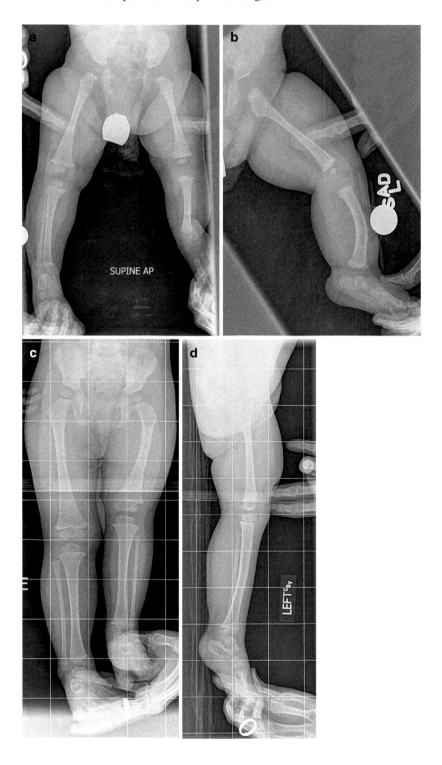

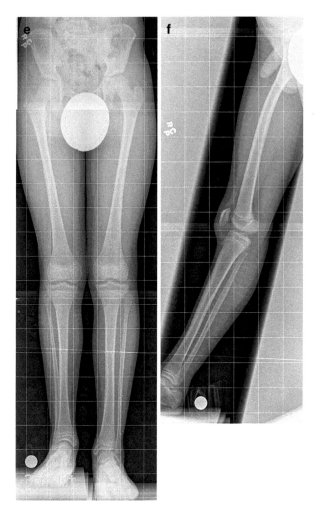

Fig. 1 (continued)

end, classifications are simply educational tools intended to highlight important components of the pathology at hand. While some are closer than others to directing treatment, classifications should not be used as a cookbook. The only recipe for success in complex congenital deformity is an in-depth understanding of the pathology, investing appropriate time to understand the patient's/family's goals, and careful execution of surgical techniques. Where the goals of treatment are function based, classification systems are required that evaluate the potential functional contributions of each component of fibular hemimelia rather than encouraging myopic focus on individual variations.

Coventry and Johnson developed the first classification system for fibular hemimelia and separated their cohort into three groups (Fig. 2) [15]:

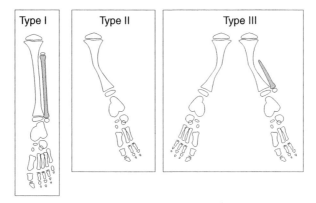

Fig. 2 Coventry and Johnson classification of fibular hemimelia: Type 1: unilateral fibular deficiency (partial), mild bowing and/or shortening, and mild-to-no foot deformity. Type 2: total or near total fibular absence, skin dimpling at the apex of the anterior tibial bow, deformed foot and ankle with absent rays. Type 3: bilateral Type 1 or Type 2 deformities, or association with other congenital differences. (Copyright 2020, Rubin Institute for Advanced Orthopedics, Sinai Hospital of Baltimore)

- Type 1: Partial unilateral absence of fibula; normal or slight bowing of the tibia with some shortening of the limb; the foot is normal or slightly deformed.
- Type 2: Fibula is completely or almost absent; anterior bowing of the tibia with skin dimpling; deformed ankle joint; deformed foot with absent rays.
- Type 3: Bilateral Type 1 or 2.

While this classification highlights a subset of known pathology present in fibular hemimelia, the focus on the amount of fibula present is of historical interest only. Perhaps the most important component is the focus on the amount of deformity in the foot/ankle.

The Achterman and Kalamchi classification, proposed in 1979, moved even further away from a functional assessment of the limb (Fig. 3) [16]. The simplicity of the classification system makes it attractive to orthopedists who do not routinely evaluate FH, but the utility is questionable. They divided the patients into two groups with one subdivision:

- Type 1: Incomplete fibular deficiency

  - 1A: Proximal fibular epiphysis distal to proximal tibial epiphysis, distal fibular physis proximal to dome of talus
  - 1B: 30–50% shortening of the fibula without a distal talofibular articulation.

- Type 2: Complete fibular deficiency, with or without a small distal fibular remnant

In 2003, Stanitski and Stanitski proposed the first functional classification of fibular hemimelia (Fig. 4) [17]. While it focuses on radiographic components, the system was an important move toward functional evaluation. The system requires evaluation of each of four components:

Normal
3-year-old child Type IA Type IB Type II

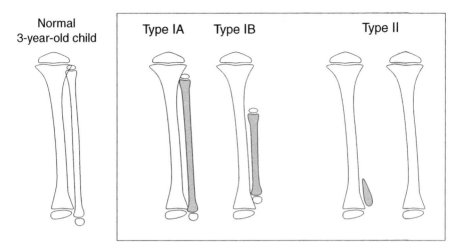

Fig. 3 Achterman and Kalamchi classification of fibular hemimelia: Type 1: partial fibular deficiency, subdivided into 1A and 1B. Type 1A: Proximal fibula distal to proximal tibial physis, distal fibular physis proximal to ankle joint. Type 1B: 30 to 50% fibular deficiency, no talofibular articulation. Type 2: Total absence of fibula, possible fibular anlage/remnant. (Copyright 2020, Rubin Institute for Advanced Orthopedics, Sinai Hospital of Baltimore)

1. Fibula: Normal, partially absent, or completely absent
2. Ankle joint: According to the morphology of the tibiotalar joint: horizontal, valgus, or ball-and-socket joint
3. Tarsal bones: Tarsal coalition present or absent
4. Foot: Numbers of rays

Moving closer to a direct functional evaluation, Birch et al. proposed a system focused on the clinical evaluation of the affected foot and severity of expected limb length discrepancy (Fig. 5) [18]. As the classification system evolved, the indications for reconstruction widened to some degree [3, 19]. Built in a retrospective manner, the original classification sought to evaluate what was done and determine if predictive factors may have been present. The three-ray "cutoff" was not intended to be used as a standalone metric, but it was reported that it did often reflect the overall status of the foot (personal communications with John G. Birch, November 20, 2020).

- Type 1: The primary feature of Type 1 is a functional foot, which can function as a stable weight-bearing platform. While exceptions certainly occurred, this criterion was most often met when three or more rays of the foot were present. After the foot is evaluated, the implications of leg length discrepancy are considered:

  - Type 1A: <6% leg length inequality; the treatment is orthosis or contralateral epiphysiodesis.
  - Type 1B: Six to 10% leg length inequality; the treatment is epiphysiodesis ± lengthening.

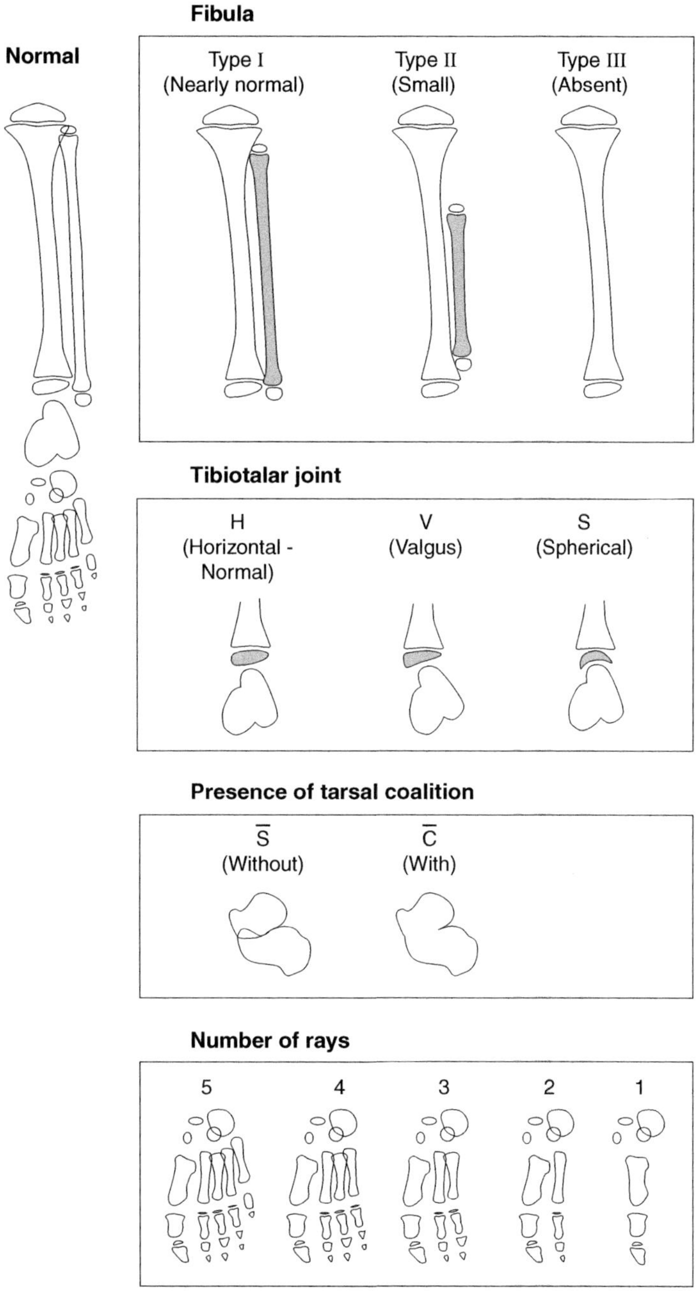

Fig. 4 Four components of the Stanitski classification: (1) Fibula: normal, partially absent, or completely absent. (2) Tibiotalar joint: Ball-and-socket, valgus, neutral. (3) Presence or absence of tarsal coalition. (4) Foot: numbers of rays. (Copyright 2020, Rubin Institute for Advanced Orthopedics, Sinai Hospital of Baltimore)

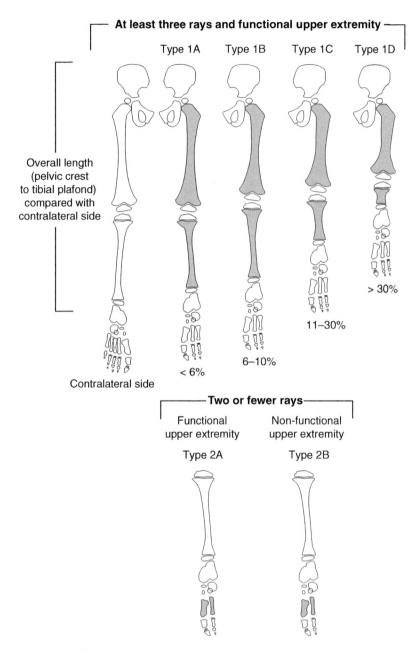

Fig. 5 Birch classification of fibular hemimelia. Type 1: foot in stable weight-bearing position, three or more rays. Type 1 is further broken down by percentage of limb length discrepancy. Type 1A: <6% limb length difference; Type 1B: 6% to 10% limb length difference; Type 1C: 11% to 30% limb length difference; Type 1D: >30% limb length difference. Type 2: nonfunctional foot (fewer than three rays, poor position). Type 2 is subdivided into Types 2A and 2B according to the functionality of the upper extremity. Type 2A: functional upper extremity; Type 2B: nonfunctional upper extremity. (Copyright 2020, Rubin Institute for Advanced Orthopedics, Sinai Hospital of Baltimore)

 – Type 1C: 11 to 30% leg length inequality; the treatment is one or two lengthening procedures ± epiphysiodesis or extension orthosis.
 – Type 1D: >30% leg length inequality; the treatment proposed is more than two lengthening procedures or amputation or extension orthosis.

• Type 2: Nonfunctional foot. Type 2 is subdivided into Types 2A and 2B according to the functionality of the upper extremity.

 – Type 2A: Upper extremities are functional; therefore, the treatment proposed is early amputation.
 – Type 2B: Upper extremities are nonfunctional, and foot amputation is contraindicated, as the foot must act as a replacement for the upper extremity.

The system did not evaluate the future potential of the foot after reconstruction, which remains to be demonstrated in future research. As it stands, the Birch classification represents the most important effort to evaluate the functional potential of the foot and ankle in fibular hemimelia and represents a critical moment in the understanding of congenital deformity treatment.

A more recent classification proposed by Paley focuses primarily on surgical treatment and subclassification of pathology centered around the ankle joint (Fig. 6) [20, 21]. The classification differentiates fibular hemimelia based on four hindfoot/ankle components:

• Type 1: Stable normal ankle.
• Type 2: Dynamic valgus ankle.
• Type 3: Fixed equinovalgus ankle. Type 3 is divided into four subtypes according to the location of the valgus deformity.

 – Type 3a: Ankle type
 – Type 3b: Subtalar type
 – Type 3c: Combined ankle and subtalar type
 – Type 3d: Talar body type

• Type 4: Fixed equinovarus ankle (clubfoot).

In this classification system, each type indicates a certain reconstruction approach:

• Type 1: Tibial lengthening, tendo Achilles lengthening as needed, depending on ankle examination.
• Type 2: Supramalleolar reorientation osteotomy, tibial lengthening, tendo Achilles lengthening.
• Type 3: Classic SUPERankle Reconstruction: peroneal tendon/Achilles lengthening, fibular anlage resection, reorientation osteotomies of the distal tibia/hindfoot as needed.

 – 3a: Supramalleolar osteotomy
 – 3b: Subtalar osteotomy
 – 3c: Supramalleolar and subtalar osteotomy
 – 3d: Opening wedge osteotomy of talar body

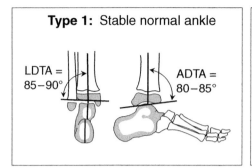

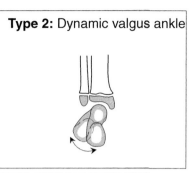

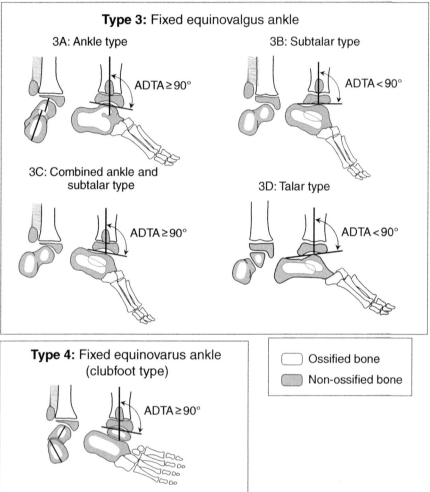

Fig. 6 Paley classification of fibular hemimelia. Type 1: normal ankle. Type 2: dynamic valgus ankle. Type 3: rigid equinovalgus ankle. Type 3 is further subdivided according to the location of the valgus into 3A (ankle), 3B (subtalar), 3C (combined ankle and subtalar), and 3D (talar). Type 4: clubfoot type (equinovarus). (Copyright 2020, Rubin Institute for Advanced Orthopedics, Sinai Hospital of Baltimore)

- Type 4: Initial Ponseti casting following typical technique and progression. This treatment protocol will often convert a Type 4 into a Type 3 and is then treated with a SUPERankle procedure at 12–18 months of age.

A thoughtful surgeon will interpret the Paley classification in the setting of anticipated outcomes of reconstruction, as well as other factors including family preference and the care environment. When focusing on reconstructive surgery for the foot and ankle, we use the Paley classification and will do so for the remainder of the chapter.

3   Clinical Assessment of a Child with FH

Children with fibular hemimelia should be seen in the neonatal period to allow the surgeon to begin discussing treatment options with the parents; a few patients will present with a prenatal diagnosis [22]. Unfortunately, a large percentage of parents do not have accurate information about the diagnosis and prognosis and also feel significant guilt about their child's condition. It is imperative that adequate time be allotted to the family in clinic so that all questions are answered.

The initial physical examination is important. A complete orthopedic exam should be completed, including overall height/length measurements, upper extremities, and cervical/thoracic/lumbar spine with evaluation of signs of neuraxial abnormalities. The range of motion of the hips must be assessed, as well as the alignment and stability of the knee. Obviously, the foot and ankle will be a critical component of the examination, focusing on range of motion, neurologic status, and deformity.

Based on clinical and radiographic evaluation, an outline or life plan should be made of various surgical options, including prosthetic and reconstructive pathways. The family should leave the initial visit with a basic understanding of the risks and benefits of each pathway that are specific to the child. Depending on their level of comfort and understanding, clinical follow-up prior to the child's first birthday may be necessary to revisit the decision-making process.

4   Radiographic Assessment of a Child with FH

In the neonatal period, radiographs of the foot and ankle will be of limited value, but a supine anteroposterior (AP) radiographic view of the legs can aid the surgeon in predicting future leg length discrepancy, which is a core component of decision-making. During the first year of life, a supine AP view radiograph of the legs is often enough to generate a rough outline for the family. If a decision has been made for reconstruction, a long lateral view radiograph can be helpful to evaluate foot position, knee laxity, and/or contracture. These radiographs should be assessed for evidence of knee and hip pathology in addition to detailed analysis of leg length discrepancy. The child's length/height can be used to predict adult height, but this should be done cautiously as small errors will be magnified significantly. While questions have been raised about the accuracy of the multiplier method for prediction of leg length discrepancy for treatment with epiphysiodesis, we use this method for initial evaluation as it is simple and allows prediction without multiple radiographs temporally spaced [23–25]. The Multiplier app is available as a free download through the Apple App Store and Google Play. For predicting adult height, we reference the height based on the long leg.

The combination of anticipated leg length discrepancy and predicted adult height is helpful for building a treatment framework for the family. The predicted leg length discrepancy generates a ballpark estimate of lengthening/epiphysiodesis options, and predicted adult height creates an environment in which the family can consider the effects of either strategy on adult height.

In older children, the initial radiographic examination includes full-length standing AP and lateral view radiographs. The AP film should be obtained with an adequately sized lift under the short leg to level the pelvis (Fig. 7). Ideally, the lateral view radiograph is obtained in full extension, though this can be technically difficult. In older patients, standing long leg films are more dependable for leg length discrepancy determination, as well as evaluation of coronal and sagittal deformity. As demonstrated by Manner et al., various degrees of tibial spine deficiency on the coronal view indicate likely knee instability and may be accompanied by subluxation on the long leg lateral view (Fig. 8) [26].

Typical findings in mild cases include valgus alignment of the extremity, generally driven by a hypoplastic lateral condyle. This is not universal, however, and the temptation to skip formal deformity analysis including the tibia should be resisted. In our practice, a complete deformity analysis is conducted on each radiograph according to the system described in *The Art of Limb Alignment* [27]. An anteromedial tibial bow may contribute to the overall valgus alignment, as can the proximal tibial physis. A skin dimple on the anteromedial surface of the tibia is a common clinical sign of the radiographic anteromedial bow (Fig. 9).

The radiographic appearance of the hindfoot varies widely depending on age. Nearly all children with fibular hemimelia have a tarsal coalition, most commonly between the talus and calcaneus. This coalition can be in a near-anatomic position (Fig. 10) or a side-by-side position (double-barrel shotgun appearance, (Figs. 11 and 12) indicating a need for subtalar osteotomy. The surgeon should avoid the temptation to rule out tarsal coalition on the radiographs of a young child (Fig. 13), as this near universal association becomes more obvious with increasing age. The anatomy of the forefoot has been shown to be more varied than previously outlined. The classical teaching that ray deficiencies are lateral in fibular hemimelia has been called into question [5]. The prognostic importance of this finding remains to be determined.

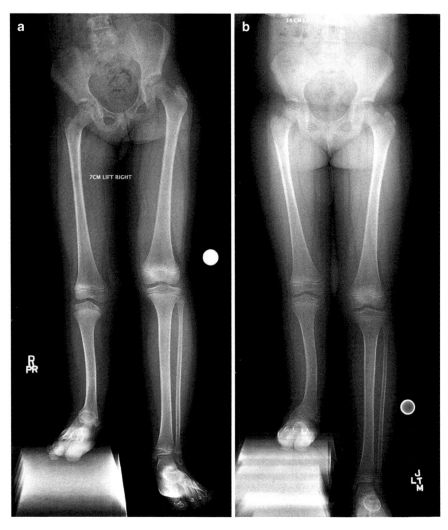

Fig. 7 In older children, the AP view radiograph should be obtained with an adequately sized lift under the short leg to level the pelvis. (**a**) An inadequate lift was used when obtaining this radiograph, but it was accepted as no surgery was planned before the next follow-up visit. (**b**) At the next follow-up visit, the previous film was used to guide proper lifting, which allows for easier evaluation of leg length discrepancy as well as more accurate assessment of acetabular coverage. (Used with permission from the Rubin Institute for Advanced Orthopedics, Sinai Hospital of Baltimore)

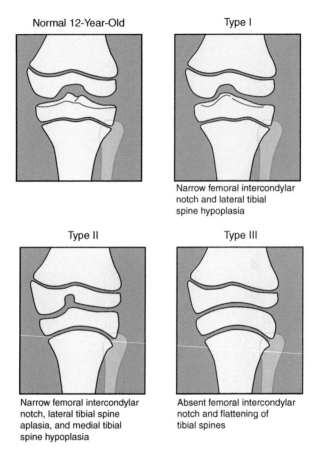

Fig. 8 Radiographic findings of ligamentous deficiency of the knee in fibular hemimelia. Type 1: narrowing of intercondylar notch and hypoplasia of the lateral tibial spine. Type 2: further narrowing of the intercondylar notch (with decreased notch height), aplasia of lateral tibial spine, hypoplasia of medial tibial spine. Type 3: absence of femoral notch, flattening of tibial spines. (Copyright 2020, Rubin Institute for Advanced Orthopedics, Sinai Hospital of Baltimore)

Magnetic resonance imaging (MRI) can be useful in evaluating the knee and ankle in fibular hemimelia, particularly during the first years of life. The primary utility lies in the ability to accurately evaluate unossified portions of the ankle and hindfoot, though useful information regarding the anatomic location of neurovascular structures and knee anatomy is also available (Figs. 14 and 15) [28]. Further information can be garnered intraoperatively using ankle arthrography, which generates a smooth "reference line" for the orientation of the ankle joint on the AP and lateral views during reorientation osteotomy. This can help to differentiate between ankle valgus and subtalar valgus (Fig. 16).

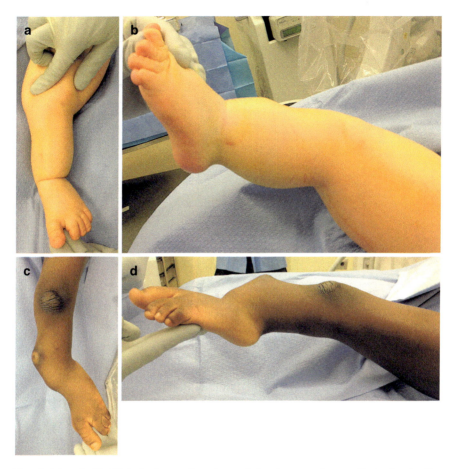

Fig. 9 (**a**) and (**b**) Clinical photos of moderate deformity secondary to fibular hemimelia. Equinovalgus of the foot and skin dimple at the apex of an anteromedial tibial bow. (**c**) and (**d**) More severe deformity secondary to fibular hemimelia, with apical dimple and equinovalgus foot deformity. (Used with permission from the Rubin Institute for Advanced Orthopedics, Sinai Hospital of Baltimore)

5   Principles of Treatment

Comprehensive treatment of the child affected by fibular hemimelia is required to optimize outcomes, either with reconstruction or prosthetic-mediated plans. Through the reconstructive route, the goals of treatment are to create a lower limb with a stable hip, knee, and ankle:

1. Correct the foot (typically equinovalgus) into a stable, plantigrade position.
2. Equalize lower limb lengths by skeletal maturity.

Fig. 10 Lateral radiograph of the tibia and foot shows the hindfoot in near normal orientation (vertically stacked), suggesting supramalleolar valgus. (Used with permission from the Rubin Institute for Advanced Orthopedics, Sinai Hospital of Baltimore)

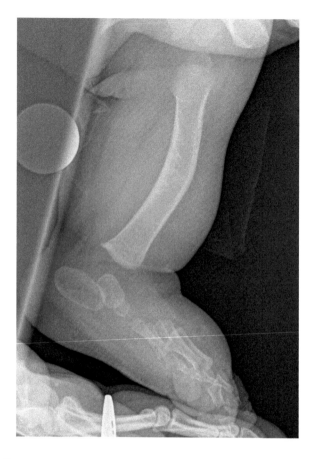

3. Restore normal limb alignment.
4. Ligamentous reconstruction of the unstable knee.

In reconstruction-mediated treatment, the ankle remains the center of attention. A general rule is that a stiff ankle remains stiff throughout treatment and, in fact, will get stiffer. The central goal is to obtain and maintain a plantigrade position. A plantigrade foot with minimal motion can remain functional for a long time, as evidenced by outcomes from ankle fusion in other patient populations [29, 30]. Whether a stiff ankle and foot is better than the absence of a foot and ankle should likely be left up to the family to decide.

As implied by the Birch classification, the total amount of leg length discrepancy predicted at adulthood is a factor in counseling families regarding the expected course of reconstruction. As a rule of thumb, each lengthening can be estimated to gain 5 cm, though it is often possible to exceed this goal at experienced centers. In both small and large discrepancies (<5 cm and >20 cm), contralateral epiphysiodesis can be a useful component to achieve the desired outcome.

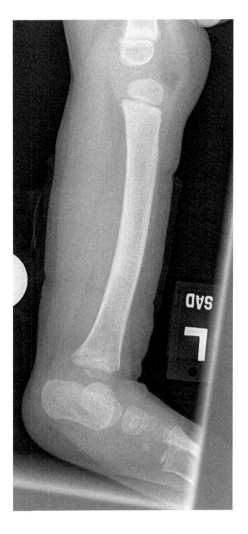

Fig. 11 Lateral radiograph of the tibia and foot shows the talus and calcaneus superimposed, suggesting a subtalar origin of the valgus deformity. (Used with permission from the Rubin Institute for Advanced Orthopedics, Sinai Hospital of Baltimore)

Outside of correction of the anteromedial bow, our center has moved away from large lengthening at the time of ankle reconstruction, as the immobilization of the hindfoot during lengthening appears to exacerbate postoperative stiffness. Correction of a large anteromedial bow is accomplished with an Ilizarov-type fixator with an oblique hinge or with hexapod frames. The majority of severe anteromedial bows are associated with very stiff hindfeet. In less severe anteromedial bows, the correction can be achieved with the shortening osteotomy realignment distal tibia (SHORDT) procedure. Based on extrapolation from adult trauma literature, caution is advised if more than 1–2 cm of shortening is required to correct the deformity, as the soft tissues may not tolerate the abrupt change [31, 32]. It is certainly possible that the safe limit is even lower for limbs that have "dense" tissue. Figure 17 shows radiographs of a patient after undergoing shortening osteotomy

Fig. 12 AP view tibia and ankle radiograph demonstrates the talus and calcaneus side by side, suggesting subtalar valgus deformity. (Used with permission from the Rubin Institute for Advanced Orthopedics, Sinai Hospital of Baltimore)

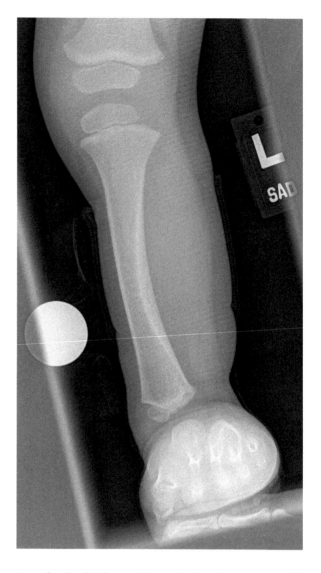

with deformity correction at another institution, with resultant soft-tissue necrosis and physeal closure. We tend to use the SHORDT procedure mainly for Paley Type 2 FH with mild to moderate deformity only (Figs. 18 and 19).

Depending on the total amount of length needed, this outline can be followed:

First Lengthening Plan for frame/device applied and removed prior to 4 years of age (typically initiating treatment shortly after third birthday). This ensures that the child will have no memory of this first lengthening. This lengthening is not included when planning treatment for mild cases. Currently, there are no viable surgical options for this first lengthening other than external fixation, though internal plates may eventually be small enough to help reduce the fixator-related complications in this group.

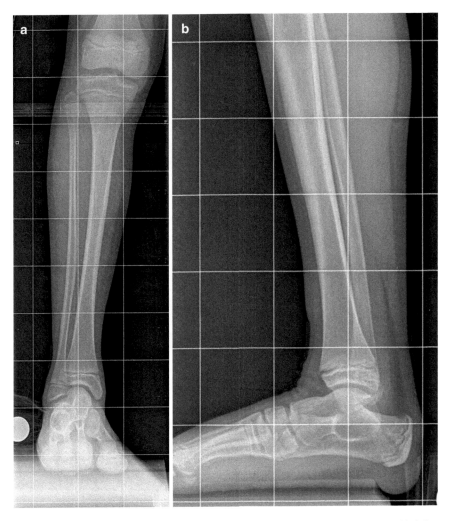

Fig. 13 (**a**) AP view radiograph of the tibia to include the foot shows ball-and-socket ankle joint. The coalition becomes more obvious as ossification progresses during normal development. (**b**) Lateral view radiograph with the classic "C" sign of the talocalcaneal coalition. A talonavicular coalition is also present. (Used with permission from the Rubin Institute for Advanced Orthopedics, Sinai Hospital of Baltimore)

Second Lengthening Initiated after age 8 years to allow involvement of the patient in the decision-making progress. The key psychological milestone that we assess for in our clinic is the ability to understand the concept of a short-term loss in exchange for a long-term gain – meaning that the patient understands the setback of surgical procedures in exchange for a longer leg.

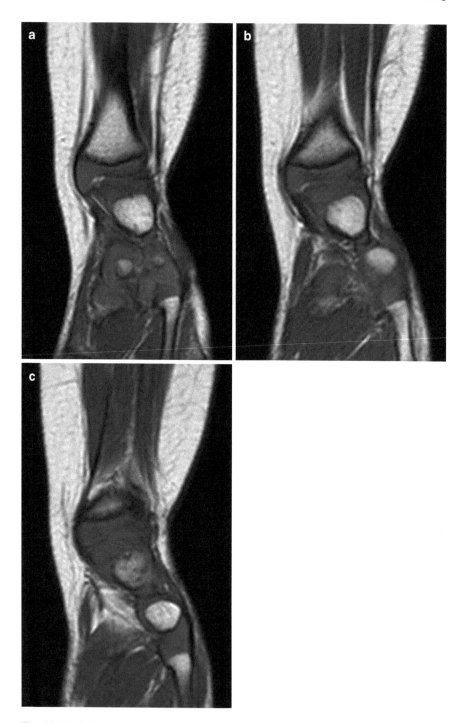

Fig. 14 (**a–c**) Supramalleolar valgus demonstrated on sequential magnetic resonance imaging evaluations (Paley Type 3A – ankle type). (Used with permission from the Rubin Institute for Advanced Orthopedics, Sinai Hospital of Baltimore)

Fig. 15 Subtalar valgus demonstrated on sequential magnetic resonance imaging scans (Paley Type 3B). (Used with permission from the Rubin Institute for Advanced Orthopedics, Sinai Hospital of Baltimore)

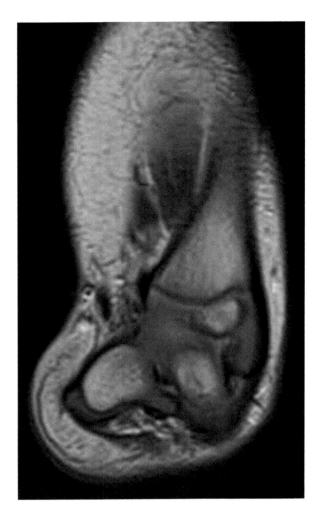

Subsequent Lengthening Procedures Depending on the goals in each case, additional lengthening can be done in 2- to 4-year intervals, allowing the soft tissue (and family) to rest and recover. Delaying the final lengthening until after physeal closure allows for internal lengthening, which has been shown to be the preferred option for patients, along with decreased minor complications [33, 34]. Importantly, the incidence of major complications from internal lengthening procedures is not less when compared to external fixator-mediated correction, indicating that these procedures should remain in the hands of experienced centers despite wide familiarity with the surgical technique of intramedullary rodding [34–36].

During lengthening, the surgeon must pay careful attention to the regenerate as it forms, initially appearing at 3- to 4-week post-osteotomy. In addition to managing the regenerate, the surgeon and physical therapy team need to pay very close attention to the position and range of motion of the knee and ankle during lengthening.

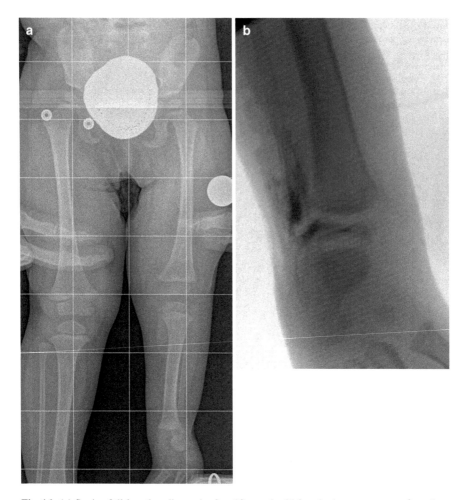

Fig. 16 (**a**) Supine full-length radiograph of an 18-month-old female demonstrates equinovalgus position of the foot. (**b**) An ankle arthrogram obtained in the operating room demonstrates supra-malleolar valgus. (Used with permission from the Rubin Institute for Advanced Orthopedics, Sinai Hospital of Baltimore)

The knee more than the ankle is subject to forces strong enough to lead to disloca-tion, and this risk can be mitigated by extension bracing, close monitoring, and specialized physical therapy. The knee range of motion must be assessed at every clinical evaluation. During femoral and tibial lengthening, we use a custom knee device to maintain full extension, as flexion contracture is a harbinger of impending knee dislocation [37]. This is of particular importance in femoral lengthening. Tibial lengthening adds risk of ankle equinus, and therapy along with splinting is an important factor to minimize the occurrence.

Fig. 17 Care should be taken to avoid extensive exposure and soft-tissue stripping during reconstruction. Patient shown underwent concurrent medial and lateral approaches to the ankle for the shortening osteotomy realignment distal tibia (SHORDT) procedure at another institution. Resultant skin necrosis and physeal closure can lead to a more complex reconstructive plan or amputation – depending on patient and family preferences. (Used with permission from the Rubin Institute for Advanced Orthopedics, Sinai Hospital of Baltimore)

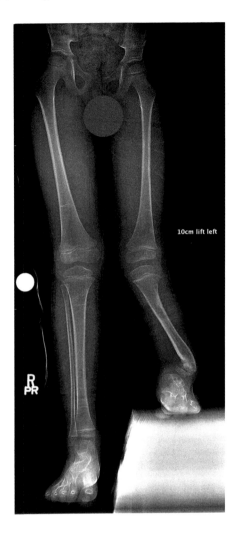

6 Surgical Techniques for FH

6.1 Lengthening for Paley Type 1

Mild cases of FH are amenable to standard lengthening techniques, with less need for soft-tissue management procedures. All children and adults with FH have some tightness of the Achilles tendon, and limb lengthening will increase this tightness. At the time of tibial lengthening, we recommend performing a triceps surae lengthening procedure. We recommend an open Vulpius procedure and a prophylactic anterior compartment fasciotomy (Fig. 20). The posterior tibial neurovascular

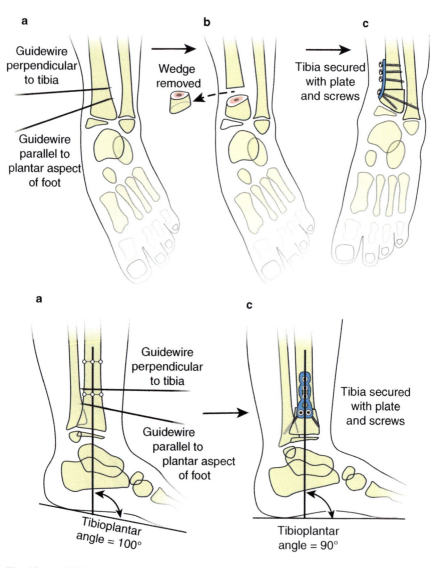

Fig. 18 (**a–c**) Illustration shows the shortening osteotomy realignment distal tibia (SHORDT) procedure. (Copyright 2020, Rubin Institute for Advanced Orthopedics, Sinai Hospital of Baltimore)

bundle is often in close proximity to the triceps surae tendon, so this procedure must be done under direct vision, not percutaneously. The fasciotomy decreases but does not eliminate the risk of compartment syndrome (a known complication of tibial osteotomy). An additional benefit of anterior compartment fasciotomy is that it allows the anterior compartment musculature to bulge out, especially if the longitudinal incision in the fascia is combined with a short, transverse cruciate incision.

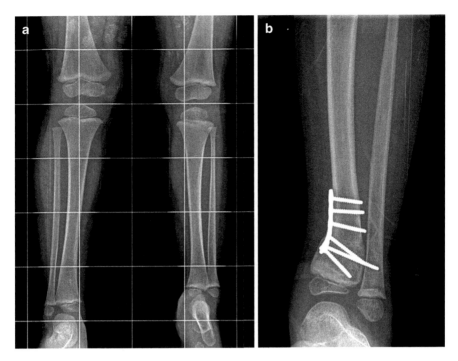

Fig. 19 (**a**) Preoperative radiograph of fibular hemimelia. Note the shortening of the fibula relative to the tibial plafond. (**b**) Postoperative radiograph obtained 3 months after shortening osteotomy realignment distal tibia (SHORDT) procedure. Note the position of the fibular physis relative to the ankle joint line. (Used with permission from the Rubin Institute for Advanced Orthopedics, Sinai Hospital of Baltimore)

This bulging of the anterior compartment musculature will create the impression of a larger diameter calf, which is desirable because all patients with FH have a smaller ipsilateral calf due to the combined bone and soft-tissue hypoplasia.

The fixator may need to be extended to include the foot to prevent ankle equinus during lengthening. If the surgeon elects to avoid fixator extension to the foot, a temporary extra-articular screw (from the calcaneus to the tibia, posteriorly) or a lateral plate may be used. Therapy is also an option and can serve as the primary preventative measure [38]. The surgeon must maintain a watchful eye and be willing to intervene if equinus develops in the absence of internal or external bridging. If the frame is extended to the foot, it may be removed to minimize stiffness after the lengthening goal is obtained, provided there is no unresolved flexion contracture of the knee.

Monolateral fixators are not appropriate for lengthening in fibular hemimelia, due to a high rate of iatrogenic deformity secondary to tight lateral structures and a tendency to drift into valgus [39]. While technical modifications can be made to limit this complication, the near universal availability of ring external fixation

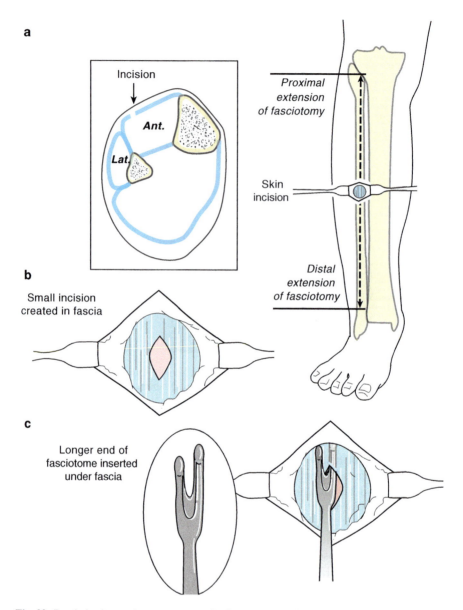

Fig. 20 Prophylactic anterior compartment fasciotomy may reduce the risk of compartment syndrome; the anterior prominence of the muscle may be desirable from a cosmetic standpoint. (**a**) A 1- to 2-cm incision is made just lateral to the tibial crest. (**b**) Fascia is opened after exposure with blunt dissection. (**c**) Fasciotome is then inserted under the fascia. (**d**) Fasciotome is advanced proximally. The fasciotome should remain as medial as possible (right of the crest). Ant., anterior compartment; Lat., lateral compartment. (Copyright 2020, Rubin Institute for Advanced Orthopedics, Sinai Hospital of Baltimore)

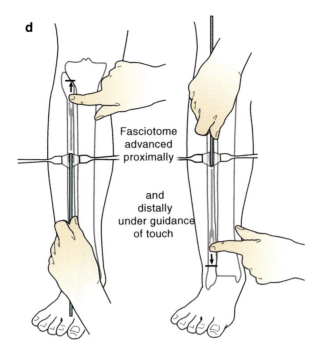

d

Fasciotome
advanced
proximally

and
distally
under guidance
of touch

Fig. 20 (continued)

systems, and their versatility, argues against the use of monolateral fixation for tibial lengthening.

Figure 21 shows a typical lengthening with external fixation for FH. In most pure external fixation cases, three pins/wires are used proximally, three pins/wires are used in the distal segment, and foot fixation may be included. The proximal and distal rings should be placed so that there is plenty of room to allow for better recruitment of soft tissue into the lengthening. The greater the distance between fixation points, the more soft tissue is available to accommodate the lengthening (less soft tissue strain, defined as the amount of tissue change required along the direction of force divided by the initial ring spacing).

For skeletally mature patients in whom there is no longer a viable proximal tibial growth plate, it is attractive to use intramedullary (IM) telescopic nails. Two systems, the PRECICE (NuVasive, Inc., San Diego, CA, USA) and the FITBONE (Orthofix, Lewisville, TX, USA), are now widely available. An important technical point of intramedullary distraction osteogenesis is to make the multiple drill holes in preparation for osteotomy prior to reaming the canal for nail placement. This is in an effort to encourage the reamings to exit anteriorly to stimulate new bone formation at the lengthening site.

In the developing world, implantable telescopic lengthening nails are generally unavailable, so the lengthening over nail (LON) technique is useful. The external

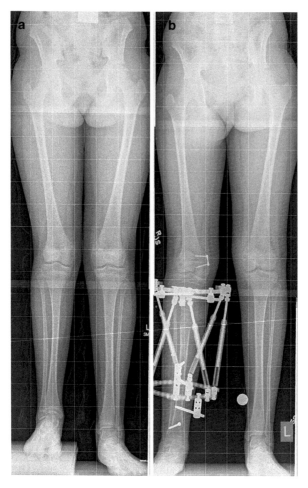

Fig. 21 Standing long leg films of a 12-year-old girl (**a**), after distraction osteogenesis of the tibia and distal femoral guided growth (**b**), after frame removal (**c**), and after neutralization of the axis through growth modulation (**d**). (Used with permission from the Rubin Institute for Advanced Orthopedics, Sinai Hospital of Baltimore)

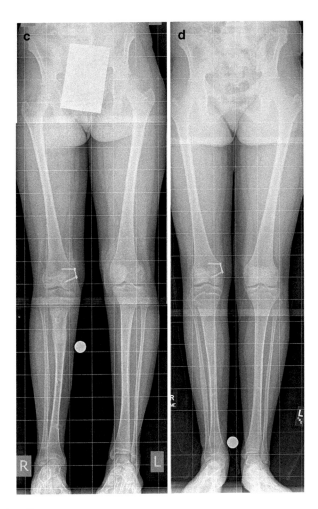

Fig. 21 (continued)

fixator that is applied for the LON technique can be a simple frame with two points of fixation at either end (Fig. 22). The rate of lengthening is adjusted according to bone formation. After lengthening is achieved, the patient undergoes distal locking and frame removal (performed in that order in the operating room to prevent shortening). The majority of the consolidation phase then occurs under the protection of the nail, without need for an external fixator. It is important to place the external fixation points outside the planned pathway of the nail and to maintain the lengthening axis of the fixator parallel to the nail axis to minimize the risk of mechanical interference.

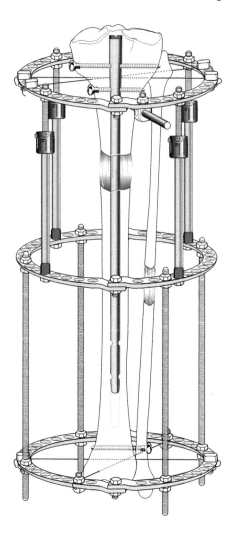

In both internal lengthening nails and LON, blocking screws (Poller screws) can be used to prevent mechanical axis deviation during lengthening. If needed in the LON technique, these screws can be inserted at the time of frame removal. Figure 23 shows lengthening with a PRECICE using a posterior blocking screw in the proximal fragment to prevent procurvatum. The recent development of an internal lengthening plate allows avoidance of external fixators for tibial lengthening prior to skeletal maturity (Fig. 24).

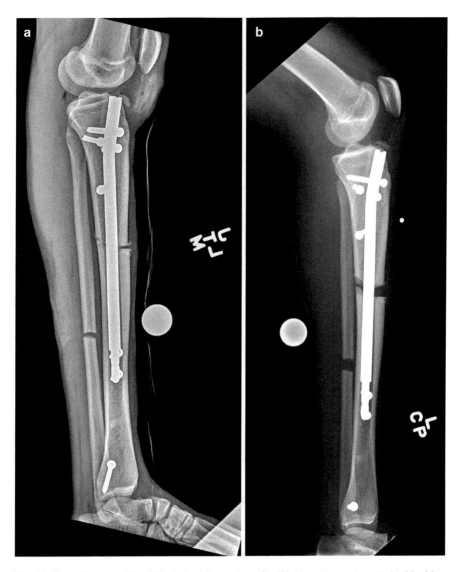

Fig. 23 Lateral views of the tibia during distraction of a tibial osteotomy. A posterior blocking screw is present in the proximal fragment to drive the nail into the anterior cortex, limiting the risk of procurvatum deformity. (**a**) Immediate postoperative radiograph. (**b**) Radiograph obtained 2 weeks postoperative. (**c**) Radiograph obtained 6 months after the procedure. (Used with permission from the Rubin Institute for Advanced Orthopedics, Sinai Hospital of Baltimore)

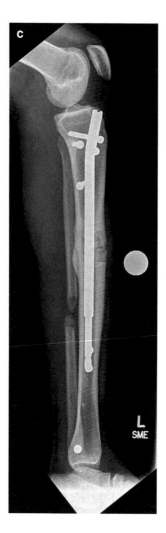

Fig. 23 (continued)

6.2 Lengthening Plus Ankle Realignment for Paley Type 2

The flexible valgus deformity of the ankle should be corrected prior to lengthening to avoid complications of asymmetric muscle pull during lengthening. Reorientation osteotomy of the supramalleolar distal tibia should be completed prior to lengthening (Fig. 25). In the same setting, intramuscular lengthening of the peroneal tendons can help to rebalance the soft tissues around the ankle.

A supramalleolar rotational dome osteotomy is appropriate in mature patients. The SHORDT procedure is more appropriate for younger children with remodeling

Fig. 24 Internal lengthening with the PRECICE plate. In this case, the anterolateral soft tissues allowed adequate coverage of the implant, and the position resists tendency toward valgus in tibial lengthening. (**a**) Immediate postoperative radiograph. (**b**) One-month postimplantation with 7-day latency. (Used with permission from the Rubin Institute for Advanced Orthopedics, Sinai Hospital of Baltimore)

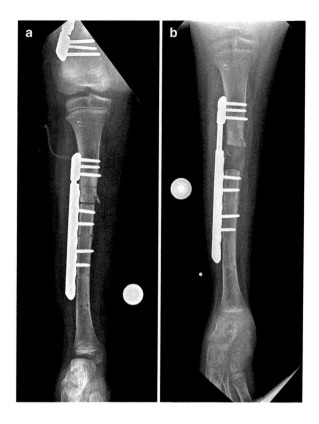

potential, but long-term outcomes are unknown (Fig. 18). From a soft-tissue stand-point, the medial osseous shortening generates a relative lengthening of the posterior tibialis muscle; at the same time, the peroneal tendons are stretched during the reorientation. For this reason (among others), we reserve the SHORDT correction for mild cases.

6.3 Lengthening Plus SUPERankle Reconstruction for Paley Type 3

For the rigid equinovalgus type, we use a modified Paley SUPERankle approach. Children can undergo this surgery as young as 1 or 2 years of age. The goal is to create a plantigrade foot and realign the foot relative to the distal tibia. The ankle joint and its ligaments are not opened during this extra-articular reconstruction.

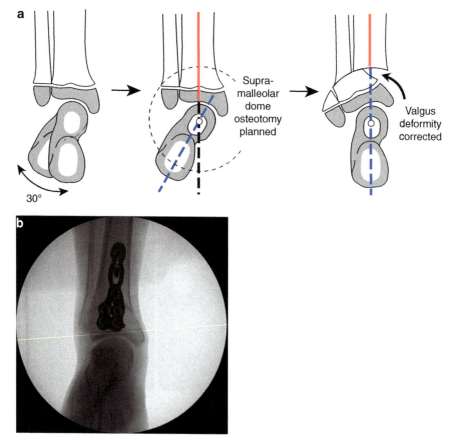

Fig. 25 (**a**) Focal dome osteotomy of the distal tibia and fibula allows realignment of the dynamic valgus ankle in patients who are deemed too skeletally mature to undergo surgical correction that requires joint remodeling (shortening osteotomy realignment distal tibia [SHORDT]). Copyright 2020, Rubin Institute for Advanced Orthopedics, Sinai Hospital of Baltimore. (**b**) Supramalleolar rotational dome osteotomy in a skeletally mature individual with fibular hemimelia. (Used with permission from the Rubin Institute for Advanced Orthopedics, Sinai Hospital of Baltimore)

6.3.1 Surgical Technique for Type 3a (Figs. 26 and 27)

Positioning

Supine position, bump under the ipsilateral sacrum, and tourniquet control.

Surgical Approach

Longitudinal (straight) incision is made laterally from the mid-calf to just above the sole of the foot. The peroneal tendons are cut with a Z-technique and later repaired

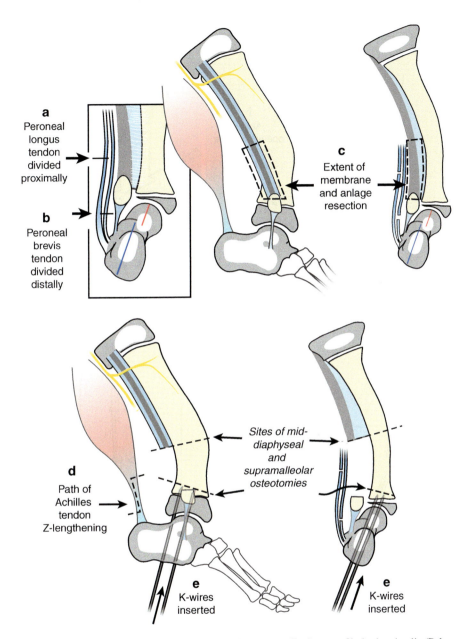

a
Peroneal longus tendon divided proximally

b
Peroneal brevis tendon divided distally

c
Extent of membrane and anlage resection

d
Path of Achilles tendon Z-lengthening

Sites of mid-diaphyseal and supramalleolar osteotomies

e
K-wires inserted

e
K-wires inserted

Fig. 26 (**a–m**) SUPERankle surgical technique for supramalleolar type fibular hemimelia (Paley Type 3A – ankle type). PRN, when necessary. (Copyright 2020, Rubin Institute for Advanced Orthopedics, Sinai Hospital of Baltimore)

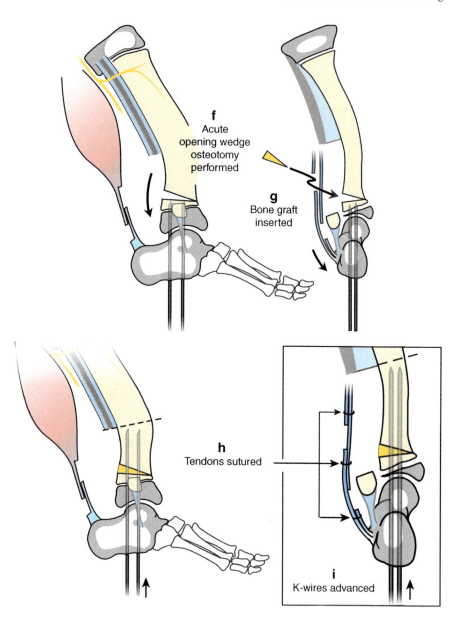

Fig. 26 (continued)

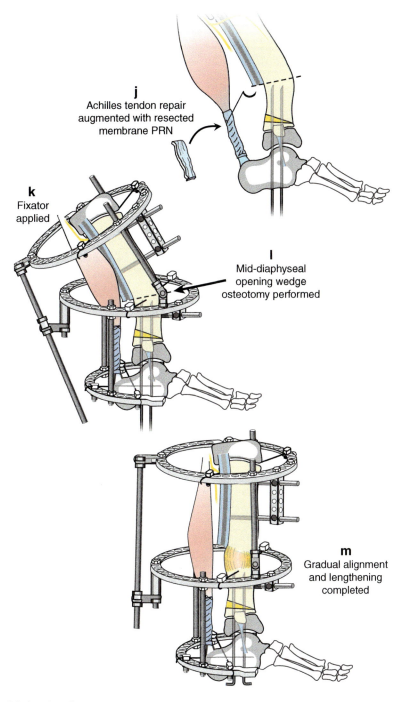

j
Achilles tendon repair
augmented with resected
membrane PRN

k
Fixator
applied

l
Mid-diaphyseal
opening wedge
osteotomy performed

m
Gradual alignment
and lengthening
completed

Fig. 26 (continued)

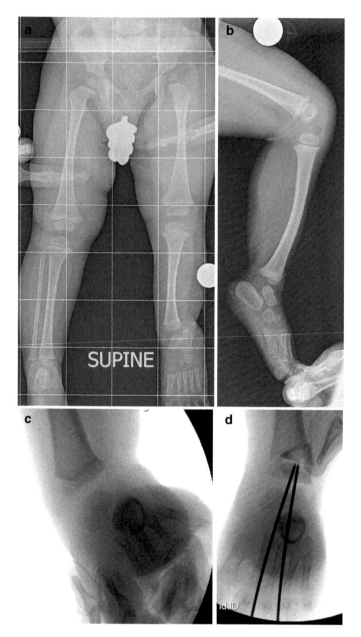

Fig. 27 Case example of an 18-month-old boy with Paley Type 3A fibular hemimelia. (**a**) and (**b**) Preoperative AP (**a**) and lateral (**b**) view radiographs showing equinovalgus foot/ankle deformity with anterior tibial bowing. (**c**–**e**) Distal tibial osteotomy of SUPERankle procedure. (**f**) Hinge position outside the convexity to allow lengthening and deformity correction. (**g**) and (**h**) Postoperative imaging of the SUPERankle procedure. (**i**) and (**j**) Two-week postoperative imaging showing correction and lengthening. (**k**) and (**l**) AP (**k**) 3-month postoperative imaging after frame removal. Note the complete correction of the tibia and the ankle. (Used with permission from the Rubin Institute for Advanced Orthopedics, Sinai Hospital of Baltimore)

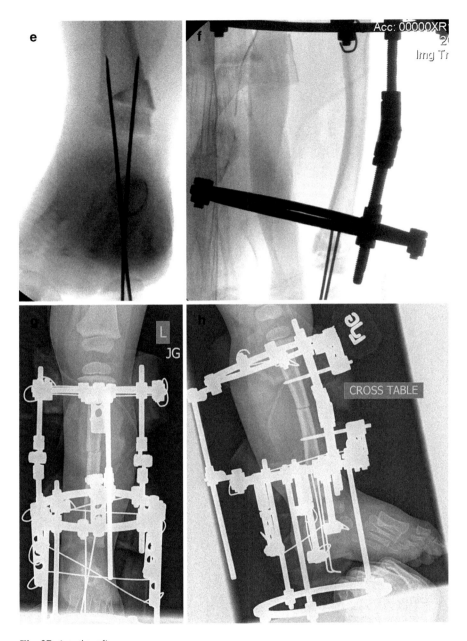

Fig. 27 (continued)

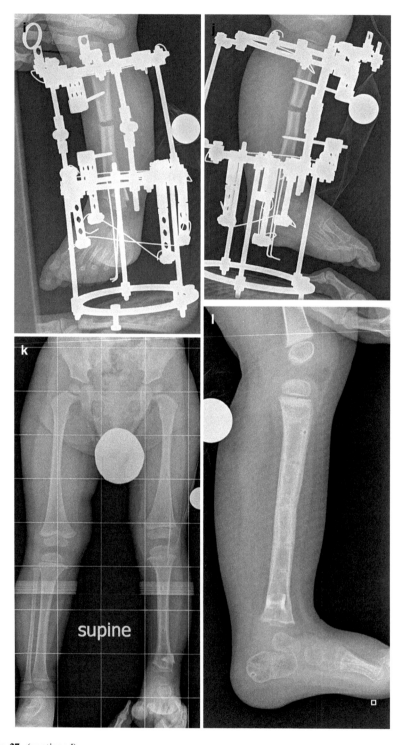

Fig. 27 (continued)

in the lengthened configuration. In some cases, only one peroneal tendon is present. If there is a distal anlage of the fibula, it may be left in place. Anterior compartment fasciotomy is performed. The superficial peroneal nerve is identified and protected. The anterior compartment muscles are dissected off of the fibular cartilage anlage and off of the intermuscular septum.

The intermuscular septum is resected from the ankle proximally up to the midportion of the tibia at the apex of the anterolateral bow. The resected intermuscular septum is placed in a sterile specimen cup and covered with saline, as it may be needed for repair and elongation of the Achilles tendon. There is no need to resect the anlage proximal to the anterior tibial bow, nor is there any need to decompress the peroneal nerve proximally.

The sural nerve is identified and protected. The Achilles tendon and posterior tibial neurovascular bundle are also identified. Avoid damage to the posterior tibial nerve, which is often in close proximity to the Achilles tendon. In some cases, the posterior tibial nerve is quite large – a nerve stimulator can help distinguish tendon from nerve. Do not be tempted to lengthen a structure before finding all of the tendons, nerves, and blood vessels. The flexor hallucis longus is identified and used as a guide to the posterolateral corner anatomy. Through this posterolateral approach, the posterior tibial nerve is decompressed into the tarsal tunnel distally as far as it can be visualized. The Achilles tendon is very short; the tendon available for lengthening can be made longer by scraping the distal muscle belly proximally to expose more of the tendon and prepare it for Z-lengthening. Despite this, it is sometimes necessary to create a tendon graft from the resected intermuscular septum to obtain sufficient Achilles tendon elongation. The foot is then placed into the maximum equinus and valgus position. Two 1.8-mm diameter Kirschner wires (K-wires) are inserted from the plantar surface of the heel, across the calcaneus and talus, across the ankle joint, and approximately 5–10 mm into the distal tibia. This pins the ankle in the maximum valgus/equinus position.

Osteotomy

A distal tibial subperiosteal dissection is performed. Great care should be taken to avoid damage to the growth plate's perichondrial ring. Mini-Hohmann retractors are placed anteriorly and posteriorly. An oscillating saw is used to make an oblique cut from posterolateral to anteromedial, but the anteromedial cortex is left intact. To correct the equinovalgus position of the hindfoot, the osteotomy is levered open from the posterolateral direction with an osteotome or laminar spreader. The osteotomy is held open with a cortical allograft (e.g., small piece of fibular allograft). The two K-wires are passed across the osteotomy and up into the distal half of the tibia, stopping just short of the anterolateral bow in the apex of the diaphysis. The K-wires are bent outside the skin of the heel and can be incorporated into the frame (if planned) or left outside the skin for removal if the frame is not going to be used. The foot is now corrected and plantigrade relative to the distal tibia.

The tourniquet can be let down for the closure. The Achilles and peroneal tendons are repaired in their lengthened configuration. The incision is closed over a small drain to prevent compartment syndrome and wound hematoma. At this point, the operation can conclude and a long leg, bivalved cast can be applied. The cast and pins are removed in 6 weeks, and then the patient can attend physical therapy sessions for the ankle.

Frame Application

Four to 6 months after the initial procedure, the tibia can be lengthened with an Ilizarov or hexapod external fixator through an osteotomy made at the apex of the anterolateral bow. Alternatively, the fixator may be applied at the same time as the SUPERankle reconstruction and used to correct the apex anteromedial bow with 1–2 cm of lengthening. The frame is removed after healing of the diaphyseal corticotomy is achieved, and a long leg cast is applied for 3–4 weeks. After cast removal, the patient undergoes mobilization and rehabilitation of the ankle to try to regain as much motion as possible.

6.3.2   Surgical Technique for Type 3b (Figs. 28 and 29)

Positioning and Surgical Approach

The positioning and approach are the same as described for Type 3a.

Osteotomy

An oblique subtalar osteotomy is performed. The osteotomy should initiate in the sinus tarsi, exit medially in the region of a typical talocalcaneal joint, and terminate posteriorly just anterior to the Achilles insertion. The cartilaginous anlage of the fibula is dissected and excised around. After the osteotomy is complete and the surgeon is able to fully mobilize the hindfoot, K-wires are initially inserted in a similar manner to Type 2A with the foot in the maximally deformed position (equinus and valgus). The distal half of the calcaneus and foot is translated medially and angulated to make the K-wires face directly upward toward the talus. The reduction of the "side-by-side" position of the talocalcaneal block reduces the overall valgus position of the foot. A bone graft can be placed posteriorly to improve the equinus position. A large piece should not be used, as it adds to overall soft-tissue tension. The fixation is then driven across the osteotomy into the talus. In some cases, sufficient purchase is available in the talus. For very young children, better purchase can be achieved by driving the wires across the ankle joint into the distal tibia. The tourniquet is released, and the closure proceeds as described for Type 3A, including external fixator application to correct the mid-diaphyseal deformity.

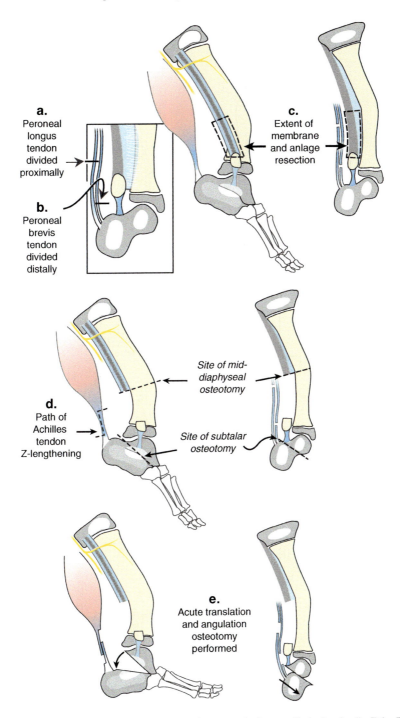

a. Peroneal longus tendon divided proximally

b. Peroneal brevis tendon divided distally

c. Extent of membrane and anlage resection

Site of mid-diaphyseal osteotomy

d. Path of Achilles tendon Z-lengthening

Site of subtalar osteotomy

e. Acute translation and angulation osteotomy performed

Fig. 28 (a–l) SUPERankle surgical technique used to treat subtalar type fibular hemimelia (Paley Type 3B). PRN, when necessary. (Copyright 2020, Rubin Institute for Advanced Orthopedics, Sinai Hospital of Baltimore)

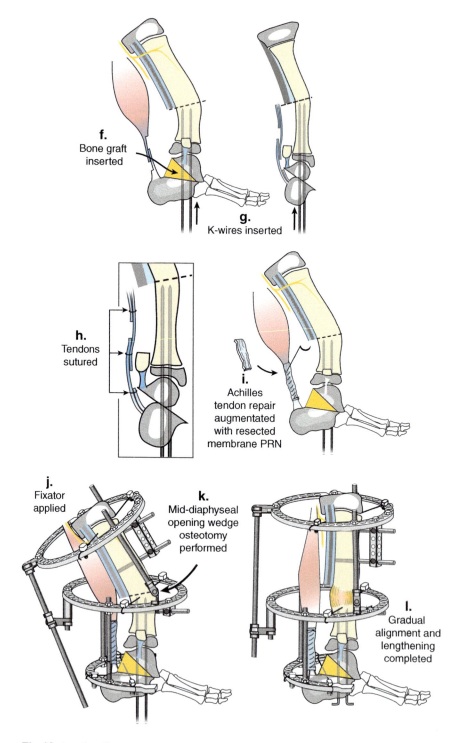

Fig. 28 (continued)

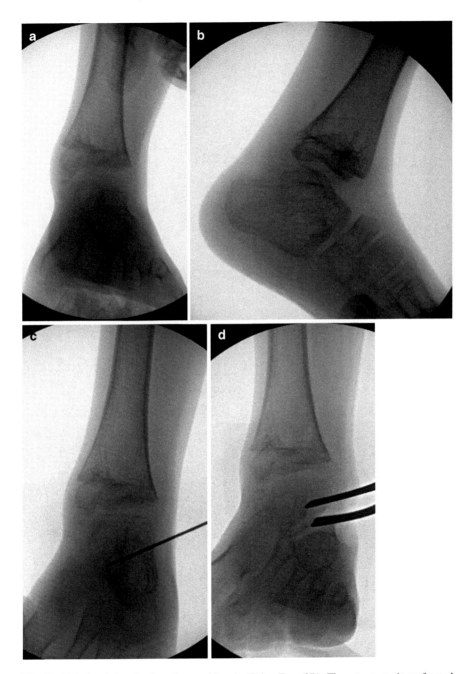

Fig. 29 Subtalar deformity in a 6-year-old male (Paley Type 3B). The osteotomy is performed through the talocalcaneal coalition. (**a**) and (**b**) AP (**a**) and lateral (**b**) views demonstrate residual valgus deformity after previous supramalleolar osteotomy at age 2 years. (**c**) K-wire guidance for planned osteotomy line. (**d**) After osteotomy completion, the distal fragment is translated medially and positioned into varus with the aid of a laminar spreader. (**e**) Fibular allograft placed to maintain correction in conjunction with retrograde K-wires. (**f**) and (**g**) Final position after deformity correction and fixation. (Used with permission from the Rubin Institute for Advanced Orthopedics, Sinai Hospital of Baltimore)

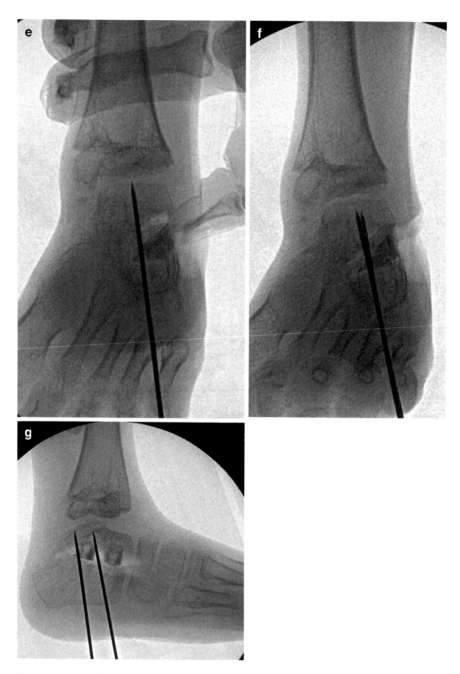

Fig. 29 (continued)

6.3.3   Surgical Technique for Type 3c (Fig. 30)

Positioning and Surgical Approach

The positioning and approach are the same as described for Type 3a.

Osteotomy

An ankle arthrogram is helpful to determine the position of the ankle joint intraoperatively. The supramalleolar osteotomy and the subtalar osteotomy are then performed. As the subtalar osteotomy can be more difficult to control, this deformity is corrected first, translating the distal fragment medially and opening posteriorly. The subtalar coalition osteotomy is provisionally held with bone graft and K-wires. The position of the ankle is then corrected, typically with a posterolateral opening wedge osteotomy to correct valgus and procurvatum of the joint surface demonstrated during the arthrogram. A fibular allograft is then introduced into the opening wedge, and the K-wires from the heel are driven into the tibia. At the completion of correction, the wires cross the subtalar coalition osteotomy, the ankle joint, and the distal tibial osteotomy. If there is too much tension on the soft tissues, the supramalleolar osteotomy may be fashioned as a closing wedge type rather than an opening wedge type. Generally this is done through the same lateral incision to limit risk for soft-tissue compromise between medial and lateral incisions.

6.3.4   Surgical Technique for Type 3d (Fig. 31)

Diagnosing Type 3d

This subtype is extremely rare and can be diagnosed in younger children through MRI evaluation or in older children through computed tomography. The distinctive feature of this deformity is a wedge-shaped talar body.

Positioning and Surgical Approach

The positioning and approach are the same as described for Type 3a.

Osteotomy

The opening wedge procedure is similar to the technique described for Type 3b (subtalar type). However, the osteotomy used in Type 3d cases does not pass completely through the medial side.

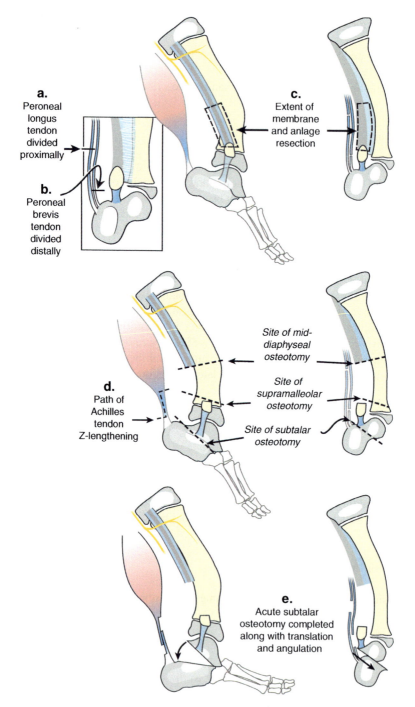

Fig. 30 (**a–o**) SUPERankle surgical technique that is used to treat combined ankle/subtalar type fibular hemimelia (Paley Type 3C). (Copyright 2020, Rubin Institute for Advanced Orthopedics, Sinai Hospital of Baltimore)

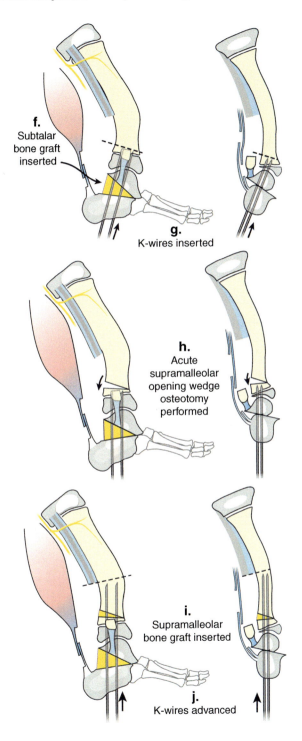

Fig. 30 (continued)

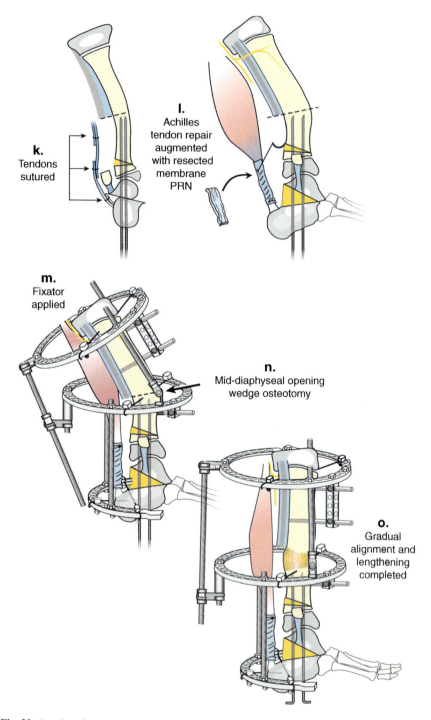

k. Tendons sutured

l. Achilles tendon repair augmented with resected membrane PRN

m. Fixator applied

n. Mid-diaphyseal opening wedge osteotomy

o. Gradual alignment and lengthening completed

Fig. 30 (continued)

Fig. 31 Surgical technique that is used to treat talar body type fibular hemimelia (Paley Type 3D). (Copyright 2020, Rubin Institute for Advanced Orthopedics, Sinai Hospital of Baltimore)

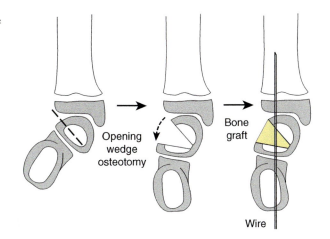

Opening wedge osteotomy

Bone graft

Wire

6.4 Initial Nonsurgical Treatment for Type 4 (Clubfoot Type)

Fewer than 15% of FH cases can be classified as Type 4; therefore, treatment must be individualized. In the authors' experience, the initial treatment is nonsurgical and should follow Ponseti principles. It is unclear why the Ponseti method is able to correct the varus and internal rotation deformity, as the Ponseti technique ostensibly works through the subtalar joint. In our experience, all children with Type 4 FH have a subtalar joint coalition. After casting and tenotomy, the deformity is converted to an equinovalgus type, which can be corrected using the SUPERankle approaches described previously.

6.5 Additional Procedures

Valgus at the knee is common in fibular hemimelia and is amenable to growth modulation as long as the physes are open. While the valgus is classically distal femoral in nature, the proximal tibia should also be evaluated to avoid creating the "bad combination" of distal femoral valgus and proximal tibial varus in the uncommon case of tibial-driven valgus. The optimal timing of growth modulation for valgus at the knee is debatable. Whether there is a long-term impact on trochlear formation is unknown. Rebound is common in younger patients [40–42]. The cause of progressive valgus has not been clearly elucidated and has been attributed to lateral femoral condyle hypoplasia traditionally. Additional factors could be the fibrous band of the fibular anlage and/or the Cozen phenomenon post-lengthening (Fig. 32).

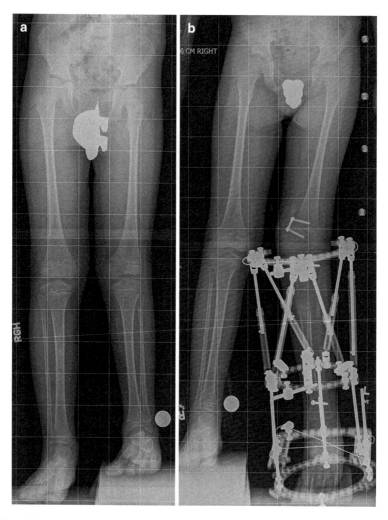

Fig. 32 (**a**) Preoperative standing full-length imaging of a 6-year-old male. (**b**) Full-length standing AP view radiograph after 6 cm of lengthening and placement of tension-band plate. Note the mild knee flexion contracture but normalized medial proximal tibial angle. (**c**) Six months after frame removal. Note the correction of the distal femur and the normalized lateral distal femoral angle. Progressive recurrence of proximal tibial valgus, possibly from a Cozen-type phenomenon. (**d**) Placement of tension-band plate on medial proximal tibia. (**e**) Improvement of proximal tibial valgus after placement of tension-band plate. (Used with permission from the Rubin Institute for Advanced Orthopedics, Sinai Hospital of Baltimore)

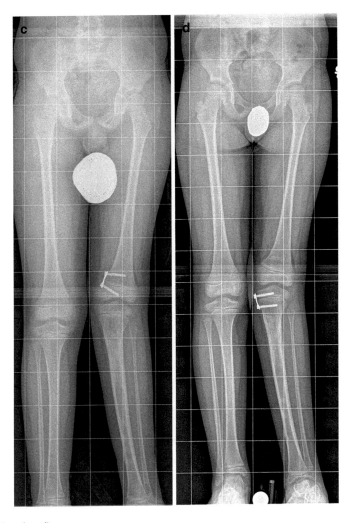

Fig. 32 (continued)

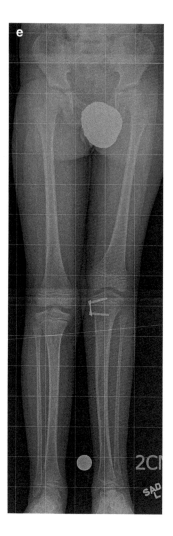

Fig. 32 (continued)

7   Postsurgical Care

The most critical component of postoperative care is physical therapy. We require 3 to 5 days per week of supervised physical therapy, depending on knee stability, family compliance, and previous lengthening experience. In addition to the supervised sessions, families are prescribed a home exercise program to help minimize complications. In tibial lengthening, these programs focus on prevention of equinus deformity (if not otherwise prevented with extra-articular screw or bridging the frame) and knee flexion contracture. Flexion contractures of the toes are also possible but have less severe consequences than knee and ankle complications. We include a splinting and stretching protocol for the toe flexors in our tibial lengthening protocol. Physical therapy continues until the completion of lengthening and restoration of normal range of motion in all joints. Nighttime extension splinting is helpful for the knee and is used for all tibial and femoral lengthening patients [37, 43]. This splinting device can be modified as needed to accommodate an external fixator.

Weight-bearing depends on the patient's size and anticipated compliance. Additional factors are choice of lengthening device. External fixators typically allow full weight-bearing as tolerated. Titanium intramedullary rods are restricted to 10 to 20 kg weight-bearing, while stainless steel intramedullary rods tolerate 65–110 kg, depending on diameter. We encourage patients to continue to use crutches for balance even if full weight-bearing is permitted.

We recommend a latency period of 7 days. If the patient experienced previous premature consolidation despite good compliance, we shorten the latency. Poor soft tissue, repeated lengthening, and a requirement for more soft-tissue dissection during osteotomy all factor into a potential decision to extend the latency period. Our typical distraction rate is 0.75–0.8 mm/day completed over three or four sessions per day depending on device used. If the ankle joint was bridged with a fixator, the foot fixation may be removed at the termination of the distraction period to allow ankle range of motion and minimize stiffness, provided there is no knee flexion contracture. If a syndesmotic wire or screw was used to maintain the ankle mortise, it should be kept in place until frame removal to avoid the potential complication of fibular shortening.

8 Outcomes

An initial single-center report by McCarthy et al. in 2000 found improved outcome scores in an amputation group when compared with a lengthening group [7]. Lengthening was done either with the Wagner device or Ilizarov method, and results were not broken down according to each strategy. Wagner lengthening has been shown to yield higher complication rates [14, 44]. Perhaps the most important distinction between the reconstructive protocol presented in this chapter and the lengthening in the study by McCarthy et al. is the presence of adjacent joint reconstruction in the modern method. McCarthy et al. reported that a valgus ankle was a risk factor for poor result in their lengthening patients, but it does not appear that ankle correction was pursued pre-lengthening [7]. Prior to the McCarthy et al. article, several other single-center studies reported similar findings [11, 45].

Reconstruction management for mild fibular hemimelia is well established as a realistic option with good to excellent outcomes [8, 12, 46–49]. Oberc and Sulko evaluated 31 patients who had undergone a variety of treatments for fibular hemimelia [12]. Overall, they found improved outcomes in patients treated with amputation instead of reconstruction; however, the group with the best outcomes was in fact a subset of the reconstruction patients. They found the highest satisfaction and functional scores were in patients treated with a combination of lengthening and epiphysiodesis, resulting in nearly equal leg lengths. The authors did note that in the lengthening-only cohort, residual leg length discrepancy exceeding 5 cm appeared to be a major factor in functional outcomes. In their series, a "nonfunctional" foot was considered an indication for amputation, though the definition was somewhat unclear [12].

In 2010, El-Sayed et al. reported the results of their comprehensive reconstruction protocol that focused on the Ilizarov lengthening method and centralization of the ankle [48]. A total of 157 patients with Kalamchi Type 2 fibular hemimelia were reviewed, with an average lengthening gain of 13.6 cm. Patient outcomes were reported by means of a distributed satisfaction survey. Of the 119 surveys returned, 70 (59%) reported excellent results, and good results were reported in an additional 49 (41%). They reported that two patients with psychiatric conditions refused to participate in the survey, likely indicating that the authors felt the reported outcome would have been poor if the survey had been completed. Twenty-two patients either declined to participate or returned incomplete surveys and could not be included. All parents were reported to be happy with the final results. While cultural factors play a large role in family acceptance of amputation, this study highlights the possibility of good results in severe cases with a comprehensive reconstruction protocol.

Catagni et al. have reviewed their experience in two reports [9, 46]. Catagni et al. presented their modifications of the Delmonte classification as follows:

- Grade I – mild shortening of fibula associated with tibial shortening, mild deformity, and stable knee/ankle joints.
- Grade II – Severe fibular shortening, no functional lateral malleolus, equinovalgus foot deformity with ray deficiencies. Tibial and femoral deformities may also be present.
- Grade III – Absent fibula, severe deformity and shortening, equinovalgus foot, and/or dislocated ankle, with femoral involvement.

Each grade was treated with a specific approach, including lengthening alone for Grade I and initial brace management followed by initiation of deformity correction at age 10–12 years for Grade II. For Grade III, treatment included initial ankle soft-tissue release at 3–6 months of age followed by a series of lengthening procedures initiating at age 5–8 years. The details of their reconstructive protocol are shown below:

- Grade I: Simple lengthening, no bridge to foot.
- Grade II:
    - Stage 1 – Ankle orthosis with shoe lift after walking age.
    - Stage 2 – Tibial deformity correction and lengthening at age 10–12 years, with foot included in the frame. Foot fixation was included for stability and gradual reduction of the deformity. Fibular transport was also included as needed. The authors noted that lengthening should be less aggressive with more severe foot deformity.
    - Stage 3 – Second lengthening, bridging to femur if double-level lengthening is planned.

- Grade III:
  - Stage 1 – Ankle release at 3–6 months of age with correction of deformity.
  - Stage 2 – Lengthening at 5–6 years of age, bridge to foot, with correction of deformity and more conservative lengthening if foot deformity present.
  - Stage 3 – Lengthening at 8–10 years of age, with or without femoral lengthening.

In their initial report, 29 patients with Grade I were treated with a range of lengthening from 4 to 37 cm [46]. In the initial series, they reported good joint function in all patients, with all patients satisfied with functional and cosmetic results. Seven Grade II patients had competed treatment. Complication rates were higher in Grade II, but all patients were reported to have met the goals of treatment. Four Grade III patients had completed treatment, complications were again higher, and outcomes were not specifically reported [46].

A follow-up study in 2011 reviewed outcomes of 32 patients with Grade III fibular hemimelia [9]. Outcomes were scored based on limitation of function (on a 4-point scale) and pain (on a 5-point scale). Most patients had moderate limitation of activity and minimal to no pain. Twenty-four of 32 patients were satisfied. In the end, 17 patients were reported to have a satisfactory outcome in the surgeons' interpretation (no need for braces and no residual need for surgical care), and an additional 8 patients had relatively good outcomes (still required brace wear for daily activity). Two patients underwent late Syme amputation. The authors noted that the majority of patients were "quite active" with minimal pain, but the details of activity level were not clearly defined. Ankle valgus deformity was noted to be a risk factor for poor outcome [9].

The use of the above described SUPERankle procedure has been evaluated as a means to limit the effect of ankle valgus deformity on reconstructive outcomes [50]. Twenty-nine consecutive patients were managed according to the Paley classification. Excellent results were reported in 55%, good results in 22%, fair results in 15%, and poor results in 7%. The authors attributed improvements in outcomes when compared to historical controls to management of the ankle deformities with pre-lengthening reconstruction [50].

A 2019 comparison between amputation and reconstruction published by Birch et al. reviewed the outcomes of amputation-mediated treatment and reconstructive surgery for fibular hemimelia [13]. Both institutions involved were highly specialized: one with an on-site prosthetics department and the other with a very high concentration of surgical experience with congenital pathology. Minor differences were identified but felt to be clinically insignificant between the outcomes of each approach. Self-selected walking speed was 1.13 m/s in the reconstruction group versus 1.20 m/s in the amputation group. Both differed significantly from control patients at 1.25 m/s. This difference, though statistically significant, was not felt to be of clinical importance. Paired with the evidence by Pate et al. that outcomes trend toward control subjects with increasing age in fibular hemimelia [51], this is a very positive indication for the long-term health of patients affected by fibular hemimelia. Based on data presented by Birch et al., fears regarding the long-term impact of multiple procedures on quality of life for children appear to be groundless, as reported mental health outcomes in both groups were equivalent [13]. Whether these results can be reproduced outside of highly specialized centers is not clear based on available evidence.

9 Summary

A wide range of complications can occur with reconstruction and lengthening of limbs affected by fibular hemimelia. Pin infections are common. Residual leg length discrepancy, delayed union, joint stiffness, refractures, knee subluxation, residual foot deformities, and psychological impacts have all been reported. In the end, at least when performed in experienced centers, the outcomes of reconstruction are generally comparable to amputation, while avoiding the need for lifelong prosthetic care [13]. As might be expected for a rare pathology, this may not be reproducible in the more generalized experience [52]. Patients and families should be counseled carefully regarding surgical and nonsurgical treatment options, ideally at experienced centers. Outcomes data are emerging to support either reconstruction or amputation-mediated treatment, but overly rosy or dark representation of either method is unjustified. Both amputation and reconstruction have meaningful risks and benefits when managed properly; to be fair to our patients, we must represent both in a complete and unbiased discussion.

References

1. Bedard T, Lowry RB, Sibbald B, Kiefer GN, Metcalfe A. Congenital limb deficiencies in Alberta-a review of 33 years (1980-2012) from the Alberta Congenital Anomalies Surveillance System (ACASS). Am J Med Genet A. 2015;167A:2599–609.
2. Stevens PM, Arms D. Postaxial hypoplasia of the lower extremity. J Pediatr Orthop. 2000;20:166–72.
3. Birch JG, Lincoln TL, Mack PW, Birch CM. Congenital fibular deficiency: a review of thirty years' experience at one institution and a proposed classification system based on clinical deformity. J Bone Joint Surg. 2011;93:1144–51.
4. Rodriguez-Ramirez A, Thacker MM, Becerra LC, Riddle EC, Mackenzie WG. Limb length discrepancy and congenital limb anomalies in fibular hemimelia. J Pediatr Orthop B. 2010;19:436–40.
5. Reyes BA, Birch JG, Hootnick DR, Cherkashin AM, Samchukov ML. The nature of foot ray deficiency in congenital fibular deficiency. J Pediatr Orthop. 2017;37:332–7.
6. Calder P, Shaw S, Roberts A, Tennant S, Sedki I, Hanspal R, et al. A comparison of functional outcome between amputation and extension prosthesis in the treatment of congenital absence of the fibula with severe limb deformity. J Child Orthop. 2017;11:318–25.
7. McCarthy JJ, Glancy GL, Chang FM, Eilert RE. Fibular hemimelia: comparison of outcome measurements after amputation and lengthening. J Bone Joint Surg Am. 2000;82:1732.
8. Changulani M, Ali F, Mulgrew E, Day JB, Zenios M. Outcome of limb lengthening in fibular hemimelia and a functional foot. J Child Orthop. 2010;4:519–24.

9. Catagni MA, Radwan M, Lovisetti L, Guerreschi F, Elmoghazy NA. Limb lengthening and deformity correction by the Ilizarov technique in type III fibular hemimelia: an alternative to amputation. Clin Orthop. 2011;469:1175–80.
10. Patel M, Paley D, Herzenberg JE, McCarthy JJ, Glancy GL, Chang FM, et al. Limb-lengthening versus amputation for fibular hemimelia. J Bone Joint Surg Am. 2002;84:317–9.
11. Naudie D, Hamdy RC, Fassier F, Morin B, Duhaime M. Management of fibular hemimelia: amputation or limb lengthening. J Bone Joint Surg Br. 1997;79:58–65.
12. Oberc A, Sulko J. Fibular hemimelia – diagnostic management, principles, and results of treatment. J Pediatr Orthop B. 2013;22:450–6.
13. Birch JG, Paley D, Herzenberg JE, Morton A, Ward S, Riddle R, et al. Amputation versus staged reconstruction for severe fibular hemimelia: assessment of psychosocial and quality-of-life status and physical functioning in childhood. JBJS Open Access. 2019;4:e0053.
14. Choi I, Kumar S, Bowen J. Amputation or limb-lengthening for partial or total absence of the fibula. J Bone Joint Surg Am. 1990;72:1391–9.
15. Coventry MB, Johnson EW. Congenital absence of the fibula. J Bone Joint Surg Am. 1952;34(A):941–55.
16. Achterman C, Kalamchi A. Congenital deficiency of the fibula. J Bone Joint Surg Br. 1979;61-B:133–7.
17. Stanitski D, Stanitski C. Fibular hemimelia: a new classification system. J Pediatr Orthop. 2003;23:30–4.
18. Birch JG, Lincoln TL, Mack PW. Functional classification of fibular deficiency. In: Herring JA, Birch JG, editors. The child with a limb deficiency. Rosemont: American Academy of Orthopaedic Surgeons; 1998. p. 161–70.
19. Hamdy RC, Makhdom AM, Saran N, Birch J. Congenital fibular deficiency. J Am Acad Orthop Surg. 2014;22:246–55.
20. Herzenberg JE, Paley D, Gillespie R. Limb deficiency. In: Staheli LT, editor. Pediatric orthopaedic secrets. 2nd ed. Philadelphia: Hanley & Belfus, Inc.; 2003. p. 406–16.
21. Paley D. Surgical reconstruction for fibular hemimelia. J Child Orthop. 2016;10:557–83.
22. Radler C, Myers AK, Hunter RJ, Arrabal PP, Herzenberg JE. Prenatal diagnosis of congenital femoral deficiency and fibular hemimelia. Prenat Diagn. 2014;34:940–5.
23. Aguilar JA, Paley D, Paley J, Santpure S, Patel M, Herzenberg JE, et al. Clinical validation of the multiplier method for predicting limb length discrepancy and outcome of epiphysiodesis, part II. J Pediatr Orthop. 2005;25:192–6.
24. Mills G, Nelson S. An improved spreadsheet for calculating limb length discrepancy and epiphysiodesis timing using the multiplier method. J Child Orthop. 2016;10:313–9.
25. Makarov MR, Jackson TJ, Smith CM, Jo C-H, Birch JG. Timing of epiphysiodesis to correct leg-length discrepancy: a comparison of prediction methods. J Bone Joint Surg Am. 2018;100:1217–22.
26. Manner HM. Dysplasia of the cruciate ligaments: radiographic assessment and classification. J Bone Joint Surg Am. 2006;88:130.
27. Standard SC, Herzenberg JE, Conway JD, Siddiqui NA, McClure PK, Assayag MJ. The art of limb alignment. 9th ed. Baltimore: Rubin Institute for Advanced Orthopedics, Sinai Hospital of Baltimore; 2020.
28. Laor T, Jaramillo D, Hoffer FA, Kasser JR. MR imaging in congenital lower limb deformities. Pediatr Radiol. 1996;26:381–7.
29. de l'Escalopier N, Badina A, Padovani JP, Harroche A, Frenzel L, Wicart P, et al. Long-term results of ankle arthrodesis in children and adolescents with haemophilia. Int Orthop. 2017;41:1579–84.
30. Trichard T, Remy F, Girard J, Soenen M, Duquennoy A, Migaud H. [Long-term behavior of ankle fusion: assessment of the same series at 7 and 23 year (19–36 years) follow-up]. Rev Chir Orthop Reparatrice Appar Mot 2006;92:701–7.
31. El-Rosasy MA. Acute shortening and re-lengthening in the management of bone and soft-tissue loss in complicated fractures of the tibia. J Bone Joint Surg Br. 2007;89:80–8.

32. Mahaluxmivala J, Nadarajah R, Allen PW, Hill RA. Ilizarov external fixator: acute shortening and lengthening versus bone transport in the management of tibial non-unions. Injury. 2005;36:662–8.
33. Landge V, Shabtai L, Gesheff M, Specht SC, Herzenberg JE. Patient satisfaction after limb lengthening with internal and external devices. J Surg Orthop Adv. 2015;24:174–9.
34. Black SR, Kwon MS, Cherkashin AM, Samchukov ML, Birch JG, Jo C-H. Lengthening in congenital femoral deficiency: a comparison of circular external fixation and a motorized intramedullary nail. J Bone Joint Surg Am. 2015;97:1432–40.
35. Laubscher M, Mitchell C, Timms A, Goodier D, Calder P. Outcomes following femoral lengthening: an initial comparison of the Precice intramedullary lengthening nail and the LRS external fixator monorail system. Bone Joint J. 2016;98-B:1382–8.
36. Szymczuk VL, Hammouda AI, Gesheff MG, Standard SC, Herzenberg JE. Lengthening with monolateral external fixation versus magnetically motorized intramedullary nail in congenital femoral deficiency. J Pediatr Orthop. 2019;39(9):458–65.
37. Bhave A, Shabtai L, Ong P-H, Standard SC, Paley D, Herzenberg JE. Custom knee device for knee contractures after internal femoral lengthening. Orthopedics. 2015:e567–72.
38. Belthur MV, Paley D, Jindal G, Burghardt RD, Specht SC, Herzenberg JE. Tibial lengthening: extraarticular calcaneotibial screw to prevent ankle equinus. Clin Orthop. 2008;466:3003–10.
39. Leyes M, Noonan KJ, Forriol F, Cañadell J. Statistical analysis of axial deformity during distraction osteogenesis of the tibia. J Pediatr Orthop. 1998;18:190–7.
40. Westberry DE, Carpenter AM, Prodoehl J. Correction of genu valgum in patients with congenital fibular deficiency. J Pediatr Orthop. 2020;40:367–72.
41. Boakes JL, Stevens PM, Moseley RF. Treatment of genu valgus deformity in congenital absence of the fibula. J Pediatr Orthop. 1991;11:721–4.
42. Leveille LA, Razi O, Johnston CE. Rebound deformity after growth modulation in patients with coronal plane angular deformities about the knee: who gets it and how much? J Pediatr Orthop. 2019;39:353–8.
43. McGrath MS, Mont MA, Siddiqui JA, Baker E, Bhave A. Evaluation of a custom device for the treatment of flexion contractures after total knee arthroplasty. Clin Orthop Relat Res. 2009;467:1485–92.
44. Dahl MT, Fischer DA. Lower extremity lengthening by Wagner's method and by callus distraction. Orthop Clin North Am. 1991;22:643–9.
45. Cheng JC, Cheung KW, Ng BK. Severe progressive deformities after limb lengthening in type-II fibular hemimelia. J Bone Joint Surg Br. 1998;80:772–6.
46. Catagni MA, Bolano L, Cattaneo R. Management of fibular hemimelia using the Ilizarov method. Orthop Clin North Am. 1991;22:715–22.
47. Başbozkurt M, Yildiz C, Kömürcü M, Demiralp B, Kürklü M, Ateşalp AS. Fibular hemimelia: Ilizarov sirküler eksternal fiksatörü ile tedavi sonuçlari [Management of fibular hemimelia with the Ilizarov circular external fixator]. Acta Orthop Traumatol Turc. 2005;39:46–53.
48. El-Sayed MM, Correll J, Pohlig K. Limb sparing reconstructive surgery and Ilizarov lengthening in fibular hemimelia of Achterman-Kalamchi type II patients. J Pediatr Orthop Part B. 2010;19:55–60.
49. El-Tayeby HM, Ahmed AARY. Ankle reconstruction in type II fibular hemimelia. Strateg Trauma Limb Reconstr. 2012;7:23–6.
50. Kulkarni RM, Arora N, Saxena S, Kulkarni SM, Saini Y, Negandhi R. Use of Paley classification and SUPERankle procedure in the management of fibular hemimelia. J Pediatr Orthop. 2019;39:e708–17.
51. Pate JW, Hancock MJ, Tofts L, Epps A, Baldwin JN, McKay MJ, Burns J, Morris E, Pacey V. Longitudinal fibular deficiency: a cross-sectional study comparing lower limb function of children and young people with that of unaffected peers. Children (Basel). 2019;6:45.
52. Elmherig A, Ahmed AF, Hegazy A, Herzenberg JE, Ibrahim T. Amputation versus limb reconstruction for fibula hemimelia: a meta-analysis. J Pediatr Orthop. 2020;40:425–30.

Brachymetatarsia: Surgical Management with Internal and External Fixation

Noman A. Siddiqui

1 Introduction

Brachymetatarsia is a term used to describe a shortened metatarsal in the foot. This condition can be congenital or acquired and occurs due to premature closure of the metatarsal epiphysis [1]. Sarrafian described a normal pedal protrusion of metatarsal length with the second metatarsal being the longest and the fifth being the shortest [2]. This protrusion creates a parabolic arch described by Lelie'vre [3]. In brachymetatarsia one or more (brachymetapodia) metatarsals are shortened with respect to this normal pedal metatarsal positioning. This condition can be unilateral or bilateral and has a higher predilection in females by almost 5:1 [4–6] and occurs in less than 1 in 1000 [1].

The most common metatarsal affected by this condition is the fourth [6–8], followed by the first metatarsal [6, 7]. Jones et al. noted in a meta-analysis of 771 metatarsals that underwent surgical intervention; the fourth metatarsal was affected 73% of the time followed by the first metatarsal (19%) [6]. Congenital conditions were implicated as the primary reason for surgical intervention in the review. Other case reports have identified certain conditions and syndromes such as Trisomy 21, monosomy X, pseudohypoparathyroidism, pseudopseudohypoparathyroidism, Adams-Oliver syndrome, Cohen syndrome, diastrophic dysplasia, and many other disorders [5, 9, 10].

Acquired brachymetatarsia occurs due to premature epiphyseal closure due to trauma, infection, idiopathic, and iatrogenic causes [1]. This type of

N. A. Siddiqui (✉)
International Center for Limb Lengthening/Rubin Institute for Advanced Orthopedics, Sinai Hospital of Baltimore, Baltimore, MD, USA
e-mail: nsiddiqu@lifebridgehealth.org

E. Wagner Hitschfeld, P. Wagner Hitschfeld (eds.), *Foot and Ankle Disorders*,
https://doi.org/10.1007/978-3-030-95738-4_12

273

brachymetatarsia presentation is more common and will often present as unilaterally. Idiopathic causes such as trauma or shortening of the first metatarsal from overzealous tarsometatarsal arthrodesis or shortening from hallux valgus correction are other sources of brachymetatarsia of the first metatarsal (Fig. 8a).

2 Anatomy

The metatarsals are important for toe off and help distribute the weight of the limb equally as gait progresses. The metatarsals form from the mesoderm approximately 5 weeks after fertilization from the lateral condensation. This continues to form primary ossification centers by week 9 until birth [2]. The secondary ossification centers are usually visualized by age 3 and ossify by 17–21 years of age.

Since the first and fourth metatarsals are most commonly involved in this condition, it is important to be familiar with some important anatomic features. The first metatarsal is a long bone that articulates proximally with the medial cuneiform and in some cases with the second metatarsal. The distal end of the metatarsal articulates with the hallux. In terms of overall size, it is the shortest metatarsal but critical for function of the foot. It has an independent axis of rotation which allows it the most mobility compared to the lesser metatarsals. The first metatarsal has intrinsic muscular attachments from the abductor hallucis muscle medially, extensor hallucis brevis, and the dorsal interosseus muscle laterally. Extrinsic tendons of the peroneus longus and tibialis anterior tendon attach directly to the base plantar and dorsally, respectively. The arterial supply of the metatarsal is robust, and it receives perfusion from the distal branches of the dorsalis pedis and medial plantar artery. The interconnections between the dorsal metatarsal arteries, plantar metatarsal arteries, and deep perforating branches provide a network of flow that supplies blood to the base, shaft, and metatarsal head. The nerve supply to the first metatarsal is provided by the sensory branches of the superficial peroneal nerve to the dorsum of the first metatarsal, the terminal aspect of the great saphenous nerve, and medial plantar nerve. Motor branches from the deep peroneal and medial plantar nerve provide function to the muscular attachments to the intrinsic muscles of the foot.

The fourth metatarsal is a long bone that articulates proximally with the cuboid and fifth metatarsal laterally, the lateral cuneiform and third metatarsal medially. At the metatarsophalangeal joint, it articulates with the proximal phalanx. Its intrinsic muscular attachments include the dorsal and plantar interosseous muscles. The arterial supply of the metatarsal receives perfusion from the dorsal and plantar metatarsal arteries. The nerve supply to the fourth metatarsal is provided by the sensory branches of the superficial peroneal nerve to the dorsum of the metatarsal, along with the lateral plantar nerve.

3 Diagnosis

The diagnosis of brachymetatarsia is made clinically and radiographically. Clinical presentation of brachymetatarsia becomes apparent with a shortened digit as the foot develops (Fig. 1). However, a thorough history and physical exam is necessary since some patients with brachymetatarsia may present with other skeletal conditions seen with syndromes mentioned above and will require co-management with

Fig. 1 An AP image of a female patient with brachymetatarsia of the fourth metatarsal

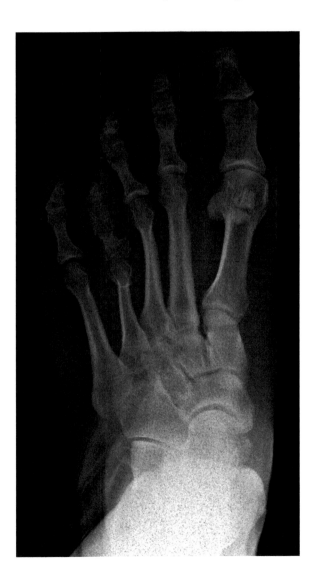

other specialties. The patient may or may not complain of pain, but in both cases one of the complaints is the appearance [4, 7, 9]. In the author's experience, juvenile patients do not complain of pain but present with a parent concerned of the appearance and the long-term effect of the shortened digit. In many of these cases, the parents may feel the cosmetic appearance will be concerning as the child transitions to adolescence and adulthood. The meta-analysis by jones revealed that 93% of the patients requiring surgical intervention have been female; thus cosmetic appearance in open toe footwear can be a concern.

The severity of the shortening can be quantified in terms of length radiographically and has been described as a deviation of the original parabola defined by Lelie'vre [3, 4, 11]. Other methods, such as the Maestro criteria, have been described, in which, metatarsal length declines in a geometric pattern by a factor of two. Deviation from this result is considered a shortening from the normal progression [12]. However, the author uses a simple reproducible approach of connecting a line from the metatarsal head of the second to the fifth metatarsal on a calibrated plain anterior-posterior radiograph (Fig. 2). The distance from this line to the shortened digit will be the amount of lengthening needed to restore a "patient normal" length. This technique can be applied to all metatarsals even in cases of brachymetapodia, acute or gradual correction, and a shortened first metatarsal by using a normal metatarsal parabola angle [12].

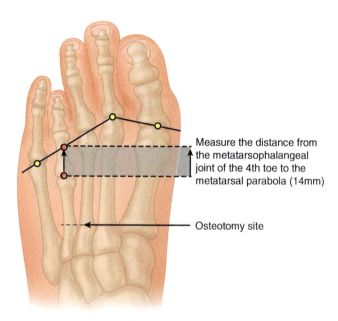

Measure the distance from the metatarsophalangeal joint of the 4th toe to the metatarsal parabola (14mm)

Osteotomy site

Fig. 2 A simple radiographic method to calculate the length needed for correction of brachymetatarsia. (Modified with permission from Rubin Institute for Advanced Orthopedics, Sinai Hospital of Baltimore, 2018)

4 Conservative Management

Brachymetatarsia can result in various forms of digital discomfort that can be alleviated with nonoperative intervention. A contracted or overriding digit at the metatarsophalangeal joint will create callosities and hyperkeratotic lesions that are irritated dorsally in shoe gear. Adjacent digits can deviate into the direction of the shortened toe and can form hammer digit deformities, and even hallux valgus, that further create difficulty with ambulation or shoes. Metatarsalgia of the adjacent metatarsals can be painful and worsen the symptoms of the foot. Padding in the shoes with felt or silicone padding can alleviate some of these painful symptoms. Additionally, these various complaints can be managed with over the counter or custom foot orthoses depending on the degree of deformity. Brachymetapodia can be managed in a similar fashion, however, poses additional challenges due to the involvement of multiple digits and metatarsals.

5 Surgical Planning/Treatment

Operative intervention of this condition requires a thorough exam of the foot. Noting adequate perfusion to the foot is critical to prevent neurovascular compromise to the digit during acute or gradual correction. Some key components to pay attention to during the physical exam is the appearance of a hypoplastic digit that will often accompany the shortened metatarsal. In some cases, despite achieving normal metatarsal length, the hypoplastic digit may give the impression of inadequate correction. Evaluation of the range of motion of the digit and determining the flexible versus a rigid contracture will be important to restoring normal metatarsophalangeal joint (MTPJ) relationship. A Kelikian push-up test is an easy method to evaluate for contracture of the MTPJ [13].

Radiological evaluation is the most important component in surgical intervention. In bilateral cases, the author utilizes the method described earlier of connecting a line from the second metatarsal head to the fifth metatarsal. When addressing unilateral cases, one can obtain standard anterior posterior, oblique, and lateral weight-bearing images. The author will obtain bilateral images despite unilateral involvement to demonstrate to the patient certain radiographic features of this condition. In many cases of brachymetatarsia, the associated digit phalanges will appear hypoplastic when compared to the contralateral foot. This associated digital hypoplasia may give the digit a smaller appearance despite restoration of normal metatarsal length, and this is discussed in the preoperative visit to prevent postsurgical disappointment. An additional benefit of bilateral foot radiographs is the absolute length of the normal and abnormal side metatarsal can be obtained. The differences can be calculated, and the surgeon can have an anatomic blueprint to lengthen the metatarsal of the affected side. However, if one chooses not to obtain bilateral films, or has prior radiographs from the patient, then the method described above can be utilized. Surgical intervention can be performed by either acute or gradual methods [14]. Acute lengthening is advised in cases of less than 1 cm [14]. However, in the review offered by Jones et al., it revealed that the mean length gained by a variety of interposition grafting methods was 13 mm. The author has had similar success and has routinely performed acute lengthening in patients under <16 mm (Fig. 3).

The technique includes the following steps:

1. 5 cm incision made on the dorsum of the fourth metatarsal (can be centralized over adjacent metatarsals if multiple require lengthening).
2. Blunt dissection is taken to the extensor tendon and a Z lengthening of the tendon is performed.

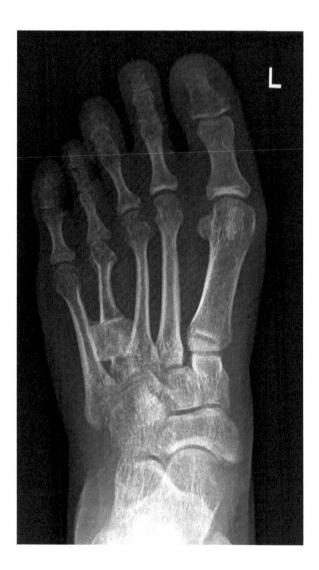

Fig. 3 An example of an acute correction of 14 mm of the fourth metatarsal with iliac crest autograft

3. Under image intensification the appropriate metatarsal is confirmed, and minimal/focal periosteal elevation.
4. Two 0.62 K-wires are inserted into the base and shaft of the metatarsal perpendicular to its long axis.
5. A transverse osteotomy is completed at the met-diaphysis of the deformed bone, and gradual correction is performed with a Hintermann distractor until the desired lengthening is completed.
6. A 0.62 K-wire is antegraded through the medullary canal to the level of the MTPJ. The dorsally displaced digit is reduced, and the pin is advanced through the proximal phalanx until the proximal end of the wire is not visible at the osteotomy (a dorsal capsulotomy and flexor tenotomy may be required to allow manual reduction of the digit).
7. An iliac crest autograft is sized based of the desired lengthening and tamped into the distraction osteotomy site. If autograft is not obtained, the author will utilize fresh frozen iliac crest allograft that has soaked in bone marrow aspirate concentrate.
8. While maintaining control of the graft, the medullary wire is retrograded into the graft and traverses into the cuboid. (prior to final placement, the Hintermann distractor can be manipulated to angulate the moving segment of the metatarsal to align the direction of the metatarsal to avoid excessive adduction/abduction.
9. If the graft does not feel stable, an additional wire can be placed in a transverse manner into the adjacent third or fifth metatarsals for stability.
10. The author has utilized placing a low-profile locking plate in cases where patient compliance with remaining protected non weight-bearing is a concern (Fig. 4).

The first described method of acute correction was by McGlamry and Cooper utilizing a calcaneal autograft [15]. Additional methods have been authored, such as an oblique osteotomy and interpositional grafting [16–20]. Myerson described application of interpositional grafting for brachymetatarsia correction and reported obtaining up to 18 mm of correction in a single stage without ischemia of the digits [20].

One of the benefits of acute lengthening is it is accomplished in a single setting without the need of external fixation. Lengthening of up to 15 mm can be performed, and many patients on average are lengthened 13 mm [6, 17]. Patients can return to activity sooner since healing is dependent on graft incorporation and not regenerate consolidation, based on the mean healing index as analyzed by Jones et al.

Disadvantages of this method are donor site morbidity in cases of autograft harvest. Additionally, lengthening greater than 15 mm can risk vascular compromise [17, 21]. Malunion, nonunion, hardware failure, MTPJ stiffness, and graft absorption are some of the reported concerns [6, 17, 21]. However, in a cohort of 41 feet, Giannini reported 100% union with the use of a metatarsal allograft with K-wire fixation with a follow-up of 3 years [17]. Patient AOFAS scores improved from 37 to 88, and none of the complications mentioned earlier were seen in this cohort. The

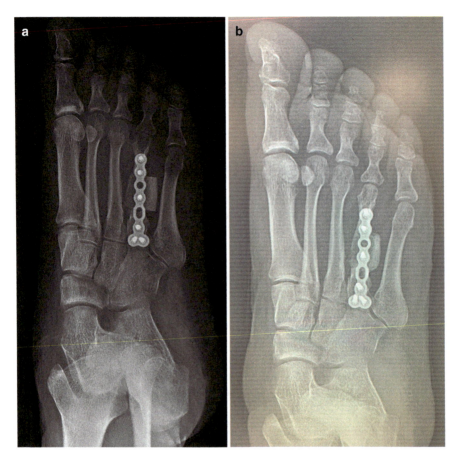

Fig. 4 (**a/b**) An acute correction with Iliac crest allograft soaked in bone marrow aspirate concentrate. (**a**) The graft was plated with a low-profile seven-hole locking plate. (**b**) Healed and well incorporated union of allograft

author has seen similar outcomes with allograft and more recently has converted to utilizing fresh frozen iliac crest allograft that is soaked intraoperatively in bone marrow aspirate concentrate (BMAC). Under correction is a possibility in the acute setting and can create dissatisfaction for the patient. Therefore, it is critical to be careful when selecting patients greater than 13–15 mm of length in one stage to avoid disappointment.

The alternative to acute lengthening is gradual lengthening with a mini external fixator via distraction osteogenesis. This method is utilized in cases of lengthening greater than 1 cm (1, Scher). Multiple descriptions of this technique are available and demonstrate an open approach to osteotomy and fixator application. The author prefers a modified percutaneous method as described by Lamm [8]. Briefly, a systematic application of the external fixator is applied in the following steps (Fig. 5a–e):

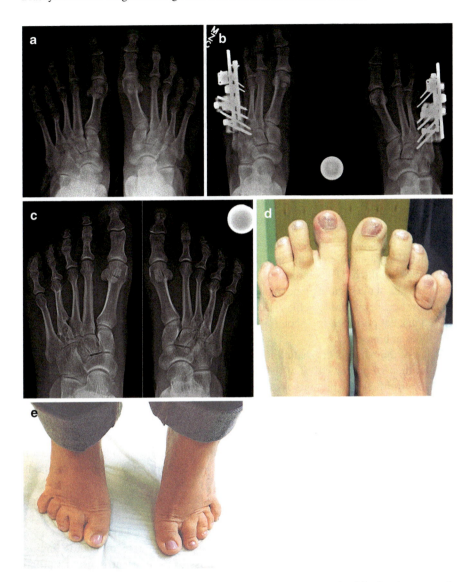

Fig. 5 (**a**) An example of a young female with bilateral brachymetatarsia of the fourth metatarsal. (**b**) A gradual correction with monolateral external fixator. The fourth MTPJ has been spanned with a fixator to distract the MTPJ. (**c**) Correction achieved and consolidation noted of the regenerate. (**d**) Clinical presentation of the fourth digit preoperatively. Note the hypoplastic appearance and dorsally contracted position of the digit. (**e**) The final corrected position of the fourth digit. This patient was able to obtain excellent function of the fourth digit full dorsiflexion at the MTPJ

- All half-pins are inserted percutaneously, perpendicular to the metatarsal shaft in a bicortical fashion, under fluoroscopic control. The key feature is to align the proximal and distal half pins in a manner to ensure the vector of lengthening does not create impingement against the adjacent metatarsal heads in the final position.

- A percutaneous osteotomy is performed with a high torque low-speed burr as close to the metatarsal metaphyseal-diaphysis.
- Acute distraction of 3–5 mm is performed (decreases time in frame).
- A 1-cm incision is made on the posterolateral aspect of the calcaneus and blunt dissection is carried down to the lateral calcaneal wall.
- A small trephine is used to harvest a bone plug. Additional curettage and graft can be obtained if needed, but a small trephine harvest provides plenty of graft in most cases.
- The autograft is packed into the distracted osteotomy site to "supercharge" the lengthening site during the 5–7 days latency period.
- Lengthening is initiated after 5–7 days at 0.5–0.75 mm/day until appropriate radiographic position of the metatarsal head is obtained.
- The affected digit is pinned while reduced during the distraction to prevent dislocation.

Once the patient obtains the length needed to correct the deformity, the digital pin traversing the MTPJ is removed. The patient is given range of motion exercises of the MTPJ in the sagittal plane to prevent stiffness. The external fixator is removed once the regenerate bone achieves consolidation. Upon removal, the foot is protected in a flat postoperative shoe for 2–4 weeks. Full activity is allowed in supportive shoes at this stage.

One of the benefits of gradual lengthening is the patient can have a deformity greater than 15 mm or <40% of the original length [1, 6, 8, 21, 22]. This expands the opportunities for patients with significant deformity to undergo correction. Another benefit is the ability to ambulate immediately compared to immobilization for 6–8 weeks. The most common drawback with callus distraction is stiffness of the MTPJ and infection of the pin site [6]. Pin site infections are most often managed by oral antibiotics and have not been reported to lead to any deep infections [6]. The stiffness of the MTPJ is concerning, and different methods have discussed trans-articular pinning and early range of motion along with joint spanning fixation [8, 23, 24]. However, no specific method has demonstrated decreasing the potential of joint stiffness and arthrosis. The author has attempted the various methods for joint ROM preservation, and none have shown to have superiority in preserving function. Given this, the author recommends having patients understand the limitations and the possibility of arthrosis and limited range of motion.

6   Brachymetapodia

A less common yet challenging condition is brachymetapodia. In this scenario, multiple metatarsals are shortened with respect to the normal metatarsal parabola. Surgical corrections utilizing acute and gradual methods have been attempted.

Indications for acute and gradual correction are based on the length needed and the ability to maintain vascularity to the digits. In the author's experience, adjacent metatarsals with less than 15 mm of length required for correction can be corrected in a single stage. However, it is critical to monitor the digit for blanching due to the stress on the distal digital vessels. Therefore, the author prefers multiple monolateral fixators on the dorsum of the foot. The slow distraction rate and the ability for the patient to ambulate immediately make this a desirable method (Fig. 6a–c).

7 Lengthening Recommendations

When performing brachymetatarsia lengthening with gradual distraction, an important aspect of the patient education is discussion of a timeline to full healing. As mentioned earlier the author prefers a distraction rate of 0.5–0.75 mm per day. The rate is dependent on multiple factors such as age, general health, medical comorbidities, smoking status, the amount of lengthening, and the stage of lengthening. Certain stages of lengthening require the rate to be decreased or increased. For example, pediatric or juvenile patients have the capacity to distract at a faster rate versus adults due to the rapid healing seen in children. Conversely, if the patient has slower forming regenerate or pain with lengthening, the rate can be decreased to allow for patient comfort and the regenerate to improve radiographically.

8 Postoperative Protocol

The author prefers a 0.5 mm/day distraction rate, and the patient is given a general timeline. The following can be utilized as a template for lengthening based of 0.5 mm of distraction daily for 15 mm of lengthening:

- Day 1: Osteotomy and frame application.
- Latency period 6 days.
- Day 7: Distraction initiated 0.5 mm daily (0.25 mm twice a day). This will be performed for 30 days.

Fixator removal at 14–18 weeks [8].

The patient will be seen every 2 weeks to ensure proper alignment and signs of regenerate formation. The patient is full weight-bearing in a protective flat surgical shoe. The patient is allowed to resume daily showers and pin care after the first postsurgical visit (day 7). Pin care is minimal, and emphasis is placed on wrapping a single roll of gauze/Kling around the pin sites in a circular manner to

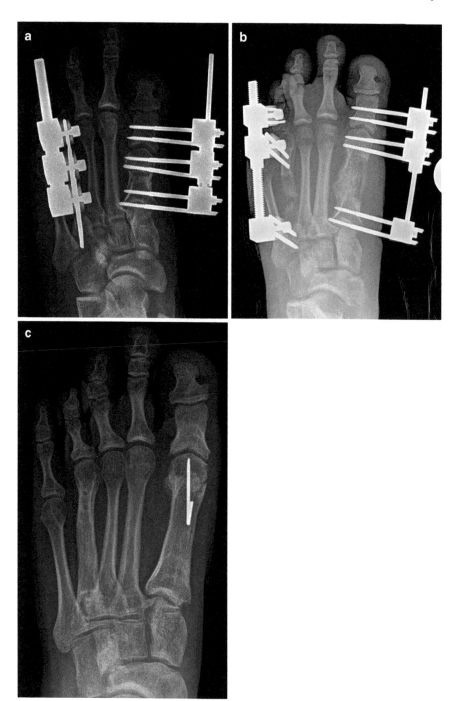

Fig. 6 (**a**) Brachymetapodia of the first and fourth metatarsals. (**b**) Abundant regenerate formation with gradual correction. (**c**) Final outcome with restoration of alignment of the first and fourth metatarsal

prevent soft tissue pistoning on the pin site, which can increase the likelihood of a soft tissue infection. A broad-spectrum first-generation cephalosporin (cephalexin) prescription is given prophylactically in the event of a perioperative pin site infection. Instructions are also given regarding symptoms of pin site infections such as pain, redness, drainage, streaking, and inability to ambulate without discomfort.

The fixator is maintained until signs of bony consolidation are noted on two views via plain radiographs. As a general rule, the author will relate to the patient the removal of the fixator will be three times the amount of the distraction phase. Thus, based off our earlier example of 30 days, removal would be at 90 days post-distraction or almost 16 weeks after the index operation. This general rule falls within the time period that has been described by other surgeons [6, 8].

9 Pitfalls to External Fixation

One of the common concerns and complications is delayed union or lack of regenerate consolidation (Fig. 7). Various methods are available to manage this during treatment. The first step is to rule out a metabolic or nutritional deficiency which can inhibit bone formation. Bone stimulation via stimulators are an alternative nonsurgical option that can be helpful. For direct manipulation, the author has utilized alternating reverse compression followed by distraction of the regenerate to stimulate healing. In some instances, the fixator itself needs to be gradually weakened to allow the bone regenerate to progressively share the load. In cases the regenerate fails to consolidate, the author's preferred method of treatment is conversion to open plating and autogenous or allograft bone grafting (Fig. 8a–e). If there is no active pin infection, the patient is taken to the operating room for frame removal, and a dowel-shaped bone graft is harvested from the ipsilateral calcaneus. The dowel is placed within the regenerate sleeve, and a standard 1/3 tubular low-profile locking plate is utilized that spans the metatarsal from the neck to the base to provide stability to the bone. Alternatively, the author has utilized iliac crest allograft soaked in BMAC to span the defect when there are no signs of regenerate formation. This is plated with a low-profile locking plate to facilitate earlier weight-bearing during the recovery. With these methods the author has not had any nonunions, and the appropriate length and alignment are secured. Lamm et al. described an alternative approach of temporary medullary fixation for delayed healing to improve regenerate consolidation [24]. In this technique an Ilizarov wire is inserted into the medullary canal from the dorsal aspect of the neck of the metatarsal and across the regenerate until bony consolidation is noted. In the small cohort of patients, all achieved bony consolidation.

Fig. 7 A potential
complication of gradual
correction is lack of
regenerate formation

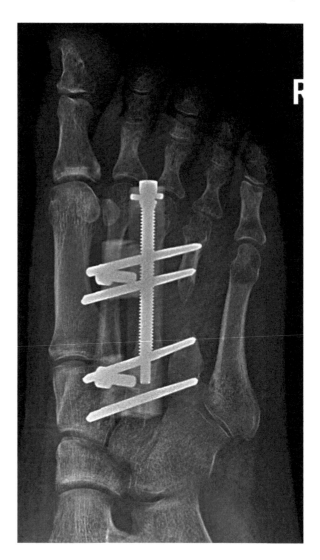

10   Final Thoughts

Brachymetatarsia is a challenging pathology, and acute and gradual correction
methods have been described. Acute and gradual corrections have both demonstrated to be effective in resolving the limb length deficits in metatarsals. The fourth
metatarsal is the most common followed by the first metatarsal. Gradual correction
has demonstrated to be effective at obtaining greater amounts of correction, however, has a greater number of potential complications [6]. Acute correction has less

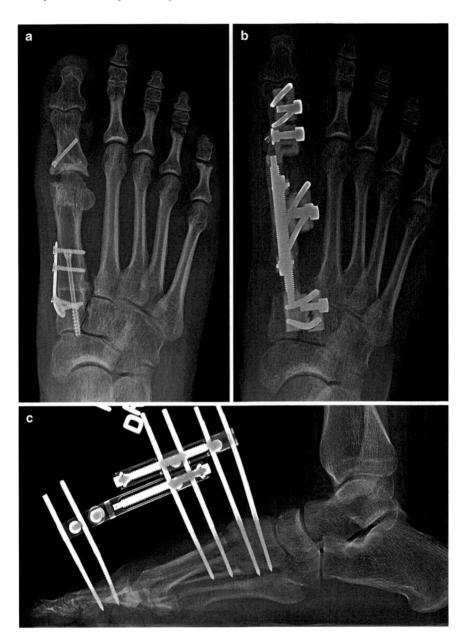

Fig. 8 (**a/b**) In this example the patient had an overzealous tarsometatarsal arthrodesis with 1.8 cm shortening. He underwent gradual correction and due to slow regenerate formation required grafting and plating with iliac crest bone allograft and locked plating. (**c**) Lateral view of the foot with appropriate axial distraction of the shortened metatarsal. (**d**) AP and (**e**) Lateral views of plating of the consolidating regenerate, demonstrating maintenance of length and regenerate consolidation

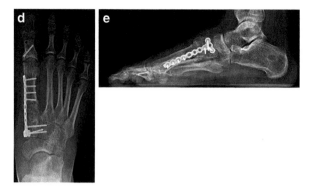

Fig. 8 (continued)

potential for complications but has shown to have a limitation in the amount of correction that can be obtained in a single setting. Regardless of method the patient needs to understand the benefits of improved cosmetic appearance, but not necessarily improved function given the high degree of stiffness noted at the MTPJ post correction [6]. In the author's experience, both methods have their merits, when applied appropriately, and patients report high levels of satisfaction.

Conflict of Interest Although none of the authors has received or will receive benefits for personal or professional use from a commercial party related directly or indirectly to the subject of this article.

References

1. Davidson RS. Metatarsal lengthening. Foot Ankle Clin. 2001;6:499–518.
2. Kelikian AS, Sarrafian SK, eds. Sarrafian's anatomy of the foot and ankle: descriptive, topographic, functional. 3rd edition. Philadelphia, PA: Wolters Kluwer; 2011.
3. Lelie've J. Pathologie du pied [Pathology of the foot]. Paris: Masson; 1971.
4. Urano Y, Kobayashi A. Bone-lengthening for shortness of the fourth toe. J Bone Joint Surg Am. 1978;60:91–3.
5. Concheiro Barreiro G, Gadañón García A, Giráldez Domínguez JM. Percutaneous foot surgery for the treatment of brachymetatarsia: a case report. Foot Ankle Surg. 2017;23:e1–5.
6. Jones MD, Pinegar DM, Rincker SA. Callus distraction versus single-stage lengthening with bone graft for treatment of brachymetatarsia: a systematic review. J Foot Ankle Surg. 2015;54(5):927–31.
7. Magnan B, Bragantini A, Regis D, Bartolozzi P. Metatarsal lengthening by callotasis during the growth phase. J Bone Joint Surg Br. 1995;77:602–7.
8. Lamm BM. Percutaneous distraction osteogenesis for treatment of brachymetatarsia. J Foot Ankle Surg. 2010;49(2):197–204.
9. Schimizzi A, Brage M. Brachymetatarsia. Foot Ankle Clin. 2004;9:555–70.
10. https://hpo.jax.org/app/browse/term/HP:0010743
11. Tachdjian MO. Pediatric orthopedics. 2nd ed. Philadelphia: WB Saunders; 1990. p. 2633–7.
12. Besse JL. Metatarsalgia. Orthop Traumatol Surg Res. 2017;103(1S):S29–39.

13. Rozbruch R, Hamdy R. Limb lengthening and reconstruction surgery case atlas. Foot and ankle; metatarsal reconstruction case 79 Brachymetatarsia 563–570.
14. Shecaira AP, Fernandes RMP. Brachymetatarsia: one-stage versus two-stage procedures. Foot Ankle Clin. 2019;24(4):677–87.
15. McGlamry ED, Cooper CT. Brachymetatarsia: a surgical treatment. J Am Podiatr Assoc. 1969;59:259–64.
16. Choudhury SN, Kitaoka HB, Peterson HA. Metatarsal lengthening: case report and review of the literature. Foot Ankle Int. 1997;18:739–45.
17. Giannini S, Faldini C, Pagkrati S, et al. One- stage metatarsal lengthening by allograft-interposition: a novel approach for congenital brachymetatarsia. Clin Orthop Relat Res. 2010;468:1933–42.
18. Kashuk KB, Hanft JR, Schabler JA, et al. Alternative autogenous bone graft donor sites in brachymetatarsia reconstruction: a review of the literature with clinical presentations. J Foot Surg. 1991;30:246–52.
19. Singh D, Dudkiewicz I. Lengthening of the shortened first metatarsal after Wilson's osteotomy for hallux valgus. J Bone Joint Surg Br. 2009;91(12):1583–6.
20. Myerson M. Management of metatarsalgia. In: Myerson M, Kadakia A, eds. Reconstructive foot and ankle surgery: Management of complications. 2nd edition. Philadelphia, PA: WB Saunders/Elsevier; 2010:123–33.
21. Kim HT, Lee SH, Yoo CI, et al. The management of brachymetatarsia. J Bone Joint Surg Br 2003;85-B:683–90.
22. Scher DM, Blyakher A, Krantzow M. A modified surgical technique for lengthening of a metatarsal using an external fixator. HSS J. 2010;6(2):235–9.
23. Masada K, Fujita S, Fuji T. Complications following metatarsal lengthening by callus distraction for brachymetatarsia. J Pediatr Orthop. 1999;19:394–7.
24. Lamm BM, Moore KR, Knight JM, Pugh E, Baker JR, Gesheff MG. Intramedullary metatarsal fixation for treatment of delayed regenerate bone in lengthening of brachymetatarsia. J Foot Ankle Surg. 2018;57(5):987–94.

Lesser Toe Deformities

Carlos Pargas and Pablo Wagner Hitschfeld

Summary The most frequent deformities that affect the lesser toes in pediatric population are called curly toes, hammer toes, overlapping toes, polydactyly, and macrodactyly. The first three diagnoses are mainly due to tendons imbalance and, therefore, are many times corrected through soft tissue procedures. The last two are congenital abnormalities that include anatomical differences (soft tissue and bone tissue) that need to be addressed more aggressively. It is important to follow these patients given the deformity relapse risk.

1 Introduction

The growth and development of the lesser toes in children can present multiple variations that need only observation and time to resolve or normalize. However, there are certain congenital and developmental lesser toe abnormalities that can be approached and managed in a straightforward and practical manner.

The most frequent deformities that affect the lesser toes in pediatric population are called curly toes, hammer toes, overlapping toes, polydactyly, and macrodactyly. The first three diagnoses are mainly due to tendons imbalance and, therefore, are many times corrected through soft tissue procedures. The last two are congenital abnormalities that include anatomical differences (soft tissue and bone tissue) that need to be addressed more aggressively. It is important to follow these patients given the deformity relapse risk.

C. Pargas (✉)
Sinai Hospital of Baltimore, Baltimore, MD, USA

P. Wagner Hitschfeld
Orthopedic Surgery Department, Clínica Alemana de Santiago - Universidad del Desarrollo, Hospital Militar de Santiago – Universidad de los Andes, Santiago, RM - Santiago, Chile

© The Author(s), under exclusive license to Springer Nature Switzerland AG 2022
E. Wagner Hitschfeld, P. Wagner Hitschfeld (eds.), *Foot and Ankle Disorders*, https://doi.org/10.1007/978-3-030-95738-4_13

This chapter will include the diagnosis and management of curly toes, hammer and claw toes, overlapping toes, polydactyly, and macrodactyly.

2 Curly Toes

This term refers to a flexion and adduction deformity of a lesser toe with concurrent external rotation. This deformity is typically attributed to a congenital contracture of the toe at the proximal and distal interphalangeal joints.

The pathophysiology is a contracture of the flexor digitorum longus and most often concurrent contracture of the flexor digitorum brevis tendon. The tendons subluxate to the tibial side of the toe resulting in adduction/varus of the toe with external torsion along with the main flexion contracture (Figs. 1 and 5). The varus occurs at the level of the PIP and DIP joints. Some authors state that this deformity does not occur in the second toe; however, Turner [5] described a variant of curly toe resulting in a flexion and valgus deformity of the second toe and overlapping third toe.

The incidence of curly toes is noted to be 2.8% (84 toes per 1588 live births) in a Canadian study [4] and 3.2% (38 toes per 1167 live births) in a South Korean study [1]. No associated syndromes or chromosomal anomalies are associated with this lesser toe deformity.

Unresolved curly toes can result in painful callosities on the end of the toe, nail plate problems, and pressure issues on the adjacent toe. Turner cited 10% of patients with curly toes complained of discomfort with shoe wear [5]. Studies differ on the most commonly affected toe. Cho et al. stated the fourth toe is the most commonly affected digit (68%) [1]. However, Hamer et al. [2] found an even distribution of the

Fig. 1 Fifth curly toe. The toe is externally rotated in 90° degrees

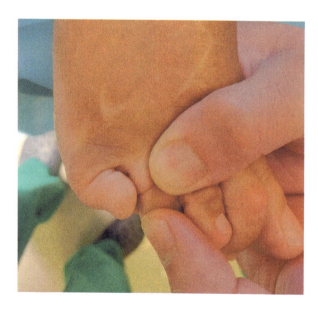

involvement of the third and fourth digits (47.8%). Interestingly, most authors state the second toe is not involved, but Turner reported a 25% incidence of second toe involvement. Bilaterality is common (up to 80%) with the same toe effected on each foot but with varying severity [5]. The flexion contracture is present at birth but can go unnoticed unless it is moderate to severe. Most families present after the child has started to stand and cruise. The parents complain of either the curled toe or the cock-up appearance of the adjacent toe. Diagnosis is simply made with observation of the contracted toe on standing and the incomplete full extension of the toe with passive stretch. The toe that appears contracted but is able to be fully extended passively is a dynamic type or positional curly toe. This type of positional curly toes either resolves spontaneously or responds to stretching and strapping treatments in the author's experience. Ross and Menelaus [3] state the importance of delineating a true curly toe from other causes of a fixed flexion deformity of the toe. A curly toe by definition is a deformity caused by the foreshortening or contracture of the flexor tendons. Menelaus stated that observing full extension of the PIP and DIP joints with MTP joint flexion confirms the contracture of the flexor tendons [3]. This type of toe deformity will resolve with elongation of the flexor tendons. The severity of the deformity can be graded by the following:

Grade 0	No deformity
Grade 1	Mild curl with no concurrent adduction or external rotation
Grade 2	Grade 1 + adduction with overlapping of adjacent toe
Grade 3	Grade 2 + increased flexion where the toenail cannot be seen when looking down on the dorsum of the foot

Conservative management of curly toes consist of observation, stretching, and strapping/taping the contracted digit. It should be noted that reports have cited spontaneous resolution of the curly toe in 25–50% of patients [4]. Many authors reference Sweetnam's study who stated in 1958 that strapping and taping methods did not alter the natural history of this congenital deformity. Other authors have demonstrated 68% [5] to 94% [4] success rate with strapping methods. However, after the strapping was discontinued, an incidence of 62.5% loss of improvement was noted. The other limitations on the success of the strapping/taping method appears to be the initiation of the treatment within the first few weeks of life. The prolonged time of strapping (3–12 months) and skin irritation were other problems noted with this treatment method.

Definitive surgical treatment has been recommended for unresolved curly toes [2, 3]. The incidence of true long-term problems with unresolved curly toes has not been completely elucidated. Cho et al. reported symptoms in adults with unresolved curly toe deformity [1]. The most common symptom was the sensation of "stepping on the toe" and callosity formation on the interphalangeal joint. The author has noted painful callosities on the tip of the contracted toe in adolescent patients. The two most common surgical techniques for correction of curly toe deformity are simple flexor tenotomy and flexor tendon transfer to the extensor tendon. Initially, the curly toe deformity was believed to be caused by a paresis of the flexor muscles creating an imbalance between the flexor structures and the extensor structures. Intuitively, a flexor release and transfer to the extensor mechanism was the surgical technique recommended. However, there has been no definitive evidence of paresis or other neurological causes of the typical curly toe deformity. Also, Hamer et al. demonstrated no significant difference in success between the two techniques in a randomized, double-blinded study [2]. Ross and Menelaus demonstrated a success rate of 95% with simple flexor tenotomy of both the long and short flexor tendons. The 5% poor results were due to postoperative contracture of longitudinal incisions that crossed the flexor crease or a missed slip of the flexor tendon. The recommendations are an open release with a transverse incision [3].

2.1   Author's Preferred Approach to Curly Toe

Observation and gentle stretching are the simplest forms of treatment in the first few months of life. If the child is under 1 year of age, I encourage the family to stretch the curly toe and strap the toe at night. Most mild or dynamic forms of curly toe will resolve. If the deformity persists or presents after the child is walking, then I recommend a simple flexor tenotomy as an outpatient procedure. I wait until the child is walking and the foot is large enough to safely perform an open tenotomy. Since one of the most common complications of curly toe release is recurrent scar formation with recurrent contracture, I perform the tenotomy with a V to Y skinplasty. This allows lengthening of both the tendon and skin structures with excellent healing and minimal scar formation.

The incision is a V shape with the apex pointing distal and just proximal to the flexion crease of the MTP joint. After the incision is created, the soft tissues are spread in line with the neurovascular bundle and retracted exposing the tendon sheath. The tendon sheath is incised longitudinally, and the three tendon strips are lifted with a micro hemostat and sharply released. The toe should maintain an extended position. With the toe extended, the V incision is converted into a Y and closed with simple absorbable sutures. A typical sling dressing of gauze is placed holding the toe in an extended position. A short leg semirigid walking cast is placed on patients between 2 and 4 years of age, and a simple soft dressing is applied to patients 5 and older. The dressing is maintained for 7–10 days and removed at the follow-up appointment. The incision site is covered with a simple band aid if needed, and the patient is allowed to advance to full activities as tolerated. In older patients (adolescent), tenotomy will not be enough to correct this rotational deformity. A Butler's procedure is the recommended technique for these cases (Fig. 2).

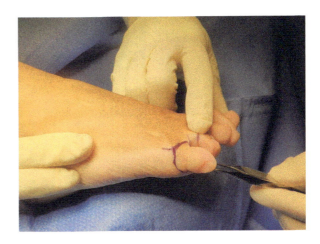

Fig. 2 Fifth curly toe. Planning of a Butler procedure

3 Hammer and Claw Toes

These are common deformities of the lesser toes although rarely studied in children. Epidemiology, physiopathology, and clinical features of these deformities in pediatric patient have been barely reported with details.

Each deformity has a particular combination of joint affectation. Hammer toe is characterized by excessive flexion of proximal interphalangeal (PIP) joint accompanied by extension of distal interphalangeal (DIP) joint. The metatarsophalangeal (MTP) joint used to be normal, however, depending of the severity of the deformity could show some levels of subluxation by hyperextension [6]. The hammer toe is most common between the second and fourth toe with significant predilection for the second [8]. Otherwise, claw toe is characterized by flexion of PIP and DIP joint as well as hyperextension at the MTP joint (Figs. 3 and 4).

These deformities are subject of loss of balance between extrinsic and intrinsic muscles flexors and extensors. Also, insufficient plantar capsule and extensions of the plantar aponeurosis to keep the dynamic balance of the joint. Adherences may develop that subsequently exacerbate the deformities [11].

3.1 Treatment

The nonsurgical management of hammer and claw toes is very similar. The only purpose is relief the pressure and subsequent pain of the involved areas. In hammer toes the dorsal aspect of PIP is the most affected and should be the most padded area. In children that already use shoes, we recommend high and wide toe box of the shoes. In cases where the deformity is severe and compromise the MTP joint, high pressure could be appreciated with a callus in the plantar area of the metatarsal head. In this case we recommend metatarsal pads placed proximal to the metatarsal

Fig. 3 Preoperative
hammer toes on second
and fourth. Flexible
deformity

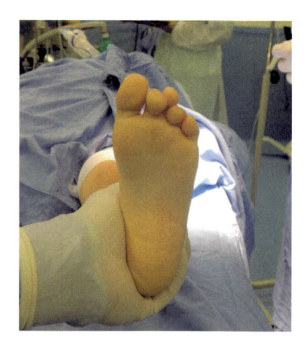

Fig. 4 Postoperative flexor
tenotomies hammer toes
on second and fourth.
Flexible deformity

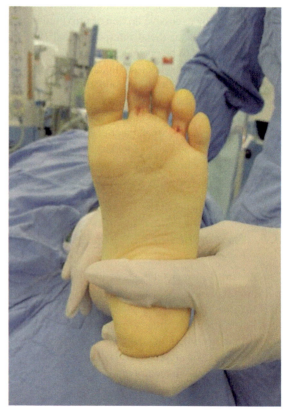

head. In claw toes in addition to dorsal PIP padding, we also recommend nail padding protection to avoid irreversible nail deformities.

Surgical options go from release, lengthening, or transfer of soft tissue to bone procedures that include joint resection, arthrodesis, or even bone shortening (Gonzalez-Rincon). However, before moving on with surgical management, some variables should be considered such as age of the patient, severity, associated disease, flexible, or fixed deformity [10]. The deformity is considered flexible when it is corrected during plantar flexion movement of the ankle, while fixed deformity does not correct with any change of position. Flexor digitorum longus (FDL) tenotomy or transfer is recommended in flexible deformities. Otherwise, fixed deformity requires PIP resection or fusion. Patients with severe deformity, without remnant growth, and associated disease as neurologic problems could benefit from performing bone procedures if the soft tissue does not allow complete correction.

Ross and Menelaus reported FDL tenotomy for hammer and curly toes was successful with only 5% of poor results, and it was more related with scar problems. In addition, they claimed that the open flexor tenotomy was preferred because it allows you to identify appropriately the flexor tendon [3]. Jacobs also concluded that open flexor tendon lengthening in hammer toes is a safe and reliable procedure. They recommend a transverse skin incision and Z-lengthening of the flexor digitorum longus [7].

If bone shortening is going to be performed in a fixed deformity, just consider that some issues related to excessive bone resection (shortening) have been reported and it is recommended to start with less bone resection (only resection of the head of proximal phalangeal) [9].

3.2   Complications

Complications may be present in any surgery, and these deformity corrections are not the exceptions. Some of the most feared complication involved the vascular insufficiency resulting the tension placed in the vessels during acute correction or collapse of vessel during shortening. Close monitoring of toe irrigation should be considered after correction [6]. Otherwise, scar contraction with recurrence of deformity or partial restriction of movements also could happen, and it is one of the most common [3]. On the other hand, general complications observed in others surgery as infection, nerve injuries, no union, or malalignment are latent.

3.3   Summary

1. Determine if the deformity is flexible (nonsurgical or soft tissue procedure as treatment) or fixed (soft and/or bone procedure).
2. The Hammer toe and claw toe share similar nonsurgical and surgical management in pediatric patient.

3. Surgical treatment as first step is the soft tissue characterized by FDL tenotomy or transfer.
4. Be careful with irreversible complication (neurovascular bundle damage).
5. Primary goal is to obtain toes without pain, fit into the shoe, and have acceptable appearance.

4   Overlapping Toe

It is a congenital deformity represented by overriding of the fourth toe by the fifth toe. This deformity has not gender predilection and usually bilateral although this remain controversial. Previous studies reported 20–30% of bilateral overriding toes. Low incidence of 1.8% was described in a population of 3100 children by Gonzalez-Rincon.

The MTP joint is the apex of the tri-planar deformity. It is characterized by adduction in the transverse plane, hyperextension in the sagittal, and external rotation in the coronal plane developing a subluxation dorsal-medial of MTP joint; the PIP and DIP usually are normal. The more acceptable cause of this pathology is the retraction of soft tissues mainly shortening and adduction of extensor digitorum longus with capsular adhesions at the metatarsal head [5, 6] (Fig. 5).

The most frequent complaint in this patient is pain, accompanied by formation of callus in the dorsal area of the fifth toe due to wear of tied shoes. On the other hand, cosmesis plays a relevant role in female patient. 50% of the patient could present dysfunctional gait [6].

Fig. 5 Image showing a combination of a fifth overlapping toe and a fourth curly toe

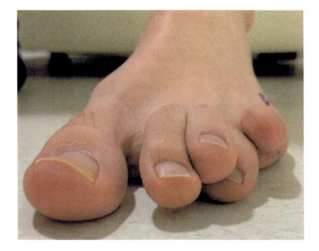

4.1 Treatment

The first treatment options in pediatric patient is nonsurgical. Stretching passive exercises, use of corrective soft wrap, or orthosis is well tolerated in younger patients. However, in adolescent wearing of orthosis is less tolerated. Indication of wide and confortable shoes becomes a better option.

When the nonsurgical treatment fails, multiple surgical procedures take the place. These range from skin to bone techniques. V or Y shape of fifth toe skin is performed with poor results due to scar retraction, syndactyly of fourth and fifth toes described by McFarland [17] with often unacceptable cosmetic results, and EDL transfer from fifth toe to the neck of fifth metatarsal or abductor digiti quinti tendon [15, 16].

Butler's technique makes adjustment in different soft tissue (mainly rotational) areas with good results reported by many authors [13, 14]. This requires a racquet incision with a plantar handle inclined laterally and a dorsal handle following the EDL tendon. Subsequent, EDL and dorsal medial and volar capsule release to allow the deformity correction. No fixation is used (however, the author recommends a temporal k-wire to hold the reduction), and skin flap from lateral to dorsal side of the foot is sutured [12, 14]. Soft tissue surgery is less common, but arthroscopic technique has been reported to have good results which stabilize the plantar plate anchored to EDL tendon and reduce the MTP joint, release of dorsal-medial capsule, and plication of lateral capsule [18].

On the other hand, bone surgeries have been described with partial success, however are not common in pediatric population. These involve bone shortening of metatarsal or proximal phalanges (diaphysis), distal metatarsal osteotomy (Weil technique), or total resection of proximal phalanges. Gonzalez-Rincon described good results in 82.9% of the patient in a report of proximal phalangeal shortening.

4.2 Summary

1. The overriding toes is a complex multiplanar MTP joint deformity that is common bilaterally.
2. The goal of the treatment is to obtain a pain-free toe with acceptable appearance.
3. Try as first line of treatment passive stretching exercises and soft padding in young patient; wide shoes are recommended.
4. The clue in the surgical treatment obtains a balance between the soft tissue previously contracted (EDL and capsule).

5 Polydactyly

Foot polydactyly is the most common malformation of the forefoot that results from defective development during pre- or postaxial patterning of developing limb [19]. This is categorized as excessive malformation and characterized by more than five digits with a wide variation in its clinical presentation going from a minor protuberance to a complex malformation compromising midfoot/forefoot to duplicate bone, sometimes, sharing the same bone, neurovascular bundle or just skin (syndactyly).

This could be related to syndromic problems, new single isolated event, or other body malformation, being the hand, the most common involved [20, 21]. Foot polydactyly causes functional limitation (pain) and cosmesis problems [21, 22].

The incidence of foot polydactyly is a 1.7 per 1000 live births. Ethnicity rates are highest in Afro-American population 3.6–13.9 per 1000 live births whereas in Caucasian is around 0.3–1.3 per 1000 live births [20, 23]. According to gender, the reports are not conclusive. There is an increased tendency to involve the left foot rather than the right [19]. Considering the anatomy area, the lateral ray is more common (79%), while medial column is 15–17% and central toes in just 4–6% of incidence [20, 21].

5.1 Etiology and Pathophysiology

Etiology has not been fully known. However, continuing efforts in researches have achieved some progress. Genetic areas have been able to identify some responsible gene of polydactyly such as GLI3 which is associated with Greig cephalopolysyndactyly syndrome, sonic hedgehog gene (SHH), fibroblast growth factor (FGF), homeobox protein aristaless-like 4 (ALX4), homeobox D (5'-HoxD), ZNF141, MIPOL1, IQCE, and PITX1 [24].

The pathophysiology is not completely clear. One theory is related to disorder in the programmed cell death during fetal limb development, and another is the genetic mutations in some gene loci.

Some signals are responsible of promote development and growth of limbs. The zone of polarizing activity (ZPA, posterior portion of mesenchyme) which is mediates by the sonic hedgehog (SHH) molecule and the atypical ectodermal ridge (AER, distal portion del ectoderm) that expresses fibroblast growth factors (FGF) could lost the balance and induce the formation of extra digits [25].

5.2 Anatomy, Classification, and Diagnosis

Polydactyly mainly has been classified by multiples authors according to anatomy: Temtamy and Mckunsick categorized these as preaxial (first ray or hallux), central (middle rays, second, third, and fourth), and postaxial (fifth ray) [20]. Venn-Watson

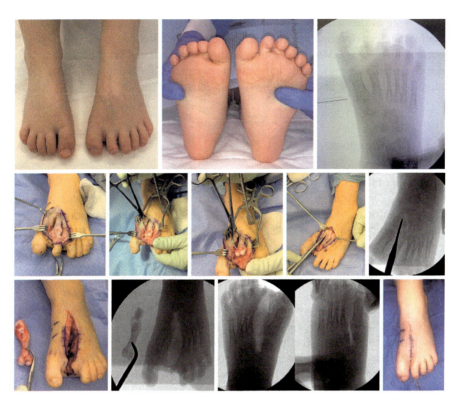

Fig. 6 Left foot central polydactyly. Preoperative and postoperative clinical and radiological images are shown. Operative sequence of a second ray excision

described a classification based in the anatomy configuration of the metatarsal: (1) normal metatarsal with distal duplication, (2) block metatarsal, (3) Y-shaped metatarsal, (4) T-shaped metatarsal, (5) normal metatarsal shaft with a wide head, and (6) ray duplication [20, 23]). Also, Watanabe et al.'s classification was based in the segment involved: (1) tarsal type (with one subtype), (2) metatarsal type (with three subtypes), (3) proximal phalangeal type (with five subtypes), and (4) distal phalangeal type (with six subtypes) (Fig. 6).

Although, this classification gives us an idea where the deformity is located, its surgical planning is not clear enough. For that reason, Seok et al. classified the foot polydactyly focused in practical surgical orientation to avoid the common complications as axis deviation, skin issues, or remaining lesion of the extra digit. They divided this in three main variables (SAM): syndactylism, axis deviation, and metatarsal extension (with three subtypes for each variable) [26].

The diagnosis starts with an accusative general physical examination. In these patients, even if the extra digit is obvious, we should be alert due to syndromic association. On the other hand, the extra toe sometimes hides complex deformity beyond the forefoot. Therefore, soft tissue (skin), axial deformities, and nail should be evaluated and considered for an appropriated diagnosis and plan.

Imaging evaluations are considered when bony connection is suspect; this normally is indicated around the first year of age to allow time for the bony ossification nucleus to show up. Most of the time, radiographic AP and lateral are enough to decide a plan. However, we do not rule out the use of CT scan or MRI [20, 23]) for more complex associated deformities in mid-/hind foot (Fig. 6).

5.3 Management

Treatment of this condition is wide as well as its variability presentation. This could be from no surgical in mild undeveloped extra toes where the patient does not refer any discomfort or cosmesis problems to a surgical treatment in more complex deformities or simply functional and cosmesis complaint. Surgical treatment is indicated mainly around the first year of age to avoid any walk developmental delay due to use of cast, orthosis, or any psychological issue related to cosmesis [23]. However, Ozren and Darko did not find any significant differences related to age of foot polydactyly surgery (Ozren).

The main goal of surgery treatment in foot polydactyly should be create a better shape of the foot to fit well into a shoe, comfortable and with acceptable appearance that allows the patient to feel good about themselves. In order to get this, the surgeon must make excision of extra digit(s), consider making an osteotomy of associated bone duplication and an appropriated skin coverage without forgetting to maintain alignment, joint stability, and soft tissue balance [23].

The tendency in surgical treatment is saving the most dominant ray and/or digit. Though, in some cases the dominant extra toe(s) could have some associated deformity, hypertrophic condition, or related skin problems which lead you to think about making an excision of this. The debate shows up when both digits are very similar. In this case, it is relevant to consider the risks of vascularity, foot stability, and soft tissue coverage.

In simple case, when the extra digit is attached to a thin soft tissue, suture ligation (occlusion of artery) is an option. However, some complications related to neuroma formation or remnant of skin could become symptomatic requiring a second procedure. In patient with extra digit attached to a dense soft tissue, racquet-type excision is recommended with neurovascular bundle visualization to decrease the possibility of a neuroma formation.

On the other hand, when the extra lateral digit (postaxial) is attached with the metatarsal and had created a real articulation, a disarticulation of lateral digit is required. Careful collateral ligament dissection and reattachment are essential to avoid joint instability. Sometimes temporal k-wire fixation could be necessary. When the metatarsal head is wide or with Y or T shape, cartilage remodeling (physiolysis) or osteotomies could be necessary to obtain an appropriated alignment. The recommendation always is focused toward removing the most lateral toe.

The complex preaxial foot deformities have worse outcomes than postaxial deformities. Poor outcomes are mainly secondary to hallux varus (incidence 40–87%) [20, 21] caused by inadequate bone resection, soft tissue reattachment, or presence of epiphyseal – physis deformation (bracket). Adequate treatment should include removing the extra medial rudimentary toe, lateral metatarsophalangeal ligament repair and a first metatarsal osteotomy [20, 21, 23].

Central polydactyly has some additional challenges such as requiring a dorsal and plantar approach. However, we do not recommend the plantar approach to avoid painful scars. Longitudinal approach could be used during central excision of one toe and Z-plasty when it is going to be more than one. The most relevant consideration during central toe excision is the width of the foot; for that reason central cuneiform bone resection is sometimes necessary. Also reconstruction of intermetatarsal ligaments using suture, wire, or cerclage helps create a narrow foot (Fig. 6).

In addition, periosteum or cartilage of extra digit should be removed completely to avoid recurrence.

5.4 Summary

1. Foot polydactyly is the most common forefoot deformity than could be associated with other syndromes.
2. Careful physical examination should be performed. The diagnosis is usually easy normally requiring foot X-rays.
3. The most used classification is preaxial, central, and postaxial. However, the developing of SAM gave us more surgical planning orientation.
4. The trend is excision of medial of lateral toes in preaxial or postaxial, respectively. Saving the dominant toe.
5. Preaxial has more complications than post-axial deformities.
6. Be careful with remaining foot width in cases of central polydactyly. Appropiate intermetatarsal ligament reconstruction and cuneiform excision are necessary.
7. During the surgery remember excision, soft tissue balance, and joint alignment.
8. The final goals of treatment are pain-free foot and an acceptable foot appearance.

6 Macrodactyly

Macrodactyly is a rare condition characterized by enlargement of every part of the toe(s) [27]; it involves an extensive variety of clinical features which in some cases even the metatarsal could be compromised [28]. This condition could cause many problems as pain, difficulty with shoe wear, psychological and cosmetic problems and diffculty with gait development, between others. If there is an asymmetric bone growth, secondary deformities as flexion/extension contraction or valgus/varus deviation appear. Macrodactyly sometimes could be associated with syndactyly (23%) and polydactyly (4%) [29].

Incidence is 1 in 18,000 live births with no clear gender difference [29, 30]. Multiple digits are more affected than isolated toes (2:1) with preference for mid-line digits.

Macrodactyly can be classified in: Primary which is characterized by congenital overgrowth no related to syndrome, usually involving soft and bony tissue and secondary or syndromic which is associated with external conditions as overgrowth secondary to tumors (neurofibromatosis, lymphangioma, hemangioma, etc.) or as part of disorders (Proteus, Klippel-Trenaunay syndrome). In this secondary group, the soft tissues are mainly affected. Also, macrodactily can be classified as static when there is only an initial toe(s) overgrowth (evident at birth) followed by a normal growth in the following years, and as progressive if there is an increased toe growth during childhood [29, 30].

6.1 Etiology

The etiology remains to be elucidated. It is believed not related to inheritance. Some theories have been mentioned in isolated macrodactyly such as abnormal nerve stimulator signals to the affected digit causing thickening of the nerve, whereas others believe that it is more related to increased blood supply in the area [31]. On the other hand, some theories related to PIK3CA mutations have been mentioned; however, this mutation is also related to some tumors [29].

6.2   Management

In most cases, surgical treatment is preferred by orthopedic surgeons. The main goal is to develop a functional shoeable foot. Cosmesis is considered especially in female foot. Surgical management often involves bone and soft tissues. Due to wide variability, the orthopedic surgeon should prepare different techniques that include skin/subcutaneous resection/reconstruction, neurolysis, epiphysiodesis, osteotomies, arthrodesis, and/or amputations.

Treatment options depend on the degree of compromise of soft tissue and/or bone.

Some reports with isolated soft tissue surgeries have had poor results due to subsequent secondary procedures [28, 32, 33]. For that reason, we just recommend soft tissue procedures in patients with mild macrodactily an age close to skeletal maturity.

In cases where isolated phalange(s) affectation is present, techniques such as amputation of phalanges, epiphysiodesis, and shortening have been described. All of them are accompanied by soft tissue debulking. Chang et al. [28] referred skin problems in cases of amputation. Epiphysiodesis has a shortening risk given that it is not possible to calculate the exact timing for that procedure.

Epiphysiodesis also could be applied when metatarsal bone is affected. There is risk of over shortening; however, with the development of new devices, temporal epiphysiodesis decreased that risk. Also, acute diaphysis shortening of the metatarsal bone with internal fixation can achieve good correction, but in immature patient, secondary shortening could be required. The most important disadvantage with these techniques is the limitation to decrease the width of the foot. For that reason, some authors have inclination for ray resection accompanied by soft tissue debulking. Dedrick and Kling [33] recommended ray resection when the foot is wider than two standard deviation of a normal foot. Chang et al. [28] recommended ray resection when intermetatarsal angle exceeds the normal side by >10 degrees. In mild cases, shortening and repeat debulking may be an option. In central toes macrodactyly, the recommendation is central ray amputation which decreases the intermetatarsal angle. Plantar and dorsal approach is recommended to help with appropriated bone and soft tissue resection.

Same indications are recommended when the great toe is involved except for ray amputation. The first metatarsal has an important role in weight-bearing and gait. Exceptional cases could be considered.

Treatment algorithm can be summarized as follows:

If there is only soft tissue compromise: soft tissue debulking vs amputation (if severe compromise). If there is a combination of soft tissue and bone: soft and bone tissue debulking (shortening osteotomy, ostectomy, partial resection) vs amputation (if severe compromise). Epiphysiodesis is a treatment option with mild correction power. If chosen, always associate it with debulking (Figs. 7, 8, 9, 10, 11, and 12).

Fig. 7 Second toe macrodactyly. Clinical image

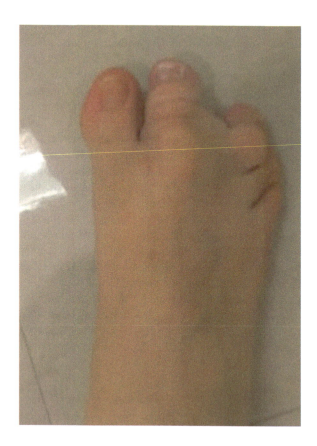

Fig. 8 Second toe macrodactyly. Preop planning

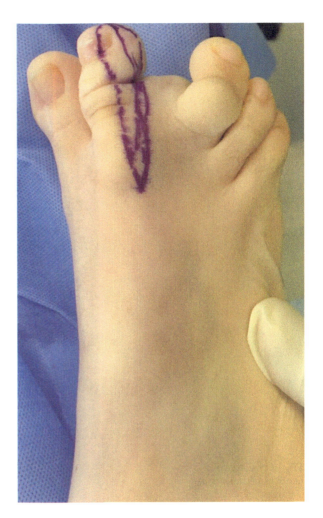

6.3 *Summary*

1. Macrodactyly is a rare condition characterized by enlargement of every part of the toe sometimes involving all ray(s).
2. Can be classified as static or progressive being central toes the most common affected.
3. Unknown etiology with stronger theory related to abnormal nerve stimulator signal. Overgrowth related to nerve territory distribution.
4. Multiple treatment options from soft tissue resection to amputations, with some other options as epiphysiodesis or shortening.
5. Final treatment goals are to reduce the foot size, cosmesis and be able to fit shoes.

Fig. 9 Second toe macrodactyly. Preop X-ray

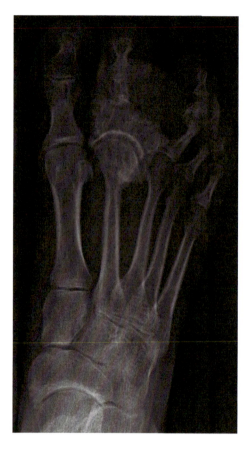

Fig. 10 Second toe macrodactyly after bone and soft tissue debulking

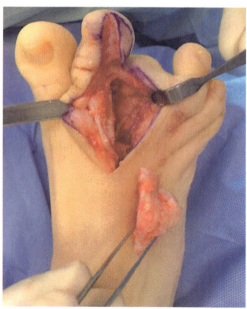

Fig. 11 Second toe
macrodactyly. Postop
clinical image

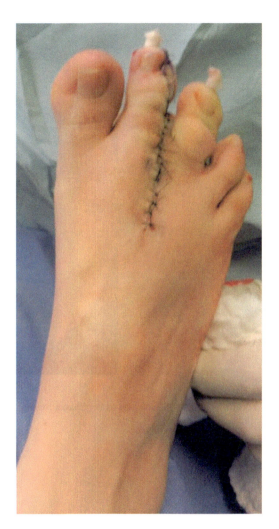

Fig. 12 Second toe
macrodactyly. Postop
X-ray

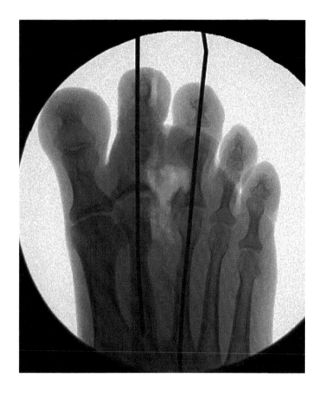

Acknowledgments Thank you to Dr. Shawn Standard, MD, for his help with images and text
edition.

References

1. Cho JY, Park JH, Kim JH, Lee YH. Congenital curly toe of the fetus. Ultrasound Obstet
   Gynecol. 2004;24(4):417–20. https://doi.org/10.1002/uog.1087. PMID: 15343596.
2. Hamer AJ, Stanley D, Smith TW. Surgery for curly toe deformity: a double-blind, randomised,
   prospective trial. J Bone Joint Surg Br. 1993;75(4):662–3. https://doi.org/10.1302/0301-620
   X.75B4.8331129. PMID: 8331129.
3. Ross ER, Menelaus MB. Open flexor tenotomy for hammer toes and curly toes in childhood.
   J Bone Joint Surg Br. 1984;66(5):770–1. https://doi.org/10.1302/0301-620X.66B5.6501376.
   PMID: 6501376.
4. Smith WG, Seki J, Smith RW. Prospective study of a noninvasive treatment for two common
   congenital toe abnormalities (curly/varus/underlapping toes and overlapping toes). Paediatr
   Child Health. 2007;12(9):755–9. https://doi.org/10.1093/pch/12.9.755. PMID: 19030460;
   PMCID: PMC2532862.
5. Turner PL. Strapping of curly toes in children. Aust N Z J Surg. 1987;57(7):467–70. https://
   doi.org/10.1111/j.1445-2197.1987.tb01399.x. PMID: 3475061.
6. Shirzad K, Kiesau CD, DeOrio JK, Parekh SG. Lesser toe deformities. Am Acad Orthop Surg.
   2011;19(8):505–14.

7. Jacobs R, Vandeputte G. Flexor tendon lengthening for hammer toes and curly toes in paediatric patients. Acta Orthop Belg. 2007;73(3):373–6. PMID: 17715729.
8. González-Rincón JA, Valle-de Lascurain G, Oribio-Gallegos JA. Diafisectomía de la falange proximal en el quinto dedo supraducto y dedo en martillo en niños [Diaphysectomy of the proximal phalanx in quintus varus supraductus and hammer toe in children]. Acta Ortop Mex 2013;27(2):103–8. Spanish. PMID: 24701761.
9. Janecki CJ, Wilde AH. Results of phalangectomy of the fifth toe for hammertoe. The Ruiz-Mora procedure. J Bone Joint Surg Am. 1976;58(7):1005–7. PMID: 977609.
10. Angirasa AK, Augoyard M, Coughlin MJ, Fridman R, Ruch J, Weil L. Hammer toe, mallet toe, and claw toe. Foot Ankle Spec. 2011;4(3):182–7. https://doi.org/10.1177/1938640011409010.
11. Scheck M. Etiology of acquired hammertoe deformity. Clin Orthop Relat Res. 1977;123:63–9. PMID: 856521.
12. Simões R, Alves C, Tavares L, Balacó I, Sá Cardoso P, Pu Ling T, Matos G. Treatment of the overriding fifth toe: Butler's arthroplasty is a good option. J Child Orthop. 2018;12:36–41. https://doi.org/10.1302/1863-2548.12.170099.
13. De Boeck H. Butler's operation for congenital overriding of the fifth toe: retrospective 1–7-year study of 23 cases. Acta Orthop Scand. 1993;64(3):343–4. https://doi.org/10.3109/17453679308993641.
14. Cockin J. Butler's operation for an over-riding fifth toe. J Bone Joint Surg Br. 1968;50(1):78–81. PMID: 4868030.
15. Lantzounis LA. Congenital subluxation of the fifth toe and its correction by a periosteocapsuloplasty and tendon transplantation. J Bone Joint Surg. 1940;22(I):147–50.
16. Lapidus PW. Transplantation of the extensor tendon for correction of the overlapping fifth toe. J Bone Joint Surg. 1942;2(4):555–9.
17. McFarland B. Congenital deformities of the spine and limbs. In: Platt H, editor. Modem trends in orthopedics. New York: P B Hoeber; 1950. p. 107–8.
18. Lui TH. Arthroscopic-assisted correction of claw toe or overriding toe deformity: plantar plate tenodesis. Arch Orthop Trauma Surg. 2006;127(9):823–6. https://doi.org/10.1007/s00402-006-0224-4.
19. Al Amin ASM, Carter KR. Polydactyly. In: StatPearls [Internet]. Treasure Island: StatPearls Publishing; 2021; 2021 Jan–. PMID: 32965966.
20. Turra S, Gigante C, Bisinella G. Polydactyly of the foot. J Pediatr Orthop B. 2007;16(3):216–20. https://doi.org/10.1097/01.bpb.0000192055.60435.31. PMID: 17414786.
21. Phelps DA, Grogan DP. Polydactyly of the foot. J Pediatr Orthop. 1985;5(4):446–51. https://doi.org/10.1097/01241398-198507000-00012. PMID: 4019759.
22. Kubat O, Antičević D. Does timing of surgery influence the long-term results of foot polydactyly treatment? Foot Ankle Surg. 2018;24(4):353–8. https://doi.org/10.1016/j.fas.2017.04.001. Epub 2017 Apr 13. PMID: 29409237.
23. Kelly DM, Mahmoud K, Mauck BM. Polydactyly of the foot: a review. J Am Acad Orthop Surg. 2021;29(9):361–9. https://doi.org/10.5435/JAAOS-D-20-00983. PMID: 33443388.
24. Umair M, Ahmad F, Bilal M, Ahmad W, Alfadhel M. Clinical genetics of polydactyly: an updated review. Front Genet. 2018;9:447. https://doi.org/10.3389/fgene.2018.00447. PMID: 30459804; PMCID: PMC6232527.
25. Bouldin CM, Harfe BD. Aberrant FGF signaling, independent of ectopic hedgehog signaling, initiates preaxial polydactyly in Dorking chickens. Dev Biol. 2009;334(1):133–41. https://doi.org/10.1016/j.ydbio.2009.07.009. Epub 2009 Jul 17. PMID: 19616534.
26. Seok HH, Park JU, Kwon ST. New classification of polydactyly of the foot on the basis of syndactylism, axis deviation, and metatarsal extent of extra digit. Arch Plast Surg. 2013;40(3):232–7. https://doi.org/10.5999/aps.2013.40.3.232. Epub 2013 May 16. PMID: 23730599; PMCID: PMC3665867.
27. Khanna N, Gupta S, Khanna S, Tripathi F. Macrodactyly. Hand. 1975;7(3):215–22. https://doi.org/10.1016/0072-968x(75)90056-x. PMID: 1205357.

28. Chang CH, Kumar SJ, Riddle EC, Glutting J. Macrodactyly of the foot. J Bone Joint Surg Am. 2002;84(7):1189–94. https://doi.org/10.2106/00004623-200207000-00015. PMID: 12107320.
29. Chen W, Tian X, Chen L, Huang W. Clinical characteristics of 93 cases of isolated macro-dactyly of the foot in children. J Orthop Surg Res. 2021;16(1):121. https://doi.org/10.1186/s13018-020-02196-2. PMID: 33557883; PMCID: PMC7869226.
30. Hardwicke J, Khan MA, Richards H, Warner RM, Lester R. Macrodactyly – options and out-comes. J Hand Surg Eur. 2013;38(3):297–303. https://doi.org/10.1177/1753193412451232. Epub 2012 Jun 26. PMID: 22736742.
31. Dennyson WG, Bear JN, Bhoola KD. Macrodactyly in the foot. J Bone Joint Surg Br. 1977;59(3):355–9. https://doi.org/10.1302/0301-620X.59B3.893515. PMID: 893515.
32. Megalodactylism RK. Report of 7 cases. Acta Orthop Scand. 1967;38(1):57–66. https://doi.org/10.3109/17453676708989619. PMID: 6035453.
33. Dedrick D, Kling TF, jr. Ray resection in the treatment of macrodactyly of the foot in children. Orthop Trans. 1985;12:40–6.

Neurologic Foot

Gino Martínez and Gonzalo Chorbadjian

1 Introduction

The neuromuscular diseases of childhood frequently compromise the locomotive system and its development, among which infant cerebral palsy, peripheral neuropathies, and myopathies stand out [1, 2]. The foot is frequently affected in its normal function as well as in its structural development during the skeletal growth, deteriorating in diverse magnitude the capacity of standing, walking, and performance in recreational and sport activities. The eventual concomitant deterioration of other anatomical segments further aggravate the patient global motor function [3, 4].

In this chapter, the main neuromuscular diseases of childhood that impact the locomotor system, specifically the foot and ankle, will be analyzed. The physiopathology of each disease, its natural history, and current treatments available will be detailed. In addition, the main morphological and functional alterations of the foot derived from these diseases will be analyzed with the options of orthopedic and surgical treatment, detailing the most used techniques depending on each particular case.

G. Martínez (✉)
Clínica Universidad de Los Andes, Santiago, Chile

Instituto Teletón, Santiago, Chile

G. Chorbadjian
Clínica Alemana – Universidad del Desarrollo, Santiago, Chile

Hospital Clínico San Borja Arriarán, Santiago, Chile

1.1 Neuromuscular Diseases in Childhood

Numerous neuromuscular diseases can affect the development of the child and especially his or her locomotive system. These conditions can have a congenital or acquired origin. They can globally compromise the psychosensory and/or motor faculties of the child. The motor involvement can have an increased or decreased muscle tone, depending on the primary condition. Both conditions have a very different therapeutic strategy [5, 6].

The main neurological diseases affecting the locomotor system in children are:

- Infant cerebral palsy
- Charcot-Marie-Tooth peripheral neuropathy
- Spinal dysraphia
- Muscular dystrophies

1.2 Infant Cerebral Palsy (ICP)

It is the most important cause of disability in childhood, affecting 2–2.5 /1000 live births. It corresponds to a set of clinical syndromes derived from damage to the central nervous system during its development, characterized by various patterns of motor and posture abnormalities. By definition, it is a nonprogressive encephalopathy resulting from a damage in the immature brain but whose clinical manifestations and on the locomotive system are evolving as the central nervous system and locomotive system develop. Its etiology is varied and sometimes multifactorial, being associated mainly to preterm births and low birth weight, which makes newborns more susceptible to damage on the central nervous system (CNS). The injuries can be ischemic, hemorrhagic, infectious, or of unknown etiology in a significant percentage of children. The motor disorders of cerebral palsy are often associated with alterations in sensitivity, perception, cognitive ability and communication, epilepsy, and motor swallowing disorders.

According to the type of motor disorder, it can be classified as spastic, ataxic, dystonic, athetotic, and mixed, depending on the area of CNS damaged. The most frequent is spastic, in which the damage is produced at the level of the first motor neuron, where hypertonia is developing as a mechanism of self-regulation and protection of the motor area involved, which generates an increase in muscle tone fundamentally triggered by muscle-tendon stretching [7].

According to the topographic area involved, it can be classified as:

- Quadriplegia: Compromise of the four extremities, usually by severe and diffuse damage of the CNS, usually with important cognitive-sensorial affection.
- Diplegia: Mainly affects the lower limbs (LL) and in a lesser grade the upper limbs (UL). Usually due to internal capsule involvement by periventricular leukomalacia, consequence of intraventricular hemorrhage. The motor involvement

is usually moderate to severe, with different degrees of cognitive impairment, and there may be self-sufficient patients in adult life.

- Hemiplegia: Damage of the motor area of a cerebral hemisphere, usually due to ischemic or punctual hemorrhagic lesions. The motor disorder is unilateral, with different degrees of functional compromise depending on the extension of the lesion. The patients usually do not present cognitive compromise and are self-sufficient [7].

Spasticity has important effects on the locomotor system development. In addition to causing movement disorders and limbs dysfunction, it causes anatomical changes in the muscles, joints, and bones. These changes can be primary, secondary, or tertiary. Primary changes refer to the direct effect of spasticity on muscle length and trophism, which generates a relative muscle shortening and decreases the joint range of the affected segments; this causes abnormal postures, gait disorders and a low functional performance of the UL, between others. Secondary changes originate in the persistence of muscle shortening that becomes structural and irreversible, which causes irreducible joint contractures and a greater degree of functional compromise. In turn, the muscle contractures generate bone deformities as the skeleton grows, which further aggravates the situation by causing joint dislocations and disorders of the lever arms necessary for efficient walking. Tertiary changes are adaptive disorders of the articular segments adjacent to the affected one, as compensation for primary and secondary alterations, which can lead to other deformities that are not originally the result of spasticity [8, 9].

The foot and ankle are frequently affected in ICP. In ambulatory children it can compromise the efficiency of walking and a lower performance in sports activities, along with difficulties in normal footwear. In nonambulatory children foot deformities can generate problems for the adequate use of orthoses and footwear, also causing skin injuries and local hygiene problems [10, 11].

For an efficient gait the foot must be plantigrade, painless, and with a rotational profile as close as possible to neutral (forward). In the stance phase, there should be an initial contact with the heel and then a stable monopodal support, with the rearfoot aligned and with the gastro-soleous complex with sufficient strength and length to stop the advance of the tibia and passively extend the knee (plantiflexor knee extension couple). Gastrocnemius should have enough power for the subsequent takeoff of the heel. For all these stages, a mobile ankle and a stable and aligned forefoot are essential.

In the swing phase, the foot must be in adequate dorsiflexion to avoid the toes touching the ground and tripping.

Foot disorders may involve different stages of walking or all of them, depending on anatomical and functional involvement. The clinical analysis then includes the clinical history (degree of functional impairment, use of orthoses, spasticity management, previous treatments, etc.), observational analysis of the gait, general and specific physical orthopedic examination of the foot, radiological study, and laboratory analysis of gait if necessary [12–14].

The observational analysis of the gait is fundamental, to evaluate the dynamics of the foot in all its phases and the alterations in other segments of the LL. The foot is analyzed by segments, determining if there are deformities of the hindfoot, midfoot, or forefoot. In standing we can observe two main patterns of deformity: planovalgus and cavus-varus. We must analyze the articular ranges, especially the ankle and subtalar (the ankle is usually affected in PC by spasticity and/or gastro-soleus shortening, generating equinus). We also must look for evidence of skin lesions by pressure or abnormal contact with the ground. Finally, we have to evaluate if the deformities of the foot are flexible or rigid (degree of manual correction) and to evaluate the extrinsic muscular power and degree of spasticity [15].

The radiographic study allows us to evidence the structured deformities of the foot, in the PA and LAT plane with load, and also of the hindfoot by means of the Saltzman view. This is fundamental for making decisions about the most appropriate treatment for the different deformities [16].

If necessary and there are larger segments involved that require correction, the laboratory gait analysis can provide us with the elements of judgment to decide which procedures to carry out on the foot and lower limbs [17].

Below we will describe the main alterations:

1.3   Equinus

Plantar flexion of the ankle due to spasticity and/or shortening of the sural triceps, which may be the first detectable alteration on physical examination. It may initially cause an abnormal initial contact on the ground, which alters the dynamics of the walk, hyperextending the knee in early stages by the generation of a force vector in front of the knee on contact with the ground. In later stages, a permanent equinus with compensatory flexion of knees and hips is produced to maintain the center of gravity in the sagittal plane, which increases energy requirements and pressure on the patella and extensor apparatus. In the foot, injuries are produced by anterior overload and metatarsalgia. It is important to differentiate if the equinus is only due to the involvement of the soleus or of the whole triceps sural by means of the Silfverskiöld test, which determines the treatment to follow: if the equinus is reducible with the knee flexed, the involvement is only of the gastrocnemius; if it is not, it is because the soleus is also shortened (Achilles contracture) [15].

1.4   Equinus-Cavus-Varus

Deformity produced as a consequence of overactivity of plantar flexors (gastrosoleus) and foot inverters (mainly posterior tibial). Initially a flexible dynamic deformity is produced, with manually reducible equinus and varus of the

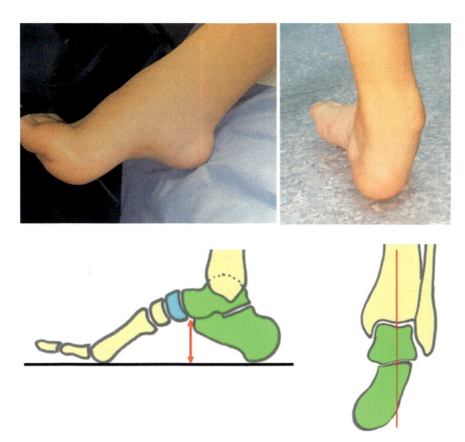

Fig. 1 Deformity in equinus-cavus-varus: increased height of the longitudinal arch, equinus of the ankle and varus of the hindfoot

hindfoot. With time the equinus and varus get stiff; in turn a cavus of the forefoot is added as a result of the traction of the plantar structures and the long peroneal tendon. The cavus added to a greater traction of the toes and hallux flexors generate a claw toe and hallux cock-up deformities (proximal phalanx hyperextension and interphalangeal flexion) (Fig. 1).

As mentioned above, initially this deformity is flexible, mainly due to the influence of the extrinsic muscles. In the swing phase, there may be an inversion of the foot generated by overactivity of the tibialis anterior, causing an initial support of the foot with the lateral border, which aggravates the hindfoot varus [18].

This deformity is frequent in patients with spastic hemiplegia and initial cases of spastic diplegia (they can evolve to plano-valgus with skeletal growth).

In patients with quadriplegia, it is common to see precocious and severe development of equinus-cavus-varus that makes standing and orthotic handling difficult [19].

1.5   Equinus-Plano-Valgus

Deformity produced as consequence of overactivity of the plantar flexors (gastrosoleus) and evertors of the foot (peroneus). This deformity is caused initially by a flexible valgus flat foot accompanied by equinus of the rearfoot, with elevation of the calcaneus. It progresses to a midfoot collapse with talonavicular subluxation and forefoot eversion (Fig. 2). The impossibility to generate an adequate take off (structured equinus and everted and unstable forefoot) leads to a "false dorsiflexion" at Chopart's joint level, which is known as "midfoot break" that aggravates the structural condition of the foot [20] (Fig. 3).

Initially, the deformities can be reduced manually, but with time they become more severe and stiff, also evolving to degenerative changes at the subtalar and talonavicular levels. Even a secondary ankle valgus can be a consequence. In the most severe cases, the weakness and shortening of the gastro-soleus complex lead to an anterior inclination of the tibia in the stance phase along with a knee

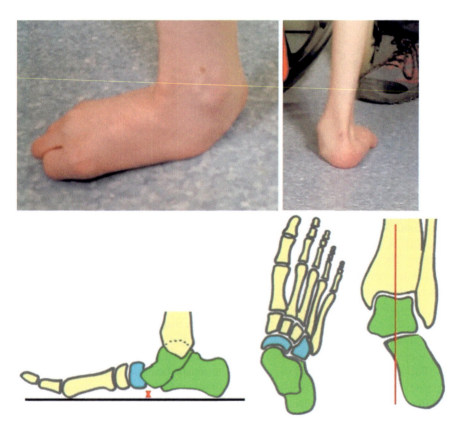

Fig. 2 Flatfoot valgus: collapse of the longitudinal arch + equinus of the calcaneus, abduction of the midfoot + talonavicular subluxation and severe valgus of the hindfoot

Fig. 3 Midfoot break: collapse of the midfoot and subluxation of the Chopart's joint, due to the limitation of the dorsiflexion of the ankle and the absence of an aligned and stable forefoot

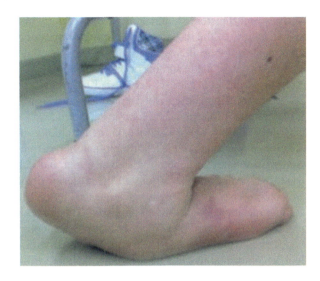

extension deficit (plantiflexor-extensor coupling failure), which generates a crouch gait.

This type of deformity is frequently seen in spastic diplegia, and usually causes severe disorders in the lever arms necessary for the generation of an efficient gait, in addition to other angular and torsional deformities of the lower limbs bones [21].

1.6   Charcot-Marie-Tooth Neuropathy

It corresponds to a hereditary sensory-motor polyneuropathy, of which there is a great variety of genetic subtypes and severities. It is the most frequent hereditary neuropathy (1/2500 persons), being one of the most frequent causes of cavus-varus foot in children and adults.

Within all the subtypes there are two main ones:

- Type 1: 2/3 of the patients, with abnormal axonal myelination and slowed conduction to electromyography (EMG). Its transmission is autosomal dominant.
- Type 2: about 1/3 of the patients, with abnormal axonal function and normal myelinization, so EMG shows normal conduction velocity but with lower magnitude of potentials. Its transmission is autosomal recessive.

Compromised nerves show progressive axonal degeneration. The involvement of the peripheral motor branches generates atrophy and muscle weakness of the extremities, mainly appendicular, where the feet are the most affected. Less frequently, the sensory nerves are also affected, which aggravates the clinical condition [22].

The clinical history should emphasize the family history. In most cases there is a known history of the disease, with varying degrees of penetrance and severity. The great majority present cavus-varus foot, but others may have mild manifestations such as repetitive ankle sprains or only claw toes.

In general, the disease is manifested by progressive distal involvement of the lower extremities mainly involving the leg muscles and the intrinsic foot muscles. Initial atrophy of the intrinsic foot musculature leads to the initial development of claw toes and pes cavus. The weakness is initially greater in the muscles of the anterior compartment of the leg (tibialis anterior, peroneus brevis, and toe extensor), which contributes to generate a steppage gait and ankle instability. On the other hand, the greater relative activity of the posterior tibial and peroneus longus (they are compromised more slowly) generates a varus of the hindfoot and a descent of the first metatarsal, aggravating the cavus. The gastro-soleus complex can be compromised late, generating equinus by atrophy and contracture.

As mentioned, the main deformity generated with the CMT is the cavus-varus foot, accompanied by claw toes. Initially flexible, with the skeletal growth and progression of neuropathy, it becomes more severe and rigid, eventually generating joint incongruencies and degenerative changes. The cavus is initially driven by a pronated forefoot (first metatarsal descent), which generates a secondary varus of the hindfoot, aggravated by the instability of the ankle due to muscle weakness. To test whether the hindfoot varus is reducible, we use the Coleman test, which consists of a block under the fifth metatarsal head. If the hindfoot varus aligns into neutral or mild valgus, the rearfoot varus is driven by a pronated forefoot. With time, the hindfoot varus becomes rigid, generating a secondary rigid hindfoot varus deformity.

It is very important to examine the extrinsic muscular strength, mainly the capacity to evert and dorsiflect the foot (peroneus brevis and tibialis anterior), that is frequently severely compromised muscles.

Often there are associated skin injuries: lateral hyperkeratosis at the base of the fifth metatarsal secondary to lateral overload, metatarsal head plantar hyperkeratosis (especially at the first and fifth metatarsals), and dorsal interphalangeal hyperkeratosis secondary to claw toes. The eventual sensory involvement can aggravate these lesions generating deep ulcers and infections.

Electrodiagnosis is fundamental to confirm the disease and define its prognosis, together with the respective genetic study [5, 23].

1.7   Spinal Dysraphia

Concept that groups congenital defects of the neural tube closure, which can involve only a hidden spina bifida by defects of the posterior arch closure and herniation of the peridural fat (lipomeningocele), of the duramadre (meningocele), or of the roots of the spinal cord together with all the anterior structures (myelomeningocele). Myelomeningocele is the most common of the neural tube closure defects, being a major cause of disability as it is compatible with life. The incidence is 1/1000 live births, being the most frequent location in the lumbosacral region. The herniation of the lower spinal roots leads to a series of disorders by peripheral denervation, causing sensory-motor paralysis and bladder and intestinal dysfunction. In addition, it is frequently associated with hydrocephalus and other neural tube malformations such as diastematomyelia or syringomyelia, which further aggravate the neurological deficit.

Its etiology is strongly associated with the deficit of folic acid intake during the first trimester of pregnancy, so its incidence has decreased significantly in countries where regular supplementation of this compound has been implemented in pregnant women. It is also associated with genetic factors and exposure to chemical substances, among which valproic acid stands out, commonly used as an antiepileptic. On the other hand, the prenatal diagnosis of neural tube anomalies has led to the elective interruption of pregnancies, as well as to the development of intrauterine surgery for the closure of these defects, which has made it possible to partially improve the motor function of these patients [24].

They are classified according to the motor level involved, with the lower levels being less affected and having a better functional prognosis:

1. High thoracic-lumbar: lack of activation of quadriceps (only hips flexion)
2. Low lumbar: lack of activation of the gluteus medius and maximum. Partial quadriceps and hamstring activity (knee extension)
3. Sacrum: complete activation of quadriceps and gluteus medius (knee extension and flection)

   - High sacrum: lack of gastro-soleus activation (dorsiflect ankles)
   - Lower sacrum: gastro-soleus activation (active ankle flexion)

   - The prognosis of independent walking depends on the motor level, commonly achieving walking with the assistance of orthotics and canes if there is active knee extension capacity (low lumbar level). The lower the level, the less external support is required for walking. The low lumbar and sacral levels are the most frequent, so the great majority of these patients have a great potential for independent walking with adequate orthotic support.

   - The foot is compromised in all cases. Denervation produces muscular atrophy and progressive fibrous retraction, which causes early skeletal deformities accompanied by local sensory deficits, which facilitates the appearance of skin lesions due to pressure, ulcers, local infections, and osteomyelitis [25, 26] (Fig. 4).

The most frequent deformities are:

- Clubfoot: equinus-cavus-varus: 44% (low lumbar level). It can often present as a severe "clubfoot" in the newborn, difficult to manage (usually associated with other lesions of the spine).
- Calcaneal varus and cavus foot: 25% (low lumbar and sacral level). Cavus and adductus of the forefoot plus varus of the hindfoot without significant equinus.
- Calcaneal foot: 12% (sacral level). Vertical calcaneus and ankle dorsiflexion. Elongated Achilles.

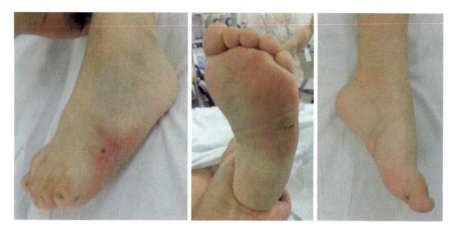

Fig. 4 Foot equinus-cavus-varus in patient with myelomeningocele, low lumbar level, with important cutaneous injury secondary to lateral hyperpressure, painless by local insensibility

Less frequent:

- Vertical talus (high levels). Total sensory and motor paresis below the knee
- Plano-valgus (low sacral level)
  Isolated equinus (when there are lesions of the spine)

The deformity of the feet is added to the rest of the lower extremity depending on the level affected. In levels above L3, there are often contractures in knee flexion, significant rotational disorders of the lower extremities, and hip instability [27].

1.8 Muscular Dystrophies

They correspond to a heterogeneous group of genetic diseases that cause degeneration and muscle weakness. The genetic defect causes some muscle protein to be defective or not to be produced in the amount needed for normal function. This causes the muscle tissue to degenerate and be replaced by nonfunctional fibrous tissue, causing lack of strength and muscle atrophy, resulting in joint retractions and skeletal deformities of varying magnitude, depending on the severity of the condition.

In some, other tissues are also affected, such as the heart or brain. The vast majority of genetic defects are identified, and the pattern of inheritance is known. The prognosis varies according to the type of dystrophy and the speed of progression. Some are mild and evolve slowly, allowing a relatively normal life expectancy, while others are more severe and cause severe functional disability. All worsen as the muscles degenerate and become progressively weaker. Most patients eventually lose the ability to walk. Life expectancy depends on the degree of muscle weakness and respiratory or cardiac involvement.

Its most common forms in boys, Duchenne and Becker muscular dystrophies, affect about 1 in 3500–5000 boys [28].

Duchenne dystrophy is the most common; it is due to the alteration of the dystrophin protein gene resulting in the absence of the protein. Linked to the X chromosome, females are carriers, and only males manifest the disease. It is rapidly progressive, causing the loss of the gait around the age of 12–14 years, and then they present cardiopathy and respiratory failure. Usually, they do not exceed 20 years of age.

Muscle involvement initially generates proximal weakness, so patients lose strength in the trunk and large muscle groups around the hips and shoulder girdle. At this stage, the sign of Gowers is characteristic, in which children have great difficulty in standing up when sitting on the floor, helping themselves with their four extremities to be able to stand up. Over time, the muscles are affected distally, and muscular atrophy and fibrosis begin to occur. This causes the patient to lose his gait and deformities appear in knee flexion and equinus-varus feet, due to the retraction of the gastro-soleus and tibialis posterior. The muscles of the extremities are infiltrated with fat, especially in the posterior region of the leg, which gives the impression that they are larger (pseudohypertrophy) [29].

Becker's dystrophy is the second most frequent. It is a milder variant than Duchenne, because of the partial but poor function of the dystrophin protein. The manifestations start around 10–11 years and then progress slowly. The deterioration of the gait is slow and variable, and not all patients lose the ability to walk completely. The cardiac and respiratory deterioration is also milder, so that the life expectancy is much higher, exceeding 40 years for the vast majority [30].

Among the other less frequent dystrophies, it is worth mentioning Emery-Dreyfus Dystrophy, the scapulohumeral fascia, and the congenital one; the latter can be very severe with early mortality.

The diagnosis is made by clinical suspicion, compatible electromyographic study, elevated blood levels of creatine phosphokinase, muscle biopsy, and corresponding genetic study.

2   Conservative Treatment

For the correct approach, we must first evaluate the foot in its global aspect, as well as clearly differentiate each one of the segments that compose it. The interrelationship between rearfoot, midfoot and forefoot, and the way in which they develop the compensations must be analyzed in detail. Hand in hand with the above should be a thorough knowledge of the anatomy of the foot and the various structures that compose it.

In addition, in the context of a foot with neurological affectation, we must consider all those variables that will condition the result, not only anatomical factors but also a correct classification of the functional level and of the biopsychosocial determinants [31], as well as an adequate control of variables such as spasticity and dystonia, among others.

On the other hand, the different alterations can be grouped by levels of deformity, as proposed by Davis according to the degree of flexibility or rigidity of the foot, and whether their appearance is primary (effect of the base pathology), secondary (as a response to the primary), or tertiary (as a compensation to the secondary). This guides the decision-making process in a comprehensive manner [10].

The use of orthotic elements is useful in those deformities that are flexible, where their use will prevent the progression and/or structuring of these deformities. In those cases in which the deformities are structured, their use is contraindicated, since they will not contribute to the correction of the deformities.

Among the orthotic alternatives available on the market, the most widely used is the ankle-foot orthosis or AFO. It consists of a plastic splint made to measure for the patient and respecting his anatomy, which covers from the infrapatellar area including the foot in its entirety. It is possible to add diverse complements that block the normal tendency of the foot toward the deformity, as well as elements of padding that avoid the appearance of pressure ulcers [32–34] (Fig. 5).

Other conservative measures such as pharmacological (botulinum toxin, baclofen) and physical therapies (physiotherapy, acupuncture, among others) contribute to modify the primary variables in order to avoid the appearance of subsequent deformities [35].

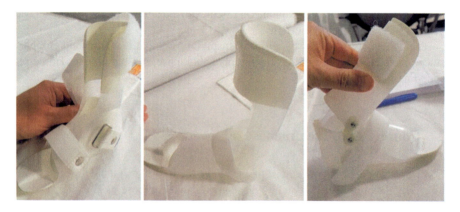

Fig. 5 Types of ankle-foot orthosis: simple or AFO (only to maintain aligned and stable position of the foot and ankle). Ground force reaction or GRAFO (to avoid anterior translation of the tibia in mid support, helping the knee to extend). Dynamic (articulated, to allow active mobilization of the ankle)

2.1   Equinus Foot

It is probably the deformity that we will find most often in patients with CP.

It must be certified in detail if the equinus origin is at the ankle or midfoot. In the first case, we must evaluate the contribution of gastrocnemius and soleus to the deformity, as well as if it is flexible or structured (Silfverskiöld test).

The initial approach includes physical therapy as a method of stretching in flexible/reducible cases prior to structuring. In spastic patients, infiltration with botulinum toxin prior to rehabilitation is useful. In addition to infiltration, some patients benefit from the placement of corrective casts; in this way a greater amount of correction is achieved [36–38]. If normal range of motion cannot be restored, the next step involves surgical lengthening.

2.2   Equinus-Plano-Valgus

In order to consider a conservative management, we must value its flexibility as well as other factors that could influence the anomalous position of the foot, like the external tibial torsion. It should be borne in mind that the correction of equinus in certain patients will condition their loss of gait (form equinus gait will end up in a crouch gait).

The use of corrective braces (insoles, plantar inserts, or similar) is useful as a first option. Although some components of the valgus plane are susceptible to containment by orthosis, the equinus will necessarily require correction to ensure a plantigrade and efficient footprint and thus avoid the appearance of cascading deformities. However, there is no evidence that conservative treatment has a proven role in preventing the natural evolution of the deformity; there are even detractors based on the lack of development of the various muscle groups with the use of orthosis.

Identified muscular imbalances due to "hyperactivity," these muscle groups are susceptible to local pharmacological management (botulinum toxin).

2.3   Equinus-Cavus-Varus

It is probably one of the most complex deformities, due to the multiplicity of elements involved and by the appearance of compensations.

We must consider each of the elements separately, as well as the respective compensations. In the clinical assessment, it is necessary to determine and differentiate those components of the deformity that are reducible and those that are structured.

Once this level of deformity has been reached, it is very likely that the different components have some degree of irreducibility, which will mean that conservative

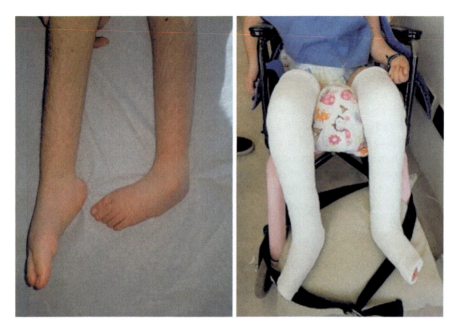

Fig. 6 Serial casts for correction of clubfoot, after local infiltration with botulinum toxin

treatment will only succeed in preventing the progression of the deformities. At an early age, these deformities can be totally or partially be corrected by the use of serial casts, to allow an adequate fit of orthosis or to lessen the magnitude of an future surgical interventions [39] (Fig. 6).

The equinus is frequently the initial deformity, and at this stage it is already structured, so a conservative approach will not correct it. The varus of the hindfoot must be assessed for its flexibility by means of the Coleman test, according to which it must be defined if it will be susceptible to conservative management or if it will require a corrective hindfoot osteotomy. For cases where standing is difficult or the patient is uncooperative, unloading assessment methods have been described.

Forefoot pronation is often a secondary compensation of the deformity. It can be exacerbated by increased activity of the peroneus longus tendon. Assessing its contribution is crucial when planning treatment. If this is the case and the deformity is reducible, we should consider elongation by means of physical therapy or complementary management with botulinum toxin injection [5, 40].

3 Surgical Treatment

It should be borne in mind that the ideal time to perform any foot surgery is one in which it is possible to avoid the appearance of secondary and tertiary deformities, being a timely treatment that achieves the best result and avoids such compensation.

This is not always possible in clinical practice, and we are often faced with complex and progressive deformities. If more radical procedures such as arthrodesis are necessary, it is desirable that they be performed after the age of 8, considering that the important thing is to achieve correct alignment. This last one is the fundamental condition for the maintenance of the result in the long term.

Depending on the underlying pathology, it is relevant to consider the overall management of certain conditions such as dystonia or spasticity, as a fundamental pillar of treatment. A global mismanagement could affect the effectiveness or durability of the result achieved after a surgical intervention.

A useful way of dividing the procedures is to group them into procedures aimed at correction and procedures aimed at maintaining the correction. Within the first group, we have all those procedures that are necessary to obtain an anatomical restoration of all the segments of the ankle-foot (usually tenotomies, joint releases, osteotomies, arthrodesis), while in the second group, we find those procedures that seek in a static or dynamic way the maintenance of this correction (mostly muscle balance) [41].

On the other hand, some patient's foot deformities may be associated with other alterations of the lower extremities that must be identified and treated in the same surgical act in order to optimize functional results (multilevel surgery) [42].

3.1   Clubfoot

Once the structuring of the deformity is achieved, it is necessary to correct it to avoid the appearance of secondary deformities. The equine as a unique deformity has different alternatives for surgical treatment depending on the level of alteration and structure involved.

The posterior region of the leg is divided into three zones, which define the type of lengthening procedure and the structures on which they act.

We must divide the deformities in those in which the equinus remains both in flexion and extension of the knee (gastrocnemius and soleus involvement, Achilles involvement), from the equinus only happening in extension of the knee (Silfverskiöld + gastrocnemius involvement). In the first scenario, the correction should be made at the Achilles tendon level (zone 3) if the equinus is severe (equinus >15°) or at the myo-tendinous junction (zone 2) if the equinus is maintained around 5–10°; while in the second scenario, we should perform procedures that maintain the soleus indemnity according to the reducibility in the clinical evaluation.

Among the alternatives to be performed, we have the disinsertion of the medial to proximal gastrocnemius muscle head (Barouk's procedure), Bauman's surgery (muscular aponeurotic recession of medial gastrocnemius), Strayer or similar (distal myo-aponeurotic recession of gastrocnemius), and to lengthen the Achilles tendon the open Z-tenotomy as the percutaneous triple hemitenotomy (Hoke) [43, 44] (Fig. 7).

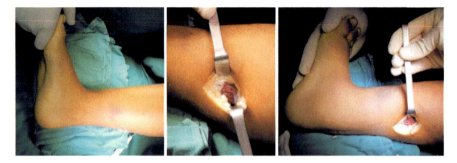

Fig. 7 Strayer's technique for equinus foot: aponeurotic elongation of the gastrocnemius (intact soleus under the sectioned aponeurosis), gaining 30° of dorsiflexion without losing muscular strength and allowing mobilization after a few weeks

In any of the techniques used, it is recommended that a cast be kept on for the first 3 weeks (with indication for discharge), followed by another 3 weeks with partial immobilization, allowing weight bearing and begining a program of progressive muscle strengthening.

Special mention should be made at this point to the deformity called "apparent equinus." In advanced stages of certain neurological alterations, a pseudoequinus appears as a functional response to a knee and hip flexion. In this scenario, a surgical elongation of the gastro-soleus complex would be contraindicated. Achilles lengthening for these cases would end up in crouch gait, with absolute loss of independent gait.

3.2 Equinus-Plano-Valgus

There is consensus that the moment to recommend foot surgery is when the deformity alters its role as a stable base of support or when pain appears. Each one of the components of the deformity must be individualized, and then the origin of each one of them must be determined. We must also assess whether there is instability of the ankle or of the midfoot (especially talonavicular).

The approach then will be to make a sequential correction of each deformity, using the principles of stage therapy. For the release of the equinus component, the same guidelines detailed in the previous sections should be followed.

The correction of the plano-valgus component seeks to restore correct tripod support of the foot, trying to preserve the mobility of adjacent joints (especially in patients with adequate functional demand). For this, it must be identified if any of the components is flexible or due to compensation for another deformity (which could aggravate it by correcting the original alteration). The lengthening of the lateral column, whose classic procedure is the Evans osteotomy (later modified by V. Mosca), seeks to restore the alignment of the osseous structures, without sacrificing articular mobility [45, 46]. It is indicated in patients with moderate functional demand and

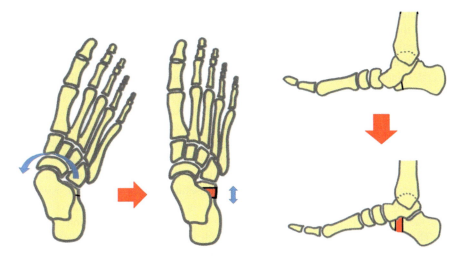

Fig. 8 Evans osteotomy: lateral column lengthening for the treatment of severe flexible flatfoot. Note the simultaneous correction of the planus and abductus (interposed structured bone graft, in red) with the subsequent reduction of the talonavicular joint

relatively good motor control (Fig. 8). A talonavicular arthrodesis can be added if this joint is very unstable or presents degenerative changes, especially in adolescents [47]. Subtalar arthrodesis will anatomically correct the alignment of the hindfoot, having the inconvenience of overloading the neighboring joints; therefore, it would be indicated only in patients with low functional demand or severe deformities.

Once the hindfoot has been corrected, the persistent deformity in the midfoot should be assessed, as well as areas of hypermobility. This is how shortening osteotomies of the internal column (subtractive wedges of the medial cuneiform), talonavicular arthrodesis could be indicated in the case of an abducted forefoot. In cases of pathological midfoot instability, a plantar midfoot wedge could help with midfoot collapse and regain sagittal plane stability [4].

The triple arthrodesis should be reserved as the last therapeutic option, by transferring all the biomechanics of the hindfoot to the ankle and forefoot. Although there are reports of good long-term results, we do not recommend it as a first line treatment except for patients nearing preadolescence and with low or no functional demand [21].

3.3   Equinus-Cavus-Varus

This deformity is very demanding from a functional point of view, since it usually occurs in patients who are ambulatory. This is how we will find feet that have various areas of hyperpressure, which will guide areas where anatomical restoration will be essential.

In the correction algorithm, we must begin by releasing the equinus to correctly assess the effect on other deformities. Due to the structuring of the equinus, a Z lengthening of the Achilles tendon may be necessary.

Then, and depending on what was obtained in the Coleman test, we proceed to correct the hindfoot, by means of a calcaneous valgus osteotomy [48]. Here, diverse alternatives exist (wedge resection or sliding osteotomies) according to the type of necessary correction. In this point it is possible to make special mention to those cases in which the equinus is slight, which could be corrected together with the hindfoot varus through an osteotomy of lateral and superior slide of the posterior calcaneal tuberosity. It is necessary to evaluate the role of the posterior tibialis tendon in the deformity. A decision has to be made to carry out a tibialis posterior lengthening or a transfer (as procedure of maintenance). As a useful parameter, we must assess in radioscopy the correct talocalcaneal divergence, an adequate talonavicular coverage, and the restoration of the Meary's angle in the frontal and lateral projection.

The midfoot cavus is usually associated with a forefoot adduction and pronation. The need for correction will depend on the reducibility once the primary deformities are corrected. Among the therapeutic alternatives are superficial medial and deep talonavicular release and osteotomies of the medial column [23].

For the forefoot correction, it should be evaluated if pure pronation exists (which increases the cavus) and/or if an adductus exists. For the first case, the subtractive dorsal wedge osteotomy of the first metatarsal or medial cuneiform is useful. A plantar additive wedge osteotomy of the medial cuneiform is an option as well. If there is a residual forefoot adductus, it should be addressed before the pronation

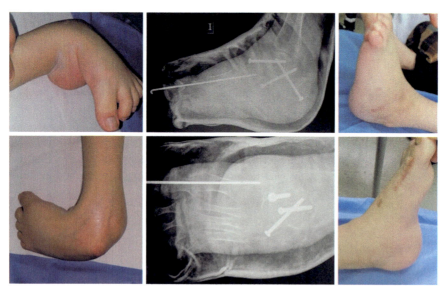

Fig. 9 Severe equinus-cavus-varus feet in adolescent with spastic quadriplegia, treated with mid and hindfoot osteotomies plus arthrodesis and soft tissue release (flexor tendons, tibialis posterior, and Achilles), achieving a plantigrade foot to recover orthotic-assisted standing

correction. Midfoot osteotomies that shorten the external column (cuboid subtractive osteotomy) are useful here. In adolescent patients with low functional capacity
and complex structured deformities, "a la carte" osteotomies and arthrodesis are an
alternative to obtain a plantigrade foot that allows standing [49] (Fig. 9).

References

1. Dobbe A, Gibbons P. Common paediatric conditions of the lower limb. J Paediatr Child Health. 2017;53(11):1077–85.
2. Lovell W, Winter R. In: Morrissy R, Weinstein S, editors. Pediatric orthopaedics. 6th ed. Philadelphia: Lippincott Williams & Wilkins; 2006.
3. Tachdjian M. The child's foot. Philadelphia: W B Saunders Co; 1985.
4. SEOP. Parálisis cerebral infantil. In: Martínez I, Abad J, editors. Manejo de las alteraciones músculo-esqueléticas asociadas. Madrid: Ergon; 2015.
5. Neumann J, Nickisch F. Neurologic disorders and cavovarus deformity. Foot Ankle Clin. 2019;24(2):195–203.
6. Butterworth M, Marcoux J, editors. The pediatric foot and ankle. Diagnosis and management. Springer; 2020.
7. Patel D, Neelakantan M, Pandher K, Merrick J. Cerebral palsy in children: a clinical overview. Transl Pediatr. 2020;9(suppl1):s125–35.
8. Miller F, editor. Cerebral palsy. Springer; 2005.
9. Graham K, Selber P. Musculoskeletal aspects of cerebral palsy. J Bone Joint Surg (Br). 2003;85-B:155–66.
10. Davids JR. The foot and ankle in cerebral palsy. Orthop Clin North Am. 2010;41(4):579–93.
11. Bennet G, Rang M, Jones D. Varus and valgus deformities of the foot in cerebral palsy. Dev Med Child Neurol. 1982;24:499–503.
12. Gage J, Schwartz M, Koop S, Novacheck T. In: Hart H, editor. The identification and treatment of gait problems in cerebral palsy. 2nd ed. London: Mac Keith Press; 2009.
13. Keenan W, Rodda J, Wolfe R, Roberts S, Borton D, Graham K. The static examination of children and young adults with cerebral palsy in the gait analysis laboratory: technique and observer agreement. J Pediatr Orthop B. 2004;13(1):1–8.
14. Chang F, Rhodes J, Flynn K, Carollo J. The role of gait analysis in treating gait abnormalities in cerebral palsy. Orthop Clin N Am. 2010;41:489–506.
15. Devinney S, Prieskorn D. Neuromuscular examination of the foot and ankle. Foot Ankle Clin. 2000;5(2):213–33.
16. Lamm B, Stasko P, Gesheff M. Normal foot and ankle radiographic angles, measurements, and reference points. J Foot Ankle Surg. 2016;55(5):991–8.
17. Davids J, Bagley A. Identification of common gait disruption patterns in children with cerebral palsy. J Am Acad Orthop Surg. 2014;22:782–90.
18. Michlitsch M, Rethlefsen S, Kay R. The contributions of anterior and posterior tibialis dysfunction to varus foot deformity in patients with cerebral palsy. J Bone Joint Surg. 2006;88-A:1764–8.
19. Ziebarth K, Krause F. Updates in pediatric cavovarus deformity. Foot Ankle Clin N Am. 2019;24:205–17.
20. Dare D, Doswell E. Pediatric flatfoot: cause, epidemiology, assessment, and treatment. Curr Opin Pediatr. 2014;26(1):93–100.
21. Kadhim M, Miller F. Pes planovalgus deformity in children with cerebral palsy: review article. J Pediatr Orthop. 2014;23(5):400–5.
22. Jani-Acsadi A, Ounpuu S, Pierz K, Acsadi G. Pediatric Charcot-Marie-Tooth disease. Pediatr Clin N Am. 2015;62(3):767–86.

23. Lin T, Gibbons P, Mudge A, Cornett K, Menezes M, Burns J. Surgical outcomes of cavovarus foot deformity in children with Charcot-Marie-Tooth disease. Neuromuscul Disord. 2019;29:427–36.
24. Swaroop V, Dias L. Orthopedic management of spina bifida. Part I: hip, knee and rotational deformities. J Child Orthop. 2009;3:441–9.
25. Swaroop V, Dias L. Orthopedic management of spina bifida-part II: foot and ankle deformities. J Child Orthop. 2011;5:403–14.
26. Akbar M, Bresch B, Seyler T, Wenz W, Bruckner T, Abel R, et al. Management of orthopaedic sequelae of congenital spinal disorders. J Bone Joint Surg Am. 2009;91:87–100.
27. Gunay H, Celal Sozbilen M, Gurbuz Y, Altinisik M, Buyukata B. Incidence and type of foot deformities in patients with spina bifida according to level of lesion. Childs Nerv Syst. 2016;32(2):315–9.
28. Mercuri E, Bönnemann C, Muntoni F. Muscular dystrophies. Lancet. 2019;394(10213): 2025–38.
29. Apkon S, Alman B, Birnkrant D, Fitch R, Lark R, Mackenzie W, et al. Orthopedic and surgical management of the patient with Duchenne muscular dystrophy. Pediatrics. 2018;142(Suppl 2):s82–9.
30. Flanigan K. Duchenne and Becker muscular dystrophies. Neurol Clin. 2014;32(3):671–88.
31. Martínez Caballero I, Chorbadjian Alonso G, Egea Gámez R, et al. Evaluación funcional y de factores limitantes del tratamiento de los trastornos de la marcha en la parálisis cerebral infantil: desarrollo del sistema de clasificación de niveles de deambulación funcional. Rev Neurol. 2020;71(7):246–52.
32. Aboutorabi A, Arazpour M, Ahmadi Bani M, Saeedi H, Head JS. Efficacy of ankle foot orthoses types on walking in children with cerebral palsy: a systematic review. Ann Phys Rehabil Med. 2017;60(6):393–402.
33. Bjornson K, Zhou C, Fatone S, Orendurff M, Stevenson R, Rashid S. The effect of ankle-foot orthoses on community-based walking in cerebral palsy: a clinical pilot study. Pediatr Phys Ther. 2016;28(2):179–86.
34. Degelaen M. Effect of ankle-foot orthoses on motor performance in cerebral palsy. Dev Med Child Neurol. 2019;61(2):119–20.
35. Sees J, Miller F. Overview of foot deformity management in children with cerebral palsy. J Child Orthop. 2013;7:373–7.
36. Dursun N, Gokbel T, Akarsu M, Dursun E. Randomized controlled trial on effectiveness of intermittent serial casting on spastic equinus foot in children with cerebral palsy after botulinum toxin – a treatment. Am J Phys Med Rehabil. 2017;96(4):221–5.
37. Park E, Rha D, Yoo J, Kim S, Chang W, Song S. Short-term effects of combined serial casting and botulinum toxin injection for spastic equinus in ambulatory children with cerebral palsy. Yonsei Med J. 2010;51(4):579–84.
38. Blackmore A, Boettcher-Hunt E, Jordan M, Chan M. A systematic review of the effects of casting on equinus in children with cerebral palsy: an evidence report of the AACPDM. Dev Med Child Neurol. 2007;49:781–90.
39. Janicki J, Narayanan U, Harvey B, Roy A, Ramseier L, Wright J. Treatment of neuromuscular and syndrome-associated (nonidiopathic) clubfeet using the Ponseti method. J Pediatr Orthop. 2009;29(4):393–7.
40. Kedem P, Scher D. Foot deformities in children with cerebral palsy. Curr Opin Pediatr. 2015;27(1):67–74.
41. Rehbein I, Teske V, Pagano I, Cúneo A, Pérez ME, Von Heideken J. Analysis of orthopedic surgical procedures in children with cerebral palsy. World J Orthop. 2020;11(4):222–31.
42. Martínez I, Lerma S, Ramírez A, Ferullo M, Castillo A. Multilevel surgery for gait disorders in cerebral palsy. Quantitative, functional and satisfaction outcomes measurement. Trauma. 2013;24(4):224–9.

43. Dreher T, Buccoliero T, Wolf S. Long-term results after gastrocnemius-soleus intramuscular aponeurotic recession as a part of multilevel surgery in spastic diplegic cerebral palsy. J Bone Joint Surg Am. 2012;94(7):627–37.
44. Shore B, White N, Graham K. Surgical correction of equinus deformity in children with cerebral palsy: a systematic review. J Child Orthop. 2010;4(4):277–90.
45. Andreacchio A, Orellana C, Miller F, Bowen T. Lateral column lengthening as treatment for planovalgus foot deformity in ambulatory children with spastic cerebral palsy. J Pediatr Orthop. 2000;20:501–5.
46. Kadhim M, Holmes L, Church C, Henley J, Miller F. Pes planovalgus deformity surgical correction in ambulatory children with cerebral palsy. J Child Orthop. 2012;6:217–27.
47. Turriago C, Arbelaez M, Becerra L. Talonavicular joint arthrodesis for the treatment of pes plano valgus in older children and adolescents with cerebral palsy. J Child Orthop. 2009;3:179–83.
48. Dwyer F. Osteotomy of the calcaneus for pes cavus. J Bone Joint Sur [Br]. 1959;41-B:80–6.
49. Mubarak S, Van Valin S. Osteotomies of the foot for cavus deformities in children. J Pediatr Orthop. 2009;29(3):294–9.

Pediatric Diaphyseal Tibia and Distal Tibia Fractures

Cristian Olmedo Gárate and Cristian Artigas Preller

1 Introduction

Tibial diaphysis fractures are the third most common long bone fracture in the pediatric patient [1, 2]. In the diaphysis of the tibia, 40% of the fractures occur [1], and the anatomical distribution within the same diaphysis varies, being more frequent those of the distal third with approximately 50% of the total diaphyseal fractures. This is followed by mid-diaphyseal fractures with 39% and finally by fractures of the proximal third of the tibia with 11% [2, 3]. In the context of the polytraumatized patient, it is the third most frequent fracture after femur and humerus fractures. Up to 10% of diaphyseal tibia fractures are exposed.

On the other hand, metaphyseal fractures of the distal tibia are infrequent; their incidence varies in the different series from 0.35% to 0.45% [4].

C. Olmedo Gárate (✉)
Clinica Alemana de Santiago, Santiago, Chile

Hospital Clínico San Borja Arriarán, Santiago, Chile

Hospital Padre Hurtado, Santiago, Chile
e-mail: colmedo@alemana.cl

C. Artigas Preller
Universidad de Chile, Santiago, Chile

Hospital de Niños Roberto del Río, Santiago, Chile

2   Etiology: Pathophysiology

Due to its anatomical location, the leg is constantly exposed to various traumas. Sports and traffic accidents are the main cause of tibia fractures in patients between 4 and 14 years of age [5, 6]. Torsional forces are the cause of approximately 80% of fractures with an intact fibula, producing a characteristically oblique or spiral feature [7].

Most isolated tibia fractures occur from direct blows, while more than 50% of ipsilateral tibia and fibula fractures are caused by traffic accidents [8, 9].

Finally, unfortunately, the tibia is the second most frequent long bone fracture in the child with non-accidental injuries, varying between 11% and 26% depending on the series [10].

3   Anatomy

The tibia is a bone of subcutaneous location in its medial part, which makes it very susceptible to exposed fractures, being the most frequent exposed fracture in the pediatric population [11]. The tibia has a triangular shape, but its endomedullary canal remains round which makes it a long bone susceptible to interlocking.

Tibia and fibula are joined by the interosseous membrane; as the child grows, the fibula takes a more posterior position in relation to the tibia. The indemnity or presence of fibular fracture will determine the tendency to deviation of the fracture by the insertions of the muscles of the anterior and lateral compartments of the leg. It is relevant to know the muscular compartments of the leg; there are four of these, the anterior, lateral, and the two posterior (superficial and deep), since the fractures of this segment can present in their evolution an acute compartment syndrome [1, 3, 9].

4   Diagnosis

These patients present clinically with pain, inability to bear weight, and in severe cases segmental deformity. In preschool children, they may present only with gait claudication. Remember that in the context of polytraumatized children, it is a frequent fracture, so in these scenarios we must perform thorough primary and secondary evaluations according to the protocols of Advanced Vital Trauma [12, 13].

It is oriented by the mechanism of trauma, either direct or indirect. Special consideration should be given to the presence of skin injury and soft tissue damage to the leg, using the Gustilo and Anderson classifications and/or the AO classification [14, 15].

Making a clinical diagnosis of neurovascular indemnity is relevant, in addition to having a high index of suspicion of compartment syndrome, with disproportionate pain being a cardinal symptom in the pediatric population [16].

Consider in the initial diagnosis simple radiography with anteroposterior and lateral orthogonal projections of the leg including the knee and ankle, being relevant to consider ipsilateral ankle involvement, there being an association with triplanar fractures, so we should add projections of the ankle and eventual evaluation of the ankle with computed axial tomography (CT) [17]. Remember the study of other segments in polytraumatized patients according to our primary and secondary evaluation [18].

5 Conservative Treatment

In order to determine which type of treatment is the most appropriate for a patient, it is necessary to study and assess the necessary to study and evaluate the different variables of the case:

(a). Of the patient: age and size, remaining growth potential, quality of the bone involved (pathological bone metabolic diseases), activity level (e.g., high-performance athlete), and functional capacity (e.g., neurological diseases).
(b). Fracture: affected area, stability, and comminution.
(c). Trauma: amount of energy involved, involvement of adjacent soft tissues, neurovascular involvement, and involvement of other systems or associated injuries.

In general, these are contraindications for orthopedic treatment:

– Polytraumatized
– Floating knee
– Neurological and/or vascular compromise
– Significant soft tissue involvement, suspected compartment syndrome.

Relative contraindications for orthopedic treatment:

– Large, obese patients
– Segmental fractures
– Exposed fractures
– Features difficult to control with a cast, e.g., varus greater than 10° with intact fibula [19]

Conservative treatment of tibial fractures using an in situ cast or closed reduction and a cast has proven to be a useful and cost effective tool [6, 9]. Sarmiento laid the foundation for defining the parameters and limits of orthopedic management of diaphyseal tibial fractures in the adult patient [20, 21]. Based on this and subsequent studies, the parameters and limits for the management of these fractures in pediatric patients are detailed in Table 1 [1, 22].

Table 1 Acceptable alignment of diaphyseal fractures of the tibia in the pediatric patient according to Henrich and Mooney [1]

Age	< 8 y/o	> 8 y/o
Varus	10°	5°
Valgus	5°	5°
Apex anterior angulation	10°	5°
Apex posterior angulation	5°	0°
Shortening	10°	5°
Rotation	5°	5°

In distal tibia fractures, angulation tends to occur mainly in recurvatum, so it is important to leave the foot in plantar flexion for 3–4 weeks. The criteria for tolerable angulation are similar and applicable to distal tibial fractures.

Embarking on orthopedic treatment implies assuming continuous and direct care of the patient's evolution, with successive weekly controls initially and then more sporadic until the end of skeletal growth. The casting technique must be precise and the molding established according to the fracture pattern.

Once the diagnosis has been made and the decision made to perform orthopedic management, this can be done in three different ways:

1. Cast in emergency box, consultation or procedure room – reserved for low-energy fractures, with little soft tissue involvement, and acceptable alignment according to described parameters that do not require reduction maneuvers. Patients usually cooperate effectively and may be accompanied by their parents.
2. Reduction and cast under sedation – for fractures that require some reduction gesture to achieve acceptable alignment parameters and thus will require maneuvering and casting of the cast which may cause significant pain to the patient. This directly influences the casting technique. It is a sine qua non condition to have an adequate procedure room to perform these procedures, with institutional protocols and personnel trained in sedation and cast placement assistance.
3. Reduction and cast under general anesthesia – involves hospitalization of the patient and use of the ward. Reserved for fractures that require more intense reduction and traction maneuvers or for patients in whom the installation of the cast and molding is technically more difficult (obese).

It is very important to have trained personnel. The assistance of a second traumatologist and/or a cast technician is key to the success of the reduction and cast installation. There are several factors to take into account during the procedure, e.g., control of rotation and axes, adequate three-point support, cast bandage tension, and soft tissue care. If only one person tries to cover all this, it is highly probable that he/she will be distracted from some of the aspects, and this could have a direct impact on the final result of the treatment (Images 1 and 2).

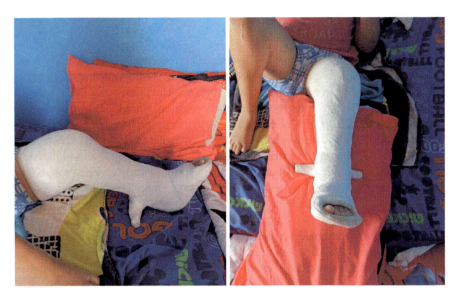

Images 1 and 2 Long boot cast in initial treatment of leg fracture. Includes bar to prevent rotation

Some recommendations to keep in mind for orthopedic treatment are:

- The patient's position is of vital importance for a good result. We recommend leaving the leg hanging on the edge of the stretcher during the reduction and installation of the cast; in this way the same force of gravity helps in the traction and alignment of the segments.
- It is necessary to protect adequately with synthetic padded bandage the skin and soft parts of injuries that can produce the cast, especially in areas where there are bony prominences.
- Casting should be performed according to the pattern and deformity of the injury, with three-point support and taking care of the position of the foot. We strongly recommend using the palms of the hands without the fingers during casting to avoid protrusions that could injure the skin.
- Once the first half of a long boot (which is a short boot) is installed and completed, three or four 1–2 cm unloading incisions should be made with a plaster scissors on the proximal edge to avoid a constriction ring in this area.
- In patients younger than 2 years, the cast may slip, so a knee flexion at 90 degrees plus an ankle flexion at 90 degrees achieves an effective locking of the cast preventing it from coming out.
- During the installation of the second half (thigh), it is important to make a good molding in the supracondylar area of the femur. The idea of this molding is to avoid slippage of the cast, especially in younger children.
- We recommend a leg X-ray after cast installation to have a starting point for follow-up and effective comparison with future images during follow-up.

5.1 Yesotomies

Yesotomy is a technique that allows for minor corrections in orthopedically managed fractures that have partially lost reduction during control. It is useful for angular corrections in the coronal and/or sagittal plane. The plaster cast is limited to a
correction of 15° and requires the patient's cooperation, since the manipulation can
cause discomfort and pain. Corrections greater than this could generate soft tissue
injuries or even compartment syndrome. We reiterate that the idea of a plaster cast is
not to achieve an anatomical reduction but to recover an acceptable axis of the limb.

   It is necessary to carry out a thorough planning prior to the plaster cast with radiographs in strict anteroposterior and lateral projections, more oblique as needed. See
Fig. 1. It is necessary to take into account in the design of the plaster cast that the
wedge can be of opening or closing, which will influence the length of the segment.
Once the wedge is designed, a cut is made between ½ and ¾ of the circumference.
Once the wedge is made, a smooth and controlled reduction is performed until the
desired correction is achieved. When the wedge is open, it is kept open with wooden
plugs cut to size, and then it is stabilized with one or two more plaster bandages [23].

5.2 Postreduction Handling

Once the cast is installed, the long boot should be maintained for 3–4 weeks. Then
a short boot should be changed to a short boot for a total of 6–8 weeks. Depending
on the stability of the feature, loading may be initiated by moving to a short boot in

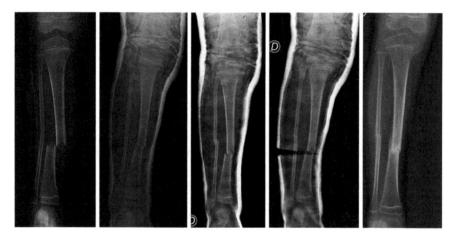

Fig. 1 5-year-old patient who suffers blunt force trauma to the leg. Fracture of the tibia and fracture of the fibula. Orthopedic reduction that evolves with valgus dislocation. It was decided to
perform a lateral opening wedge plaster cast. Final result with good alignment

stable fractures or eventually deferred until a more generous callus is obtained at around 6 weeks in more unstable fractures. Loading in older patients, able to use canes, is initiated with progressive partial loading, whereas in younger children who cannot use canes, it is initiated with the short boot cast. It is also possible in stable fractures to switch from a long boot cast to a walking boot, which is usually more comfortable for the patient, allowing skin care and grooming.

5.3   Rehabilitation

Rehabilitation is usually not necessary in healthy younger patients. There are a small number of patients who benefit from physical therapy. Gait, muscle trophism, and joint range are restored with the return to activities of daily living.

In older patients and adolescents, targeted physical therapy is necessary for reeducation of gait, joint range, lower extremity strengthening, balance, and equilibrium.

6   Surgical Treatment

Surgical management will be chosen depending on the age of the patient and the initial displacement or subsequent displacement to perform an adequate orthopedic reduction with an appropriate casting technique, especially during the first 3 weeks of evolution.

There are multiple osteosynthesis to be used, ideally trying to achieve a closed reduction. Among the surgical techniques, we can use elastic endomedullary nails, rigid endomedullary nails, plates with traditional or minimally invasive technique, external fixators in their multiple forms (monolateral, hybrid or circular), Kirschner wires, or even mixtures of these.

The final choice will depend on the surgeon's experience, the patient's age, if the fracture is open or closed, the fracture comminution and its location.

Strict indications for surgical management are considered to be the concomitance of a compartment syndrome of the leg, the presence of vascular lesions, and the presence of floating knee or in the context of polytraumatized patients. When we are faced with open fractures, it is important to first perform an extensive cleaning and debridement; it should be noted that in recent years good results has been shown in open fractures treated with cleaning and debridement in the emergency room through minimal exposure in addition to antibiotic treatment initiated during the first 3 hours of the fracture [11, 24]. See Fig. 2.

In polytraumatized patients, the systemic compromise and the need for emergency surgery (abdominal, thoracic, cerebral, etc.) should be the first problems to solve [13]. For open fractures, acute management with surgical cleaning during the first 24 hours and the early indication of antibiotics according to known protocols can be accompanied by definitive osteosynthesis with any of the techniques already

342 C. Olmedo Gárate and C. Artigas Preller

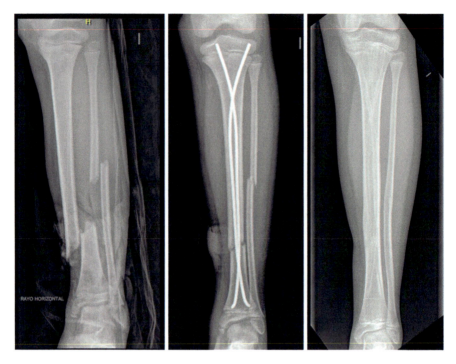

Fig. 2 Exposed fracture of the tibia and fibula Gustilo II with oblique feature and comminution due to run over in an 11-year-old patient. After surgical cleaning, osteosynthesis is performed with closed reduction of the focus. Final result after removal of the endomedullary nails with good alignment

mentioned. It is possible to perform treatment with molded casts and cast windows (in cases of minimal exposures to perform wound care through the cast) for stable fractures.

The tibia is a long bone that is susceptible to interlocking. The stable elastic interlocking technique is the most widely used for the management of tibial diaphyseal fractures in children and was popularized by Metaizeau [25]. The adequate placements of these nails, with prestressing and three-point support, are the most relevant points for them to be successful and achieve the expected result. See Fig. 3.

The surgical technique begins with the patient in the supine position, the proximal physis of the tibia is marked with fluoroscopy, and distal to it an anteromedial

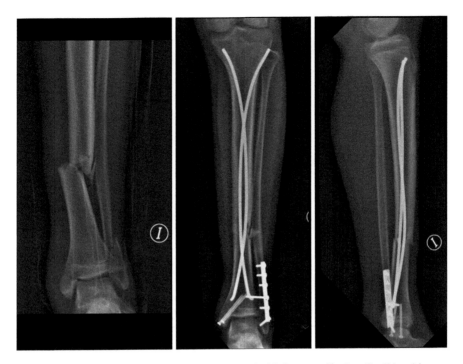

Fig. 3 Fracture of the distal third of the leg associated with fracture of both malleoli in a 14-year-old patient due to a traffic accident as a passenger. Closed reduction with flexible titanium endo-medullary nails (TEN) and osteosynthesis of both malleoli were performed

and anterolateral incision is made. Two proximal holes are created as entry points for the elastic nails. The diameter of each nail should be 40% of the width of the endomedullary canal, so that 80% of the width of the canal is occupied when two elastic nails are used. The nails should be prebend in a C shape prior to insertion, in order to achieve greater cortical contact at the height of the fracture, thus achieving optimal three-point support. The prebend nails are inserted at the entry points, the fracture is reduced, into the distal fragment, after the fracture is reduced. They should be left 1-2 cm proximl to the distal tibial physis. After obtaining an adequate reduction, the nails are cut proximally, not leaving too short in order to be able to remove them when the fracture is healed. Finally, postoperative immobilization with a cast is used.

If the technique is used correctly, it can be used in the great majority of diaphyseal fractures, especially if we are faced with simpler and not complex fracture patterns [26, 27].

The use of rigid endomedullary nails is reserved for adolescents close to skeletal maturity, being able to use some radiological parameters of the proximal tibia to consider their use [28]. See Fig. 4.

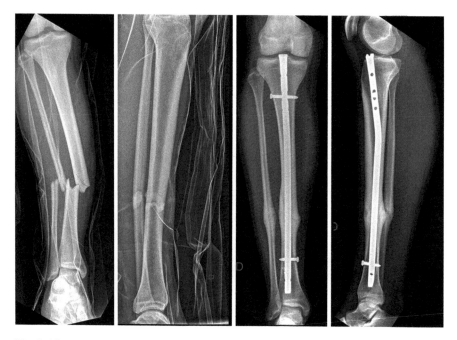

Fig. 4 15-year-old patient who is kicked during a soccer game. He evolves with a displaced leg fracture. Due to age it was decided to treat with a solid tibia nail. She evolves with satisfactory shafts and consolidation

The use of an external fixator is considered in the treatment of open fractures and in polytraumatized patients due to the rapidity of its installation [29, 30].

Plates, mainly locked, are preferred in very comminuted features, or affecting very distal or very proximal segments, ideally with minimally invasive techniques in order to preserve the biology of these fractures [31, 32] (Fig. 5).

6.1 Surgical Treatment of Distal Tibial Fractures

More distal fractures pose a significant surgical challenge, and there are modifications to the classic technique (Metaizeau) of stable elastic endomedullary nailing, with the use of divergent nailing [33], nail rolling (placement of nails in the opposite direction to the initial deformity), or more than two nails [34].

Likewise, it is a segment in which in children older than 12 years, we could use locked LCP plates with minimally invasive technique or in younger children the use of crossed Kirchner wires [35].

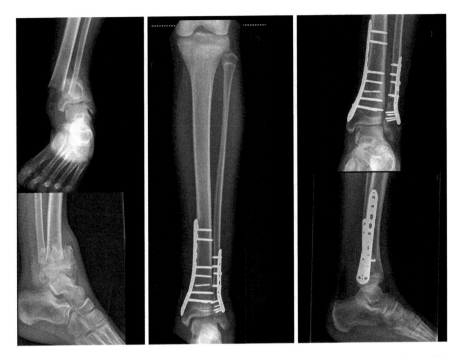

Fig. 5 Patient 13 years old. Fall from height. Distal metaphyseal fracture of the leg with medial exposure of 1 cm. Deep and superficial peroneal hypoesthesia associated with pale foot, no capillary refill and no foot pulse. Urgent reduction was performed plus cleaning and osteosynthesis with LCP plates. It evolves satisfactorily with good axes, adequate consolidation and function

6.2 Postoperative Protocol

Depending on the stability achieved with our osteosynthesis and the type used, we can perform early weight bearing (from the first weeks). At least three cortices must be healed to allow full weight bearing [36].

Passive mobility of the ankle and knee can be initiated very early if we achieve stable osteosynthesis, even from the first postoperative week.

Gait reeducation and more intense exercises under physical therapy supervision will be performed when an advanced bone callus is achieved. Intense and risky sports activities should be avoided during the first 6 months postoperatively, especially in adolescents. Children under 10 years of age will probably not require rehabilitation, since the usual demand of children's games at this age allow patients to quickly recover their muscular trophism and motor skills.

During the first 4–6 postoperative weeks, clinical and imaging controls should be performed biweekly to analyze radiological parameters and be alert to loss of reduction (especially when a stable construct was not achieved surgically).

7 Treatment Complications

We have divided the complications according to the treatment option.

A. Conservative treatment (cast)

(a) Compartment syndrome
(b) Pressure ulcers
(c) Neuropraxias
(d) Joint stiffness
(e) Malunion
    I. Angular malalignment
      1. Varus-valgus
      2. Pro-recurvatum
    II. Rotation
    III. Length discrepancy

B. Surgical treatment

(a) Compartment syndrome
(b) Infection
(c) Delayed consolidation/nonunion
(d) Symptomatic osteosynthesis
(e) Malunion
    I. Angular malalignment
      1. Varus-valgus
      2. Pro-recurvatum
    II. Rotation
    III. Length discrepancy

Acute compartment syndrome can have devastating long-term sequelae, so early diagnosis and a high index of suspicion are relevant; risk factors such as age older than 14 years, exposed fractures with significant soft tissue involvement, and the use of endomedullary nailing are described. Increased anxiety and increased analgesia requirements are relevant symptoms in the pediatric population; the measurement of intracompartmental pressure is cumbersome in practice, and there are no clear values in the pediatric population [37, 38].

Emergency fasciotomy is the treatment of choice and can be performed through two approaches to open the four compartments of the affected leg; the closure of this fasciotomy can be performed 5–7 days after it is performed if the skin allows it [39].

Malunions should be detected early in the postoperative period. If a malunion is detected, the deformity apex should be identified by using appropiate xrays (long leg xrays) to determine the correction site and surgical method. We must remember that axial malunions (malrotations) do not remodel with time. The surgeon must stay alert to this deformity in the postoperative period [3, 27, 40, 41].

Acute and chronic bone and soft tissue infections should be treated aggressively with surgical cleanings and/or bone resection until infection-free edges are obtained. In addition, adequate antibiotic treatment (according to bone cultures) with duration according to the context and under the supervision of a infectious disease specialist is mandatory. Soft tissue coverage is of utmost importance, so early coverage helps prevent or treat bone infections [42, 43].

Delayed or non unions are not common in the pediatric population. If they occur, mechanical and/or biological causes must be identified to address all of them during treatment [27]. Overgrowth is not as frequent in tibia fractures as in femur fractures, but it is important to monitor this situation especially in children under 10 years of age [44].

Osteosynthesis can be symptomatic, proximally with elastic nails, anteriorly at the knee with rigid nails, and medially at the ankle with distal tibia plates. In these cases, removal is recommended when complete bone healing is achieved. Hopefully hardware removal should be performed before 1 year postoperative, since bone growth can make this removal very difficult if performed after 1 year [40, 45]. This can be even faster with titanium material.

References

1. Mooney J, Hennrikus W. Fractures of the shaft of the tibia and fibula. In: Flynn JM, Skaggs DL, Waters PM, editors. Rockwood and Wilkins fractures in children. 8th ed. Philadelphia: Wolters Kluwer Health; 2014. p. 1874–932.
2. Larsen P, Elsoe R, Hansen SH, Graven-Nielsen T, Laessoe U, Rasmussen S. Incidence and epidemiology of tibial shaft fractures. Injury. 2015;46(4):746–50. Epub 2015 Jan 16.
3. Raducha JE, Swarup I, Schachne JM, Cruz AI Jr, Fabricant PD. Tibial shaft fractures in children and adolescents. JBJS Rev. 2019;7(2):e4. https://doi.org/10.2106/JBJS.RVW.18.00047.
4. Cravino M, Canavese F, De Rosa V, et al. Outcome of displaced distal tibial metaphyseal fractures in children between 6 and 15 years of age treated by elastic stable intramedullary nails. Eur J Orthop Surg Traumatol. 2014;24(8):1603–8.
5. Mellick LB, Reesor K, Demers D, et al. Tibial fractures of young children. Pediatr Emerg Care. 1988;4:97–101.
6. Shannak AO. Tibial fractures in children: follow-up study. J Pediatr Orthop. 1988;8:306–10.
7. Cheng JCY, Shen WY. Limb fracture pattern in different pediatric age groups: a study of 3350 children. J Orthop Trauma. 1993;7:15–22.
8. Hansen BA, Greiff S, Bergmann F. Fractures of the tibia in children. Acta Orthop Scand. 1976;47:448–53.
9. Hogue GD, Wilkins KE, Kim IS. Management of pediatric tibial shaft fractures. J Am Acad Orthop Surg. 2019;27(20):769–78.
10. Pandya NK, Baldwin K, Wolfgruber H, et al. Child abuse and orthopaedic injury patterns: analysis at a level I pediatric trauma center. J Pediatr Orthop. 2009;29(6):618–25.
11. Nandra RS, Wu F, Gaffey A, Bache CE. The management of open tibial fractures in children: a retrospective case series of eight years' experience of 61 cases at a paediatric specialist centre. Bone Joint J. 2017;99-B(4):544–53.
12. Advanced Trauma Life Support for Doctors. ATLS student manual. 8th ed. American College of Surgeons; 2008. p. 225–57.
13. Kay RM, Skaggs DL. Pediatric polytrauma management. J Pediatr Orthop. 2006;26(2):268–77.

14. Gustilo RB, Anderson JT. Prevention of infection in the treatment of one thousand and twenty-five open fractures of long bones: retrospective and prospective analyses. J Bone Joint Surg Am. 1976;58(4):453–8.
15. Volgas DA, Harder Y. Preoperative assessment and classification of soft-tissue injuries. In: Manual of soft-tissue management in orthopaedic trauma. Stuttgart, New York: Georg Thieme Verlag; 2011. p. 54–77.
16. Lin JS, Samora JB. Pediatric acute compartment syndrome: a systematic review and meta-analysis. J Pediatr Orthop B. 2020;29(1):90–6.
17. Sheffer BW, Villarreal ED, Ochsner MG 3rd, Sawyer JR, Spence DD, Kelly DM. Concurrent ipsilateral tibial shaft and distal tibial fractures in pediatric patients: risk factors, frequency, and risk of missed diagnosis. J Pediatr Orthop. 2020;40(1):e1–5.
18. Miele V, Di Giampietro I, Ianniello S, Pinto F, Trinci M. Diagnostic imaging in pediatric poly-trauma management. Radiol Med. 2015;120(1):33–49.
19. Sarmiento A, Sharpe FE, Ebramzadeh E, et al. Factors influencing the outcome of closed tibial fractures treated with functional bracing. Clin Orthop Relat Res. 1995;315:8–24.
20. Sarmiento A. On the behavior of closed tibial fractures: clinical/radiological correlations. J Orthop Trauma. 2000;14:199–205.
21. Sarmiento A, Gersten LM, Sobol PA, et al. Tibial shaft fractures treated with functional braces. Experience with 780 fractures. J Bone Joint Surg Br. 1989;71:602–9.
22. Mashru RP, Herman MJ, Pizzutillo PD. Tibial shaft fractures in children and adolescents. J Am Acad Orthop Surg. 2005;13:345–52.
23. Böhler L. Verbandlehre für Schwestern, Helfer, Studenten und Ärzte. Wien: Wilhelm Maudrich; 1943. German.
24. Godfrey J, Choi PD, Shabtai L, Nossov SB, Williams A, Lindberg AW, Silva S, Caird MS, Schur MD, Arkader A. Management of pediatric Type I open fractures in the emergency department or operating room: a multicenter perspective. J Pediatr Orthop. 2019;39(7):372–6.
25. Ligier JN, Metaizeau JP, Prévot J. L'embrochage élastique stable à foyer fermé en trauma-tologie infantile [Closed flexible medullary nailing in pediatric traumatology]. Chir Pediatr. 1983;24(6):383–5.
26. Goodbody CM, Lee RJ, Flynn JM, Sankar WN. Titanium elastic nailing for pediatric tibia fractures: do older, heavier kids do worse? J Pediatr Orthop. 2016;36(5):472–7.
27. Pennock AT, Bastrom TP, Upasani VV. Elastic intramedullary nailing versus open reduction internal fixation of pediatric tibial shaft fractures. J Pediatr Orthop. 2017;37(7):e403–8.
28. O'Connor JE, Bogue C, Spence LD, Last J. A method to establish the relationship between chronological age and stage of union from radiographic assessment of epiphyseal fusion at the knee: an Irish population study. J Anat. 2008;212(2):198–209.
29. Myers SH, Spiegel D, Flynn JM. External fixation of high-energy tibia fractures. J Pediatr Orthop. 2007;27(5):537–9.
30. Iobst CA. Hexapod external fixation of tibia fractures in children. J Pediatr Orthop. 2016;36(Suppl 1):S24–8.
31. Özkul E, Gem M, Arslan H, Alemdar C, Azboy I, Arslan SG. Minimally invasive plate osteo-synthesis in open pediatric tibial fractures. J Pediatr Orthop. 2016;36(4):416–22.
32. Radhakrishna VN, Madhuri V. Management of pediatric open tibia fractures with supracutane-ous locked plates. J Pediatr Orthop B. 2018;27(1):13–6.
33. Harly E, Angelliaume A, Lalioui A, Pfirrmann C, Harper L, Lefèvre Y. Divergent intramedul-lary nailing (DIN): a modified intramedullary nailing technique to treat paediatric distal tibial fractures. J Pediatr Orthop. 2019;39(10):e773–6.
34. Shen K, Cai H, Wang Z, Xu Y. Elastic stable intramedullary nailing for severely displaced distal tibial fractures in children. Medicine (Baltimore). 2016;95(39):e4980.
35. Brantley J, Majumdar A, Jobe JT, Kallur A, Salas C. A biomechanical comparison of pin configurations used for percutaneous pinning of distal tibia fractures in children. Iowa Orthop J. 2016;36:133–7.

36. Jenkins MD, Jones DL, Billings AA, Ackerman ES, France JC, Jones ET. Early weight bearing after complete tibial shaft fractures in children. J Pediatr Orthop B. 2009;18:341–6.

37. Livingston KS, Glotzbecker MP, Shore BJ. Pediatric acute compartment syndrome. J Am Acad Orthop Surg. 2017;25(5):358–64.

38. Flynn JM, Bashyal RK, Yeger-McKeever M, Garner MR, Launay F, Sponseller PD. Acute traumatic compartment syndrome of the leg in children: diagnosis and outcome. J Bone Joint Surg Am. 2011;93(10):937–41.

39. Herman MJ, Martinek MA, Abzug JM. Complications of tibial eminence and diaphyseal fractures in children: prevention and treatment. J Am Acad Orthop Surg. 2014;22(11):730–41.

40. Gordon JE, Gregush RV, Schoenecker PL, Dobbs MB, Luhmann SJ. Complications after titanium elastic nailing of pediatric tibial fractures. J Pediatr Orthop. 2007;27(4):442–6.

41. Dwyer AJ, John B, Krishen M, Hora R. Remodeling of tibial fractures in children younger than 12 years. Orthopedics. 2007;30:393–6.

42. Glass GE, Pearse M, Nanchahal J. The orthoplastic management of Gustilo grade IIIB fractures of the tibia in children: a systematic review of the literature. Injury. 2009;40(8):876–9. Epub 2009 May 5.

43. Berkes M, Obremskey WT, Scannell B, Ellington JK, Hymes RA, Bosse M, Southeast Fracture Consortium. Maintenance of hardware after early postoperative infection following fracture internal fixation. J Bone Joint Surg Am. 2010;92(4):823–8.

44. Lee SH, Hong JY, Bae JH, Park JW, Park JH. Factors related to leg length discrepancy after flexible intramedullary nail fixation in pediatric lower-extremity fractures. J Pediatr Orthop B. 2015;24(3):246–50.

45. Bakhsh WR, Cherney SM, McAndrew CM, Ricci WM, Gardner MJ. Surgical approaches to intramedullary nailing of the tibia: comparative analysis of knee pain and functional outcomes. Injury. 2016;47(4):958–61. Epub 2016 Jan 18.

Ankle Transitional Fractures

Matias Sepulveda (ID) **and Estefania Birrer** (ID)

1 Introduction

Fractures of the distal tibia constitute the third most frequent site of physeal fractures, approximately 11% of them, with this physis being the most frequently injured in the lower extremities [1]. The complex growth of the distal tibia predisposes the presentation of specific fracture patterns for certain age groups. Thus, during the last years of development of the distal tibia segment, there are two unique fracture patterns of adolescence that are called "transitional fractures," since they occur during the transition process from adolescence to adulthood. These correspond to intra-articular and transphyseal fractures of the distal tibia. They occur immediately prior to the end of growth in this segment, usually between 12 and 15 years of age in girls and between 13 and 18 years of age in boys [2]. Two types of transitional fractures are described: the juvenile Tillaux and the triplanar fracture. The juvenile Tillaux usually presents as a Salter-Harris III fracture, while the triplanar fracture corresponds to a Salter-Harris III fracture in anterior-posterior view and Salter-Harris II fracture in lateral view. The pattern of these fractures will be determined by the size of the physeal closure at the time of injury and the force vectors

M. Sepulveda (✉)
Universidad Austral de Chile, Valdivia, Chile

Hospital Base de Valdivia, Valdivia, Chile

AO Foundation, PAEG Expert Group, Davos, Switzerland
e-mail: contacto@matiassepulveda.com

E. Birrer
Universidad Austral de Chile, Valdivia, Chile

Hospital Base de Valdivia, Valdivia, Chile
e-mail: ebirrer@ortopediaytraumatologia.org

© The Author(s), under exclusive license to Springer Nature
Switzerland AG 2022
E. Wagner Hitschfeld, P. Wagner Hitschfeld (eds.), *Foot and Ankle Disorders*,
https://doi.org/10.1007/978-3-030-95738-4_16

351

associated with the trauma. Proper diagnosis and management of these injuries will seek to restore joint congruence, reducing the risk of early osteoarthritis.

2 Physiology and Physeal Anatomy

Initially, the distal physis of the tibia is a transverse, linear structure (Fig. 1). As it develops, ripples begin to appear in the tibia from the age of 12 months. Within the first year of life, the secondary ossification center appears, with a central presentation, which is distributed homogeneously until it gives shape to the tibial plafond, like a wedge toward the lateral face (Fig. 2). Between the ages of 6 and 7 years, ossification advances toward the medial malleolus, which is completed at the end of adolescence (Fig. 3) [3]. Both ossification of the distal tibia and its physeal closure begin from the anteromedial area, progressing toward the posterior and lateral areas

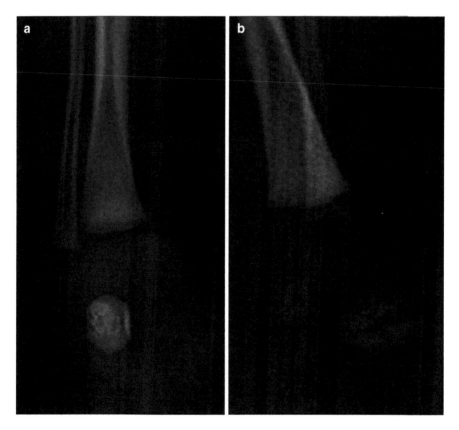

Fig. 1 Anteroposterior (**a**) and lateral (**b**) X-ray views of the right ankle of a 1-day-old girl. The presence of the physis is observed in a horizontal linear fashion. Secondary ossification nucleus has not yet appeared

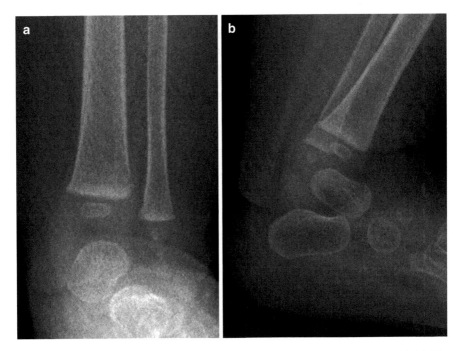

Fig. 2 Anteroposterior (**a**) and lateral (**b**) X-ray views of the left ankle of a 9-month-old girl. The secondary ossification nucleus can be seen in the distal tibial epiphysis, central, with a wedge shape (medial base)

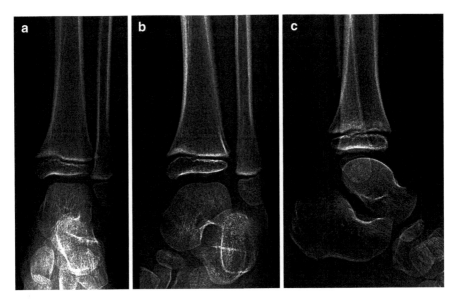

Fig. 3 Anteroposterior (**a**), mortise (**b**), and lateral (**c**) X-ray views of the left ankle of a 6-year-old child. The beginning of ossification of the medial malleolus and the presence of a distal tibial "wavy" physis are visualized

(Fig. 4). The distal fibula physis continues its growth after tibial physis closure. Prior to the tibial physeal closure, there is a ripple in the distal tibial physis, in the anteromedial area, called "Poland hump" or "Kump's hump" (Fig. 5), from where closure progresses to medial and then to posterior and lateral [4]. This growth pattern has been confirmed by magnetic resonance imaging [5], which shows that physeal closure begins in girls between 11 and 12 years of age and in boys between

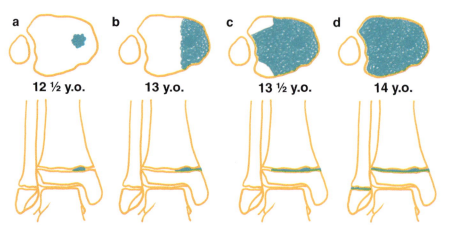

Fig. 4 Physeal closure sequence for the distal tibial physis. Starts with the closure of the "Poland hump" at the anteromedial area (**a**), from where it progresses to medial (**b**), then to lateral (**c**), to complete the closure (**d**)

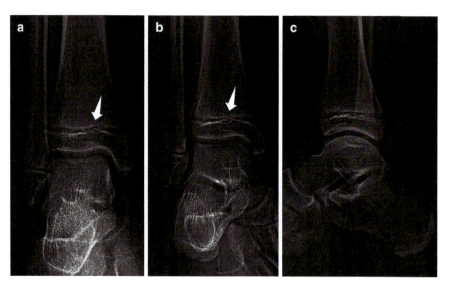

Fig. 5 Anteroposterior (**a**), mortise (**b**), and lateral (**c**) X-ray views of the right ankle of a 12-year-old boy, showing the beginning of the physeal closure at the level of the "hump of Poland" (arrow), and the complete ossification of the medial malleolus

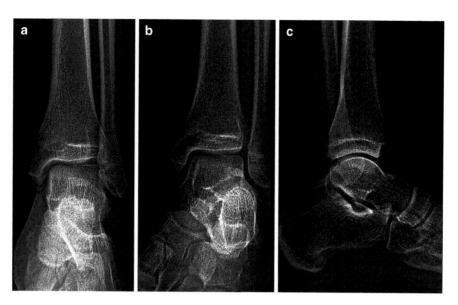

Fig. 6 Anteroposterior (**a**), mortise (**b**), and lateral (**c**) X-ray views of the left ankle of a 14-year-old girl. The physiological closure has been completed, achieving the adult ankle anatomy

12 and 13 years of age. The growth given by the distal physis will correspond to approximately 45% of the length of the tibia [6].

The process of physeal closure can last up to 17 years in girls (average 14 years) and 20 years in boys (average 16 years), in a process that usually takes 18 months (Fig. 6) [7]. The distal tibia physis is the first of the lower extremity to close. Given the long period that elapses during this physeal closure, the distal tibia is susceptible to this type of fractures [8].

3   Juvenile Tillaux Fracture Pathophysiology

Paul Jules Tillaux (1834–1904) described in a cadaver specimen in 1892 the isolated avulsion of the lateral margin of the distal tibia by means of a forced abduction mechanism, without mentioning the presence of physis and demonstrating a different triangular lateral fragment than that found in adolescents [9]. From this description, the term juvenile Tillaux was born, to refer to the fracture of the distal anterior tubercle of the tibia in adolescents, without being exactly the same as what is today known as Juvenile TIllaux. However, Cooper in 1822, was the first to describe the fracture pattern [10].

This fracture is secondary to a foot abduction and external rotation mechanism or internal rotation of the tibia with the foot fixed on the ground. In this way the fibula is moved posteriorly, causing tension of the anterior tibiofibular ligament and avulsion of the distal anterolateral tibial tubercle, which is susceptible to fracture because it is narrower in the anteroposterior plane (Fig. 7).

Fig. 7 Juvenile Tillaux
fracture. The square-
shaped fragment
corresponds to the distal
anterior tubercle of the
tibia. With external rotation
of the ankle (or internal
rotation of the tibia with
the foot fixed to the
ground), the fibula moves
posteriorly, pulling the
distal anterior tibial tuber
through the anterior
tibiofibular ligament

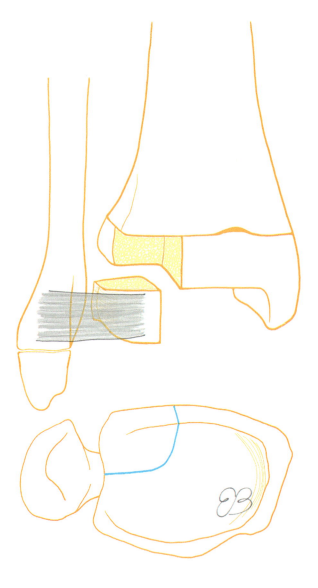

Juvenile Tillaux occurs in adolescents when the medial portion of the distal physis of the tibia has closed but laterally is still open. It usually consists of a Salter-
Harris III type pattern, with a horizontal component through the physis and a vertical
one in the epiphysis, creating a square bone fragment (Fig. 8). In cases closer to the
growth end, a Salter-Harris IV type pattern may occur, with a small lateral triangular metaphyseal fragment, similar to the adult Tillaux lesion [2].

There are no specific classifications for this type of fracture, since the anatomical
description is enough, and they are usually specified as a group of independent
fractures [11, 12].

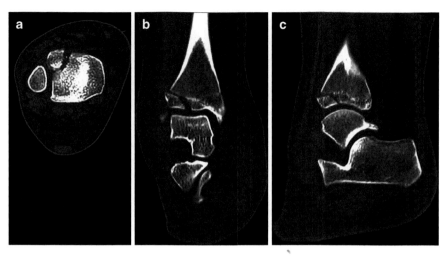

Fig. 8 Computerized tomography (CT) scan of the right ankle of a 15-year-old boy, showing a juvenile Tillaux. The square-shaped fragment is observed in the axial (**a**) and coronal (**b**) views and the coronal line in the sagittal view (**c**)

They correspond to 3–5% of all ankle fractures in children [13]. The usual age of presentation is between 11 and 15 years of age, with an average of 13 years. It occurs more frequently in girls, in a ratio of 2:1 [2].

4   Triplanar Fracture Pathophysiology

The triplanar fracture occurs in three planes: coronal, transverse, and sagittal. In the transverse plane, it corresponds to a physeal fracture, in the coronal plane a metaphyseal fracture, and in the sagittal plane an epiphyseal fracture [14].

These injuries were described in 1957 by Johnson and Fahl in their classification of ankle fractures in children [15], while the term "triplanar fracture" was developed by Lynn in 1972 [16].

The triplanar fracture is secondary to a twisting mechanism of the ankle in which the "hump of Poland" is present. This hump stabilizes the medial portion of the physis causing a sagittal fracture at the epiphyseal level, which can be medial (only some published cases) or lateral to it (most cases). Physeal closure does not need to be started; nevertheless, the hump (of Poland) must be present.

Its classic presentation consists of an epiphyseal sagittal fracture, lateral to the "hump of Poland," accompanied by a posterolateral metaphyseal coronal fracture line. Both are connected by a transverse fracture through the physis. This would correspond to a Salter-Harris IV type pattern but is usually described as a Salter-Harris III pattern in the anteroposterior view and a Salter-Harris II pattern in the lateral projection (Fig. 9). This pattern is very variable, determining different

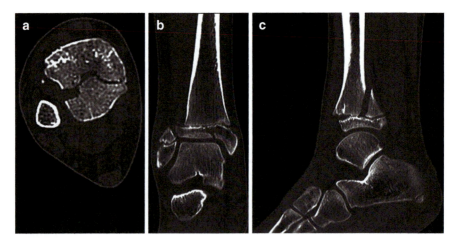

Fig. 9 CT scan of the right ankle of a 12-year-old girl, with a triplanar fracture, showing a metaphyseal coronal plane fracture line in the axial view (**a**), a physeal and sagittal epiphyseal fracture line in the coronal view (**b**), and a physeal and coronal metaphyseal fracture line in the sagittal view (**c**)

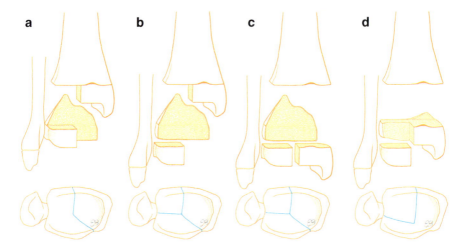

Fig. 10 A schematic of the main patterns of triplanar fractures with joint involvement: lateral epiphyseal in two parts (**a**), lateral epiphyseal in three parts (**b**), lateral epiphyseal in four parts (**c**), medial epiphyseal in three parts (**d**)

presentations in relation to the epiphyseal fragment [17]: lateral epiphyseal in two parts, three parts, and in four parts and medial epiphyseal in three parts (Fig. 10). Extra-articular epiphyseal patterns are also described (Fig. 11), in which the fracture line is directed to the medial malleolus [18] (Fig. 12).

Triplanar fractures correspond to 4–10% of ankle fractures in children and 7–20% of fractures of the distal physis of the tibia [14]. The usual age of

Fig. 11 Schematic of an
extra-articular triplanar
fracture presentation
pattern

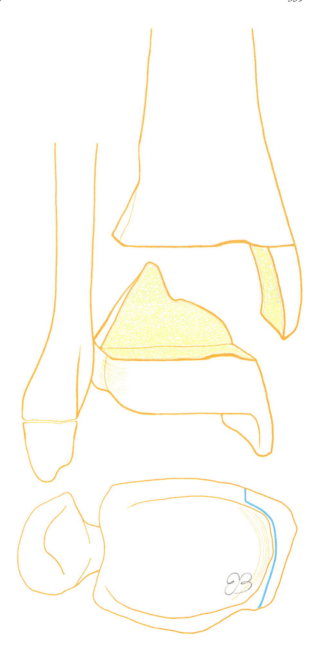

presentation in girls is 11–12 years and in boys 13–14 years. This age corresponds to the beginning of pubertal growth spurt and the beginning of the distal
tibial physis closure. The younger the patient, the more medial the epiphyseal
fracture line.

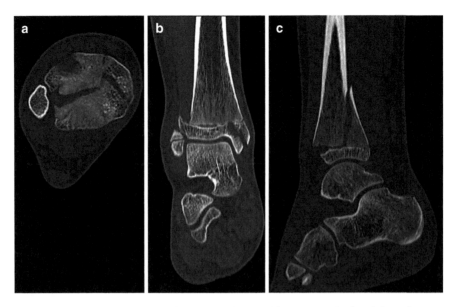

Fig. 12 CT scan of the left ankle of a 13-year-old girl with an extra-articular triplanar fracture. The sagittal fracture line involving the medial malleolus is seen in the axial (**a**) and coronal (**b**) views. The sagittal view (**c**) shows the metaphyseal-physeal fracture line

5 Diagnosis

For the diagnosis of transitional fractures, we must have the suspicion of this type of injury in adolescent patients, when the injury mechanism is present.

In the juvenile Tillaux type, a moderate extremity edema will appear in the anterolateral ankle, with pain on compression and dorsiflexion limitation. The physical examination of a triplanar fracture will be variable, depending on the mechanism and force of the traumatic injury. In high-energy injuries, the presence of soft tissue involvement can be found, including a compartment syndrome [13].

The study with simple X-ray should include the anteroposterior, mortise, and lateral projections [13]. In these projections, a widening of the medial clear space can be seen in 86% of cases, depending on the separation of the fracture segments [19], as well as a widening of the affected physis (Fig. 13).

In the juvenile Tillaux, the lateral projection may show an incongruity in the anterior aspect of the distal tibia, or even no alteration at all. The mortise projection is essential in order to see the juvenile Tillaux lesions that are occasionally hidden behind the fibula in the anteroposterior (AP) view [8]. In the AP projection, a vertical fracture line from the physis to the joint will be evident in most cases (Fig. 14). The fracture location will depend on the amount of medial physeal closure that

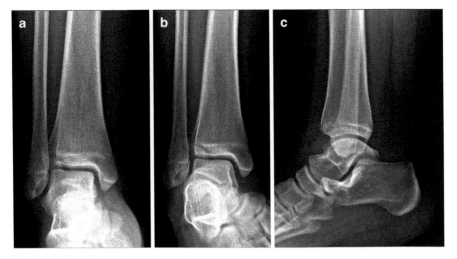

Fig. 13 X-ray views of the right ankle of a 12-year-old girl, with a juvenile Tillaux. The fracture line is evident in the anteroposterior (**a**) and mortise (**b**) views. In the lateral view (**c**), a subtle incongruence is observed on the anterior aspect of the distal tibia

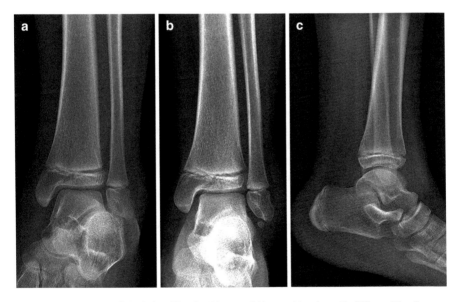

Fig. 14 X-ray views of the left ankle of a 14-year-old boy, with a juvenile Tillaux. The fracture line is subtle in the anteroposterior view (**a**) but is more clearly seen in the mortise view (**b**). No evidence of a fracture in the lateral plane (**c**) due to slight displacement

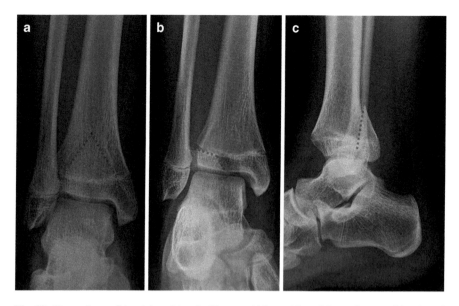

Fig. 15 X-ray views of the right ankle of a 13-year-old boy with a triplanar fracture (blue dotted line). In the anteroposterior view (**a**), the metaphyseal fracture is evident as a "Gothic arch." In the mortise view (**b**) the epiphyseal fragment is observed. In the lateral view (**c**), the metaphyseal feature is more clearly seen

occurred at the time of the injury. The greater the closure, the more lateral the location of the fracture line. Usually the study with simple X-rays is enough to evaluate these injuries, detecting lesions greater than 1 mm; however, their displacement can be better evaluated with computed tomography (CT) [20].

For triplanar fractures, the three fracture lines can be seen in the AP view, if the displacement of the fragments is significant. The epiphyseal sagittal line can be intra-articular or deviated to the medial malleolus as an extra-articular fracture [21, 22]. The coronal metaphyseal line can be evidenced as a "Gothic arch" in this image. Occasionally the sagittal fracture line is oblique, being better evaluated in the mortise projection. In the lateral projection we can better visualize the coronal metaphyseal line and see if it reaches the joint, which would condition a fracture in three parts (Fig. 15).

The study with CT is recommended for all triplanar fractures diagnosis and treatment planning, especially to precisely analyze the axial plane [14, 23]. A classic description of this axial view is a three-pointed star sign, "Mercedes-Benz sign" (Fig. 16). Computed tomography allows to specify the number and size of fragments and their displacement and to plan the appropriate treatment [24, 25]. CT assessment influences the surgical indication [26]. The use of magnetic resonance imaging has been described to support the diagnosis and characterization of these lesions; however, the higher cost, dubious value in treatment, and time of acquisition limit its use [13, 14].

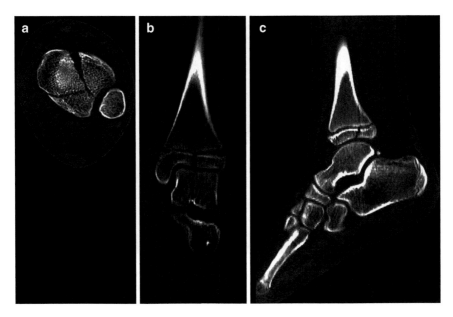

Fig. 16 CT scan of the left ankle of a 14-year-old boy. The "Mercedes-Benz" sign can be seen on the axial view (**a**). He has a triplanar fracture in three parts, with an intra-articular fracture line visible in the coronal (**b**) and sagittal (**c**) views

6 Treatment

The main goal of treatment is the restoration of joint congruence in order to preserve the functionality of the ankle joint.

The patient presenting with a transitional ankle fracture will be at the beginning of the physeal closure, so the risk of growth arrest secondary to physeal damage is minimal, especially in the case of a juvenile Tillaux. Most authors define a joint line displacement of up to 2 mm as acceptable [18] and can be treated conservatively, i.e., non-weight-bearing in a walking boot for 4 weeks followed with progressive weight-bearing for 2–4 weeks. Displacements greater than 2 mm are not consistent with good long-term results [27], associated with arthritic changes, usually asymptomatic, between 6 and 9 years after the injury [28]. Conservative treatment can also be performed on extra-articular triplanar fractures with small displacement [14], with excellent results (Fig. 17).

If the fracture is a juvenile Tillaux with a displacement greater than 2 mm, it is necessary to reduce and stabilize this fragment. This is achieved by internal rotation of the foot. If the reduction is achieved, verified in a mortise image, definitive stabilization can be carried out with a cannulated compressive screw, through a percutaneous approach. If reduction is not achieved, an ankle arthroscopy or an anterolateral approach should be performed to allow adequate visualization of the joint surface (Fig. 18). During the surgical approach, the joint capsule must be minimally opened

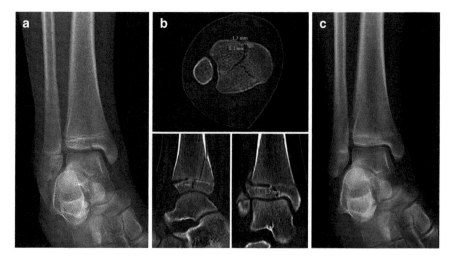

Fig. 17 Radiological images of the right ankle of a 13-year-old girl with a triplanar fracture. Initial X-ray AP view (**a**) demonstrates the intra-articular fracture line. CT scan of the ankle (**b**) confirms a triplanar fracture, displaced less than 2 mm. Conservative treatment is decided. Radiographic control at 3 months shows bone healing without joint gap (**c**)

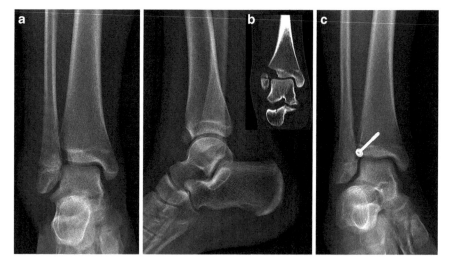

Fig. 18 Radiological images of the right ankle of a 14-year-old girl. Anteroposterior and lateral X-ray views (**a**) demonstrate a displaced juvenile Tillaux. CT scan (**b**) shows significant articular compromise. Surgical management is performed by open reduction and stabilization with cannulated screw (**c**)

avoiding injuring the tibiofibular ligament. Interposition of tissue or periosteum is rare, since in this type of fracture the metaphysis is usually not affected. Once fracture anatomic reduction has been achieved, it is stabilized with a compression screw.

The decision on surgical treatment should in the first week, given that healing process will be advanced by 7–10 days [13].

In the case of triplanar fractures, adequate understanding of the number and size of the bone fragments, the direction of the fracture lines, and their displacement is required for treatment decision and planning. We recommend the evaluation with CT for all triplanar fractures. Surgical management is usually indicated for fractures with more than 2 mm of articular line displacement. Some authors recommend a stricter limit of 1 mm. In addition, it is fundamental to evaluate the congruence of the syndesmosis that could be unstable if there is an associated fibular fracture, which occurs in approximately 50% of cases [29]. Significant displacements of the fibula or shortenings greater than 2 mm should be reduced and anatomically stabilized [30]. Some authors recommend surgical treatment only after the reduction maneuver has been performed (under sedation or general anesthesia) [31], broadening the indication for conservative treatment if adequate reduction of the fragments is achieved.

If surgical treatment is decided for a triplanar fracture, the goal of therapy will be an anatomic reduction of all articular fracture lines. Extra-articular fractures do not require anatomical reduction [32]. The reduction maneuver is performed starting with sustained traction of the foot in plantar flexion and internal rotation for lateral fractures or external rotation for medial fractures. Afterward, anterior translation and maximum dorsiflexion of the ankle should be performed [14]. If the reduction is achieved in a closed manner with this maneuver, the stabilization of the fragments can be done with percutaneous compression screws (Fig. 19). If open reduction is to be considered, the surgical approach will depend on multiple considerations, including the fracture pattern and the soft tissue condition [1]. Typically, medially displaced triplanar fractures will be approached anteromedially, while laterally displaced fractures are approached anterolaterally [14]. To achieve adequate joint

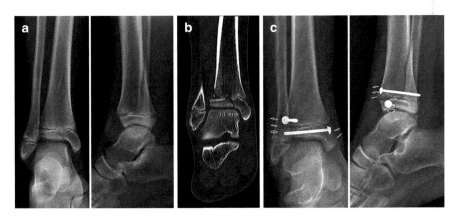

Fig. 19 Radiological images of the right ankle of a 13-year-old child. Anteroposterior and lateral X-ray views (**a**) demonstrate a triplanar, with Gothic arch sign and joint involvement. CT scan (**b**) shows a joint step greater than 2 mm. Surgical treatment is performed by closed reduction and percutaneous fixation with screws (**c**)

congruence, reduction of the anterolateral fragments should be carried out first, followed by the posteromedial fragments. There are no long-term differences in secondary joint deformities between open fixation treatment and percutaneous fixation [33].

Using ankle arthroscopy for fracture visualization and reduction has been described with good results [14, 34]. This technique limits the aggressiveness of the approach and the soft tissue injury, obtaining a direct visualization of the joint. However, it is a technique that requires a learning curve in order to obtain its maximum benefit.

Postoperative period consists of non-weight-bearing in a removable walking boot for 3–4 weeks, followed by rehabilitation therapy for 3–6 weeks. Return to sport is indicated at 9–12 weeks.

7   Complications

In juvenile Tillaux there are no complications related to growth alterations, angular deformities, or avascular necrosis of bone. Residual joint incongruence can lead to joint stiffness, pain, and early onset osteoarthritis and should therefore be avoided [19, 35]. Occasionally, there may be discomfort associated with symptomatic osteosynthesis. If osteosynthesis is to be removed, it should be done early since implants that remain in the area for more than a year are difficult to remove [36]. As for triplanar fractures, their prognosis will be determined by the age of presentation, the type of injury, and the treatment performed. The earlier the presentation, the more likely it is that there will be growth alterations due to physeal damage. A compartment syndrome should be sought directly both preoperatively and postoperatively [37]. Without doubt the most frequent complication of triplanar fractures is persistent pain, due to edema and degenerative changes, which have been described in up to one out of three cases, associated with a noncongruent reduction of the joint surface [1, 29]. For this reason, anatomic reduction of these fractures is of paramount importance.

8   Summary

Transitional fractures are common traumatic injuries to the ankle in adolescents at the end of growth, usually between 12 to 15 years in girls and 13 to 18 years in boys. Given its characteristics, they require an early diagnosis, adequate radiological study including the use of computerized tomography in triplanar fractures, and surgical treatment for joint defects greater than 2 mm. An anatomic reduction is required to obtain good clinical results.

References

1. Peterson HA. Chapter 11: Distal tibia. In: Peterson HA, editor. Epiphyseal growth plate fractures. Berlín Heidelberg: Springer; 2007. p. 273–388.
2. Olgun ZD, Maestre S. Management of pediatric ankle fractures. Curr Rev Musculoskelet Med. 2018;11:475–84.
3. Ogden JA, McCarthy SM. Radiology of postnatal skeletal development VIII. Distal tibia and fibula. Skelet Radiol. 1983;10:209–20.
4. Mac Nealy GA, Rogers LF, Hernandez R, Poznanski AK. Injuries of the distal tibial epiphysis: systematic radiograph evaluation. AJR Am J Rad Roentgenol. 1982;138:683–9.
5. Chung T, Jaramillo D. Normal maturing distal tibia and fibula: changes with age at MR imaging. Radiology. 1995;194:227–32.
6. Birch JG. Growth and development. In: Herring J, Tachdjian MO, editors. Tachdjian's pediatric orthopaedics. 4th ed. Philadelphia: Saunders; 2008. p. 3–22.
7. Hansman CF. Appearance and fusion of ossification centers in the human skeleton. Am J Roentgenol. 1962;88:476–82.
8. Mosca VS. Techniques of operative reduction and fixation of triplane and juvenile Tillaux fractures in adolescents. Oper Tech Orthop. 1995;5:171–7.
9. Tillaux P. Traité d'Anatomie Topographique avec Applications à la Chirurgie, 7th edn [French]. Paris: Asselin et Houzeau; 1892.
10. Ogden JA. Chapter 23: Tibia and fibula. In: Ogden JA, editor. Skeletal injury in the child. 3rd ed. Nueva York: Springer-Verlag; 2001. p. 990–1090.
11. Dias LS, Giegerich CR. Fractures of the distal tibial epiphysis in adolescence. J Bone Joint Surg. 1983;65A:438–44.
12. Tachdjian MO. Fractures and dislocations. In: Pediatric orthopaedics. 2nd ed. Philadelphia: WB Saunders; 1990. p. 3013–373.
13. Wuerz TH, Gurd DP. Pediatric physeal ankle fracture. J Am Acad Orthop Surg. 2013;21(4):234–44.
14. Schnetzler KA, Hoernschemeyer D. The pediatric triplane ankle fracture. J Am Acad Orthop Surg. 2007;15(12):738–47.
15. Johnson EW Jr, Fahl JC. Fractures involving the distal epiphysis of the tibia and fibula in children. Am J Surg. 1957;93:778–81.
16. Lynn MD. The triplane distal tibial epiphyseal fracture. Clin Orthop. 1972;86:187–90.
17. Hadad M, Sullivan B, Sponseller P. Surgically relevant patterns in triplane fractures. A mapping study. J Bone Joint Surg Am. 2018;100:1039–46.
18. Shea K, Frick S. Chapter 32: Ankle fractures. In: Flynn J, Skaggs D, Waters P, editors. Rockwood and Wilkins' fractures in children. 8th ed. Philadelphia: Wolters Kluwer Health; 2015. p. 1173–224.
19. Gourineni P, Gupta A. Medial joint space widening of the ankle in displaced tillaux and triplane fractures in children. J Orthop Trauma. 2011;25:608–11.
20. Horn BD, Crisci K, Krug M, Pizzutillo PD, MacEwen GD. Radiographic evaluation of juvenile Tillaux fractures of the distal tibia. J Pediatr Orthop. 2001;21:162–4.
21. Feldman DS, Otsuka NY, Hedden DM. Extra-articular triplane fracture of the distal tibial epiphysis. J Pediatr Orthop. 1995;15(4):479–81.
22. Denton JR, Fischer SJ. The medial triplane fracture: report of an unusual injury. J Trauma. 1981;21:991–5.
23. Schneidmueller D, Sander A, Wertenbroek M, Wutzler S, Kraus R, Marzi I, Laurer H. Triplane fractures: do we need cross-sectional imaging? Eur J Trauma Emerg Surg. 2014;40:37–43.
24. Eismann E, Stephan Z, Mehlman C, Denning J, Mehlman T, Parikh S, Tamai J, Zbojniewicz A. Pediatric triplane ankle fractures: impact of radiographs and computed tomography on fracture classification and treatment planning. J Bone Joint Surg Am. 2015;97:995–1002.

25. Kim JR, Song KH, Song KJ, Lee HS. Treatment outcomes of triplane and tillaux fractures of the ankle in adolescence. Clin Orthop Surg. 2010;2:34–8.
26. Liporace FA, Yoon RS, Kubiak EN. Does adding computed tomography change the diagnosis and treatment of Tillaux and triplane pediatric ankle fractures? Orthopedics. 2012;35:e208–12.
27. Rapariz JM, Ocete G, Gonzalez-Herranz P, et al. Distal tibial triplane fractures: long-term follow-up. J Pediatr Orthop. 1996;16:113–8.
28. Crawford A. Triplane and tillaux fractures: is a 2 mm residual gap acceptable? J Pediatr Orthop. 2012;32:S69–73.
29. Ertl JP, Barrack RL, Alexander AH, VanBuecken K. Triplane fracture of the distal tibial epiphysis: long-term follow-up. J Bone Joint Surg Am. 1988;70:967–76.
30. Thordarson DB, Motamed S, Hedman T, et al. The effect of fibular malreduction on contact pressures in an ankle fracture malunion model. J Bone Joint Surg Am. 1997;79:1809–15.
31. Manderson EL, Ollivierre CO. Closed anatomic reduction of a juvenile Tillaux fracture by dorsiflexion of the ankle. A case report. Clin Orthop Relat Res. 1992;276:262–6.
32. Tan ACB, Chong R, Mahadev A. Triplane fractures of the distal tibia in children. J Orthop Surg. 2013;21(1):55–9.
33. Zelentya W, Yoonb RS, Shabtaid L, Choid P, Martine B, Hornf D, Feldmang DS, Otsukac NY, Godfrieda DH. Percutaneous versus open reduction and fixation for Tillaux and triplane fractures: a multicenter cohort comparison study. J Pediatr Orthop B. 2018;27:551–5.
34. McGillion S, Jackson M, Lahoti O. Arthroscopically assisted percutaneous fixation of triplane fracture of the distal tibia. J Pediatr Orthop B. 2007;16:313–6.
35. Landln L, Danlelsson L, Jonsson K, Pettersson H. Late results in 65 physeal ankle fractures. Acta Orthop Scand. 1986;57:530–4.
36. Peterson HA. Metallic implant removal in children. J Pediatr Orthop. 2005;25(1):107–15.
37. Patel S, Haddad F. Triplane fractures of the ankle. Br J Hosp Med. 2009;70(1):34–40.

Part III
Adult Orthopaedics: Forefoot

Hallux Valgus

Pablo Wagner Hitschfeld and Emilio Wagner Hitschfeld

1   Introduction

The hallux valgus (HV) or bunion is the valgus deviation of the great toe and a medial deviation of the first metatarsal. This toe deviation is often associated with pronation (internal rotation) of the first metatarsal [1]. This deformity is usually progressive, evolving into a metatarsophalangeal subluxation. Occasionally, due to the lateral pressure exerted by the hallux, secondary pathologies develop in lesser toes and the sole of the foot. Among these are claw and mallet toes, metatarsalgia (plantar pain in the head of the metatarsals), synovitis, and intermetatarsal neuropathies.

About 90% of the patients are female, who have been carrying the deformity for a long time and request medical evaluation when it begins to limit their daily functional activity. A prevalence of 20–30% of hallux valgus is described [2, 3]. Historically, in the nineteenth century, it was part of the general knowledge that bunions were produced by increased volume of soft tissue or bone [4]. Clinically, it manifests itself with medial pain over the head of the first metatarsal as this area becomes more prominent due to the valgus deviation of the great toe. The skin becomes erythematous and sensitive due to the constant pressure that footwear exerts on it, and ulcers may form. High-heel shoes are the ones that generate more pressure on the area of the first metatarsophalangeal joint. This is why most patients with symptomatic hallux valgus are women. The ratio of women to men is estimated at 3:1 [3].

P. Wagner Hitschfeld (✉)
Orthopedic Surgery Department, Clínica Alemana de Santiago - Universidad del Desarrollo, Hospital Militar de Santiago – Universidad de los Andes, Santiago, RM - Santiago, Chile

E. Wagner Hitschfeld
Orthopedic Surgery Department Clínica Alemana de Santiago - Universidad del Desarrollo, Santiago, RM - Santiago, Chile

E. Wagner Hitschfeld, P. Wagner Hitschfeld (eds.), *Foot and Ankle Disorders*,
https://doi.org/10.1007/978-3-030-95738-4_17

371

2 Normal Anatomy

Anatomy is fundamental to understand the elements involved in the deformity. Regarding bones, the first metatarsal articulates with the base of the proximal phalanx and proximally with the medial cuneiform (Figs. 1, 2, and 3). The metatarsal head rests on two bones, medial and lateral sesamoids. These articulate with the metatarsal head on two sesamoid facets that are separated from each other by the

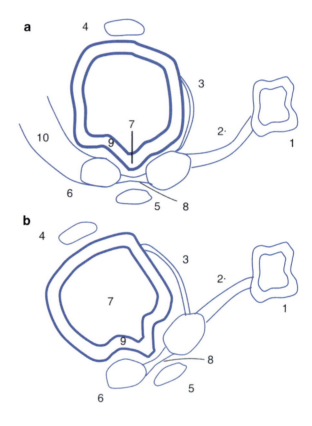

Fig. 1 Diagram of periarticular metatarsosesamoid ligaments: coronal cut. (**a**) Non pronated metatarsal. (**b**) Pronated first metatarsal. 1. Second metatarsal. 2. Intermetatarsal ligament. 3. Metatarsosesamoid ligament. 4. Extensor hallucis longus tendon. 5. Flexor hallucis longus tendon. 6. Medial sesamoid. 7. First metatarsal intersesamoid crista. 8. Intersesamoid ligament. 9. Metatarsal sesamoid facet. 10. Flexor hallucis brevis medial head (insertion in medial sesamoid)

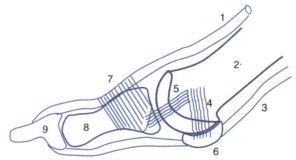

Fig. 2 Diagram of first metatarsophalangeal ligaments: sagittal cut. 1. Extensor hallucis longus tendon. 2. First metatarsal. 3. Flexor hallucis longus tendon. 4. Metatarsosesamoid ligament. 5. Collateral ligament. 6. Sesamoid. 7. Extensor hood. 8. Proximal phalanx. 9. Distal phalanx

Fig. 3 Diagram of first metatarsophalangeal soft tissues: axial cut. 1. Adductor hallucis tendon. 2. Adductor hallucis oblique head. 3. Adductor hallucis transverse head. 4. Abductor hallucis tendon. 5. Flexor hallucis brevis tendons inserting in sesamoids. 6. Medial sesamoid. 7. First metatarsal. 8. Proximal phalanx

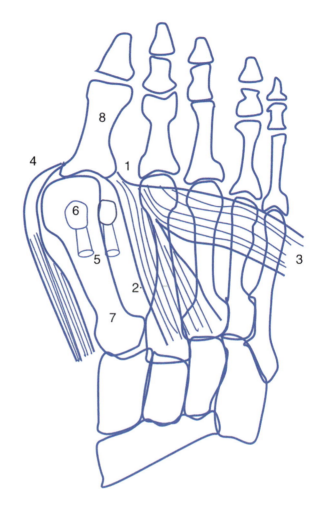

intersesamoid crest or "crista." The sesamoid bones can be bipartite in 20–30% of cases. One or both may be congenitally absent. The sesamoids have various functions, including flexor hallucis longus (FHL) tendon protection from weight load, lever arm increase for flexor muscles (flexor hallucis brevis tendons), and load-bearing surface (load up to 50% body weight and up to 300% body weight during impulse), among others [5–8] (Fig. 1).

Regarding soft tissues surrounding the hallux metatarsophalangeal (MTP) joint, multiple ligaments and tendon structures are present. Beginning with plantar structures, besides being weight-bearing loading bones, the sesamoids are accessory ossicles in the path of the short flexor muscle tendons of the hallux (flexor hallucis brevis, FHB). The FHB has a distal plantar insertion into the hallux proximal phalanx. The flexor hallucis longus (FHL) tendon runs between the FHB tendons and the respective sesamoids. The FHL inserts at the distal phalanx of the hallux. The FHL is contained in a ligament sheath protected by the sesamoids. The adductor hallucis muscle has two heads, the oblique and the transversal head. They are inserted distally into the lateral sesamoid bone and in the lateral corner of the proximal phalanx. The hallux abductor muscle, on the other hand, is inserted medially into the medial corner of the hallux proximal phalanx. It is the adductor antagonist. Finally, the extensor hallucis brevis (EHB) and extensor hallucis longus (EHL) are inserted dorsally at the toe. The EHB runs laterally to the EHL and inserts into the dorsum of the proximal phalanx. The EHL is inserted into the dorsum of the distal phalanx of the hallux. The EHL and EHB are kept centered and attached to the proximal phalanx and distal metatarsal by the extensor hood. This sheath has both medial and lateral insertions at the proximal phalanx and first metatarsal, as well as metatarsophalangeal capsular insertions (Fig. 1).

The ligaments surrounding the metatarsophalangeal joint are multiple. Among the most important are the medial and lateral metatarsophalangeal collateral ligaments, the suspensory or metatarsosesamoid, intersesamoid, intermetatarsal, and sesamoid-phalangeal ligaments. These determine, together with the sesamoid bones and flexor tendons, a "hammock" (e.g., plantar plate) or hanging surface that participates in the stability and load capacity of the metatarsophalangeal joint [5–8] (Fig. 2).

Irrigation of the first metatarsal originates from a nourishing artery that enters at the lateral diaphysis of the metatarsal at the junction of the distal third and the two proximal thirds. This artery divides endomedullary into a short distal branch and a long proximal branch. The short distal branch anastomoses with short epiphyseal vessels. This artery is at risk when performing a distal Chevron osteotomy eventually causing avascular necrosis of the metatarsal head, if the anastomosis of this branch is insufficient. The proximal branch has an extensive anastomosis with a large network of proximal epiphyseal vessels [8, 9] (Figs. 1, 2, and 3).

3 Etiology: Physiopathology

Identifying the cause of HV has not been without controversy. Multiple theories have been postulated, but none has been unanimously accepted by the medical community. Among the intrinsic causes that would explain its development can be mentioned: cuneometatarsal instability, medial column malrotation with the consequent metatarsophalangeal instability, and sesamoid complex malalignment causing deviation of the hallux, insufficiency of the metatarsophalangeal ligament complex, muscular imbalance around the hallux including long and short flexors and long and short extensors of the hallux, and instability of the entire medial column, among others [10, 11]. Genetics plays a clear role in HV, although an exact cause has not yet been found. A prevalence of HV of up to 94% has been described in mothers of children with HV [12]. There is no doubt that the most important extrinsic factor in HV is the use of narrow shoes [13]. This became evident after World War II when the incidence of HV in Japanese women increased as they began to wear pointed and heeled shoes [14].

There are important anatomical considerations in hallux valgus that determine the occurrence of the deformity. Already mentioned and described in detail in Roger Mann's 1987 book Surgery of the Foot [7], they have shown validity over time in subsequent studies. The shape of the metatarsophalangeal joint is one of them. The square shape has less risk of hallux valgus than the rounded shape [15]. As previously mentioned, the initial trigger of the deformity is under discussion; however, a combined instability of the medial foot column appears to be the most likely cause for progressive deformity of the first metatarsal [11]. As the varus deviation of the metatarsal progresses, the first metatarsal pronates, and the hallux deviates into valgus. The most likely theory of this process starts as follows: due to the strong ligamentous attachment of the sesamoid complex to the second metatarsal and the base of the proximal phalanx of the hallux, a varus deviation of the first metatarsal does not change the sesamoid complex position. The stability of the plantar plate is further enhanced by the musculature of the adductor hallucis which functions as a post-anchoring the sesamoids and proximal phalanx to the lesser metatarsals. The sesamoid-plantar plate is attached to the metatarsal sesamoid facets through its metatarsosesamoid ligaments, which attach at the plantar surface of the metatarsal. Due to the strong attachment between the sesamoid-plantar plate and the rest of the forefoot, a varus deviation of the first metatarsal derives in an inevitable pronation of the metatarsal, given that its plantar half is fixed to the plantar plate, but not the dorsal half. This rotational motion occurs not only in the metatarsal but also in the medial cuneiform [10, 11] (pronation of the entire medial column). The tarsometatarsal joint does not demonstrate rotational instability in the majority of hallux valgus patients (except in severe, advanced cases or patients with collagen disease). The metatarsal continues to medialize and pronate as the severity of the deformity increases. The rotational deformity is a factor that further contributes to a rapid worsening of the bunion. Due to the progressive varus and rotation of the medial column, the flexor tendons (FHB and FHL) trajectory is lateral to the center of the metatarsal head; hence, the action of these muscles increases the valgus vector of the great toe or the so-called dynamic deforming force [7, 16–18]. This progressively positions the phalanx into more valgus and thus worsens the vicious circle of hallux valgus deformity. This is why it is said that the muscles play a predominant role in the progression of the deformity. In conclusion, not only the skeletal alignment should be considered of great importance when treating this pathology but also the dynamic stability (Fig. 1).

There is a moment when the plantar plate and the suspensory ligaments loose adhesion to the metatarsal. This is manifested by a real dislocation of the sesamoids and plantar plate of the metatarsal, even with erosion or even total loss of the intersesamoid crest, with loss of the articular relationship of the sesamoid facets with the sesamoids [1, 19]. When the metatarsosesamoid congruency is lost, the lateral tethering effect the plantar plate has over the metatarsal is lost too, and a decrease in pronation and an increase in metatarsal varus can be observed. Sometimes even a complete correction of the pronation deformity can occur, with a concurrent increase in metatarsal varization. The latter would occur because there is no longer a fixation of the metatarsal to the lateral ligament structures. By dislocating the plantar plate off the sesamoid facets, a significant relief can be observed from the pain coming from pronation and metatarsosesamoid arthritis [19]. This is evident in patients when they report that bunion pain has suddenly subsided, even though the deformity increased considerably.

Hallux valgus has other consequences from a mechanical point of view. The hallux itself is frequently pronated (internal rotation) as well. A keratosis will often be observed at the plantar medial side of the hallux at the interphalangeal joint level. This is secondary to the medial ray pronation. Inefficient flexion (secondary to a rotated toe), valgus, and pronation of the hallux lead to an altered gait. This, together with the insufficient medial column and the imbalance of the flexor-extensor muscles, produces a relative increase in the load and impact on the lesser metatarsals (which could end up in transfer metatarsalgia). Also, the hallux valgus will cause a lateral deviation of the lesser toes, contributing even more, to the lesser MTP joints instability. These mechanical consequences will be dealt with in the chapter on metatarsalgia.

4   Clinical Presentation

History and physical examination: It is important to find out the patient's occupation, since this changes and determines to a great extent the treatment that will be recommended. Frequently, patients need to be on their feet all day at work, wear pointed and high-heel shoes, and walk constantly, among others. This must be evaluated very well before considering therapeutic options. Usually, the patient has not fully perceived the limitations caused by HV, because the symptomatology is very insidious and not disabling. Common limitations found in the patient's history include stopping to wear shoes of his own choice, avoiding certain social activities, and stopping certain sports to avoid pain in the affected foot. Some people say that the pain is not disabling, being their main reason for consulting that they are ashamed of their feet. They say that they hide them when they are in public or at the beach. As the reader can see, it can be a painful pathology, not only from a physiological point of view but also from a psychological one.

The physical examination is a determining factor in the type of treatment the patient will need. The most obvious is the medial protrusion at the level of the first metatarsal head; however, it is probably the least important. Among other aspects, flexibility of the hallux in flexoextension and the presence of pain in the midrange of movement, both of which are important in order to rule out associated osteoarthritis, should be ascertained. The presence of metatarsalgia (2–5 MTP) (whether or not associated with plantar keratosis, "corns"), pain and/or deformity of the lesser toes (claw or mallet deformity), pain and deformity of the foot attributable to a flat foot, or a short gastrocnemius-soleous complex should also be evaluated during physical examination. We refer readers to the corresponding chapters on metatarsalgia or lesser toe deformities for further study regarding these pathologies.

5 Diagnostic Imaging

Standing X-ray is the most widely used diagnosis method worldwide. It is essential to measure the deformity in order to plan the best treatment. Lateral projection X-rays are useful to detect any evidence of osteoarthritis or instability (step or asymmetry) at the tarsometatarsal joint (TMT) that might change the surgical plan. The standard sesamoid axial projection is not performed under load and does not represent the physiological position of the components of the MTP joint [20]. Weight-bearing axial sesamoid view [17, 21, 22] is not comfortable for the patient as it includes dorsiflexion of the toes in addition to an ankle equinus. In this projection it is possible to see the sesamoid-metatarsal relationship, evaluating whether there is a dislocation of the sesamoids from their facets or a pronation of the metatarsal with sesamoids still congruent [17, 21, 22]. The image obtained with weight-bearing computerized tomography (WBCT) is the option that will provide the most detail regarding the metatarsal varus, pronation of the medial column, degree of existing arthrosis, the sesamoid-metatarsal congruence, and the metatarsophalangeal deviation, among others. The problem with WBCT is its poor availability worldwide. There are still no published studies analyzing if the additional information provided by the WBCT changes the treatment plan.

The most commonly used measurements or angles to quantify the deformity are the following: intermetatarsal (IMA), metatarsophalangeal (MTF) [23], angle to be corrected [24], sesamoid position [25], distal articular metatarsal angle (DMAA) [26], and metatarsal pronation three-level estimation [27]. These angles are measured with the AP foot weight-bearing view (Figs. 3 and 4). For the IMA, the angle between two lines drawn along the diaphysis of the first and second metatarsal is measured, with normal values up to 9 degrees [23]. The metatarsophalangeal angle is measured between the diaphyseal line representing the axis of the first metatarsal and the line forming the axis of the proximal phalanx, with a normal value of up to 15 degrees. The authors recommend measuring this last angle between the first metatarsal axis and a line drawn between the base of the proximal phalanx and the tip of the distal phalanx. This line represents more precisely the alignment of the entire hallux which is what should be corrected. The angle to be corrected [24] is measured between a line that begins at the base of the first metatarsal and ends in the midpoint between the sesamoids and another along the axis of the first metatarsal. This angle is based on the fact that the sesamoids do not change their position, and it is the metatarsal that deviates in varus and moves away from its original position. It has the limitation that the plantar plate with its sesamoids does undergo some pronation, so that they can overlap in an AP X-ray, not being possible to draw the aforementioned line. The sesamoid position [25] was separated into seven levels according to Hardy and Clapham and evaluates the position of the medial sesamoid with respect to the metatarsal axis in a standing AP X-ray. This classification cannot assess whether the sesamoids are dislocated or only congruent but pronated along with the metatarsal, although it is an aid in assessing the deformity severity [17, 25].

Fig. 4 Diagram of main hallux valgus angle to be measured. 1. Hallux valgus angle (HVA): drawn between a first metatarsal line (mid-diaphysis) and a great toe line (mid proximal phalanx to mid distal phalanx). 2. Distal metatarsal articular angle (DMAA): drawn between a line along the first metatarsal diaphysis and a perpendicular to the distal first metatarsal articular surface. 3. Intermetatarsal angle (IMA): drawn between a first metatarsal line (mid-diaphysis) and a second metatarsal line (mid-diaphysis)

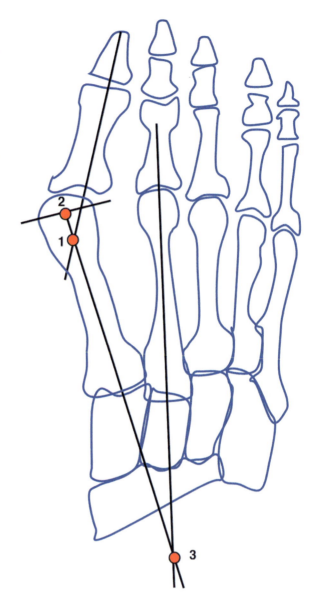

The sesamoid position is one of the factors associated with relapse of an operated bunion (factors to be treated later), so it is a valuable observation.

In a weight-bearing foot AP X-ray, it is also possible to estimate the pronation of the medial column. This is done by analyzing the shape of the lateral contour of the metatarsal head [27] (Fig. 5). The head takes on a progressively more rounded shape as it pronates (external rotation). A mild pronation (<20 degrees), is manifested by a rather "flat" or "square" lateral contour, where a mildly rounded contour proximal

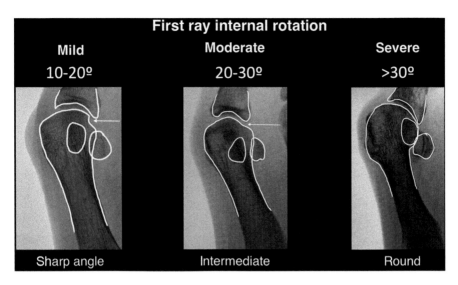

Fig. 5 First ray internal rotation stagesMild: shows a lateral metatarsal head shape that is angled laterally at the joint edge (arrow). It has a round contour proximal to the joint lateral edge. This shape can be seen when 10–20° of metatarsal pronation is present (measured with weight-bearing computerized tomography, WBCT)Intermediate: shows a lateral metatarsal head shape that has no angle or edge) but is completely round. It has a different curvature radius than the distal metatarsal joint. This shape can be seen when 20–30° of metatarsal pronation is present (measured with WBCT)Severe shows a lateral metatarsal head shape that is round. It has no difference in curvature radius comparing it with the distal metatarsal joint shape. This shape can be seen when more than 30° of metatarsal pronation is present (measured with WBCT)Stage 0 (not shown in diagram) shows a straight-flat lateral head contour. This shape can be seen when less than 10° of metatarsal pronation is present (measured with WBCT). Please check Fig. 9

to the MTP lateral corner can be found. This rounded ridge appears proximal to the metatarsophalangeal joint corner, corresponding anatomically to the lateral edge of the lateral metatarsal condyle [19, 27, 28]. A moderate pronation (20–30 degrees) is visible in the standing AP X-ray as a metatarsal head with a rounded lateral border that is continuous laterally with the MTP joint (i.e., without any corners or steps in between). Severe metatarsal pronation (>30 degrees) is manifested as a completely circular lateral head contour, representing the complete profile of the lateral metatarsal condyle as seen from a frontal view (Fig. 5). Metatarsal pronation can also be accurately measured on a WBCT [1, 19, 29], using the loading surface as a reference (floor) and measuring the angle of this line to one running from the medial edge of the medial sesamoid facet to the lateral edge of the lateral sesamoid facet (Fig. 6). The advantage of using the sesamoid facets is that this is the working axis of the metatarsal, which is determined by the plantar vectors (sesamoids and FHL), being independent of anatomical variations of the metatarsal.

Published studies measuring first metatarsal pronation show approximately 10 degrees more pronation angle in the hallux valgus population vs. controls [30, 31]. The pronation of the first ray in feet without hallux valgus varies from 0 to 15

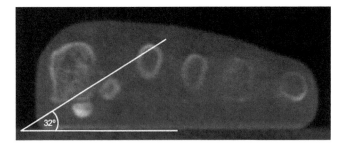

Fig. 6 Weight-bearing computerized tomography coronal cut at the metatarsosesamoid joint. First metatarsal pronation angle is shown. It is measured between a line along the weight-bearing surface and another along the metatarsosesamoid facet

Fig. 7 Bilateral AP foot weight-bearing X-ray. The dotted lines depict lateral round contours at the each first metatarsal head: they represent the metatarsal lateral condyle, which can be seen on an AP foot X-ray given the metatarsal pronation. The distal solid line follows the distal metatarsal joint surface. The joint surface is dysplastic, showing an increased DMAA

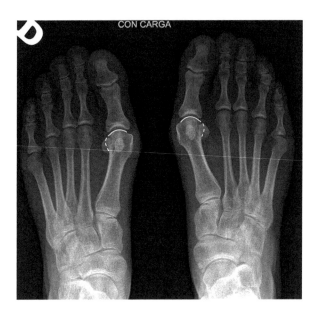

degrees [1, 30]. In cases of hallux valgus, the pronation angle shows an average of 22–29 degrees [31, 32]. Dayton et al. showed that to correct hallux valgus, it was necessary to correct 22 degrees of pronation on average. The origin of this pronation has not yet been accurately determined; however, available information shows that it occurs along the entire medial column, including the naviculocuneiform, intercuneiform, cuneometatarsal, and metatarsophalangeal joints [10]. A recent cadaveric study [11] confirmed the finding that the entire medial column pronates. Finally, the DMAA represents the orientation of the metatarsophalangeal joint with respect to the metatarsal axis. This measurement has been shown to be an essential factor in juvenile hallux valgus [26], being also present in adults [33]. It is a recognized deformity relapse factor. It is measured between a line that follows the axis of the first metatarsal and another that is parallel to the MTP joint surface. DMAA should not be confused with metatarsal pronation (Figs. 7 and 8).

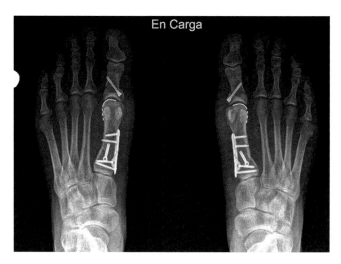

Fig. 8 Bilateral AP foot weight-bearing X-ray. Same feet shown in Fig. 7 with an operated hallux valgus using the PROMO and Akin techniques. Please note that the dotted line representing the pronation is now straight (stage 0), showing that pronation was fully corrected. Please note that the distal metatarsal joint surface is still laterally deviated as the DMAA was not corrected with a biplanar Chevron

Hypermobility of the medial column has been a topic of discussion for decades. It has been described in some studies using special devices [34], the most recent being Kimura's work using weight-bearing CT [10]. Coughlin et al. [35] published how this hypermobility of hallux valgus was corrected after corrective osteotomies (and not arthrodesis). The authors consider that this hypermobility is a product of skeletal malalignment and altered muscle balance (traction vector of FHL and EHL off-axis of the metatarsal), not constituting a causative factor in every hallux valgus. Once the skeleton and muscle traction are corrected, hypermobility disappears. However, there are exceptions where pathological hypermobility is the cause of hallux valgus [18], mainly in cases of undiagnosed hyperlaxity (idiopathic, Marfan, Ehlers Danlos). This is observed in approximately 5% of operated cases, being an intraoperative finding not identifiable in preoperative studies. In these cases, after performing the corrective technique of choice, it is observed that the intermetatarsal angle is not corrected as planned, evidencing a pathological midfoot hypermobility. This occurs both after osteotomies and after tarsometatarsal arthrodesis (TMT) techniques (modified Lapidus), because the hypermobility occurs along the entire medial column and not only at the first cuneometatarsal joint. In these cases, you should be prepared in surgery to add flexible ("suture button") or rigid (screws) fixations from the medial to the intermediate column (intercuneiform, medial cuneiform to second metatarsal or intermetatarsal 1–2). There are cases in which hyperlaxity can be identified in X-rays at the TMT joint. An asymmetry or incongruency at the TMT is the most frequent findings. In these cases, a fusion is recommended including the TMT and intercuneiform joints.

6   Conservative Treatment

Regarding conservative treatment, it is important to mention that there is no demonstration in the literature about its effectiveness in correcting the deformity; however, it can be useful in relieving the patient's pain. Conservative measures include adhesive tapes, silicone bunion protections, metatarsal silicone pads (frequently indicated for associated metatarsalgia), and night splints (sometimes painful and poorly tolerated by patients), between others. The most relevant factor is to avoid direct pressure on the bunion. This can be achieved mainly with square toe-box shoes, wide last, and preferably using cloth or flexible material. New shoes are classically more painful than old ones, because an already worn shoe is already partially molded to the deformity, thus causing less pressure on the area. In the case of men, it is frequent that changing shoes for a wider one is enough for pain relief. However, in women who wear high-heel shoes for work, it is difficult (if not impossible) for them to change their shoes. This is not accepted in today's society, where the use of fashionable shoes is required.

7   Surgical Treatment-Timing-Postoperative Protocol

Initial surgical treatments focused on resection of soft tissue (bursa) and/or prominent bone. The first surgical bone treatment was described by Reverdin in 1881, which consisted of a medial closing wedge at the metatarsal neck [4]. Today there are more than 150 surgical techniques described to correct hallux valgus [36]. They range from soft tissue procedures to amputations, fusions, and tendon transfers among many other techniques. This great variety of techniques is proof that none is appropriate for correcting all bunions. It is the consensus today that surgical treatment should be based on osteotomies and all soft tissue procedures are secondary [37–39]. All feet are different from each other, varying in factors intrinsic to hallux valgus (severity of the deformity, for example) and extrinsic (e.g., obesity, collagen disease). We see in practice patients who are dissatisfied with surgery, finding among the most frequent reasons: recurrence of the deformity, remaining pain and inability to return to sports activities, among others. It is of vital importance to mention to patients that the pain may not completely subside after surgery, that there may be some increased stiffness in their big toe, and that the possibility of a relapsed deformity exists (to be discussed in the complications section). There are certain groups of patients who should be specially advised before embarking on surgery. These are patients with skeletal immaturity and patients who make a living from sports. In the case of the infant-adolescent, the recommendation is to perform surgery, if possible, after skeletal maturity (after 15 years) to decrease the risk of recurrence [40]. However, if it is very painful, it is possible to consider surgery, but parents should be warned of the possibility of recurrence being higher than in adulthood, approximately 30% [26, 40–42].. In patients under 10 years of age, it is possible to perform a combined metatarsal and proximal phalangeal hemiepiphysiodesis [43, 44], which is an operation with minimal morbidity and demonstrated effectiveness. If the patient is an adolescent (less than 15 years), the option is to perform an osteotomy that must correct all the altered parameters with adequate power. As it will be detailed later, altered DMAA is often present in adolescents and must be corrected [26]. In the case of athletes, there must be a complete understanding by the patient that the pain of the prominence is likely to improve; however, the big toe joint will be somewhat less mobile, which should be evaluated by the athlete if it could influence future performance. It is also important to consider the patient's psychological profile. People with depressive disorders have poorer functional outcomes [45], so they should be evaluated and advised according to their expectations of the surgery.

It is important for these reasons not to operate on every hallux valgus. They are all different patients with different realities, and all feet are different from each other, so if they are operated on, it is not appropriate to solve them all with the same technique.

Objectives and considerations of hallux valgus surgery:

- To evaluate the patient's suitability for surgery.
- Master various surgical techniques that can correct the deformity.
- To know treatment options in case of complications.
- Correct completely the metatarsal varus and pronation of the first metatarsal.
- Restore the load capacity of the first metatarsal to the rest of the foot.
- Restore the muscular balances around the hallux metatarsophalangeal joint (MTTF).

7.1   Decision-Making

It is vital to have multiple options in the surgical technique cabinet to solve a hallux valgus according to its specific type.

The variables to take into account when choosing a surgical technique are:

1. Degree of deformity in the frontal plane

    It is important to make certain measurements in the radiograph (measurement technique already mentioned previously) that include the IMA and the MTP angles mainly. In cases of mild deformities, with IMA angles less than 14 degrees, a distal osteotomy (Chevron-type) would be indicated [46]. In cases of moderate deformities, with an IMA between 15 and 19 degrees, an osteotomy with greater corrective power would be recommended: long Chevron, Scarf, PROMO or Bosch-PECA-MICA (MIS variant) [46–51]. Which one to choose depends on the presence of metatarsal rotation, tarsometatarsal instability, and metatarsus adductus, between others. In cases of IMA greater than 20°, a Lapidus (tarsometatarsal fusion) is recommended [52, 53].

2. Degree of pronation of the medial column

    This requires a measurement in the WBCT or in the weight-bearing AP foot X-ray. By means of the three-level estimation, it is possible to estimate a mild, moderate, or severe pronation. In cases of mild pronation (less than 20 degrees), there is no need for pronation correction, as it falls within the normal pronation range for feet without deformity. In this case, a Chevron-type translation osteotomy, Scarf, PECA, MICA, or Bosch [46–51] can be performed. In cases of moderate (20–30°) or severe (>30°) pronation, it is advisable to perform a technique that corrects the malrotation. These include: PROMO, Lapidus, and dome osteotomy [52–59]. This degree of pronation will not be corrected with pure translation techniques such as Chevron, Scarf, PECA, etc.

3. Degree of joint surface inclination (DMAA)

    This deformity is difficult to identify in cases with associated metatarsal pronation. The pronation appearance is often mistaken for an increased DMAA and vice versa (Figs. 7 and 8). It frequently happens that, once the pronation has been corrected, the DMAA normalizes. In cases of an altered DMAA (>15 degrees), a distal osteotomy should be added to the surgery to correct the joint inclination. Currently the recommended technique is a biplanar Chevron [60].

4. Degree of metatarsus adductus

    Metatarsus adductus is a deformity that prevents complete correction of the metatarsal varus, due to the proximity of the minor metatarsals to the first metatarsal. This deformity should be evaluated and discussed with the patient. If this deformity is present and is >15 degrees [61] (Sgarlato angle), correction of the metatarsus adductus is recommended. In cases where the metatarsus adductus is not corrected, an undercorrection of the deformity may result. For cases in which the metatarsus adductus is corrected, the recommendation is to calculate the IMA with the metatarsal adductus corrected. This resulting angle is very frequently >18, being necessary in most cases to perform a Lapidus technique due to its great corrective power. The technique recommended by the authors to correct the metatarsus adductus consists of minimally invasive osteotomies (MIS acronym) of the base of metatarsals 2, 3, and 4, with a lateral closing wedge (4 mm diameter conical burr is used). Only the osteotomy of the second metatarsal is recommended to be fixed with a 2.5 mm cannulated compressive screw to maintain its position. After the metatarsus adductus correction, the Lapidus procedure is performed (Figs. 9 and 10) [62].

5. Tarsometatarsal instability or arthrosis

    Tarsometatarsal instability can be identified by a joint incongruency or by a plantar gapping. In these cases, and in patients with symptomatic TMT osteoarthritis, a Lapidus technique should be considered [63, 64].

By taking all these factors into account when choosing a surgical technique, the risk of recurrence will be minimized. An algorithm is attached that summarizes the decision-making process (Fig. 11).

Surgery objective regarding skeletal alignment:

Approximately the following immediate postoperative angular values should be obtained to have a low risk of deformity relapse:

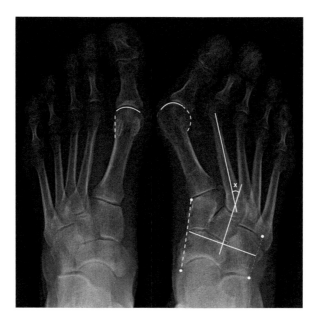

Fig. 9 Bilateral AP foot weight-bearing X-ray. Left foot shows no hallux valgus with no pronation. Note the lateral head contour with a flat shape. Right foot shows a stage 3 pronation (dotted line follows same curvature radius as distal articular solid line). Metatarsus adductus is evident on right foot. Sgarlato measurement technique is used. Method: draw a medial tarsal line between the medial first metatarsal base and proximal-medial navicular corner. The lateral tarsal line is drawn between the lateral fourth metatarsal base and the cuboid proximal lateral corner. A third line (tarsal axis line) is drawn between the medial and lateral tarsal lines midpoints. A line is drawn perpendicular to the tarsal axis line. The metatarsus adductus angle (X in the figure) is measured between the latter (line perpendicular to the tarsal axis) and a second metatarsal diaphyseal line

- Intermetatarsal angle 1–2 (IMA): < 7
- Hallux valgus angle (MTF): <5
- Mild Pronation: < 20, stage 1
- Sesamoid position <3
- Metatarsus adductus <15

7.2   Hallux Valgus Surgical Techniques

They are separated into the following types

- Exostectomy
- Soft tissue technique (McBride)
- Distal intracapsular: Chevron-Peico
- Distal extracapsular PECA-MICA
- Proximal osteotomies: PROMO, dome
- Tarsometatarsal and metatarsophalangeal arthrodesis
- Hallux phalanx osteotomy: Akin
- Postoperative dressing

Fig. 10 Right foot AP
X-ray. Same foot as from
Fig. 9. Note the corrected
metatarsus adductus
performed with a
minimally invasive second,
third, and fourth metatarsal
osteotomy. Only the
second metatarsal
osteotomy was fixed with a
cannulated compression
screw. After this correction,
a Lapidus technique was
performed, given the
increase (>20°) in
intermetatarsal angle after
the metatarsus adductus
correction. Note how the
first metatarsal had to be
shortened to be able to
correct the deformity. To
compensate for this
shortening, the surgeon
increased the plantar
flexion of the first
metatarsal to avoid transfer
metatarsalgia to the lesser
metatarsals

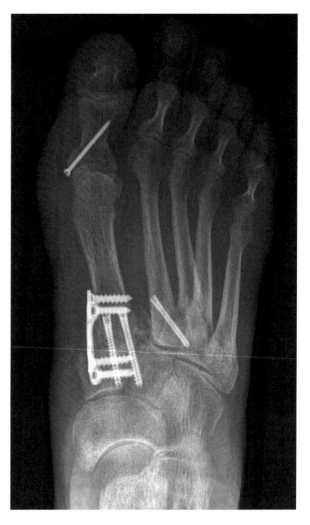

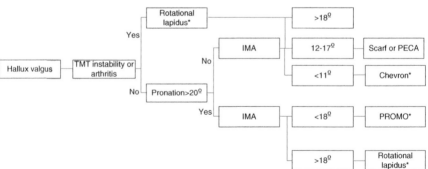

Fig. 11 Hallux valgus treatment algorithm. See text for details. *:if DMAA >10°: add biplanar
Chevron. **: if metatarsus adductus >15°: correct needed (before Hallux Valgus surgery)

7.2.1 Exostectomy

This technique is not recommended as an isolated treatment for a symptomatic bunion. It is commonly associated with other corrective techniques when there is a palpable and symptomatic prominence of the metatarsal head. There are rare occasions when this treatment can be offered to patients with hallux valgus. These cases can include very mild deformities and low functional demand patients with exclusive symptoms of exostosis rubbing against shoes, with an X-ray with a great exostosis. It should be explained to the patient that the origin of the deformity is not being treated. It is certain that the deformity will recur in the short to medium term. The advantage is the recovery that takes about 3–4 weeks compared to the rehabilitation of a formal bunion surgery that takes at least 3–4 months.

Technique: It can be done openly or minimally invasive (MIS). For the open approach, a longitudinal medial approach is recommended at the metatarsal head, approximately 2- to 3-cm long, starting 5 mm distal to the MTTP joint and advancing proximal up to the metatarsal neck. After passing through the subdermal fat, the joint capsule is exposed. Care has to be taken to protect the dorsal and plantar digital sensory branches. A straight medial longitudinal capsulotomy is then performed, exposing the head exostosis medially. It is not necessary to expose more than the medial prominence. There are different capsulotomy techniques; however, in practice they make no difference from the point of view of functionality. In theory, inverted L capsulotomy would have greater corrective power when repaired than other capsulotomies [65], but this does not seem important to the authors since its aim is not to correct the deformity but only to resect the prominence. After exposing the prominence, using an oscillating saw (which may also be an osteotome), the medial eminence is resected following the medial edge of the diaphysis up to the medial articular sulcus. Then the edges are softened with a rongeur. Capsulorrhaphy is performed by three separate stitches using a resorbable suture. Skin closure is performed using an intradermal technique.

In case of opting for the MIS approach, a 0.5 mm incision is made perpendicular to the skin, in the proximal-inferomedial corner of the metatarsal head at the level of the proximal pole of the medial sesamoid, preferably using a beaver blade. The scalpel is then inserted aiming to the center of the head at an oblique angle until it contacts the bone. Then, using a dissector or elevator, the capsule is separated from the metatarsal head until a space or pocket is created around the metatarsal head. Introduce the "Shannon" burr (usually 2 mm diameter and 12-mm-long), and using a suitable motor (high torque, speeds 3000–5000 rpm), proceed to remove the exostosis. After eminence resection, squeeze the area to help remove the resected bone through the skin incision. Irrigate thoroughly the incision with the help of a syringe. Close the skin portal with one single stitch.

It is important to note, that when the exostectomy (resection of medial head prominence) is performed, the head is being freed from any medial capsule-ligament attachment. This results in the sesamoid-plantar plate system losing its medial attachment to the head and being pulled to the side. This is evident when performing this procedure under X-rays, where it is evident how a lateral displacement of the sesamoids occurs after the capsule elevation. This, however, is not important, given that as soon as the patient activates muscles and starts to walk, sesamoids are relocated in their facets. In the 2 weeks postoperative X-ray, sesamoids are already centered under the metatarsal head [7, 8, 66].

7.2.2   Soft Tissue Techniques

The classical soft tissue technique was initially popularized by Silver and later modified by McBride and several other authors [7, 67, 68]. It consists of a dorsal approach between the first and second metatarsals and a release of the adductor tendon, the intermetatarsal ligament, and the lateral metatarsophalangeal capsule. Only if the fibular sesamoid is arthritic could its resection be considered. A resection of the medial metatarsal exostosis (bunionectomy) and a plication of the medial metatarsal capsule are then performed. The intermetatarsal space is sutured and closed using sutures between the lateral metatarsal capsule and the adductor tendon with the intermetatarsal and metatarsosesamoid ligament. This technique is currently not recommended as the sole treatment for bunion deformity [69]. It can be used as an adjunct to an osteotomy but has no scientific basis for use as an isolated technique.

Currently the recommended soft tissue release consists of a percutaneous release of the adductor tendon that attaches to the lateral base of the proximal phalanx of the hallux. This procedure can also be associated with the release of the lateral metatarsosesamoid ligament at the lateral edge of the fibular sesamoid.

Technique: via MIS, under X-rays a scalpel (ideally Beaver-type) is positioned 1 cm proximal and 1 cm lateral to the proximal lateral corner of the proximal hallux. It is introduced with an angulation of 45 degrees lateral to medial and 45 degrees proximal to distal. Checking under X-rays, the scalpel will enter the dorsolateral metatarsophalangeal capsule of the hallux. Once inside the joint, perform a lateral movement with the scalpel to section the lateral metatarsophalangeal capsule. Then follow the lateral corner of the proximal phalanx with the scalpel releasing the adductor tendon and collateral ligament. This gesture should be performed while applying varus force to the hallux. Normally, a click is felt when this release is made [66, 69].

7.2.3   Metatarsal Osteotomies

Distal Intracapsular

Chevron: The best-known distal osteotomy is the Chevron-Austin osteotomy. Described and designed by Austin in 1981 [70], this osteotomy consists of a metatarsal head V-cut, with an apex at the center of the head rotation. It is a reliable procedure, with a low complication rate and a predictable corrective power [46, 67, 69, 70]. The corrective power is approximately 5–7 degrees of IMA [46]. It should be borne in mind that this osteotomy, both in its open modality and MIS (Peico) [71], cannot correct pronation. Since they are translational and uniplanar osteotomies (like Scarf), it is geometrically impossible for them to achieve head rotation correction.

Chevron Technique: Through the same medial approach described previously, the metatarsal head is exposed up to the neck. A minimal exostectomy should be performed, which only facilitates osteotomy planning but does not remove substantial bone. The metatarsal head is exposed medially and dorsally. The center of rotation of the head is drawn on the medial side with a marker pen. The center of the osteotomy is located 3 mm proximal to the head rotation center. From this point, the vertical branch of the osteotomy is drawn perpendicular to the foot weight-bearing surface. On the dorsum of the metatarsal, the osteotomy should be perpendicular to the second metatarsal, not perpendicular to the first metatarsal (this avoids lengthening the metatarsal once the osteotomy has been displaced, which would make correction of the deformity difficult). The second branch of the osteotomy starts at the apex already described, extending proximally parallel to the foot bearing surface. It will exit at the metatarsal neck. It is frequent that once the osteotomy is complete, the lateral capsule remains attached to the head, preventing its adequate lateral displacement. It must be released with the use of an elevator, either from the dorsolateral aspect of the metatarsal or through the osteotomy. The head is then moved laterally maintaining a minimum contact of 40–50% between the bone surfaces. It is transiently fixed in the desired position with a 1.6 Kirschner wire, and the appropriate position is confirmed under X-rays. If an altered DMAA is detected, a medial base wedge resection (biplanar Chevron) can be added in this step. If the position of the metatarsal head is satisfactory, fixation is performed with a 2–3 mm diameter screw. If fluoroscopy shows that the fibular sesamoid is not correctly positioned under the metatarsal head, or that it prevents adequate displacement of the osteotomy, a soft tissue release including the adductor tendon and the metatarsosesamoid ligament should be performed. In cases where there is associated osteoarthritis or increased soft tissue tension, the metatarsal should be shortened by a 2–3 mm through bone resection at the dorsal branch of the osteotomy (Fig. 12).

Reverdin-Isham: This osteotomy was the first osteotomy described for hallux valgus. It was initially described by Dr. Reverdin in 1881 [4], as a medial base wedge with lateral cortical indemnity. It has undergone some modifications, including the approach. It is now best known for its modification called Reverdin-Isham, which is performed via MIS. This osteotomy does not significantly correct the IMA but is mainly indicated for alterations of the DMAA (joint orientation) and only slight alterations of the IMA (corrects 1–2 degrees).

Technique: The MIS burr is inserted through the same incision described in the exostectomy section. After medial eminence resection, at a 45-degree plantar-proximal to dorsal-distal angulation at the metatarsal head, an incomplete osteotomy is performed initially advancing through the dorsal cortex and then terminating at the plantar cortex. The lateral cortex should be left untouched. This technique is performed so that the osteotomy is immediately proximal to the articular surface. After the osteotomy is performed, the metatarsal head must be compressed

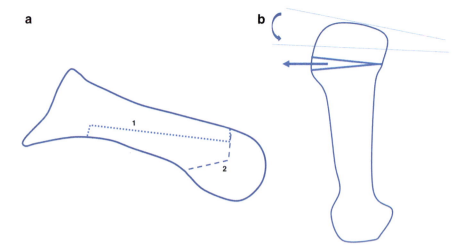

Fig. 12 First metatarsal diagram. (**a**) Sagittal first metatarsal diagram, depicting the Scarf osteotomy (dotted line, 1) and the Chevron osteotomy (dashed line, 2). (**b**) Axial first metatarsal view, showing the biplanar Chevron. Please note the medial base wedge, which after removal corrects the DMAA

proximally in order to close the gap and achieve osteoclasia, thus angulating the metatarsal head medially. Normally this technique does not require rigid fixation due to its intrinsic stability [66].

Distal Extracapsular

These types of osteotomies were grouped together because of the anatomical area where the osteotomy is performed. Extracapsular cervical osteotomies consist of Bosch variants, PECA (percutaneous extracapsular Chevron-Akin) and MICA (minimally invasive Chevron-Akin) [47, 48, 51, 72]. These are techniques performed in MIS form on the metatarsal neck (proximal sesamoid pole). The difference between these types is the shape of the osteotomy. Bosch and PECA use a single cut, straight, perpendicular to the metatarsal [47–49]. Different is the MICA which is a Chevron osteotomy, with two bone cuts angled to each other in a "V" shape [51]. The functional differences between these techniques lie in the shape of the osteotomy. Bosch and PECA, being a straight cut, allow some head rotational correction (they are able to correct mild metatarsal pronation ($<20°$). If there is more pronation ($>20°$), this technique will not be able to correct it. The MICA osteotomy is more stable than the Bosch osteotomy due to the V-shape (Chevron cut vs. single cut); however, it does not allow rotation correction due to the nature of the bone cut. Like the open Chevron or Scarf, MICA is a purely translational osteotomy. These techniques are indicated for moderate deformities, 15–19° IMA.

Original Bosch technique [48]: MIS adductor release is performed, as previously explained. A 2.5 mm Kirschner wire is then inserted 5 mm medially to the medial base of the great toenail. The wire is then advanced medially, subperiosteal to the proximal phalanx, and metatarsal head up to the metatarsal neck. Then, using a Beaver-type scalpel, a sharp incision is made at the level of the metatarsal neck (proximal sesamoid pole), located by means of radioscopy. Using a 2 mm burr, 20-mm-long, between 3000 and 8000 rpm, the burr is inserted in the metatarsal neck midline, perpendicular to the second metatarsal. Then, applying small oscillating back and forth movements, the upper half of the metatarsal is cut, taking care to maintain the perpendicularity of the metatarsal axis. This cut should not take more than 5 seconds, thus avoiding thermal injury to soft tissue and bone. Then, the osteotomy of the lower half of the metatarsal is completed. Again, this cut should take no more than 5 seconds. It should be remembered that the movement of the drill is pendulous, taking as its center of movement the skin where the drill enters. After confirming that the osteotomy is complete, an elevator or Hohmann retractor is inserted through the same approach. This instrument must move the head laterally and then enter the endomedullary canal of the metatarsal in a retrograde fashion. This will position the head over the sesamoids. Once the head has been moved sideways, the Kirschner wire is advanced into the endomedullary canal to the metatarsal base. The wire is cut 2 cm outside the skin (6 weeks postoperatively, it must be removed). This technique is called second generation MIS [71] (Fig. 13).

The technique recommended by the authors replaces the K-wire with screws. This reduces the risk of infection, MTTF joint stiffness, and discomfort for the patient during the period the wire is in position. The Bosch technique, where screws are used instead of K-wires, is called PECA (percutaneous extracapsular Chevron-Akin) [47, 71].

PECA [47, 49, 72] technique: Once the osteotomy has been completed, the metatarsal head is moved laterally with the help of an elevator, Hohmann retractor, or similar instrument that can be introduced into the metatarsal endomedullary canal. The rotation of the hallux should be adjusted so that the metatarsal head has a straight rather than a curved lateral edge under fluoroscopy (Fig. 5). Once the metatarsal head is in the desired place and the rotation is corrected, it is fixed temporarily with a 1.6 K-wire from the metatarsal to the head. Two cannulated screw wires are then positioned from proximal medial to distal lateral. To facilitate the entry of the wires into the medial cortex, it is recommended that an entry be made with the MIS drill to facilitate the maneuverability of the wires. The first wire starts 1 cm distal to the TMT and should ideally finish at the lateral cortex of the metatarsal head, crossing the lateral diaphyseal cortex previously. This wire should then be replaced by a 4.0 cannulated screw. Then, a second wire starts 1 cm distal to the first and should end in the middle of the metatarsal head. This is then replaced by a 3.0 or 3.5 mm screw (Fig. 14). A modification of this technique consists in driving the wires prior to the cervical osteotomy. This implies that once the osteotomy is performed and the head is moved to the side, the wires should only be advanced, which quickly fixes the head in the desired position. The disadvantage of this technique modification is that the wires' position is approximate. They frequently require repositioning if they do not aim to the final head position.

Fig. 13 AP foot weight-bearing X-ray showing a Bosch technique. Please note a transverse cervical osteotomy was performed. A wire is inserted starting at the hallux interphalangeal dorsomedial crease, passing adjacent to the metatarsal head, entering the metatarsal diaphysis

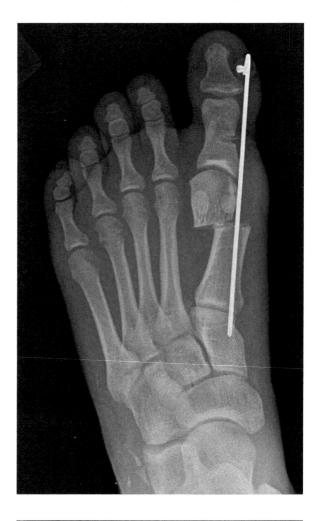

Fig. 14 Bilateral AP foot weight-bearing X-ray. Shows a bilateral PECA osteotomy. Please note how the most proximal screw traverses the head lateral cortex. This helps with the osteotomy stability

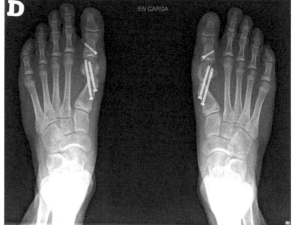

MICA [51] technique: All steps are similar to those already described. The only difference lies in the shape of the osteotomy. When entering the metatarsal neck midline with the burr, the osteotomy in the top half of the head should be angled proximally (approximately 30 degrees). Then, the plantar cut is made again angled 30 degrees proximally. The screws are then placed as previously described.
To perform this osteotomy, it is recommended that frequent radioscopic guidance be used at least in the first ten cases operated on. MIS techniques with screws have a low rate of infection but a high rate of OTS removal rate (24%) [71, 72].

Diaphyseal

Diaphyseal osteotomies are characterized by a moderate corrective power, similar to the MIS cervical osteotomies already described. Scarf osteotomy is the most widely used diaphyseal osteotomy. There are many others, including Ludloff, Mau, Mitchell, etc., but they will not be detailed in this chapter. Scarf osteotomy is translational, i.e., the distal segment of the osteotomy is lateralized in one plane. Like MICA or Chevron, it does not allow axial rotation. The indication for this technique (similar to Bosch or MICA) is a moderate deformity, with an IMA of 10–15. The shape of this osteotomy simulates an inverted "Z" that begins at the metatarsal neck dorsum and ends at the proximal-plantar base (see Fig. 12). This shape has been modified where the plantar and dorsal branches are as short as possible (5 mm), thus avoiding fractures at the ends of the osteotomy. This osteotomy was initially described as a purely lateral displacement one, but modifications have been proposed where an angulation of the distal segment is added over the proximal in addition to the translation [46, 50, 73–75]. This effect increases the corrective power of the IMA; however, when the distal segment is angulated, the DMAA (angulation of the joint surface) also increases relatively. The main limitation of the Scarf is the inability to add a biplanar Chevron in case the DMAA needs to be corrected. In addition, there is a risk of a complication called the troughing effect. This refers to what happens when two semicircular segments are placed one on top of the other; they lack intrinsic stability and can collapse. After the Scarf osteotomy is performed, two semicircular segments are produced, i.e., the plantar-proximal and dorsal-distal segments of the metatarsal bone, which can collapse into each other producing an elevation and pronation of the distal segment (Fig. 15). This is called troughing. To decrease this risk, the distal and proximal osteotomy cuts should be made as distal and proximal as possible, respectively, to have more bone density, which in turn decreases the risk of troughing. In addition, it should be recommended not to bear weight directly on the medial column in the postoperative period for approximately 1 month. This can be achieved by asking the patient to wander around carrying his or her weight on the lateral edge of the foot or on the heel. The Scarf complication rate can be as high as 50%, but with proper technique and postoperative management, it is lower and not different from the complication rate of other techniques [72–74, 76, 77].

Fig. 15 Coronal Scarf osteotomy diagram (mid-diaphyseal cut). (**a**) Shows the osteotomy in its expected position. (**b**) Shows the troughing effect. The plantar metatarsal segment impacts dorsally into the dorsal segment. This ends up in an elevated and pronated metatarsal head, which could lead to a dorsal metatarsophalangeal impingement and Hallux valgus deformity relapse

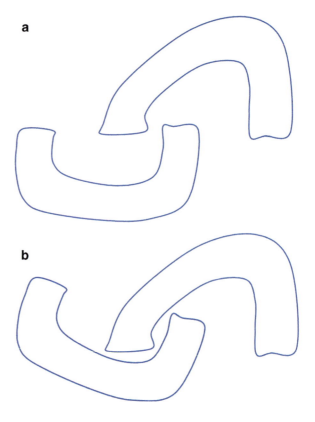

Technique: A medial longitudinal approach is performed, starting at the metatarsal base and ending at the metatarsophalangeal joint. After skin incision, the bone is exposed, maintaining adequate hemostasis. Distally, 1 cm proximal to the articular surface, a 5-mm-thick dorsal-distal osteotomy is performed. Then, the osteotomy is extended proximally along the metatarsal axis, with a slight angulation from distal-dorsal to proximal-plantar. 1 cm distal to the tarsometatarsal joint, this longitudinal branch of the osteotomy ends, and the plantar branch is performed. This plantar branch should be a maximum of 5-mm-thick. Before finishing the osteotomy, it is recommended to confirm that the plane of the osteotomy is being performed parallel to the plantar foot. This is so that once the bone segments are displaced, they should slide between them without elevating or descending. If the osteotomy is not made parallel to the sole of the foot, by moving the distal segment laterally, it can elevate or lower depending on the plane of the osteotomy. This can alter the loading pattern on the lesser metatarsals producing transfer metatarsalgia. When displacing the osteotomy, a minimum of 30–40% bone contact should be maintained between the metatarsal segments. The recommended method of fixation is using two cannulated screws 2–2.5 mm in diameter, orthogonal to the osteotomy.

Proximal

The osteotomies that will be described in this section are the PROMO and the cupuliform or dome [7, 56, 57]. The PROMO osteotomy is a technique that consists of an oblique osteotomy starting 1 cm from the base of the metatarsal. The bone is cut obliquely from distal-dorsal to plantar-proximal. This obliqueness gives this technique the characteristic that, by rotating one bone segment with respect to the other, the distal segment is also angled in its axis. In other words, this osteotomy is capable of correcting the IMA and metatarsal pronation through a single osteotomy. A wedge must not be resected to achieve this correction. The degree of obliqueness of this osteotomy determines how many degrees of IMA and pronation it can correct. The more transverse the osteotomy is to the metatarsal axis, the more pronation and the less IMA it can correct. Conversely, the more longitudinal this osteotomy is done in relation to the metatarsal, the more IMA it will correct, but the less pronation it will correct. Thus, the obliqueness of this osteotomy can correct any combination of IMA and pronation. This obliquity is obtainable from published tables and determined preoperatively. In addition, this osteotomy, being oblique, is stable under load since it closes with weight-bearing [27, 54–56].

Technique: In the preoperative period, the IMA should be measured and metatarsal pronation (mild, moderate, severe) estimated. These parameters of the hallux valgus deformity are entered into the PROMO osteotomy calculation table (Fig. 16), which will provide the angle at which the osteotomy should be performed to correct that particular foot. Through a 4-cm-long medial approach that starts at the metatarsal base and extends distally, the first metatarsal is exposed at its base and diaphysis by dorsal and plantar. A guide wire is then placed 1 cm distal to the TMT joint, parallel to the foot support surface, and perpendicular to the metatarsal. With the help of the position guide, a second wire is positioned through the hole in the guide that is marked with the metatarsal pronation measurement taken in that patient. Then, with that second wire as a guide, the osteotomy is performed at the angulation indicated by the table with the help of the osteotomy guide. Finally, once the osteotomy is completed, the rotation guide is used to mark the degrees of pronation to

		Rotation angle		
		10–19º	20–30º	>30º
Intermetatarsal angle	8–10º	38	28	13
	11–12º	47	33	18
	13–14º	55	38	23
	15–17º	55	42	28
	>17º	55	47	33

Fig. 16 Promo osteotomy calculation table. The osteotomy angulation is obtained by entering the IMA and the rotation angle measured in AP foot X-ray. Note that if more rotation and less IMA is present, the more transverse the osteotomy will need to be to correct the deformity parameters. Vice versa, if more IMA and less rotation is present, the more longitudinal the osteotomy needs to be to correct the first metatarsal deformity

be corrected. Both wires must be positioned parallel to each other so that the prona-tion and IMA measured preoperatively will be corrected. Once the osteotomy has been stabilized with two Kirschner wires, it is stabilized with a medial metatarsal locking plate plus an interfragmentary screw (Fig. 17). For more details on the tech-nique, it is recommended that the specific references be reviewed [55, 56]. For the postop period, non-weight-bearing is recommended for 4 weeks.

The dome, crescentic, or cupuliform osteotomy is performed 2 cm from the tar-sometatarsal joint. The disadvantage of this osteotomy is its intrinsic instability due to the way it is performed. When applying weight load, this osteotomy, despite being fixed, can easily lose congruence and malunite, producing an elevation of the metatarsal. Malunion is one of the most frequent complications [7, 57–59] (13%).

Technique: Through a dorsomedial approach on the base of the metatarsal, the diaphysis and base of the metatarsal are exposed. Using a curved saw blade, a 1.5 cm osteotomy distal to the TMT is marked dorsally on the metatarsal, drawing a hemicylinder looking down on the metatarsal. This will create a semicircular

Fig. 17 AP foot weight-bearing X-ray showing a PROMO and Akin osteotomy. Please note how there is no rotation present in that head (as seen as a lateral curvature at the metatarsal head)

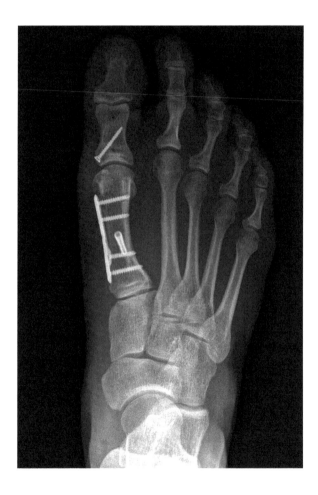

osteotomy perpendicular to the metatarsal. This allows a correction of the metatarsal varus. Originally described with a K-wire fixation, the authors recommend the use of a medial locking plate in addition to a distal-dorsal to proximal-plantar interfragmentary screw. In addition, because of the intrinsic instability of this osteotomy, it should be protected from loading for 6 weeks postoperatively.

7.2.4   Tarsometatarsal (Lapidus) and Metatarsophalangeal Arthrodesis

These techniques are indicated for severe deformities, IMA >18, hallux valgus angle >40°, TMT instability, and arthrosis.

The tarsometatarsal (TMT) arthrodesis or Lapidus technique [78–80] achieves through a TMT fusion the first ray bone alignment. This technique achieves correction in a more proximal site than the previously described osteotomies, so it has greater corrective power than them. In addition, it eliminates the risk of recurrence of the deformity that could be caused by instability of the tarsometatarsal joint. The other characteristic it has is its ability to rotate the metatarsal [31, 32, 52]. However, it has certain limitations. It can increase plantar pressure under the first ray by up to 37% in mid-support phase (due to loss of flexibility) and by 22% under the second metatarsal. The fifth metatarsal-cuboid and navicular-cuneiform joints also suffer increased joint pressure (27% and 40%, respectively) [81]. Stress fractures of minor metatarsals may also occur when the first metatarsal is shortened without sufficient plantar flexion to compensate for the shortening of the ray [82]. Remember that all Lapidus are shortened by at least 5 mm. This shortening can also have other consequences, such as metatarsalgia due to weight transfer, plantar plate rupture, appearance of shortened hallux, etc. The rate of complications in Lapidus arthrodesis is approximately 16% [83]. The sports return rate is around 30–80% [84]. The previously mentioned consequences together with the fact that a generally healthy joint is being removed should be taken into consideration when deciding to choose this procedure. For the authors, Lapidus arthrodesis is indicated in cases of clearly unstable, arthritic joints or in cases of severe deformities.

Furthermore, being an arthrodesis, its rate of fusion is lower than that of an osteotomy. Approximately the rate of nonunion is 3–10% [79, 80, 85, 86].

Technique: It can be done by open or minimally invasive technique. The open technique consists of a medial incision that begins 2 cm proximal to the tarsometatarsal and extends to the neck of the metatarsal. The TMT joint is exposed after adequate hemostasis. 2 mm of cartilage is resected at the base of the metatarsal and at the medial cuneiform using an osteotome or oscillating saw. Multiple holes should be drilled in the subchondral plate allowing for pinpoint bleeding (Paprika's sign). Metatarsal alignment correction is achieved using a distal clamp between the first and second metatarsals as a transient aid, fixing the TMT temporarily with K-wires. Always remember to perform an external rotation (supination) and axial compression of the metatarsal before positioning the transient wires (under fluoroscopy evaluate the lateral metatarsal head silhouette, so that it has a straight edge, and the sesamoids are relocated under the metatarsal head). The methods of fixation are varied. Initially, two crossed screws were described. Biomechanical studies have shown a greater stability of a medial plate [63, 87]. There is an option for fixation even with an endomedullary nail type device [88], as well as cannulated screws. We will describe the technique using a medial plate as fixation. After the bone segments are aligned, a plate is placed medially. It is recommended to have two locking holes distally and proximally, in addition to an oblong hole for the cortical screw. After the plate is fixed distally to the metatarsal with a locking screw, the cortical hole is used to place one cortical screw into the medial cuneiform. This should be placed at the proximal end of the oblong hole to obtain compression with the plate. A 3.5 mm compressive cannulated screw is then positioned outside the plate. This is normally positioned from dorsal-distal to proximal-plantar. Before this screw is tightened definitively, the plate cortical screw should be partially loosened, the cannulated compressive screw is then tightened definitely, and then the cortical plate screw is also retightened. Finally, position one more locking screw through the plate distally (to the metatarsal) and two locking screws through the plate proximally (to the medial cuneiform).

There are occasions where there is intercuneiform instability. After fixing the TMT joint, an opening of the intermetatarsal angle is observed. In these cases, there are two options. One is to add a distal Chevron (technique already described). The other option is to add stability by integrating the intermediate column into the fixation. This corresponds to the original Lapidus technique, in which the base of the one to two metatarsals are prepared and added to the arthrodesis. This can be done with screws from the first metatarsal to the base of the second metatarsal or to the intermediate cuneiform (Fig. 18).

Metatarsophalangeal fusion is a valid option in cases of very severe deformity (>50 degrees of MTP angle) or advanced MTP osteoarthritis. In these cases, alignment through the metatarsophalangeal joint corrects the hallux valgus deformity. Details of the technique will be described in the section on rheumatoid foot and hallux rigidus.

7.2.5 Phalanx Osteotomy: Akin

Akin osteotomy is a technique that orients the toe itself, resecting a small medial wedge and thus achieving a straight toe. Many times considered only a cosmetic detail, it is really a very powerful realignment osteotomy. By orienting the hallux, this osteotomy also orients the forces that balance the joint, mainly the FHL and EHL. In any joint (see chapter on transfers), it is essential to have a balance between agonists and antagonists. If this is not achieved, a deformity will certainly be created in the medium term. The same criteria apply to the hallux. This osteotomy is vital for the final tendon balance. Even a suboptimal metatarsal realignment can be compensated with an Akin, thus obtaining a satisfactory result. Relapse rates have been shown to be lower in surgeries involving Akin vs. no Akin (15% vs. 2%) [89].

Fig. 18 AP foot weight-bearing X-ray showing a Lapidus arthrodesis. In this case, a medial locking plate and a compression screw were used. In addition, a one to two metatarsal screws were used (as in a classic Lapidus). An Akin osteotomy was performed as well in these patients together with a Weil osteotomy to the second metatarsal

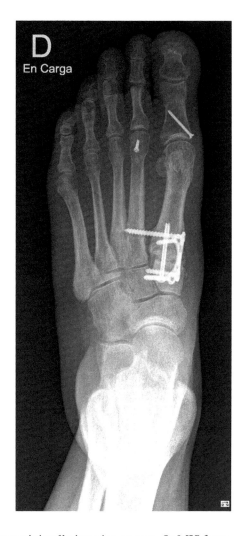

Technique: This technique can be done minimally invasive or open. In MIS form, it is performed by a percutaneous incision medial to the proximal phalanx, 5 mm distal to the metatarsophalangeal joint, guided by X-rays. Then using the 2.0 x 12 mm burr (rpm 3000–7000), the osteotomy is performed. Start by entering with the burr at the phalanx midline. The lateral cortex must be reached, but not crossed. In this position (always maintaining small pendulum movements), the upper segment of the phalanx is cut. This should not take longer than 3–5 seconds to avoid thermal injury. Then, using the same groove created, the osteotomy of the lower half of the phalanx is completed. At the end, an incomplete osteotomy of the medial half of the proximal phalanx is performed, keeping only the lateral cortex intact. With manual axial pressure on the hallux, this osteotomy must be collapsed, thus varizating the hallux. It is then fixed with a cannulated oblique screw 2.0–2.5 mm in diameter (Figs. 17 and 18).

The open technique is performed through a 3 cm medial approach starting at the base of the proximal phalanx. The base of the proximal phalanx is exposed, protecting the EHL and FHL dorsally and plantarly, respectively. Using a 1-cm-wide oscillating saw, an incomplete osteotomy is carried out, maintaining the lateral cortex unharmed, by resecting a 2 mm medial wedge. This osteotomy is then collapsed by axial compression of the hallux. This technique can be fixed with a staple and a cannulated oblique screw or even left without osteosynthesis. In the latter case, it depends on the postoperative dressing.

7.3   Postoperative Dressing

The postoperative dressing helps to control the edema and pain and can help maintain the alignment obtained. MIS techniques without osteosynthesis depend exclusively on the postoperative dressing for their stabilization, so it is of vital importance to master the technique. After hallux valgus surgery, regardless of the technique used, a long gauze is applied between the hallux and second toe. In case you want to increase the toe spread you can pass two bandages. These gauzes surround the foot medially (protecting and covering the area of the medial surgical wounds. Then pass another long gauze between the second and third toes, which also surrounds the foot medially covering the wounds. A new gauze is then wrapped around the forefoot, protecting the metatarsophalangeal joints of the hallux and the fifth toe. Then, the last gauze covers the midfoot at the base of the fifth metatarsal, proximal to the surgical wounds. Finally, the forefoot is wrapped with a protective bandage. Care should be taken when applying the final bandage not to overtension it, so as not to produce bullae or hyperpressure skin injury.

8   Complications

The main complications of hallux valgus surgery are recurrence of the deformity and hallux varus. Less frequent complications are avascular necrosis of the first metatarsal head, nonunion, malunion (metatarsus elevatus), and soft tissue compromise secondary to surgery.

Deformity relapse is the most frequent complication (up to 70%) [90–92] in the long term. There are multiple factors identified in the literature that increase the probability of its occurrence [26, 33, 62, 92–95]. As a summary:

1. Identifiable in the preoperative period: metatarsophalangeal angle >40, intermetatarsal angle (the more deformity, the more risk of recurrence); metatarsal adductus >23 degrees; pronation >20 degrees; DMAA >15 degrees; tarsometatarsal instability, sesamoid position >3.

2. Identifiable in the intraoperative period: DMAA >15; tarsometatarsal instability (identified after fixation of the procedure, the first ray diverges from the second metatarsal).
3. Identifiable in the early postoperative period (<1 month): sesamoid position >3; hallux valgus >8°, pronation >20, gap, or tarsometatarsal step-off.

In the event of a relapse, defined as hallux valgus angle >15 degrees, it should be assessed for associated symptoms. In general, it will depend on the personality and expectations of the patient, what degree of recurrence will be symptomatic, and whether it will eventually end in a reoperation.

As stated above, the published rate of recurrence of hallux valgus is 20–70% [91]. This rate is extremely high, considering that there are factors identified that when corrected can help lower that probability. Strict preoperative and intraoperative care must be taken to identify and correct any factors that may increase the risk of recurrence. When identifying a recurrence that needs to be treated, not only should the angle of hallux valgus and intermetatarsal be corrected but also the factor that was probably preponderant in the reappearance of the bunion. In case there is an alteration in the DMAA, pronation, or metatarsus adductus, a new osteotomy that can correct these factors should be considered. In case the factor is a tarsometatarsal instability, a Lapidus arthrodesis should be used. If the cause of recurrence is a nonunion of a Lapidus, the fusion should be revised. In case the medial ray has been shortened due to repeated surgeries, an allograft or bone substitute should be considered to recover medial column length, in order to avoid further shortening of the ray and the consequent mechanical consequence for the foot. In selected cases of Lapidus relapse, where bone angulation has not worsened in 1 year, an osteotomy (e.g., Chevron) to correct the deformity may be considered without revising the Lapidus (even if it has a nonunion).

Hallux varus is the second complication in frequency [96]. This is secondary to techniques that overcorrect the deformity. It is defined by a negative hallux valgus angle. From the treatment point of view, the analysis should be guided by symptoms and X-ray. If it is asymptomatic, no treatment is required. In cases where it is symptomatic (discomfort mainly due to medial rubbing of the hallux), X-rays should be analyzed to evaluate the origin of the malalignment. In the case of hallux varus secondary to metatarsal overcorrection, a reverse Chevron osteotomy is recommended. The technique and methods of fixation are the same as for the Chevron already described, only in this case the head movement is reversed (medial direction). If the varus deformity is caused by an overcorrection of an Akin, a reverse Akin should be performed, using the same technique described previously, only reverse. In case the correction of hallux varus is insufficient after the reverse Chevron, it is recommended to add soft tissue techniques. The recommended ones are EHB tenodesis and lateral synthetic ligament reconstruction. The first technique consists of sectioning the EHB at its myotendinous junction, passing it from distal to proximal under the intermetatarsal ligament and inserting it into a bone tunnel in the first metatarsal, from lateral to medial. Another technique is to use a synthetic suture reinforcement to the lateral metatarsophalangeal collateral ligament. This can be done using a suture button that augments the lateral ligaments by attaching medially at the proximal phalanx and metatarsal.

Other less frequent complications are Lapidus nonunion (3–10% of cases), metatarsal head avascular necrosis (<1% of distal osteotomies), osteoarthritis, metatarsophalangeal stiffness, and osteotomy malunion. The latter usually occurs after insufficient stabilization, early weight-bearing, poor bone quality, or incorrect technique [79, 80, 85, 86, 96, 97].

Complications of the MIS technique (13% on average) [98] include thermal necrosis of the portals, infection (same rate as open technique, 2–3%), nonunion and malunion, dysesthesia (nerve damage), aseptic nonunion due to thermonecrosis, excessive shortening, joint stiffness, and heterotopic ossification [98–102]. Most of these complications are avoidable with adequate training in MIS surgery.

Finally, the overall dissatisfaction rate of hallux valgus surgery is approximately 10% [103]. This percentage is lower than the reported complications rate, which shows that there are satisfied patients, even though their hallux valgus surgery had some problems. This is probably because surgery is effective in controlling pain and decreasing the functional limitation hallux valgus produces on patients.

9 Summary

Hallux valgus is a quite common condition, more frequently seen in women. Surgical treatment must consider every factor of each individual foot to decide the technique to be used, among others: severity of the deformity, presence of altered DMAA, first ray malrotation (pronation), metatarsus adductus, etc. We must have an adequate set of surgical techniques in order to choose one that can correct every identified factor, and not rely on just one way to solve all deformities. This is the only way to reduce the high relapse rate of hallux valgus.

References

1. Kim Y, Kim JS, Young KW, et al. A new measure of tibial sesamoid position in hallux valgus in relation to the coronal rotation of the first metatarsal in CT scans. Foot Ankle Int. 2015;36(8):944–52.
2. Nishimura A, Fukuda A, Nakazora S, et al. Prevalence of hallux valgus and risk factors among Japanese community dwellers. J Orthop Sci. 2014;19(2):257–62.
3. Roddy E, Zhang W, Doherty M. Prevalence and associations of hallux valgus in a primary care population. Arthritis Rheum. 2008;59(6):857–62.
4. Reverdin J. The deviation of hallux valgus and its treatment. De la deviation en dehors du gros orl (hallux valgus) et son traitement chirurgical. Trans Int Med Cong. 1881;2:408–12.
5. Srinivasan R. The Hallucal-sesamoid complex: normal anatomy, imaging, and pathology. Semin Musculoskelet Radiol. 2016;20(2):224–32.

6. Dedmond BT, Cory JW, McBryde A Jr. The hallucal sesamoid complex. J Am Acad Orthop Surg. 2006;14(13):745–53.
7. Capítulo 4: Hallux Valgus y sus complicaciones en "Cirugía del pie" de Roger Mann. Quinta edición 1987. Editorial médica panamericana S.A.
8. Mark Myerson. Chapter 9: Hallux valgus. In Foot and ankle disorders. Vol. 1. Philadelphia, Pennsylvania, USA: WB Saunders Company; 2000.
9. Tonogai I, Wada K, Higashino K, Fukui Y, Sairyo K. Location and direction of the nutrient artery to the first metatarsal at risk in osteotomy for hallux valgus. Foot Ankle Surg. 2018;24(5):460–5.
10. Kimura T, Kubota M, Suzuki N, Hattori A, Marumo K. Comparison of intercuneiform 1-2 joint mobility between hallux valgus and Normal feet using weightbearing computed tomography and 3-dimensional analysis. Foot Ankle Int. 2018;39(3):355–60.
11. Wagner E, Wagner P, Pacheco F, Villarroel C, Palma F, Guzman-Venegas R. Novel Hallux Valgus cadaveric model: role of ligament damage and tendon pull in recreating the deformit, eposter presentation at the 2020 AOFAS Annual Meeting.
12. Joseph TN, Mroczek KJ. Decision making in the treatment of hallux valgus. Bull NYU Hosp Jt Dis. 2007;65(1):19–23.
13. Coughlin MJ, Thompson FM. The high price of high-fashion footwear. Instr Course Lect. 1995;44:371–7.
14. Kato T, Watanabe S. The etiology of hallux valgus in Japan. Clin Orthop Relat Res. 1981;157:78–81.
15. Piggott H. The natural history of hallux valgus in adolescence and early adult life. JBJS. 1960;42:749–60.
16. Inman VT. Hallux valgus: a review of etiologic factors. Orthop Clin North Am. 1974;5:59–66.
17. Saltzman CL, Brandser EA, Anderson CM, Berbaum KS, Brown TD. Coronal plane rotation of the first metatarsal. Foot Ankle Int. 1996;17(3):157–61.
18. Perera AM, Mason L, Stephens MM. The pathogenesis of hallux valgus. J Bone Joint Surg Am. 2011 7;93(17):1650–61.
19. Ono Y, Yamaguchi S, Sadamasu A, et al. The shape of the first metatarsal head and its association with the presence of sesamoid-metatarsal joint osteoarthritis and the pronation angle [published online ahead of print, 2019 Jul 17]. J Orthop Sci. 2019; S0949–2658(19)30197–6.
20. Ota T, Nagura T, Yamada Y, et al. Effect of natural full weight-bearing during standing on the rotation of the first metatarsal bone. Clin Anat. 2019;32(5):715–21.
21. Talbot KD, Saltzman CL. Assessing sesamoid subluxation: how good is the AP radiograph? Foot Ankle Int. 1998;19(8):547–54.
22. Talbot KD, Saltzman CL. Hallucal rotation: a method of measurement and relationship to bunion deformity. Foot Ankle Int. 1997;18(9):550–6.
23. Coughlin MJ, Saltzman CL, Nunley JA. Angular measurements in the evaluation of hallux valgus deformities: a report of the Ad Hoc Committee of the American Orthopaedic Foot & Ankle Society on Angular Measurements. Foot Ankle Int. 2002;23(1):68–74.
24. Ortiz C, Wagner P, Vela O, Fischman D, Cavada G, Wagner E. "Angle to Be Corrected" in preoperative evaluation for hallux valgus surgery: analysis of a new angular measurement. Foot Ankle Int. 2016;37(2):172–7.
25. Hardy RH, Clapham JC. Observations on hallux valgus; based on a controlled series. J Bone Joint Surg Br. 1951;33:376–91.
26. Coughlin MJ, Roger A, Award M. Juvenile hallux valgus: etiology and treatment. Foot Ankle Int. 1995;16(11):682–97.
27. Wagner P, Wagner E. Is the rotational deformity important in our decision-making process for correction of hallux valgus deformity? Foot Ankle Clin. 2018;23(2):205–17.
28. Yamaguchi S, Sasho T, Endo J, et al. Shape of the lateral edge of the first metatarsal head changes depending on the rotation and inclination of the first metatarsal: a study using digitally reconstructed radiographs. J Orthop Sci. 2015;20(5):868–74.

29. Scheele CB, Christel ST, Fröhlich I, et al. A cone beam CT based 3D-assessment of bony forefoot geometry after modified Lapidus arthrodesis [published online ahead of print, 2019 Dec 5]. Foot Ankle Surg. 2019;S1268–7731(19)30204–8.
30. Campbell B, Miller MC, Williams L, Conti SF. Pilot study of a 3-dimensional method for analysis of pronation of the first metatarsal of hallux valgus patients. Foot Ankle Int. 2018;39:1449–56.
31. Conti MS, Willett JF, Garfinkel JH, et al. Effect of the modified lapidus procedure on pronation of the first ray in hallux valgus. Foot Ankle Int. 2020;41:125–32.
32. Dayton P, Kauwe M, DiDomenico L, et al. Quantitative analysis of the degree of frontal rotation required to anatomically align the first metatarsal phalangeal joint during modified tarsalmetatarsal arthrodesis without capsular balancing. J Foot Ankle Surg. 2016;55(2):220–5.
33. Kaufmann G, Sinz S, Giesinger JM, Braito M, Biedermann R, Dammerer D. Loss of correction after Chevron osteotomy for hallux valgus as a function of preoperative deformity. Foot Ankle Int. 2019;40(3):287–96.
34. Klaue K, Hansen ST, Masquelet AC. Clinical, quantitative assessment of first tarsometatarsal mobility in the sagittal plane and its relation to hallux valgus deformity. Foot Ankle Int. 1994;15(1):9–13.
35. Coughlin MJ, Jones CP, Viladot R, Golan'o P, Grebing BR, Kennedy MJ, Shurnas PS, Alvarez F. Hallux valgus and first ray mobility: a cadaveric study. Foot Ankle Int. 2004;25(8):537–44.
36. Smyth NA, Aiyer AA. Introduction: why are there so many different surgeries for hallux valgus? Foot Ankle Clin. 2018;23(2):171–82.
37. Trnka HJ. Osteotomies for hallux valgus correction. Foot Ankle Clin. 2005;10(1):15–33.
38. Pinney SJ, Song KR, Chou LB. Surgical treatment of severe hallux valgus: the state of practice among academic foot and ankle surgeons. Foot Ankle Int. 2006;27(12):1024–9.
39. Pinney S, Song K, Chou L. Surgical treatment of mild hallux valgus deformity: the state of practice among academic foot and ankle surgeons. Foot Ankle Int. 2006;27(11):970–3.
40. Agrawal Y, Bajaj SK, Flowers MJ. Scarf-Akin osteotomy for hallux valgus in juvenile and adolescent patients. J Pediatr Orthop B. 2015;24(6):535–40.
41. Gicquel T, Fraisse B, Marleix S, Chapuis M, Violas P. Percutaneous hallux valgus surgery in children: short-term outcomes of 33 cases. Orthop Traumatol Surg Res. 2013;99(4):433–9.
42. Chell J, Dhar S. Pediatric hallux valgus. Foot Ankle Clin. 2014;19(2):235–43.
43. Schlickewei C, Ridderbusch K, Breyer S, Spiro A, Stücker R, Rupprecht M. Temporary screw epiphysiodesis of the first metatarsal for correction of juvenile hallux valgus. J Child Orthop. 2018;12(4):375–82.
44. Chiang MH, Wang TM, Kuo KN, Huang SC, Wu KW. Management of juvenile hallux valgus deformity: the role of combined hemiepiphysiodesis. BMC Musculoskelet Disord. 2019;20(1):472. Published 2019 Oct 25.
45. Shakked R, McDonald E, Sutton R, Lynch MK, Nicholson K, Raikin SM. Influence of depressive symptoms on hallux valgus surgical outcomes. Foot Ankle Int. 2018;39(7):795–800.
46. Wagner E, Ortiz C. Osteotomy considerations in hallux valgus treatment: improving the correction power. Foot Ankle Clin. 2012;17(3):481–98.
47. Robinson P, Lam P. Percutaneous surgery for mild to severe hallux valgus. [published online ahead of print April 16, 2020]. Tech. foot ankle surg.
48. Bösch P, Wanke S, Legenstein R. Hallux valgus correction by the method of Bösch: a new technique with a seven-to-ten-year follow-up. Foot Ankle Clin. 2000;5(3):485–vi.
49. Lam P, Lee M, Xing J, et al. Percutaneous surgery for mild to moderate hallux valgus. Foot Ankle Clin. 2016;21:459–77.
50. Murawski CD, Egan CJ, Kennedy JG. A rotational scarf osteotomy decreases troughing when treating hallux valgus. Clin Orthop Relat Res. 2011;469(3):847–53.
51. Vernois J, Redfern DJ. Percutaneous surgery for severe hallux valgus. Foot Ankle Clin. 2016;21(3):479–93.
52. Klemola T, Leppilahti J, Laine V, Pentikäinen I, Ojala R, Ohtonen P, Savola O. Effect of first tarsometatarsal joint derotational arthrodesis on first ray dynamic stability compared to distal Chevron osteotomy. Foot Ankle Int. 2017;38(8):847–54.

53. Coetzee JC, Resig SG, Kuskowski M, Saleh KJ. The Lapidus procedure as salvage after failed surgical treatment of hallux valgus. Surgical technique. J Bone Joint Surg Am. 2004;86-A Suppl 1:30–6.
54. Wagner P, Ortiz C, Wagner E. Rotational osteotomy for hallux valgus. A new technique for primary and revision cases. Tech Foot Ankle. 2017;16:3–10.
55. Wagner P, Wagner E. Proximal Rotational Metatarsal Osteotomy for Hallux Valgus (PROMO): short-term prospective case series with a novel technique and topic review. Foot Ankle Orthopaed. 2018;3(3):247301141879007.
56. Wagner P, Wagner E. The use of a triplanar metatarsal rotational osteotomy to correct hallux valgus deformities. JBJS Essent Surg Tech. 2019;9(4):e43.
57. Yasuda T, Okuda R, Jotoku T, Shima H, Hida T, Neo M. Proximal supination osteotomy of the first metatarsal for hallux valgus. Foot Ankle Int. 2015;36(6):696–704.
58. Dreeben S, Mann RA. Advanced hallux valgus deformity: long-term results utilizing the distal soft tissue procedure and proximal metatarsal osteotomy. Foot Ankle Int. 1996;17(3):142–4.
59. Stith A, Dang D, Griffin M, Flint W, Hirose C, Coughlin M. Rigid internal fixation of proximal crescentic metatarsal osteotomy in hallux valgus correction. Foot Ankle Int. 2019;40(7):778–89.
60. Corte-Real NM, Moreira RM. Modified biplanar chevron osteotomy. Foot Ankle Int. 2009;30(12):1149–53.
61. Dawoodi AI, Perera A. Reliability of metatarsus adductus angle and correlation with hallux valgus. Foot Ankle Surg. 2012;18(3):180–6.
62. Aiyer A, Shub J, Shariff R, Ying L, Myerson M. Radiographic recurrence of deformity after hallux valgus surgery in patients with metatarsus adductus. Foot Ankle Int. 2016;37(2):165–71.
63. DeVries JG, Granata JD, Hyer CF. Fixation of first tarsometatarsal arthrodesis: a retrospective comparative cohort of two techniques. Foot Ankle Int. 2011;32(2):158–62.
64. Lapidus PW. Operative correction of the metatarsus varus primus in hallux valgus. Surg Gynecol Obstet. 1934;58:183–91.
65. Sever GB, Aykanat F, Cankuş C. Comparison of longitudinal and inverted L-type capsulorrhaphy in hallux valgus correction surgery. Medicine (Baltimore). 2019;98(24):e15969.
66. Mariano de Prado. Chapter 5: Hallux valgus. In: Minimally invasive foot surgery. About Your Health publishers. 2009.
67. Johnson JE, Clanton TO, Baxter DE, Gottlieb MS. Comparison of Chevron osteotomy and modified McBride bunionectomy for correction of mild to moderate hallux valgus deformity. Foot Ankle. 1991;12(2):61–8.
68. Mann RA, Pfeffinger L. Hallux valgus repair. DuVries modified McBride procedure. Clin Orthop Relat Res. 1991;272:213–8.
69. Choi GW, Kim HJ, Kim TS, et al. Comparison of the modified McBride procedure and the distal Chevron osteotomy for mild to moderate hallux valgus. J Foot Ankle Surg. 2016;55(4):808–11.
70. Austin DW, Leventen EO. A new osteotomy for hallux valgus: a horizontally directed "V" displacement osteotomy of the metatarsal head for hallux valgus and primus varus. Clin Orthop. 1981;157:25–3.
71. Del Vecchio JJ, Ghioldi ME. Evolution of minimally invasive surgery in hallux valgus. Foot Ankle Clin. 2020;25(1):79–95.
72. Lee M, Walsh J, Smith MM, Ling J, Wines A, Lam P. Hallux valgus correction comparing percutaneous chevron/akin (PECA) and open scarf/akin osteotomies. Foot Ankle Int. 2017;38(8):838–46.
73. John S, Weil L Jr, Weil LS Sr, Chase K. Scarf osteotomy for the correction of adolescent hallux valgus. Foot Ankle Spec. 2010;3(1):10–4.
74. Coetzee JC. Scarf osteotomy for hallux valgus repair: the dark side. Foot Ankle Int. 2003;24(1):29–33.
75. Barouk LS. Scarf osteotomy for hallux valgus correction. Local anatomy, surgical technique, and combination with other forefoot procedures. Foot Ankle Clin. 2000;5(3):525–58.

76. Bock P, Kluger R, Kristen KH, Mittlböck M, Schuh R, Trnka HJ. The scarf osteotomy with minimally invasive lateral release for treatment of hallux valgus deformity: intermediate and long-term results. J Bone Joint Surg Am. 2015;97(15):1238–45.
77. Lee SC, Hwang SH, Nam CH, Baek JH, Yoo SY, Ahn HS. Technique for preventing troughing in scarf osteotomy. J Foot Ankle Surg. 2017;56(4):822–3.
78. Lapidus PW. The author's bunion operation from 1931 to 1959. Clin Orthop. 1960;16:19–135.
79. Myerson M. Metatarsocuneiform arthrodesis for treatment of hallux valgus and metatarsus primus varus. Orthopaedics. 1990;13(9):1025–31.
80. Myerson M, Allon S, McGarvey W. Metatarsocuneiform arthrodesis for management of hallux valgus and metatarsus primus varus. Foot Ankle. 1992;13(3):107–15.
81. Wang Y, Li Z, Zhang M. Biomechanical study of tarsometatarsal joint fusion using finite element analysis. Med Eng Phys. 2014;36:1394–400.
82. Wong DW, Zhang M, Yu J, et al. Biomechanics of first ray hypermobility: an investigation on joint force during walking using finite element analysis. Med Eng Phys. 2014;36:1388–93.
83. Willegger M, Holinka J, Ristl R, Wanivenhaus AH, Windhager R, Schuh R. Correction power and complications of first tarsometatarsal joint arthrodesis for hallux valgus deformity. Int Orthop. 2015;39(3):467–76.
84. Fournier M, Saxena A, Maffilli N. Hallux valgus surgery in the athlete: current evidence. J Foot Ankle Surg. 2019;58(4):641–3.
85. Thompson IM, Bohay DR, Anderson JG. Fusion rate of first tarsometatarsal arthrodesis in the modified Lapidus procedure and flatfoot reconstruction. Foot Ankle Int. 2005;26(9):698–703.
86. Mani SB, Lloyd EW, MacMahon A, Roberts MM, Levine DS, Ellis SJ. Modified lapidus procedure with joint compression, meticulous surface preparation, and shear-strain-relieved bone graft yields low nonunion rate. HSS J. 2015;11(3):243–8.
87. Klos K, Gueorguiev B, Mückley T, Fröber R, Hofmann GO, Schwieger K, Windolf M. Stability of medial locking plate and compression screw versus two crossed screws for lapidus arthrodesis. Foot Ankle Int. 2010;31(2):158–63.
88. Shofoluwe A, Fowler B, Marques L, Stewart GW, Badana ANS. The relationship of the Phantom® lapidus intramedullary nail system to neurologic and tendinous structures in the foot: An anatomic study. Foot Ankle Surg. 2021;27(2):231–4.
89. Kaufmann G, Hofmann M, Ulmer H, Putzer D, Hofer P, Dammerer D. Outcomes after scarf osteotomy with and without Akin osteotomy a retrospective comparative study. J Orthop Surg Res. 2019;14(1):193.
90. Pentikainen I, Ojala R, Ohtonen P, Piippo J, Leppilahti J. Preoperative radiological factors correlated to long-term recurrence of hallux valgus following distal chevron osteotomy. Foot Ankle Int. 2014;35(12):1262–7.
91. Jeuken RM, Schotanus MG, Kort NP, Deenik A, Jong B, Hendrickx RP. Long-term follow-up of a randomized controlled trial comparing scarf to chevron osteotomy in hallux valgus correction. Foot Ankle Int. 2016;37(7):687–95.
92. Shibuya N, Kyprios EM, Panchani PN, Martin LR, Thorud JC, Jupiter DC. factors associated with early loss of hallux valgus correction. J Foot Ankle Surg. 2018;57(2):236–40.
93. Park CH, Lee WC. Recurrence of hallux valgus can be predicted from immediate postoperative non-weight-bearing radiographs. J Bone Joint Surg Am. 2017;99(14):1190–7.
94. Okuda R, Kinoshita M, Yasuda T, et al. The shape of the lateral edge of the first metatarsal head as a risk factor for recurrence of hallux valgus. J Bone Joint Surg Am. 2007;89:2163–72.
95. Okuda R, Kinoshita M, Yasuda T, et al. Postoperative incomplete reduction of the sesamoids as a risk factor for recurrence of hallux valgus. J Bone Joint Surg Am. 2009;91:1637–45.
96. Monteagudo M, Martínez-de-Albornoz P. Management of complications after hallux valgus reconstruction. Foot Ankle Clin. 2020;25(1):151–67.
97. Filippi J, Briceno J. Complications after metatarsal osteotomies for hallux valgus: malunion, nonunion, avascular necrosis, and metatarsophalangeal osteoarthritis. Foot Ankle Clin. 2020;25(1):169–82.

98. Malagelada F, Sahirad C, Dalmau-Pastor M, Vega J, Bhumbra R, Manzanares-Céspedes MC, Laffenêtre O. Minimally invasive surgery for hallux valgus: a systematic review of current surgical techniques. Int Orthop. 2019;43(3):625–37.

99. McGann M, Langan TM, Brandão RA, Berlet G, Prissel M. Structures at risk during percutaneous extra-articular chevron osteotomy of the distal first metatarsal [published online ahead of print, 2019 Dec 31]. Foot Ankle Spec. 2019;1938640019895917.

100. Arauz Y, Juan M. Treatment of minimally invasive hallux valgus surgery complications, techniques. Foot Ankle Surg. 2017;16(1):11–9.

101. Iannò B, Familiari F, De Gori M, Galasso O, Ranuccio F, Gasparini G. Midterm results and complications after minimally invasive distal metatarsal osteotomy for treatment of hallux valgus. Foot Ankle Int. 2013;34(7):969–77.

102. Frigg A, Zaugg S, Maquieira G, Pellegrino A. Stiffness and range of motion after minimally invasive Chevron-akin and open scarf-akin procedures. Foot Ankle Int. 2019;40(5):515–25.

103. Barg A, Harmer JR, Presson AP, Zhang C, Lackey M, Saltzman CL. Unfavorable outcomes following surgical treatment of hallux valgus deformity: a systematic literature review. J Bone Joint Surg Am. 2018;100(18):1563–73.

Hallux Rigidus: A Comprehensive Review

Gaston Slullitel and Valeria Lopez

1 Introduction

Hallux rigidus is a condition characterized by pain and restriction in motion of the first metatarsophalangeal joint (MTPJ), especially in dorsiflexion. Symptoms commonly associated with degenerative arthritis of the first MTPJ were initially reported by Davies-Colley in 1887, although Cotterill is credited with proposing the term hallux rigidus. According to the etiology, hallux rigidus can be classified as primary or secondary [1].

2 Etiology

Although various causes have been proposed for hallux rigidus, its exact etiology has yet to be elucidated [1]. Trauma or osteochondritis dissecans may damage the articular surfaces of the MTPJ. Several biomechanical and structural factors may play a role in the development of hallux rigidus.

G. Slullitel · V. Lopez (✉)
Instituto de Ortopedia y Traumatología Dr. Jaime Slullitel, Rosario, Santa Fe, Argentina

© The Author(s), under exclusive license to Springer Nature
Switzerland AG 2022
E. Wagner Hitschfeld, P. Wagner Hitschfeld (eds.), *Foot and Ankle Disorders*,
https://doi.org/10.1007/978-3-030-95738-4_18

2.1 Functional Hallux Limitus or the Role of the Dynamic Factor

Functional hallux limitus is a clinical condition in which the first MTPJ motion is impaired on weight-bearing conditions but not when unloaded. That means that the joint moves in an open kinetic chain, but not in a closed chain [2]. Its etiology serves as an explanation of the influence of the soft tissue structures in the genesis of the first metatarsophalangeal degenerative arthritis.

The range of motion in a weight-bearing condition depends on structures that are not within the joint itself. Among these structures, the so-called Achilles-calcaneal-plantar system and the medial column of the foot are mainly responsible for optimally setting the first MTPJ in order to provide anteromedial support of the foot during the third rocker or propulsive phase of gait; this requires adequate passive dorsiflexion of the joint while the hallux is purchasing the ground and the verticalized first metatarsal is axially loading the hallux-sesamoid complex [2]. Failure to achieve first metatarsal plantar flexion or an increase in tensile stress at the plantar fascia will limit passive first MTPJ dorsiflexion in the transition from the second rocker (plantigrade support) to the third one (forefoot support). These can impede the ideal gliding contact pattern at the first MTPJ, producing rolling contact on the dorsal margin of the joint [2].

During the second rocker, the tibia must glide forward on the ankle to allow the body's center of mass to progress from an initial position posterior to the supporting foot to a final position anterior to it. A restriction to ankle passive dorsiflexion during the second rocker (derived from a contractured gastrocnemius) will increase dorsiflexing moments at the forefoot, thus increasing tensile stress at the plantar soft tissues due to the truss and beam mechanism of the plantar vault support [2].

A cadaveric study conducted by Viehofer et al. [3] demonstrated that increased tension of the plantar fascia results in a decrease of first MTPJ dorsiflexion, and this also provides a plausible explanation for the development of functional hallux limitus.

2.2 The Structural Factor

The anatomy of the first metatarsal is unique, and its shape has been proposed to play a significant role in the development of hallux rigidus [4]. The first metatarsal head is a large transversely flattened quadrilateral structure with dorsoplantar diameter smaller than transverse [5]. The normal MTPJ has a range of motion of 110 degrees, with a plantar flexion of 35 degrees and dorsiflexion of 75 degrees. The consistency and three-dimensional geometry of the articular surfaces confer stability to the center of rotation of the joint [6].

In a normal foot, the centers of rotation are constant in motion and are on the metatarsal head, but in hallux rigidus they are located eccentrically to the metatarsal head [7]. The proximal phalanx moves gradually into a plantar position relative to the metatarsal head, resulting in progressive displacement of the center of rotation [7]. This displacement causes dorsal impingement of the joint during dorsiflexion. Cartilage lesions occur on the dorsal aspect of the first metatarsal head because of repeated compression under high stresses. This compression eventually leads to the development of dorsal osteophytes and joint degeneration [6].

Although in most patients with hallux rigidus it may be possible to objectively detect an elevation of the first metatarsal with respect to the second metatarsal in a lateral weight-bearing radiograph, in others this is not possible. In some cases, there is evidence of instability of the first metatarsocuneiform joint on the sagittal plane during clinical examination, but this may not be evident radiographically [2].

The role of metatarsus primus elevatus (MPE) in the pathogenesis of hallux rigidus has been debated since its first description by Lambrinudi in 1938, although a recent study hypothesized that with a higher grade of hallux rigidus, the plantar fascia windlass mechanism no longer works. The hallux plantar plate contracts, thus limiting hallux dorsiflexion and forcing the first metatarsal into MPE as a secondary phenomenon [8]. It has been widely debated whether the elevation of the head of the first metatarsal (Fig. 1) is the primary mechanical anomaly or whether the increase in tension in the plantar aponeurosis is the culprit [2, 9]. In the presence of either alteration, the other may end up occurring: an elevation of the head of first metatarsal will increase the tension in the plantar aponeurosis by reducing the vault's anti-collapse moment arm, while an abnormal increase in the tension of the fascia will impede the gliding motion in the first MP joint, increasing the dorsal compressive forces in the joint [2]. It changes the first MP joint motion from a gliding to a hinging type.

Flat foot as a cause of hallux rigidus has been implicated in several studies, but no demographic data were reported in any of these studies to substantiate the notion. This concept may arise from a 1948 study that reported on 3619 normal military recruits and noted that 15% of the patients had an asymptomatic depression of the

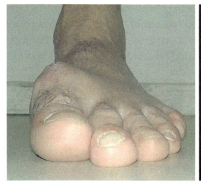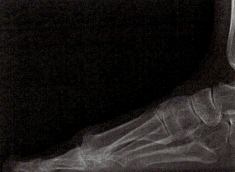

Fig. 1 Picture and radiograph depicting the elevated first metatarsal in advanced hallux rigidus patient

longitudinal arch [10]. In a case series evaluated by Coughlin et al., 11% of 140 patients had pes planus and/or excess heel valgus.

The exact role of a long first metatarsal as an associated factor in this particular entity is still controversial. Coughlin and Shurnas [10] found that a long first metatarsal was no more common in patients with hallux rigidus than in the general population. The author's perspective has been that those flat or chevron-shaped first MTPJs will be exposed to an axial overload during gait that might be the trigger factor of the degenerative process. We believe this is far more significant than the metatarsal length [11].

An increased hallux valgus interphalangeus angle has been evaluated as an associated radiographic and clinical finding of hallux rigidus [12]. This association was seen 90% of the time in the series by Coughlin and Shurnas [5, 10].

Development of degenerative changes can also be secondary to repetitive stress or inflammatory or metabolic conditions such as gout, rheumatoid arthritis [13]. Coughlin and Shurnas [10] found in their study on etiology that adolescent patients with unilateral disease are likely to have reported acute trauma. They also found in the same study that if trauma was reported, the disease was unilateral in 78% of patients regardless of age [5]. A hyperextension injury to the plantar plate and sesamoid complex (so-called turf toe) and a hyperplantar flexion injury may create compression or shear forces that then lead to chondral or osteochondral injury, capsular damage, synovitis, and adhesions and thus have been linked to the development of hallux rigidus [6].

3 Anatomy and Radiological Findings

In 1988 Hattrup and Johnson published the most common classification system used in orthopedic literature. It is based on radiographic changes of the first MTPJ on standing anteroposterior and lateral radiographic examination of the foot. Grade 1 changes consist of mild to moderate osteophyte formation with preservation of joint space. Grade 2 changes exist if there is less than 50% narrowing of joint space, subchondral sclerosis, and moderate osteophyte formation. Grade 3 changes result when there is marked osteophyte formation and more than 50% loss of visible joint space, with or without subchondral cyst formation [1]. Lately Coughlin and Shurnas have introduced a new classification method, adding a grade 4 stage, using clinical information to classify the pathology. This classification includes the assessment of pain patterns. According to this, late stages are characterized for pain in the midrange of motion of the 1 MTPJ [10] (Table 1).

Beeson et al. [14] conducted a systematic review to critically evaluate the various classification systems for hallux rigidus. The authors criticized hallux rigidus grading systems because none had undergone independent testing to assess reliability and validity. Despite this, the Coughlin and Shurnas grading scale for hallux rigidus is the most commonly used and cited. It has been suggested to be prognostic of the severity of great toe arthritis and used to guide treatment [15–17].

Table 1 Coughlin and Shurnas classification scheme

Grade	Dorsiflexion (degrees)	Radiograph	Clinical
0	40°–60	Normal	No pain. Stiffness and some loss of motion
1	30°–40°	Dorsal osteophytes Minimal joint narrowing Flattening of MTT head Periarticular sclerosis	Mild/intermittent pain Stiffness at maximal dorsiflexión/plantar flexion
2	10°–30°	Periarticular osteophytes Mild to moderate joint narrowing	Moderate/severe pain and stiffness more frequently Pain appears near end ROM
3	< 10°	Cystic changes subchondrally Sesamoid irregularities	Constant pain and stiffness Pain appears at end ROM
4	< 10°	Same as grade 3	Pain appears at midrange of ROM

Baumhauer et al. studied the relationship among the clinical factors making up this most commonly used hallux rigidus grading scale, in patients with hallux rigidus, and to explore the correlation of these factors to grade selection [15]. They failed to find a positive correlation between active dorsiflexion ROM and VAS pain scales at baseline with the Coughlin grade. More important, the Coughlin grade was only weakly correlated with the presence of remaining cartilage as observed within the joint and did not predict the success or failure of clinical treatment.

4 Diagnosis

4.1 Clinical Findings

Physical examination reveals a painful swollen MTP joint (Fig. 2) with restriction of dorsiflexion. The patient usually reports a history of pain and stiffness that worsens with activities involving an MTP dorsiflexion, such as stairs or running. Pain during walking occurs above all in lift-off phase of the gait [18]. Moreover, the patient can report numbness on the medial border of the great toe for the impingement of the medial branch of the superficial peroneal nerve from the dorsal osteophytes [17].

At this point it is particularly important to determine if pain occurs at the midrange of motion or in maximum dorsiflexion. Pain at midrange of passive motion refers to pain that is elicited not only at the extremes of passive dorsiflexion and plantar flexion of the metatarsophalangeal joint but also in between [10].

This aspect must be considered to determine the appropriate surgical technique for the patient. Osteophytes around the joint may cause a superficial bursitis, neuritis, or skin ulceration. It is possible to observe an interphalangeal joint

Fig. 2 Clinical picture
demonstrating the
swollen MTPJ

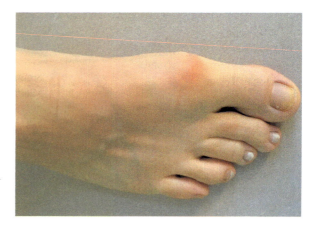

hyperextension as compensation of restricted MTPJ dorsiflexion [1]. This could eventually lead to nail disorders due to the continuous trauma with the toe box of the shoe. Pain at the tarsometatarsal joint may also occur because of this same mechanical compensation.

The inability to effectively dorsiflex the hallux during the swing phase, transfer the load to the second and probably third metatarsal. In that case complaints that lead to seek medical advice could be those of transfer metatarsalgia. When this phenomenon takes place in a load transfer could even take place in the fifth metatarsal head, producing a mixed second and third rocker hyperkeratosis. This phenomenon can also be observed when the patient adopts an antalgic supinated gait due to overpulling of the anterior tibial tendon.

5   Conservative Treatment

Conservative care is the first indication for patients with hallux rigidus, depending on the extent of arthritis and symptoms. The measures commonly used include foot orthoses, modification in shoe-wear, limitations in activity, physical therapy, and injections with corticosteroid or sodium hyaluronate [1].

Foot orthoses and modified shoe-wear are used to reduced motion and impingement at maximum dorsiflexion [19]. One clinical study found that 47% of patients responded to custom orthoses alone, while another 10% responded to simple shoe modifications [20] (Level IV evidence).

Shoe modifications include using low-heeled shoes and toe boxes that allow for accommodation of the first MTPJ.

Injections with corticosteroid or sodium hyaluronate may provide temporary relief of symptoms. Pons and colleagues [21] prospectively compared the effects of injections with either corticosteroid or sodium hyaluronate. Clinical improvement was observed in both groups at 3 months.

The results of these studies suggest that conservative treatment relieves pain associated with daily activities and constitute fair evidence (grade B recommendation).

An insole with a Morton extension [22] is commonly used in the management of hallux rigidus. Made of either spring steel or carbon graphite composite, these extensions are embedded between the layers of the sole, extending from the heel to the toe. They can be placed in nearly any type of shoe and can be used together with a rocker sole to enhance its function. The Morton extension also acts as a splint, preventing the shoe from bending and in the process limiting dorsiflexion of the big toe during gait and decreasing the forces acting through the midfoot and forefoot. The rocker sole is one of the most prevalent modifications, the main function of which is to rock the foot from heel strike to toe-off without requiring the shoe or foot to bend. A high toe box can also be used to prevent direct contact between the dorsal osteophyte and shoe [23].

Functional orthoses have been designed to reverse the windlass mechanism, allowing the first metatarsal to achieve sufficient plantar flexion in preparation for propulsion. First-ray cutouts, designed to allow plantar flexion of the first ray and pronate the forefoot and forefoot postings are other functional orthotic modifications that have been used to improve first-ray function and reduce pain [6]. In contrast, accommodative orthoses are adopted for the immobilization and for the alteration of the magnitude and temporal loading patterns of the first MTPJ. Accommodative orthoses include custom orthoses with a navicular pad and Morton extensions [6].

Physical therapy involves joint mobilization, manipulation, improving range of motion, muscle reeducation, and strengthening of the flexor hallucis longus muscles as well as the plantar intrinsic muscles of the feet to improve the stability of the first MTPJ. Gait training, together with rest, ice, compression, and elevation, has also been advocated in the reduction of pain and inflammation [6].

6   Surgical Treatment

Surgical correction of hallux rigidus is indicated when conservative treatment fails to relieve pain. At the most basic level, the surgical options involve either preservation or destruction of the articular surfaces, and the decision to pursue one option over the other hinges on the degree of articular cartilage degeneration. At moderate stages, joint-preserving procedures constitute a more rational approach. Different techniques have been proposed, but the optimal surgical procedure has yet to be defined [11].

6.1   Joint-Preserving Procedures

6.1.1   Cheilectomy

Dorsal cheilectomy can be performed for patients in early stages of hallux rigidus. This can result in good relief of their symptoms provided that it mainly consist of impingement pain and stiffness in the absence of mid-range pain and a negative grind test. It is popular as an initial treatment for hallux rigidus as it improves pain, preserves joint movement, maintains joint stability, and keeps future secondary options open [24, 25]. The traditional open dorsal cheilectomy involves removing dorsal osteophytes from both the metatarsal and phalangeal side of the joint and up to 30% of the joint surface, in order to achieve dorsiflexion of greater than 45 degrees [26].

In Coughlin and Shurnas's landmark series of 93 feet undergoing cheilectomy with a mean follow-up of 9.6 years, they noted a 92% success rate in terms of pain relief and function [10]. In a more recent investigation, Sidon et al. reported a 69% rate of patient satisfaction with a 29% of failure rate [27].

The main difficulty is selecting the correct patient suitable for dorsal cheilectomy. Most authors agree that mid-range pain with passive motion (Coughlin and Shurnas grade 4) is a contraindication for dorsal cheilectomy [25]. Easley et al. [28] reported in their series that 90% of the patients were satisfied with increased range, and there was a 40-point improvement in American Orthopaedic Foot and Ankle Society (AOFAS) score following cheilectomy at mean follow-up of 63 months. Of the 58 patients in the series of Nicolosi et al. [29], 51 (87.9%) experienced no limitations in their daily activities at an average follow-up of 7.1 years, with two patients (3.3%) subsequently requiring an arthrodesis. Teoh et al. [25] reported on a cohort of 89 patients (98 feet) which underwent minimally invasive cheilectomy followed for a mean of 50 months, with considerable improvement of VAS and self-reported outcome scores. Authors reported a 10% of grades 2 and 3 patients went onto an arthrodesis at a mean of 15 (range, 8–30) months after initial surgery, and this could be due to the fact that they offer MIS cheilectomy to a series of grade 3 patients.

6.1.2   Osteotomies

Metatarsal Osteotomies

Watermann was the first to report in 1927 a dorsal closing wedge trapezoidal osteotomy of the distal first metatarsal bone [13]. It was designed to relocate the viable plantar cartilage to a more dorsal location, allowing more dorsiflexion of the hallux. This was a relatively unstable osteotomy due to its perpendicular orientation and the resulting difficult fixation.

Decompressive osteotomy would theoretically be able to alleviate pain and improve function. A modification of this technique is the Green-Watermann, which involves decompression and offers a more stable configuration of the osteotomy.

Finally, the long-arm decompression osteotomy was proposed by Robinson and Frank as an intermediate to the distal decompression osteotomies and more proximal plantarflexory osteotomies. They reported that it offered the possibility of greater shortening and greater plantar flexion than its more distal counterparts and was also more stable than the proximal osteotomies [11].

Although it was initially conceived for a long first metatarsal, Youngswick osteotomy (Figs. 3 and 4) showed good results in both harmonic and nonharmonic formulas, at alleviating pain and improving function over the short and intermediate

Fig. 3 Youngswick osteotomy. Placed in order to obtain a longitudinal decompression of the joint by proximal translation of the metatarsal head and plantarflexing it by moving the apex of the osteotomy plantarly

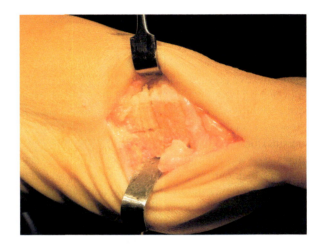

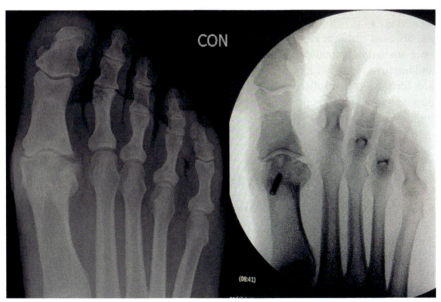

Fig. 4 Youngswick osteotomy. Placed in order to obtain a longitudinal decompression of the joint by proximal translation of the metatarsal head and plantarflexing it by moving the apex of the osteotomy plantarly

terms [30]. Its rationale is to obtain a longitudinal decompression of the joint by proximal translation of the metatarsal head and plantarflexing it as desired by moving the apex of the osteotomy plantarly, allowing the surrounding soft tissues to relax and remodel. Concerns may arise about survival of this joint-preserving procedures although Slulitell et al. published in 2019 a report zero cases of progression to MTPJ arthrodesis despite of progressive worsening (recurrence of dorsal osteophyte and joint space narrowing) of the radiographic appearance in a cohort of 61 patients followed through a mean of 54.8 months [30].

Phalangeal Osteotomies

Dorsiflexion phalangeal osteotomy, as first described by Kessel and Bonnie in 1958, is an effective procedure for remodeling an arthritic first MTPJ, restoring pain-free movement to the joint, and alleviating the pain associated with footwear irritation of dorsal and medial osteophytes of the metatarsal head [31].

Roukis conducted a systematic review of 11 studies of cheilectomy and phalangeal dorsiflexion osteotomy, with a mean follow-up period of 12 months. In 374 procedures, pain was relieved in 89%, and 77% of the patients were satisfied or very satisfied with their outcomes. Just under 5% of the patients required revision surgery [32].

This osteotomy intends to gaining dorsiflexion at the expense of plantar flexion [33] by changing the orientation of the hallux in relation to the first metatarsal for a given angle between the metatarsal and proximal phalanx and may therefore change the direction or distribution of forces at the joint [33]. In a cadaveric study by Kim et al. [33], Moberg osteotomy proved to shift the center of contact pressure plantar an average of 0.7 mm, but did not decrease the peak pressure therefore offloading the diseased cartilage of the dorsal aspect of the joint. The Moberg osteotomy has been studied in patients with advanced hallux rigidus, showing a reduction in pain and improved range of motion 2–4 years after surgery [34]. Probably the main reason for the good results obtained with this technique is that less dorsiflexion is needed at the metatarsophalangeal joint, thus not producing any dorsal metatarsal impingement.

6.2   Joint-Sacrificing Techniques

6.2.1   Metatarsophalangeal Arthroplasty

Arthroplasty has been proposed as an alternative surgical option. The main advantage of arthroplasty over arthrodesis is the preservation of movement without the risk of malunion or nonunion.

Cook and Carpenter et al. [35, 36] divided the prosthetic implants of the first MTP joint into four categories:

- First generation: silicone implants.
- Second generation: silicone implants with grommets.
- Third generation: metal implants with press-fit fixation.
- Fourth generation: metal implants with threaded stem fixation.

Silastic implants using a silicone and plastic hybrid were introduced in the 1960s, to improve the outcome of the Keller's arthroplasty [37]. They were originally single-stemmed hemi-implants. Initial studies in the 1980s, however, reported extremely high rates of complications and failure, including synovitis, migration, osteolysis, granulomas, and lymphadenopathy [38]. However those studies evaluated single-stemmed Silastic implants which are no longer commercially available.

Biomechanically, the Silastic implant is designed to act as a sloppy hinged dynamic spacer but has no inbuilt ability to correct deformity or maintain correction. It is not directly attached to the bone, allowing self-alignment in the axis of the joint. This, combined with its low modulus of elasticity, reduces stress-shielding and promotes bone loading, preventing bone reabsorption and fractures. It has viscoelastic properties and high resistance to fatigue. It is a single component; hence once encapsulation occurs, backside wear is not seen [37]. Cautions and contraindications for Silastic implants should be the same as for any arthroplasty. We would not recommend its use when there is a sizeable associated deformity such as valgus or in rheumatoid disease where the bone may be soft and/or cystic [39].

A recent systematic review suggested that arthroplasty leads to similar outcomes, satisfaction, rate of complications, and reoperation as arthrodesis [38, 39]. Despite several subsequent studies in the 1990s reporting good outcomes with the new implant with high satisfaction rates (80–90%), low rates of complication, failure, and revision [39, 40], it continues to be rarely used and remains a controversial surgical option for patients with end-stage HR [41].

There are several Silastic implants, with different stems length and angulation.

A 2020 study [39] on double stemmed Silastic implants reported a 97.2% implant survivorship at a mean 5.3 years follow-up in a 108 hallux rigidus patient population, with high satisfaction rates and considerable improvement in self-reported outcome measures. Three patients require revision (one infection and two implant fractures). A total of 25 patients (23.1%) had a complication, most were minor, responding to simple treatment, and authors stated that this did not affect the outcome. In the same scenario Van Duijvenbode et al. [42] described the results of 43 implants in 36 patients at a mean follow-up of 19 years. There was a 4% revision/reoperation rate, with one revision to a further Silastic implant at 9 years and two revisions to a Keller's procedure at 13 and 17 years. They report good to excellent patient-reported outcome measures (PROM) scores and a median satisfaction rate of 10.

There are other possibilities when replacing the first MTPJ surface. A metallic proximal phalangeal resurfacing was evaluated in a recent review which included a total of 97 implants reported survival rates of 85.6% and rates of satisfaction of 75% at a median follow-up of 5.4 years. Causes of failure included osteolysis and deep infection but most commonly persistent pain. The authors concluded that this implant should be used with caution in younger patients due to the high revision rate [43].

Some three-component implants are available. There are studies showing good early results for these implants [44]. Titchener et al., however, reported alarming results in a series of 86 Toefit-Plus implants in 73 patients with a 9.3% intraoperative fracture rate and 24% revision rate at a mean follow-up of 33 months (2–72) [45]. Gupta and Masud [46] reported the results of 47 Toefit-Plus implants with a 21% (10/47) revision rate and a further 23% (11/47) complaining of ongoing pain at a mean follow-up of 11.1 years. This field is still of ongoing investigation although some results are promising in terms of preserving first MTPJ motion for those patients with severe HR.

6.2.2 Metatarsophalangeal Hemiarthroplasty

Hemiarthroplasty consists of a unipolar implant designed to replace the articular surface of the head of the metatarsal or the proximal phalanx base. This procedure requires less bone resection and maintains the length of the first ray. Moreover, if a conversion to arthrodesis becomes necessary, it should be technically easier. Meriç et al. [47], with a mean follow-up of 24.2 ± 7.2 months, reported an improvement from a preoperative AOFAS score of 33.9 ± 9.8 points to a final follow-up score of 81.6 ± 10.1 points, VAS diminished from 8.4 ± 0.9 to 1.21 ± 1.2 and first MTPJ ROM improved from 22.8° to 69.6°. There was no implant loosening at follow-up and only one case of revision in arthrodesis due to pain and immobility.

Mermerkaya and Adli [48] have retrospectively compared outcomes of total joint arthroplasty and hemiarthroplasty of the metatarsal component to a mean follow-up of 27.1 ± 7.5 months and 29.9 ± 5.2 months, respectively. Authors have observed significant improvement in AOFAS scores and significant decreases in VAS in both groups at follow-up, with no significant between-group difference, at last, follow-up. No implant loosening, radiolucency, or subsidence was found in the cases treated.

6.2.3 Polyvinyl Alcohol Implant

Historically, the most commonly performed procedure in patients with moderate to severe HR is arthrodesis; however, this procedure leaves the patient with no motion through the first MTPJ [49]. Newer techniques have focused on procedures that maintain range of motion (ROM) and allow patients to weight-bear immediately following surgery [50].

A novel polyvinyl alcohol (PVA) hydrogel implant has recently been developed [51]. This synthetic material has water content comparable to healthy cartilage and a compressive modulus and tensile strength similar to human articular cartilage. Therefore it can withstand shear and axial load forces beyond those experienced in the great toe, without fragmentation. These biomechanical features make it an ideal material for use in hemiarthroplasty of the first MTPJ [50].

The efficacy and safety of this small PVA hydrogel implant in comparison to first MTPJ arthrodesis was recently evaluated in a prospective, randomized, clinical trial conducted at 12 centers in Canada and the United Kingdom. At the 2-year follow-up, the implant hemiarthroplasty demonstrated equivalent pain relief and functional outcomes to first MTPJ arthrodesis, with no cases of implant fragmentation, wear, or bone loss [52].

An additional study evaluated the 5-year outcome of 27 grade 2, 3, and 4 HR patients treated in 3 different centers, which were assigned to the PVA implant in a random manner and reported clinically and statistically significant improvements in patient-reported outcome measures (VAS, SF-36 FAAM-ADL) and 65% of patients rating their overall function level as normal, with a 96% implant survivorship [50]. Interestingly, range of motion through the MTP joint improved following hemiarthroplasty with the PVA hydrogel implant compared with baseline, which represents an additional benefit to these patients.

Cassinelli et al. [53], in a non-designer study, reported less favorable results in a series of 64 implants in 60 patients with 38% (24/64) being "unsatisfied" or "very unsatisfied," a 20% (13/64) reoperation rate, and an 8% (5/64) rate of conversion to arthrodesis, at a mean follow-up of 18.5 months (12–30).

6.2.4 Metatarsophalangeal Arthrodesis

First MTPJ fusion today represents the mainstay of surgical care for high-grade, advanced hallux rigidus [54]. Improvement of pain is achieved by eliminating residual degenerated cartilage layer, overstepping the subchondral bone and sacrificing the joint motion. Preparation of the surfaces may lead to the creation of complementary bone interfaces, through flat or conical molding of the metatarsal and phalangeal portions [54].

Fusion rates have been observed between 53% and 100%, depending on the type of fixation and type of pathoanatomy [55]. Chraim et al. [56] reported the long-term outcome of first MTPJ fusion using a transarticular screw and dorsal non-locked plate, with 93.3% of fusion rate and 6.7% of painless nonunion with no needed additional surgery.

Arthrodesis is particularly indicated in younger patients, with mid- or high-performance requests or more active patients, in severe pathologies, such as salvage procedure in recurrences or failed motion-sparing procedures (Fig. 5a–c). Recommended fixation of the hallux is 10°–15° of dorsiflexion and 10°–15° of valgus [57, 58].

Different fixation techniques have been described to achieve fusion [59]. Recent plating techniques yielded significant improvements in fixation stability and union rates. While plating techniques are highly successful, they necessitate a relatively large dorsal incision, which can lead to postoperative complications. The plates can also be bulky, creating subsequent symptoms during activities and showing wear over time. In contrast, arthroscopic fusion requires smaller incisions, which may

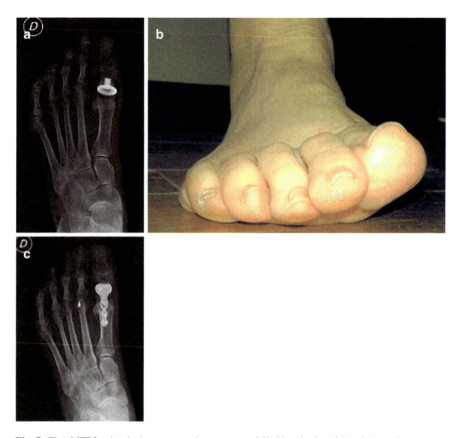

Fig. 5 First MTPJ arthrodesis as a procedure to save a failed hemiarthroplasty that was in an unacceptable hyperextension. (**a**) Radiograph depicting the hemiarthroplasty implant in position. Note the osteolysis around the implant stem. (**b**) Photograph demostrating the hyperextension of the MTPJ tha caused pain with shoe wearing. (**c**) Correct aligmnent after MTPJ arthrodesis

result in less swelling, less pain, and fewer complications. The evolution of minimally invasive techniques and instruments has enabled the arthroscopic preparation of an arthritic hallux MTPJ for arthrodesis. Fixation for arthroscopic MTPJ fusion can be achieved by crossing compression lag screw [60].

Compression lag screws were previously compared with standard dorsal plates, and standard plates were shown to be mechanically superior. Fully threaded headless screws may provide superior stability when compared with compression lag screws because the threads engage the cortex in three places, the outer cortex at the site of insertion and both cortices at the MTPJ. Standard compression lag screw threads, however, do not always engage cortical bone, depending on surgeon technique. Fully threaded screws may provide a more stable construct to allow early weight-bearing, particularly if the subchondral plate is preserved.

In a cadaveric study which compared the mechanical stability of the current generation of locking plates used in conjunction with a single compression lag screw to fully threaded headless compression screws, there was a significant difference in mean stiffness in favor of the plate plus lag screw construct; however, no significant difference was found when examining mean load to failure [60].

6.2.5 Resection and Interposition Arthroplasty

A simple resection technique of the first phalangeal base has been described in 1904 by Keller and Menger [61], for treatment of hallux valgus associated with osteoarthritis of the first metatarsophalangeal joint, without replacement of the joint space with non-tissue implants. Actually, this technique is used for decompression and restoration of range of motion of high-grade hallux rigidus, especially in those patients that refuse arthrodesis. Complications described include first MTPJ instability, cock-up deformity and transfer metatarsalgia [54]. This procedure is usually reserved for older and low demand patients.

When a traditional resection arthroplasty is combined with the insertion of a biologic spacer into the joint, it is called interposition arthroplasty. Its rationale is given by the reduction in bone loss from the proximal phalangeal base, the maintenance of length, and improving joint stability and motion. Various tissues have been utilized and described: capsular autograft, meniscus allograft, regenerative tissue matrix, and tendon autograft [62, 63].

7 Summary

Hallux rigidus is still a complex entity in which optimal treatment has yet to be defined. New developments and techniques should be in the direction of joint and motion preservation, especially in high demand or younger patients.

References

1. Migues A, Slullitel G. Joint-preserving procedure for moderate hallux rigidus. Foot Ankle Clin. 2012;17(3):459–71. https://doi.org/10.1016/j.fcl.2012.06.006.
2. Maceira E, Monteagudo M. Functional hallux rigidus and the Achilles-calcaneus-plantar system. Foot Ankle Clin. 2014;19(4):669–99. https://doi.org/10.1016/j.fcl.2014.08.006.
3. Viehöfer AF, Vich M, Wirth SH, Espinosa N, Camenzind RS. The role of plantar fascia tightness in hallux limitus: a biomechanical analysis. J Foot Ankle Surg. 2019;58(3):465–9. https://doi.org/10.1053/j.jfas.2018.09.019.
4. Coughlin MJ, Shurnas PS. Hallux rigidus: grading and long term results of operative treatment. J Bone Joint Surg Am. 2003;85:2072–88.
5. Lucas DE, Hunt KJ. Hallux rigidus: relevant anatomy and pathophysiology. Foot Ankle Clin. 2015;20(3):381–9. https://doi.org/10.1016/j.fcl.2015.04.001.
6. Kunnasegaran R, Thevendran G. Hallux rigidus: nonoperative treatment and orthotics. Foot Ankle Clin. 2015;20(3):401–12. https://doi.org/10.1016/j.fcl.2015.04.003.

7. Flavin R, Halpin T, O'Sullivan R, et al. A finite-element analysis study of the metatarsophalangeal joint of the hallux rigidus. J Bone Joint Surg Br. 2008;90(10):1334–40.
8. Cheung ZB, Myerson MS, Tracey J, Vulcano E. Weightbearing CT scan assessment of foot alignment in patients with hallux rigidus. Foot Ankle Int. 2018;39:67–74. https://doi.org/10.1177/1071100717732549.
9. Roukis TS. Metatarsus primus elevatus in hallux rigidus. Fact or fiction? J Am Podiatr Med Assoc. 2005;95(3):221–8.
10. Coughlin MJ, Shurnas PS. Hallux rigidus: demographics, etiology, and radiographic assessment. Foot Ankle Int. 2003;24(10):731–43. https://doi.org/10.1177/107110070302401002.
11. Slullitel G, López V, Seletti M, Calvi JP, Bartolucci C, Pinton G. Joint preserving procedure for moderate hallux rigidus: does the metatarsal index really matter? J Foot Ankle Surg. 2016;55(6):1143–7. https://doi.org/10.1053/j.jfas.2016.06.003.
12. Hunt K, Anderson R. Biplanar proximal phalanx closing wedge osteotomy for hallux rigidus. Foot Ankle Int. 2012;33(12):1043–50.
13. Galois L, Hemmer J, Ray V, Sirveaux F. Surgical options for hallux rigidus: state of the art and review of the literature. Eur J Orthop Surg Traumatol. 2020;30(1):57–65. https://doi.org/10.1007/s00590-019-02528-x.
14. Beeson P, Phillips C, Corr S, Ribbans W. Classification systems for hallux rigidus: a review of the literature. Foot Ankle Int. 2008;29(4):407–14.
15. Baumhauer JF, Singh D, Glazebrook M, et al. Prospective, randomized, multi-centered clinical trial assessing safety and efficacy of a synthetic cartilage implant versus first metatarsophalangeal arthrodesis in advanced hallux rigidus. Foot Ankle Int. 2016;37(5):457–69. https://doi.org/10.1177/1071100716635560.
16. Deland JT, Williams BR. Surgical management of hallux rigidus. J Am Acad Orthop Surg. 2012;20(6):347–58.
17. Hamid KS, Parekh SG. Clinical presentation and management of hallux rigidus. Foot Ankle Clin. 2015;20(3):391–9.
18. Ho B, Baumhauer J. Hallux rigidus. EFORT Open Rev. 2017;2:13–20. https://doi.org/10.1302/2058-5241.2.160031.
19. Smith RW, Katchis SD, Ayson LC. Outcomes in hallux rigidus patients treated nonoperatively: a long-term follow-up study. Foot Ankle Int. 2000;21(11):906–13.
20. Horton GA, Parks YW, Myerson MS. Role of metatarsus primus elevatus in the pathogenesis of hallux rigidus. Foot Ankle Int. 1999;20(12):777–80.
21. Pons M, Alvarez F, Solana J, et al. Sodium hyaluronate in the treatment of hallux rigidus. A single-blind, randomized study. Foot Ankle Int. 2007;28(1):38–42.
22. Sammarco VJ, Nichols R. Orthotic management for disorders of the hallux. Foot Ankle Clin. 2005;10(1):191–209.
23. Janisse DJ, Janisse E. Shoe modification and the use of orthoses in the treatment of foot and ankle pathology. J Am Acad Orthop Surg. 2008;16(3):152–8.
24. Walter R, Perera A. Open, arthroscopic, and percutaneous cheilectomy for hallux rigidus. Foot Ankle Clin. 2015;20(3):421–31.
25. Teoh KH, Tan WT, Atiyah Z, Ahmad A, Tanaka H, Hariharan K. Clinical outcomes following minimally invasive dorsal cheilectomy for hallux rigidus. Foot Ankle Int. 2019;40(2):195–201. https://doi.org/10.1177/1071100718803131.
26. Stevens R, Bursnall M, Chadwick C, Davies H, Flowers M, Blundell C, Davies M. Comparison of complication and reoperation rates for minimally invasive versus open cheilectomy of the first metatarsophalangeal joint. Foot Ankle Int. 2020;41(1):31–6. https://doi.org/10.1177/1071100719873846.
27. Sidon E, Rogero R, Bell T, McDonald E, Shakked RJ, Fuchs D, Daniel JN, Pedowitz DI, Raikin SM. Long-term follow-up of cheilectomy for treatment of hallux Rigidus. Foot Ankle Int. 2019;40(10):1114–21. https://doi.org/10.1177/1071100719859236.
28. Easley ME, Davis WH, Anderson RB. Intermediate to long-term follow-up of medial-approach dorsal cheilectomy for hallux rigidus. Foot Ankle Int. 1999;20(3):147–52. https://doi.org/10.1177/107110079902000302.

29. Nicolosi N, Hehemann C, Connors J, Boike A. Long-term follow-up of the cheilectomy for degenerative joint disease of the first metatarsophalangeal joint. J Foot Ankle Surg. 2015;54(6):1010–20.

30. Slullitel G, López V, Calvi JP, D'Ambrosi R, Usuelli FG. Youngswick osteotomy for treatment of moderate hallux rigidus: thirteen years without arthrodesis. Foot Ankle Surg. 2019:S1268-7731(19)30208-5. https://doi.org/10.1016/j.fas.2019.11.008.

31. Coutts A, Kilmartin TE. Dorsiflexory phalangeal osteotomy for grade II hallux rigidus: patient-focused outcomes at eleven-year follow-up. J Foot Ankle Surg. 2019;58(1):17–22. https://doi.org/10.1053/j.jfas.2018.06.004.

32. RoukisTS. Outcomes after cheilectomy with phalangeal dorsiflexory osteotomy for hallux rigidus:a systematic review. J Foot Ankle Surg. 2010;49:479–87.

33. Kim PH, Chen X, Hillstrom H, Ellis SJ, Baxter JR, Deland JT. Moberg osteotomy shifts contact pressure plantarly in the first metatarsophalangeal joint in a biomechanical model. Foot Ankle Int. 2016;37(1):96–101. https://doi.org/10.1177/1071100715603513.

34. O'Malley MJ, Basran HS, Gu Y, et al. Treatment of advanced stages of hallux rigidus with cheilectomy and phalangeal osteotomy. J Bone Joint Surg Am. 2013;95:606–5. https://doi.org/10.2106/JBJS.K.00904.

35. Cook KD. Capsular interposition for the Keller bunionectomy with the use of soft-tissue anchors. J Am Podiatr Med Assoc. 2005;95(2):180–2. https://doi.org/10.7547/0950180.

36. Carpenter B, Smith J, Motley T, Garrett A. Surgical treatment of hallux rigidus using a metatarsal head resurfacing implant: mid-term follow-up. J Foot Ankle Surg. 2010;49:321–5. https://doi.org/10.1053/j.jfas.2010.04.007.

37. Swanson AB, Lumsden RM, Swanson GD. Silicone implant arthroplasty of the great toe. A review of single stem and flexible hinge implants. Clin Orthop Relat Res. 1979;142:30–43.

38. Clough TM, Ring J. Silastic first metatarsophalangeal joint arthroplasty for the treatment of end-stage hallux rigidus. Bone Joint J. 2020;102-B(2):220–6. https://doi.org/10.1302/0301-620X.102B2.BJJ-2019-0518.R2.

39. Park YH, Jung JH, Kang SH, Choi GW, Kim HJ. Implant arthroplasty versus arthrodesis for the treatment of advanced hallux rigidus: a meta-analysis of comparative studies. J Foot Ankle Surg. 2019;58(1):137–43.

40. Ter Keurs EW, Wassink S, Burger BJ, Hubach PC. First metatarsophalangeal joint replacement: long-term results of a double stemmed flexible silicone prosthesis. Foot Ankle Surg. 2011;17(4):224–7.

41. Majeed H. Silastic replacement of the first metatarsophalangeal joint:historical evolution, modern concepts and a systematic review of the literature. EFORT Open Rev. 2019;4(3):77–84.

42. van Duijvenbode DC, Bulstra GH, Nijsse BA. Nineteen-year follow-up of the silastic double stemmed hinge prosthesis of the first metatarsophalangeal joint. Foot Ankle Surg. 2013;19(1):27–30.

43. Clement ND, MacDonald D, Dall GF, et al. Metallic hemiarthroplasty for the treatment of end-stage hallux rigidus: mid-term implant survival, functional outcome and cost analysis. Bone Joint J. 2016;98-B(7):945–51.

44. Tunstall C, Laing P, Limaye R, et al. 1st metatarso-phalangeal joint arthroplasty with ROTO-glide implant. Foot Ankle Surg. 2017;23(3):153–6.

45. Titchener AG, Duncan NS, Rajan RA. Outcome following first metatarsophalangeal joint replacement using TOEFIT-PLUS™: a midterm alert. Foot Ankle Surg. 2015;21(2):119–24.

46. Gupta S, Masud S. Long term results of the Toefit-Plus replacement for first metatarsophalangeal joint arthritis. The Foot (Edinb). 2017;31:67–71.

47. Meriç G, Erduran M, Atik A, Köse Ö, Ulusal AE, Akseki D. Short-term clinical outcomes after first metatarsal head resurfacing hemiarthroplasty for late stage hallux rigidus. J Foot Ankle Surg. 2015;54(2):173–8. https://doi.org/10.1053/j.jfas.2014.10.016.

48. Mermerkaya MU. Adli H.a comparison between metatarsal head-resurfacing hemiarthroplasty and total metatarsophalangeal joint arthroplasty as surgical treatments for hallux rigidus: a

retrospective study with short- to midterm follow-up. Clin Interv Aging. 2016;11:1805–13. https://doi.org/10.2147/CIA.S110865.

49. Yee G, Lau J. Current concepts review: hallux rigidus. Foot Ankle Int. 2008;29(6):637–46. https://doi.org/10.3113/FAI.2008.0637.

50. Daniels TR, Younger AS, Penner MJ, et al. Midterm outcomes of polyvinyl alcohol hydrogel hemiarthroplasty of the first metatarsophalangeal joint in advanced hallux rigidus. Foot Ankle Int. 2017;38(3):243–7. https://doi.org/10.1177/1071100716679979.

51. Younger ASE, Baumhauer JF. Polyvinyl alcohol hydrogel hemiarthroplasty of the great toe: technique and indications. Techn Foot Ankle Surg. 2013;12(3):164–9.

52. Baumhauer JF, Singh D, Glazebrook M, et al. Correlation of hallux rigidus grade with motion, VAS pain, intraoperative cartilage loss, and treatment success for first MTP joint arthrodesis and synthetic cartilage implant. Foot Ankle Int. 2017;38(11):1175–82. https://doi.org/10.1177/1071100717735289.

53. Cassinelli SJ, Chen S, Charlton TP, Thordarson DB. Early outcomes and complications of synthetic cartilage implant for treatment of hallux rigidus in the United States. Foot Ankle Int. 2019;40(10):1140–8.

54. Massimi S, Caravelli S, Fuiano M, Pungetti C, Mosca M, Zaffagnini S. Management of high-grade hallux rigidus: a narrative review of the literature. Musculoskelet Surg. 2020; https://doi.org/10.1007/s12306-020-00646-y.

55. Raikin SM, Ahmad J. Comparison of arthrodesis and metallic hemiarthroplasty of the hallux metatarsophalangeal joint: surgical technique. J Bone Joint Surg Am. 2008; https://doi.org/10.2106/JBJS.H.00368.

56. Chraim M, Bock P, Alrabai HM, Trnka HJ. Long-term outcome of first metatarsophalangeal joint fusion in the treatment of severe hallux rigidus. Int Orthop. 2016; https://doi.org/10.1007/s00264-016-3277-1.

57. Kelikian AS. Technical considerations in hallux metatarsophalangeal arthrodesis. Foot Ankle Clin. 2005;10(1):167–90.

58. McNeil DS, Baumhauer JF, Glazebrook MA. Evidence-based analysis of the efficacy for operative treatment of hallux rigidus. Foot Ankle Int. 2013;34(1):15–32. https://doi.org/10.1177/1071100712460220.

59. Migues A, Calvi J, Sotelano P, Carrasco M, Slullitel G, Conti L. Endomedullary screw fixation for first metatarsophalangeal arthrodesis. Foot Ankle Int. 2013;34(8):1152–7. https://doi.org/10.1177/1071100713483113.

60. Fuld RS 3rd, Kumparatana P, Kelley J, Anderson N, Baldini T, Younger ASE, Hunt KJ. Biomechanical comparison of low-profile contoured locking plate with single compression screw to fully threaded compression screws for first MTP fusion. Foot Ankle Int. 2019;40(7):836–44. https://doi.org/10.1177/1071100719837524.

61. Konkel KF, Menger AG. Mid-term results of titanium hemi-great toe implants. Foot Ankle Int. 2006;27(11):922–9.

62. Clews CNL, Kingsford AC, Samaras DJ. Autogenous capsular interpositional arthroplasty surgery for painful hallux rigidus: assessing changes in range of motion and postoperative foot health. J Foot Ankle Surg. 2015;54(1):29–36. https://doi.org/10.1053/j.jfas.2014.09.004.

63. Delacruz EL, Johnson AR, Clair BL. First metatarsophalangeal joint interpositional arthroplasty using a meniscus allograft for the treatment of advanced hallux rigidus: surgical technique and short-term results. Foot Ankle Spec. 2011;4(3):157–64. https://doi.org/10.1177/1938640011402821.

Sesamoiditis

Florencia Pacheco Martinez and Eduardo Fuentes Morales

1 Introduction

The term "sesamoid" was originally coined by Galen in 180 BC, due to the similarity in shape of this bone with sesame seeds. The function of each sesamoid varies according to its location in the skeleton. The sesamoids of the foot are contained in the plantar plates of the interphalangeal and metatarsophalangeal joints [1].

Specifically, the sesamoids of the first metatarsophalangeal joint play an important role in the function of the hallux. The sesamoid complex acts as a pulley to enhance the movement and flexor force of the metatarsophalangeal joint during walking. "Sesamoiditis" is a pathology that describes a wide spectrum of pathologies that have as a common factor the pain of the sesamoids under the head of the first metatarsal and can be due to diverse causes which we will analyze in this chapter.

2 Anatomy

The sesamoids begin their development in the fetus during the third month. Ossification begins at age 8 in women and 12 in men, starting with the lateral and then the medial sesamoid. There is up to 30% of the population in which the sesamoids will not complete the ossification process, giving rise to bipartite or multipartite sesamoids. This is more frequent to see in the medial sesamoid (10%) than in the lateral one, appearing bilaterally in 25% [1, 2].

The joint of the first metatarsal, in relation to the sesamoids, is compared with the patellofemoral joint. The crista divides the trochlear plantar surface from the

F. Pacheco Martinez · E. Fuentes Morales (✉)
Instituto de Seguridad del Trabajo Viña del Mar, Clínica Ciudad del Mar, Viña del Mar, Chile

© The Author(s), under exclusive license to Springer Nature   427
Switzerland AG 2022
E. Wagner Hitschfeld, P. Wagner Hitschfeld (eds.), *Foot and Ankle Disorders*,
https://doi.org/10.1007/978-3-030-95738-4_19

metatarsal head. The medial and lateral sesamoids articulate their dorsal surface covered in hyaline cartilage with the corresponding facet of the metatarsal head [2].

The sesamoids are stabilized by the intersesamoid ligament, which runs between the medial and lateral collateral ligaments, plus two accessory ligaments of the metatarsal head, called the medial and lateral metatarsal-sesamoid ligaments. However, in 13% of cases, the sesamoid can be located at the interphalangeal joint, contained within the flexor hallucis longus tendon.

The sesamoid complex is a resistant capsuloligamentous structure, in which the medial and lateral sesamoids are incorporated into the plantar plate and are joined proximally to the proximal phalanx by the medial and lateral insertion of the heads of the flexor hallucis brevis. In general, the medial sesamoid is slightly more distal than the lateral one. The latter has connections with the transverse and oblique component of the long hallux adductor, in addition to the intermetatarsal ligament which is attached to the neck of the second metatarsal and the lateral sesamoid ligament. The medial sesamoid has the insertion of the long hallux adductor and the medial sesamoid ligament (Fig. 1).

The shape of the sesamoids is variable. The medial sesamoid is longer, ovoid, and elongated compared to the lateral sesamoid which is smaller. The average size of the medial sesamoid is 13.4 mm in length and 10 mm in width, while the side measures 9 mm by 8 mm. Within the variations in size present, the medial sesamoid is longer than the lateral by 80%, similar by 15% and smaller by 5% [1].

Fig. 1 Plantar vision of the hallux anatomy. (1a) Adductor hallucis brevis: transverse belly. (1b) Adductor hallucis brevis: oblique belly. (2a) Flexor hallucis brevis: lateral belly. (2b) Flexor hallucis brevis: medial belly. (3) Intersesamoid ligament. (4) Medial sesamoid. (5) Sesamoid lateral. (6) Medial metatarsal-sesamoid ligament. (7) lateral metatarsal-sesamoid ligament. (8) Medial phalangeal-sesamoid ligament. (9) Lateral phalangeal-sesamoid ligament. (10) Flexor hallucis longus tendon

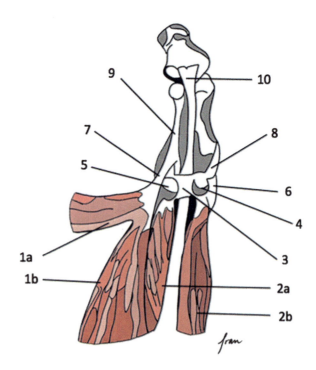

3 Circulation

The irrigation of the sesamoids is complex, and it has been seen that this is mainly extraosseous [3].

The extraosseous circulation of the sesamoids has been evaluated by several authors. Pretterklieber et al., in an arteriographic study on 29 corpses, divided the patterns into three types. The most common anatomical distribution was a branch of both the medial plantar artery and the plantar arch and was present in 52% of the specimens. 24% had an isolated branch of the plantar arch, and a similar percentage had an isolated branch of the medial plantar artery [4]. Sobel et al. found that extraosseous circulation was provided by two major vessels (proximal and plantar) and one minor vessel (distal). The proximal pole was irrigated by a branch of the first plantar metatarsal artery that entered through the insertion of the flexor hallucis brevis and irrigated the proximal 50–60% of the sesamoid [5]. The plantar vessels irrigate the distal aspect and to a lesser extent the circulation at the capsular level. This acquires importance in the presentation of pathologies like the osteonecrosis and the nonunion. The only intraosseous contribution is from proximal to dorsal. In conclusion, the main source of irrigation of the sesamoids is the plantar vessels; therefore, in case of surgical resection, these can be approached at intra or extra-articular level through medial and lateral incisions of the capsule, which seems to be a safe avascular zone, reason why the knowledge of the bony irrigation is of vital importance to avoid damaging it during the plantar approaches.

4 Biomechanics

It is speculated that the biomechanical function of sesamoids is as follows:

1. Mechanical protection for the flexor hallucis longus tendon, which moves in the intersesamoid space
2. As a pulley that promotes plantar flexion in an intrinsic way, increasing the lever arm of the intrinsic muscles of the foot
3. To dissipate forces from the metatarsal head by elevating it

The metatarsal-sesamoid complex transmits 50% of the body weight and can increase up to 300% in the take-off phase of the gait [1].

Cadaveric studies of the biomechanical effect of sesamoidectomy have reported the importance of the hallucis longus flexor as the main hallux metatarsophalangeal flexor. Aper et al. showed a significant reduction in the tendon lever arm when resecting the medial or lateral sesamoid or both [6].

Normally, there is 60–80° of dorsiflexion in this joint. The hallux supports more than two times the load of the lesser toes, which is equivalent to 40–50% of the body weight. At full extension, the sliding action gives way to compression on the dorsal surface of this joint. The stability of the joint is greater in the plantar aspect, as well as in the medial and lateral sides.

The plantar support comes from the plantar plate reinforced by the medial and lateral sesamoids and the collateral ligaments.

5   Etiology-Pathology

The pathology of the sesamoids covers 9% of ankle and foot injuries. Within the etiologies, we find stress fractures (40%), acute fractures (10%), synovitis, chondromalacia, sesamoiditis (30%), arthritis (5%), and bursitis (5%) among others. Although sesamoiditis can be seen as a separate entity from the rest of the pathologies mentioned, the definition in the literature is ambiguous and can lead to encompassing up to 50% of the sesamoid conditions depending on the classification used [1, 2].

If we base ourselves on the definition of "sesamoiditis" as any pain in the sesamoids under the head of the first metatarsal, we can differentiate this pathology according to the following division: capsuloligamentous (turf toe), soft tissues (synovitis, tenosynovitis, bursitis, nerve compression), acute fractures, stress injuries (chondromalacia, osteochondritis, osteonecrosis, stress fracture), anatomical alteration (asymmetry in size, rotational misalignment, condylar malformation), and infections (cellulitis, osteomyelitis).

6   Clinical Presentation

The sesamoid region experiences multiple forces during jumps or runs, which in situations of excess or repetitive stress can result in an inflammation of one or both sesamoids. This repetitive trauma may be secondary to increased activity, problems with footwear, or anatomical variations that generate stress under the head of the first metatarsal, such as pes cavus, hindfoot varus, or equinus. Sesamoiditis can also occur due to other conditions such as infection, inflammatory pathology, and arthrosis in the absence of repeated trauma [7].

In general, there is no history of direct trauma. An insidious onset of weeks is frequently described, with gradual progression of pain, focused edema, and discomfort to mobility, mainly to dorsiflexion. Athletes often report increased symptoms when running, jumping, or facing changes in direction. Walking on the side edge of the foot can minimize your discomfort. Claw deformity following a traumatic event may raise the suspicion of a plantar plate injury.

The physical examination begins by looking for increased focal volume in the plantar aspect of the foot. On palpation, the patient may report tenderness in relation to the involved sesamoid. In cases where there is a pes cavus associated with a first metatarsal in flexion, it may show an inflamed bursa under the head of the metatarsal.

Dermatological causes of plantar pain may be related to a painful plantar keratoma, also called untreatable plantar keratosis. Part of the physical examination includes passive and active assessment of the range of motion of the first metatarsophalangeal joint. The patient may refer increased pain to dorsiflexion in cases of sesamoid stress fractures. Secondary to chronic repetitive trauma and medial incisions secondary to hallux valgus surgical procedures, the medial plantar nerve may be compromised. We can find the positive Tinel sign just above the medial sesamoid or lateral to the fibular sesamoid.

We must differentiate tenosynovitis of the flexor hallucis longus (FHL) from sesamoid pathology. Pain at plantar flexion against resistance of the hallux interphalangeal joint leads to tendon pathology.

It is important to document the alignment of the hallux, mainly after some episode of trauma or excision of one or both sesamoids. There may be some change in alignment secondary to a muscle imbalance.

Upon examination, the position of the sesamoid can be deduced from the degree of hallux pronation. We should examine the degree of contracture of the lateral structures (adductor, lateral sesamoid ligament, and lateral capsular) and examine the range of motion in dorsiflexion and plantar flexion with the corrected position of the hallux.

Allen et al. in 2001 published a clinical test that allows isolating the dynamic components associated to the sesamoids by means of the passive axial compression maneuver (PAC test) (Fig. 2). With the patient in supine position with the leg extended, the sesamoids are located by manual palpation. Then the hallux is brought into dorsiflexion, and compression is generated just proximal to the sesamoid area. Finally, the hallux is positioned in passive plantar flexion maintaining the compression, which generates pain associated with the bony compression of the sesamoids against the base of the phalanx or head of the metatarsal, while the surrounding structures are in relaxation [8].

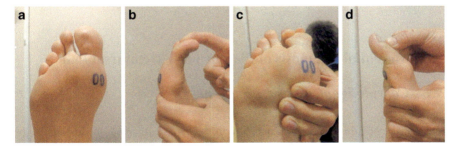

Fig. 2 Passive axial compression test. (**a**) The sesamoids are under the head of the first metatarsal. (**b**) The maximum dorsiflexion of the hallux generates distal migration of the sesamoids. (**c**) Generating compression proximal to the sesamoids stabilizes them in their more distal position. (**d**) The test is positive if passive plantar flexion generates pain

7   Imaging

Within the imaging study, we must evaluate the patient with bilateral feet weight bearing radiographs, both in the anteroposterior, lateral, and oblique planes. For a more specific evaluation of the sesamoids, we request an axial projection of the sesamoids visualizing the joint, in addition to the lateral and medial oblique projection at 40°, specific for each sesamoid separately. The axial projection of the sesamoids allows us to identify the adequate congruence of these in relation to the head of the first metatarsal, besides evidencing possible degenerative compromises of the metatarsal-sesamoid joint. However, the initial X-rays in the confrontation of sesamoiditis can be negative in up to 85% of the cases [9]. In case further imaging is required, bone scintigraphy has been classically used as a support in the diagnosis of sesamoiditis. The use of computed axial tomography (CT) allows us to better evaluate the morphology of the sesamoid bone and joint complex, while MRI guides us to the soft tissue pathology associated with the complex, in addition to evidencing bone edema as a secondary inflammatory sign. Capsuloligamentous lesions, such as turf toe, are identifiable in sagittal sections, where we can visualize the presence of discontinuity of the plantar plate or changes in the signal, both in its union with the sesamoids and in the base of the proximal phalanx. MRI also helps to differentiate between bipartite sesamoids and nonunion [10]. Currently, the use of SPECT-CT has acquired relevance in the differential diagnosis.

8   Diagnosis

The differential diagnosis of sesamoiditis is primarily clinical, identifying the area of pain under the head of the first metatarsal. However, the specification based on the etiology is necessarily associated with the imaging that provides the visualization and differentiation of the great variety of structures present in the same region [3, 11, 12].

9   Differential Diagnosis of Plantar First Metatarsal Pain

9.1   Capsuloligamentous Lesion (Turf Toe)

There must be a high index of suspicion in the capsuloligamentous lesions of the first metatarsophalangeal (MTP) joint, and we can see from a slight sprain to a complete lesion of these structures. The patient can present ecchymosis, increase in volume, and pain during loading, mainly in the take-off phase. We must palpate the collateral ligaments and the dorsal capsular area in search of pain and instability. In general, the referred pain proximal to the sesamoids suggests a low-intensity lesion, while the located distal to these can orient to a greater severity and instability [11]. Based on the extent of the involvement, Clanton in 1994 described a classification later modified by Anderson, which divides this injury into three degrees. Grade I corresponds to damage to the joint capsule without loss of continuity, without alteration of the range of motion or pain on walking. X-rays are negative for the lesion, and magnetic resonance imaging (MRI) shows soft tissue edema. Grade II shows a partial rupture of the plantar and capsular plate, associated with edema and ecchymosis. The patient presents difficulty in walking and pain when moving the hallux, and while the X-ray does not suggest injury, the MRI shows soft tissue edema and alteration of the signal in the plantar plate that does not involve the whole of it. Finally, a grade III lesion corresponds to a complete rupture of the plantar plate and capsule, with secondary findings, such as sesamoid fracture (Table 1).

9.2 Acute or Stress Fracture

The history of an acute pain episode secondary to trauma should raise suspicions of acute injury. We can differentiate it from a bipartite sesamoid by the characteristics of the feature, and at the imaging level, we can support it with scans or MRIs. The sesamoid frequently involved in fractures is the tibial, with a usually transverse trait [12].

In the case of stress fractures, this diagnosis can be suspected according to the patient's history, as a result of an alteration in his or her usual training. The pain and inflammation are related to the activity, and the X-rays are usually negative for the injury, so the MRI study is very useful [9].

Table 1 Turf toe grade description

Hyperextension (turf toe)
I. Stretching of the plantar capsular ligamentous complex. Localized tenderness, minimal swelling, and ecchymosis
II. Partial tear of plantar capsular ligamentous complex. Diffuse tenderness, moderate swelling, and ecchymosis. Restricted movement with pain
III. Frank tear of plantar capsular ligamentous complex
Severe tenderness, marked swelling, and ecchymosis. Limited movement with pain, and vertical Lachman's test.
Possible associated injuries: medial/lateral injury. Sesamoid fracture or bipartite diastasis. Articular cartilage/subchondral bone bruise

Classification system of capsuloligamentous lesions by hyperextension (turf toe) of the first phalangeal metatarsal joint. (Anderson RB)

9.3 Infection

Infection is a rare diagnosis in this area. A puncture wound that results in a direct doorway or a major skin injury could result in sesamoid involvement.

9.4 Metatarsal-Sesamoid Arthritis

It can be seen associated with hallux rigidus or the isolated metatarsal-sesamoid zone. It can be secondary to trauma or chondromalacia.

9.5 Intractable Plantar Keratosis (IPK)

This pathology is generated under the head of the metatarsal. This is related to repetitive abrasion in a load zone. It is important to differentiate a IPK from a plantar wart. The X-ray imaging study allows the detection of bone that explains the increase in pressure under a certain area.

9.6 Bursitis

The intermetatarsal or adventitious bursa may be affected. Imaging can be performed as MRI for diagnostic support and location of origin.

9.7 Nerve Compression

The digital medial and lateral plantar nerves run in relation to the sesamoids, and their irritation or compression can cause neurological symptoms.

10 Treatment

In general, the treatment of all plantar MTP and sesamoid disorders begin with general measures, which consist of unloading the first metatarso-phalangeal joint, relative joint immobilization with rocker-soled shoes or insoles with carbon fiber extension at the MTP, MTP taping, orthosis with or without first metatarsal head unloading, modifications of the patient's physical activity, anti-inflammatory measures, and decreasing load at the first MTP (avoid use of high heel shoes).

Once conservative treatment fails, surgical treatment should be considered, which will vary depending on each specific pathology. The techniques have changed over the years. In the first place, any underlying cause should be looked for, like shortening of the gastrocnemius-soleus complex or the plantar inclination of the first metatarsal that can be observed in the patients with cavo-varus feet.

Among the surgical alternatives to be considered are percutaneous fixation (in case of acute fractures) and partial or total medial or lateral sesamoidectomy. Sesamoidectomy should be considered in those cases in which there are no alterations in the alignment of the first metatarso-phalangeal joint [13].

10.1 Capsular Ligament Injuries: Turf Toe

10.1.1 Conservative Treatment

The treatment of capsuloligamentous lesions will depend on the degree of involvement of the lesions. In all of them the first line of the treatment consists of rest, local cold, elevation, and anti-inflammatory for a limited time. The conservative handling is usually sufficient for those injuries of low degree.

A gradual return to sports activity is recommended after 2–6 weeks, until dorsiflexion between 50° and 60° of the metatarsophalangeal joint of the hallux can be achieved and free of pain [12].

In moderate injuries, it is recommended that the first metatarsophalangeal joint be immobilized in plantar flexion in order to allow healing of the plantar structures (Fig. 3). Insoles do help with gradual sports return (Fig. 4). Joint infiltration with corticosteroids is not recommended since they can mask other types of injuries.

Fig. 3 Hallux phalangeal metatarsal plantar flexion immobilization systems with bandage and plaster (**a**) or functional taping (**b**)

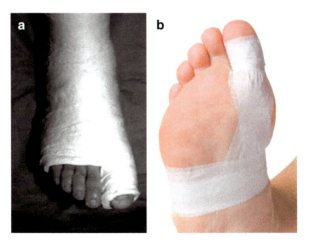

Fig. 4 Orthosis with carbon fiber extension to decrease the mobility of the hallux MTP

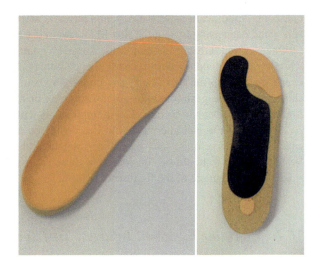

10.1.2 Surgical Treatment

In grade III injuries, with complete rupture of the capsuloligamentous apparatus, surgical treatment is recommended, with direct repair of the compromised structures, which reports good results in the literature [2, 12].

Indications for surgical treatment:

1. Large capsular avulsions with joint instability
2. Sesamoid or bipartite sesamoid fracture with diastasis or retraction
3. Vertical instability at physical examination (mini Lachman test)
4. Post-traumatic hallux valgus
5. Intra-articular free body articular cartilage injuries
6. Failure of conservative treatment

10.1.3 Types of Approach

The approach that is generally used in the surgical management of these lesions is the medial one, which can be angulated at 90° in the metatarsophalangeal fold, to increase exposure and subsequently carry out the direct repair intrasubstance with the use of anchors if there is tearing of the base of the proximal phalanx (Fig. 6).

10.1.4 Postoperative Handling

Immobilization in a plaster cast that maintains the plantar flexion of the hallux MTP between 10° and 20° or a short orthopedic boot is recommended. Start of mobilization a week after surgery to avoid arthrofibrosis, avoiding passive dorsiflexion and plantar flexion against resistance so as not to damage the repair. Maintain the discharge of the operated foot for 4 weeks in an orthopedic boot. Start the load progressively from 4 weeks with a boot, which should be discontinued at 8 weeks, and then using a rigid-soled shoe with a rigid forefoot insole in order to limit the dorsiflexion of the hallux MTP (Fig. 4).

Start kinesiotherapy to recover the joint range of hallux MTP from 8 weeks, waiting for the return to sports activity from 12 to 16 weeks.

Patient expectations should be tempered in the sense that full recovery can take up to a year and that residual pain and joint stiffness are common.

10.2 Acute and Stress Fracture of the Sesamoids

While displaced fractures suggest a break in the plantar plate and sesamoid complex requiring surgical repair, in most cases, the abundant soft tissue connections keep the fragments in relative apposition. In non-displaced or minimally displaced fractures, conservative treatment is the first line of treatment. The typical protocol involves 4–6 weeks of rigid immobilization with the hallux in plantar flexion with an additional period of protected loading and gradual return to normal activity.

It should be taken into consideration that non-displaced sesamoid fractures are difficult to differentiate from bipartite sesamoids in the radiographic study, as we have already mentioned in this chapter.

Open surgery with meticulous reconstruction of the flexor hallucis brevis tendon is mandatory to achieve good results. An alternative to open surgery is percutaneous fixation with a cannulated screw, which is placed in a retrograde fashion. Pagenstert G. and Hintermann B. [14] performed percutaneous screw fixation on eight athletes, all patients returned to their pre-injury level of sports and occupational activity within 12 weeks after surgery (Fig. 5).

Sesamoidectomy has been described in cases of persistent pain after conservative management, particularly in complex fracture patterns, comminuted fractures, failure to use bone grafting, degenerative joint disease, or avascular necrosis [12].

The risks of this procedure include the development of hallux valgus following medial sesamoid resection and hallux varus following fibular resection, claw deformity secondary to hallucis brevis flexor involvement, transfer metatarsalgia, and problems with operative wound or nerve injury. In order to avoid future deformities, sesamoid resection should be performed as localized as possible ("shelling out"), repairing the defect created including the involvement of the plantar plate and the intersesamoid ligament.

Regarding the development of hallux valgus or varus after medial or lateral sesamoidectomy, respectively (10–20% of cases), Kane et al. [15], in a study of 46 patients, observed that those with lateral sesamoid fracture had low MTP and intermetatarsal angles, which tend to decrease after fibular sesamoidectomy. Patients with medial sesamoid fractures, on the other hand, had higher than normal MTP and intermetatarsal angles preoperatively and both increased post-resection. In both cases this situation did not determine that the measurements were clinically significant.

Fig. 5 Percutaneous fixation with cannulated screw described by Pagenstert G. and Hintermann B. Use of anchors for fixation in the hallux F1

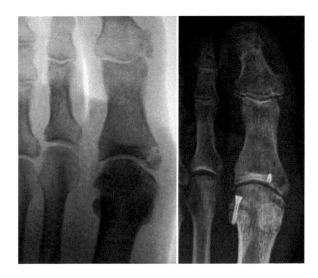

10.3 Avascular Necrosis and Bone Edema (Proper Sesamoiditis)

For patients with avascular necrosis (AVN) as well as sesamoiditis with bone edema who do not respond to conservative treatment, resolution of the disease is less likely to be achieved with correction of the underlying anatomical causes, and sesamoidectomy (partial or total) may be indicated with or without further correction of the malalignment or anatomical abnormalities.

Medial sesamoidectomy should be partial in cases of involvement of only part of the sesamoid or in cases of mild sesamoiditis. In these cases, the plantar shaving of the medial sesamoid can be considered, preferably using a direct approach. In this case, there is a low risk of MTP valgus deformity, but, if symptoms persist, a risk of a secondary surgery to perform a total sesamoidectomy exists.

In relation to total sesamoidectomy, there is consensus in the literature on the use of the medial approach, with which most orthopedic surgeons are very familiar. To perform fibular sesamoidectomy, which is a rare procedure, there are some authors in favor of dorsal [16], lateral plantar [16, 17], or medial plantar [18] (Figs. 6 and 7).

10.4 Infections

If the course of osteomyelitis of the sesamoids is proven, the indicated treatment is resection of the affected sesamoid. In neuropathic patients, with the presence of a plantar ulcer, exposure to perform sesamoidectomy can be extended. Once the resection and surgical cleaning of the area have been carried out with the corresponding taking of cultures for the diagnosis of certainty, the repair of any tendon

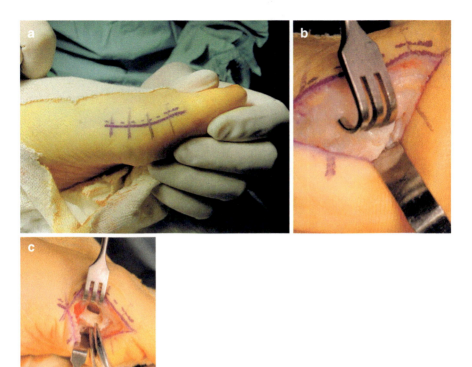

Fig. 6 The image shows the medial approach for performing tibial sesamoidectomy. (**a**) Demarcation of the medial approach to MTP from dorsal hallux to plantar skin. (**b**) Longitudinal capsulotomy and release of the tibial sesamoid. (**c**) Extraction of the sesamoid

damage present is carried out in order to avoid subsequent deformities. The removal of both sesamoids can cause the descent of the metatarsal head which alters the position of the center of rotation of the head and can lead to the development of a cock-up or intrinsic minus of the hallux [19].

10.5   Metatarso-Sesamoid Arthritis

In cases of hallux valgus-associated sesamoid subluxation showing signs of joint degeneration of the metatarso-sesamoid joint, the realignment of the head of the first metatarsal over the sesamoid apparatus in both the frontal and coronal planes must be taken into account (treated in Hallux Valgus chapter). In case there is evident arthritis causing the patient's symptoms, sesamoidectomy is the treatment of choice.

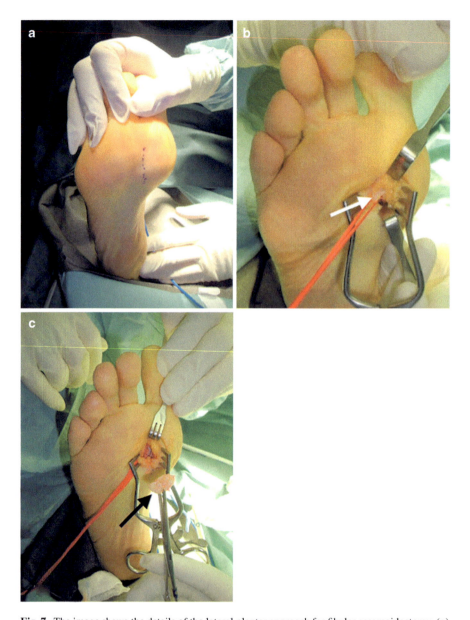

Fig. 7 The image shows the details of the lateral plantar approach for fibular sesamoidectomy. (**a**) Longitudinal incision in relation to the lateral edge of the first metatarsal fat pad. (**b**) Identification and isolation of the plantar digital branch (white arrow). (**c**) Resection of the fibular sesamoid (black arrow)

10.6   Intractable Plantar Keratosis (IPK)

Alternatives to conservative treatment include resection of the skin lesion, followed by the use of insoles to avoid areas of overload, and also avoiding the use of high-heeled shoes. For older patients with plantar fat atrophy, the use of total contact insoles should also be considered.

In cases that do not respond to conservative treatment and in the absence of plantar flexion of the first metatarsal, surgical alternatives such as sesamoid plantar shaving of 30–50% can be considered [20]. In patients diagnosed with cavus foot who present plantar flexion of the first metatarsal, elongation of the Achilles tendon (Strayer or Hoke) should be considered and/or a first metatarsal elevation osteotomy (oblique dorsal wedge resection) should be performed. This elevation osteotomy with a dorsal wedge resection is performed at the base of the first metatarsal from distal-dorsal to proximal-plantar, as appropriate [19].

11   Complications of Surgical Procedures

11.1   Turf Toe Surgery

Joint stiffness with loss of passive dorsiflexion, this can lead to joint compression, chondrolysis, and osteoarthritis.

11.2   Medial Sesamoidectomy

Injury to the medial sensory branch and the common digital nerve during the approach.

Injury of the medial tendon of the flexor hallucis brevis during sesamoid resection. Valgus and cock-up deformities are deformities associated with medial sesamoid resection, which can be avoided by reconstructing the medial soft tissues and adequately balancing the intraoperative hallux MTP. Another complication associated with the resection of the tibial sesamoid is the decrease in plantar strength of hallux MTP due to the decrease of the lever arm.

11.3   Fibular Sesamoidectomy

Injury to the lateral plantar digital branch of the hallux during the approach, painful plantar scar. Other complications include varus deformity of hallux MTP and loss of take-off force during the third rocker of the gait cycle.

11.4   Sesamoid Fracture

Complications of surgical treatment of fractures include osteoarthritis of the sesamoid metatarsal joint, avascular necrosis, and joint irritation from malposition of the fixation screw.

References

1. Atiya S. Sesamoiditis of the metatarsophalangeal joint. OA Orthopaed. 2013;1(2):19.
2. Srinivasan R. The Hallucal-Sesamoid complex: normal anatomy, imaging, and pathology. Semin Musculoskelet Radiol. 2016;20:224–32.
3. Cohen B. Hallux sesamoid disorders. Foot Ankle Clin N Am. 2009;14:91–104.
4. Pretterkleiber ML, Wanivenhaus A. The arterial supply of the sesamoid bones of the hallux. Foot Ankle. 1992;13(1):27–31.
5. Sobel M, Hashimoto J, Arnoczky SP, et al. The microvasculature of the sesamoid complex. Foot Ankle. 1992;13(6):359–63.
6. Aper RL, Saltzman CL, Brown TD. The effect of hallux sesamoid excision on the flexor hallucis longus moment arm. Clin Orthop Relat Res. 1996;325:209–17.
7. Sims A. Painful sesamoid of the great toe. World J Orthop. 2014;5(2):146–50.
8. Allen M. The passive axial compression (PAC) test: a new adjunctive provocative maneuver for the clinical diagnosis of hallucal sesamoiditis. Foot Ankle Int. 2001;22(4):345–6.
9. Greaser M. Foot and ankle stress fractures in athletes. Orthop Clin N Am. 2016;47(4):809–22.
10. Boric I. Hallux Sesamoiditis - radiological diagnostics and conservative management. RAD 540. Med Sci. 2019;48–49:27–32.
11. Clough T. Turf toe injury – current concepts and an updated review of literature. Foot Ankle Clin N Am. 2018;23(4):693–701.
12. York P. Injuries to the great toe. Curr Rev Musculoskelet Med. 2017; https://doi.org/10.1007/s12178-017-9390-y.
13. Boike A, Schnirring-Judge M, McMillin S. Sesamoid disorders of the first metatarsophalangeal joint. Clin Podiatr Med Surg. 2011;28(2):269–85.
14. Pagenstert G, Hintermann. Percutaneous fixation of hallux sesamoid fractures. Tech Foot Ankle Surg. 2008;7(2):107–14.
15. Kane J. Radiographic results and return to activity after sesamoidectomy for fracture. Foot Ankle Int. 2017;38(10);1100–106.
16. Kurian J. Dorsolateral excision of the fibular sesamoid: technique and results. Tech Foot Ankle. 2014;13:226–35.
17. Efficacy FS. Outcomes, and alignment following isolated fibular sesamoidectomy via a plantar approach. Foot Ankle Int. 2019;40(12):1375–81.
18. Harris T. Medial approach to lateral sesamoid removal and presentation of case series. Tech Foot Ankle Surg. 2018; https://doi.org/10.1097/BTF.0000000000000193.
19. Myerson MS. Foot and ankles disorders, vol. 1. Philadelphia: Saunders; 2000.
20. Loretta B. Chou. Orthopaedic knowledge update: foot and ankle, Disorders of Hallucal Sesamoids. Saul G. Trivino: Intractable Plantar Keratoma (Partial Medial Sesamoidectomy), 2018;1:393.

Metatarsalgia

Pilar Martinez de Albornoz and Manuel Monteagudo

1 Introduction

Metatarsalgia is defined as a symptom of excess pressure in the plantar region of the forefoot that causes pain and inflammation. The most frequent cause is due to mechanical alterations, while rheumatic diseases are becoming less prevalent thanks to new pharmacological therapies. In metatarsalgia there will always be an inflammatory process, but the recognition of the mechanical factor that causes it will be the key to understanding, diagnosing, and treating it correctly. There are feet with a greater susceptibility to develop metatarsalgia. The anatomical and functional factors of the leg and foot during the gait cycle can cause a patient to develop metatarsalgia. Even if a foot has a mechanically nonideal metatarsal formula (index plus minus is associated with a lower risk of developing metatarsalgia), we cannot consider it pathological as long as it is not painful.

A forefoot with a "pathological" structure can remain painless for years thanks to the biological mechanisms of adaptation and load transfer, until one day when the compensation mechanisms fail and pain appear. The "reading" of the sole of the foot allows us to identify keratoses that "speak" of their mechanical origin during the walking cycle. The visual analysis of the gait, the exploration of the Achilles-calcaneal-plantar system, the identification of the keratoses, the location of the pain within the forefoot, and the interpretation of weight-bearing X-rays of both feet allow us to know what type of metatarsalgia the patient has and to be able to indicate the most appropriate conservative and surgical treatment.

In this chapter we will give some guidelines to the reader to identify the main mechanical alterations present in the different types of metatarsalgia, and we will

P. Martinez de Albornoz (✉) · M. Monteagudo
Quironsalud University Hospital Madrid, Madrid, Spain

E. Wagner Hitschfeld, P. Wagner Hitschfeld (eds.), *Foot and Ankle Disorders*,
https://doi.org/10.1007/978-3-030-95738-4_20

443

study their consequences on the structures and tissues of the foot. We intend to establish a clear link between clinical and radiological findings with the diagnosis and the most appropriate treatment for each type of metatarsalgia.

2 Mechanics: Defining "Normal" and "Abnormal"

Not all metatarsals are the same. We can develop metatarsalgia because we walk, and if we don't understand how we walk, we can't understand how we hurt ourselves. There are several ways to explain the movement of the human body, and the theory of the walking cycle and the mechanism of the three rockers described by Perry [1], from our point of view, is the one that best explains the correlation between the visual analysis of walking that we can do in consultation and the mechanism of generation of metatarsalgia. The nature of gait provides humans a perfect mechanism to simultaneously achieve a continuous progression in movement as well as a stable support.

The gait cycle is divided into three rockers or phases:

1. During the initial support phase, the initial contact of the foot is made at the heel, over which the tibia rotates forward until the forefoot contacts the ground (first rocker or heel rocker).
2. Once the foot is planted on the ground, the tibia rotates on the talus (second rocker or ankle rocker); the supporting limb must be functionally longer to allow the contralateral limb to perform the gait clearance.
3. When the body's center of mass is anterior to the foot, the tibia rotates on the metatarsophalangeal joints (third rocker or forefoot rocker) while at the same time the foot push-off starts.

Metatarsalgia, as a mechanical disturbance, can develop during any of the three rockers, although most metatarsalgia is generated during the third rocker of the gait.

3 Pathomechanics: How We Get Injured

A foot that has remained without pain for years can become symptomatic at any moment of life. When the structure of the forefoot or the mechanical leg-ankle-foot conditions is not harmonic or ideal, the mechanisms of adaptation and compensation end up failing and producing a mechanical overload in the metatarsal region. Continuous mechanical overload produces tissue and bone stress, and this biological damage can become symptomatic at a given time. Any forefoot tissue can suffer the consequences of abnormal compression, tension, or shear forces that end up injuring it [2]. The tissue will eventually develop signs (stigmas) of this overload that will be visible to the scanner. Following the theory of the three rockers, we will explain the causes of metatarsalgia, its relationship with the gait cycle, its diagnosis, and the solutions to be considered to improve the patient.

1. First rocker: Physiologically, during the first rocker, there is no contact between the forefoot and the ground, so it would not be possible to generate first rocker metatarsalgia. However, there are patients with pathological, neurological, or post-traumatic equinus, who perform their first rocker on the forefoot instead of on the heel.

2. Second rocker: During the second rocker of gait, the foot is plantigrade with respect to the ground. Any mechanical overload on the metatarsal head during the second rocker will increase the vertical and compressive forces to the soft tissues located strictly plantar to the metatarsal head. The mechanical factors that can potentially increase plantar pressure during the second rocker with the foot planted on the ground are (i) a shortening of the gastrocnemius and/or (ii) an excessive plantar tilt of a metatarsal. These factors can act in isolation or sometimes in combination to cause metatarsalgia.

    (i) Shortening of the gastrocnemius: Under ideal mechanical conditions, in the final milliseconds of the second rocker, the knee should achieve full extension and the ankle full dorsiflexion. When a patient has a short gastrocnemius, full dorsiflexion of the ankle cannot be executed with full extension of the knee, and ground reaction forces will act on the metatarsal area causing tissue damage. If the patient develops compensation mechanisms to avoid this unfavorable mechanical situation – bouncy gait or tarsal pronation to reach plantigrade – he or she can avoid metatarsal overload and not develop second rocker metatarsalgia [3].

    (ii) Excessive plantar tilt of a metatarsal (increased metatarsal incidence angle): The anatomical and/or functional tilt of the metatarsals is crucial to ensure adequate load distribution under each metatarsal head in the frontal plane [4]. Excessive anatomical plantar flexion of one or more metatarsals (e.g., in a pes cavus), contiguous elevation of a metatarsal (such as iatrogenic elevation following a fracture or osteotomy), or inadequate adaptation at the Lisfranc joint may lead to the development of second rocker metatarsalgia.

An example that we see in consultation with some frequency of second rocker metatarsalgia is the case of painful keratosis located under the head of the 4th MT. In the exploration of these patients, we found an excessive plantar flexion of the fourth metatarsal, either constitutional or due to a lack of compensation in the sagittal plane in the Lisfranc joint and a Silfverskiöld maneuver that indicates the existence of a gastrocnemius-dependent equinus. The relative length of the metatarsals is not relevant in this phase of the gait, but it will be in the next one.

3. Third rocker: During the third rocker or propulsive phase, the ankle is subjected to progressive flexion, and the longitudinal axis of the foot is placed vertically on the ground. The body weight falls just on the front region of the plantar pad and the structures that receive a greater load are those plantar-distal to the metatarsal

head (plantar plate, fat pad, skin). Keratoses in third rocker metatarsalgia are plantar-distal to the metatarsal head and not strictly plantar as in second rocker. The mechanical factors related to a third rocker scenario would be (i) the hallux: an index minus or a hallux valgus could cause a loss of propulsive power in the first radius generating a load transfer to the lesser metatarsals, and (ii) the relative length of the lesser metatarsals within the metatarsal parabola, with a non-harmonic length causing an overload of certain metatarsal(s).

Although controversial, the metatarsal parabola described by Maestro is a good model for explaining pathology in the third rocker and for treatment planning, provided that the sagittal plane does not present constitutional anomalies. The metatarsal formula that is associated with a smaller number of patients with metatarsalgia is the index plus minus. The first metatarsal is equal to or slightly shorter than the second, and the lesser metatarsals are in a decreasing parabola, all in a dorsal projection weight-bearing feet X-ray [5]. Ideally, and in order for the first radius to be mechanically more competent, the head of the first metatarsal should be centered over the sesamoids.

All metatarsal radiological variants are considered normal as long as the foot is painless and functional. They will be considered pathological when symptoms develop. Nonharmonic metatarsal formulas have a greater tendency to develop third rocker metatarsalgia than harmonic formulas.

Depending on the phase of the gait in which the metatarsalgia is generated, we can consider in a general way (excluding the atypical cases of first rocker) [4]:

(i) Metatarsalgia of 2nd rocker or non-rocker
(ii) Metatarsalgia of 3rd rocker or propulsive

Most of the metatarsals we treat in consultation are third rocker. Tissue stress, in addition to pain, also produces deformities and histological changes such as keratoses, soft tissue inflammation, bone adaptations, and bone stress reactions. The knowledge of why and how metatarsalgias are generated will allow us to diagnose and treat them. Some patients present mixed metatarsalgia, frequent in iatrogenic cases, with signs and stigmas of second and third rocker in the same forefoot, and require combined solutions of second and third rocker in the same forefoot.

4   Diagnosis of Metatarsalgia

As explained in the previous section, the orthopedic surgeon must know how to "read" the sole of the foot, how to detect equinus, and how to "read" a bilateral feet weight bearing X-ray.

4.1 Physical Exploration

Examination ("reading") of the sole of the foot, keratoses, limb alignment, and visual analysis of the gait provide valuable information for understanding the pathomechanics of metatarsalgia. With this information, even before having the X-rays, the doctor must be able to recognize the main alterations and correlate the metatarsalgia with one of the walking rockers. Plantar keratoses are key to suspecting what type of mechanical stress is responsible for the clinical condition of each patient. Increased pressure and/or shear forces are responsible for the development of plantar calluses. The morphology and location of plantar keratoses reflect the contact pattern between the foot and the ground.

The exploration of a metatarsalgia follows the reference of the previously mentioned rockers:

- Second rocker (non-propulsive metatarsalgia): Second rocker keratoses are strictly located plantar to the metatarsal head and can be "drawn" only to the corresponding metatarsal, without tendency to coalesce with neighboring lesions. In the second rocker, the plantar plate is not damaged, and the progressive deformities that can be associated in this phase are the digital claws with subluxation (never complete dislocation) of the metatarsal-phalangeal joints. The elastic component of the gastrocnemius can play an important role in the transition from the second to the third rocker. An equinus will cause an increase in the reaction forces of the soil against the metatarsal region. The "split-second effect" describes this mechanism and its clinical consequences [3]. The Silfverskiöld test evaluates if the retraction of the gastrocnemius is the only mechanism responsible for the equinus (positive test) or if there is some other factor that causes the equinus (negative test: there is not an increase of the dorsiflexion of the ankle with the knee bent and the forefoot supinated to avoid the mediotarsal sagittal movement) [6].

Figure 1 shows sole of the foot with second rocker keratosis.

- Third rocker (propulsive metatarsalgia): During the third rocker, the foot rotates externally on the ground, and this rotation produces a shearing of the plantar fat pad located in a plantar-distal position to the lesser metatarsal heads. Keratoses appear planto-distal to the bone plane. They often fuse with neighboring keratoses, so that a single diffuse, rounded keratosis can appear, making it difficult to recognize the metatarsal(s) involved in the lesion [4].

Figure 2 is sole of the foot with third rocker keratosis.

During this phase, the metatarsal is positioned vertically to the floor, transmitting axial compressive forces on the plantar plate. The chronic overloading of the plantar plate causes its rupture, allowing the base of the phalanx to be completely dislocated dorsally, until the phalanx and metatarsal are placed parallel to each other. In addition, axial forces along the MT bone equally compress the compact/cortical and cancellous bone. Since most of the MT head is made up of cancellous bone and its modulus of elasticity is lower than the cortical bone, a transverse fracture could occur in the MT head itself, deteriorating blood flow and producing secondary

Fig. 1 Foot sole with second rocker keratosis. Patient with second rocker metatarsalgia and circumscribed plantar keratosis under the head of the fourth metatarsal

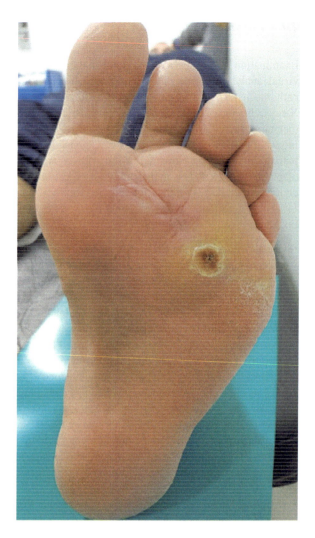

osteonecrosis (Freiberg's disease). This collapse of the metatarsal head sometimes shortens the bone to the point necessary to achieve an ideal metatarsal parabola [7].

Many patients (especially after failed surgery) may present stigmas of both types of mechanical metatarsalgia (mixed metatarsalgia), which makes the analysis and management of these cases difficult. There are some "special" metatarsalgias that we must correlate with the right gait rocker in order to plan the correct treatment.

Metatarsalgia with extensor recruitment (second rocker): When the tibialis anterior does not mechanically assist the foot in the transition from the second to the third rocker, either because of neurological dysfunction or because of a pes cavus, the extensor digitorum longus is recruited to assist in propulsion. The problem is that its activation occurs during the second rocker and is maintained during the third rocker ending up in a claw toe that can be painful by rubbing against the footwear. These claws never end up producing a complete dislocation but rather a subluxation

Fig. 2 Foot sole with third rocker keratosis. Patient with bilateral third rocker metatarsalgia and diffuse plantar keratoses in lesser metatarsals. The keratoses are not limited to a single radius

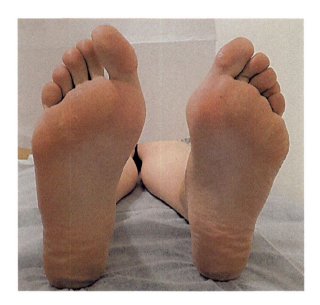

with sliding of the phalanx over the dorsal region of the head of its metatarsal. The metatarsal pain is strictly plantar to the metatarsal head. The surgical treatment consists in a extendor digitorum longus tenotomy and a secondary reinsertion into the lateral cuneiform.

Figure 3 is extensor replacement case.

Metatarsalgia with second intermetatarsal space (third rocker) syndrome: The second space syndrome is a group of signs and symptoms, including divergence of the second and third toes in a weightbearing situation (they may not be divergent non-weightbearing), with third rocker metatarsalgia. Sometimes there are neuritic symptoms similar to those produced by a third space Morton's neuroma [8]. The second space syndrome is accompanied by a third rocker keratosis. The cause is found in a second and third metatarsal that is longer than the first and fourth, thus producing a "pole effect" during the third rocker. The second and third toes diverge in an attempt to gain a greater base of support and strength for propulsion and because of metatarsophalangeal joint synovitis [9]. This is a third rocker metatarsalgia and the shortening of the second and third metatarsals until a harmonic metatarsal parabola is achieved usually cures the metatarsal pain.

Figure 4 shows second space syndrome.

4.2   Radiological Examination: How to Read a Weightbearing X-ray

The radiological study of the patient with metatarsalgia should include comparative anteroposterior and lateral feet weightbearing X-rays. In order to estimate deformities, make measurements, and plan surgical correction, the projections of the loaded

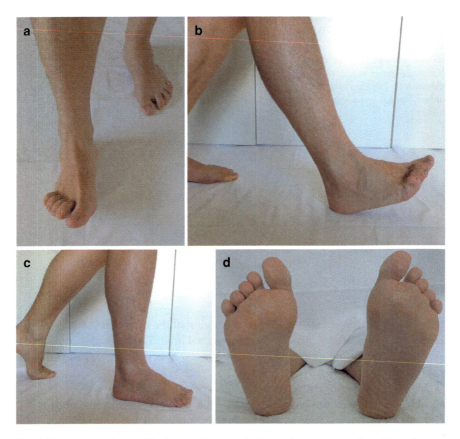

Fig. 3 Extensor recruitment. The images show a typical case of extensor recruitment by a shortening of the medial gastrocnemius. (**a–c**) In the visual examination of the gait cycle, there is an extensor substitution of the lesser toes that results in a flexible claw deformity of the toes. (**d**) In the right foot sole, he presents some mixed painful keratoses under the heads of the 2nd–third metatarsals and in the left foot some mixed keratoses under the head of the second metatarsal

radiographs must be technically accurate. The dorsal-plantar projection must be centered and focused between both feet so that the examination is reproducible and reliable. The second cuneometatarsal joint should be clearly seen (the joint should show an orthogonal projection) [10]. There should be a geometric regression from the first to the fifth metatarsal. In the ideal formula, the length of the first metatarsal should be equal to or slightly shorter than the second metatarsal (index plus minus) [5], and the head of the first metatarsal should cover both sesamoids. Maestro established [5] that the center of the lateral sesamoid and the center of the head of the fourth metatarsal should be at the same level in a dorsal-plantar projection. The lateral projection must be able to show the tibia perpendicular to the floor. Figure 5 shows normal weightbearing feet X-rays.

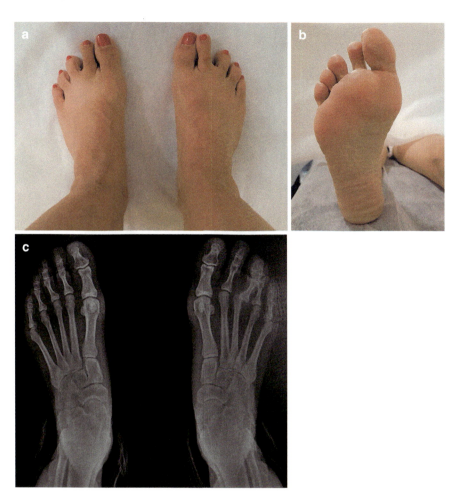

Fig. 4 Second space syndrome. The images show the case of a patient with a "second space" syndrome. (Image **a**) feet in standing position with divergence of second and third toes. (**b**) Image of the diffuse plantar keratosis around the second metatarsal. (**c**) The dorsal-plantar projection of the X-ray of the feet in load shows an index minus formula with an increased relative length of the lesser rays and a complete dislocation of the third metatarsophalangeal joint in the right foot

Second rocker (non-propulsive metatarsalgia): In most second rocker metatarsalgia, the weightbearing radiographs reveal a correct metatarsal parabola in the dorsal-plantar projection, and the problem lies in the sagittal/coronal plane due to increased plantar flexion of the metatarsal head. The surgeon must focus on the lateral projection where the alignment of the first and second metatarsal can be visualized. In an unoperated foot, the dorsal cortex of the diaphysis of both metatarsals should be (ideally) parallel. In this projection it is sometimes possible to identify a metatarsal with a different inclination to the neighbors (in dorsiflexion or

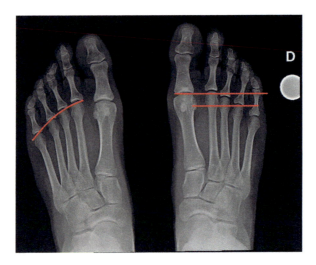

Fig. 5 Bilateral feet weightbearing X-ray and "normal" parameters. Dorsal-plantar foot projection under load. The X-ray is correctly centered and the second cuneometatarsal joint is visualized. This would be a case of "ideal foot": with index plus minus formula, in which there is a similar length of the first and second metatarsals, the head of the first metatarsal covers both sesamoids, there is a geometric regression of all rays and the center of the lateral sesamoid is centered or over the head of the fourth metatarsal

plantar flexion). The axial sesamoid projection (Walter-Müller) can be helpful to estimate the relative position of the metatarsal heads and the arthritic changes of a dysplastic head.

Third rocker (propulsive metatarsalgia): The metatarsal parabola in weightbearing X-rays, in dorsal-plant projection, is relevant in the diagnosis and management of third rocker metatarsalgia. As previously mentioned, the problem may lie in:

(a) The hallux: when the head of the first metatarsal is not centered on both sesamoids (as in a hallux valgus), or the hallux is too short (index minus), there will be a decrease in the efficiency of the mechanical work of the first radius, causing transfer metatarsalgia [11]. This scenario is especially evident when in failed hallux valgus surgery there is a shortening and elevation of the first metatarsal or its head.

(b) The length of the lesser metatarsals: The harmonic parabola with decreasing lengths of the lesser metatarsals described by Maestro correlates well with the diagnosis of third rocker metatarsalgia. In addition, we can use the same projection to measure the relative lengths of the metatarsals and perform correct preoperative planning. The amount (in millimeters) of shortening of the lesser metatarsals and the correction/translation (in millimeters) of the hallux should be calculated on weightbearing radiographs [7].

The physical examination together with weightbearing X-rays provide us with enough information to be able to diagnose and manage 90% of all cases of metatarsalgia. Rarely additional tests are required. Magnetic resonance imaging (MRI) can be helpful in assessing soft tissue, cartilage, and bone damage. MRI is useful for diagnosing and quantifying the involvement in Freiberg's disease, a stress fracture, a ruptured plantar plate, or a soft tissue tumor. Computed tomography (CT) is used for the evaluation of nonunions or malunions, loss of bone stock, subchondral cysts, osteophytes, sclerosis, and alterations in the normal contour of the metatarsal heads. The development of weightbearing CT can be helpful to accurately calculate metatarsal lengths and angles of a metatarsal with respect to its neighbors. It is a great tool in preoperative planning as well [12].

5   Treatment of Metatarsalgia

In any metatarsalgia, conservative treatment should always be attempted before surgery is indicated. Being a mechanical problem, conservative treatment solutions will also be mechanical.

5.1   Conservative

Generally, conservative treatments include pain medication, anti-inflammatory, rehabilitation devices, physical therapy, stretching exercises, insoles, and footwear.

Nonmechanical treatments (other than insoles and footwear) have a very partial and limited effect in time. But there are patients who improve with them. The explanation may be due to the decrease in inflammation and the mechanisms of compensation/transfer of the foot can once again function by entering a period of pain and functional improvement.

Insoles are the cornerstone of treatment for metatarsalgia. Usually, and in order to achieve symptomatic relief, a retrocapital pad/olive is formed (behind the metatarsal heads) and with some medial longitudinal arch support, in EVA (ethylene-vinyl-acetate)-type material [13]. In second rocker metatarsalgia, the point of highest load is located under the metatarsal head, so the templates may incorporate a fenestration (depression) under the affected metatarsal head. In third rocker metatarsalgia, the insoles will focus on improving the function of the hallux and relieving the excess load on the planto-distal region of the metatarsal fat pad. To improve hallux function, it may be helpful to incorporate a kinetic wedge under the head of the first metatarsal to passively increase dorsiflexion of the first metatarsophalangeal joint [14]. To reduce the load on the central metatarsal region, insoles can be fitted with an retrocapital pad. The increased surface area for load distribution should decreae the metatarsal heads pressure and thus relieve metatarsalgia. The retrocapital elevation also relaxes the transverse arch of the metatarsal area and allows for pain relief by decompression of the interdigital spaces [14].

The metatarsal retrocapital bars unload all metatarsal heads. In some studies they have shown greater efficacy than metatarsal retrocapital olives in reducing pain and in forefoot function [15]. Figure 6 shows insoles.

Footwear can also help a patient with metatarsalgia. A wide toe-box can relieve pain in patients with toe deformities like claw toe or Hallux Valgus. Reducing heel height in women's shoes reduces pain in propulsive metatarsalgia. Soft-soled shoes usually relieve any type of metatarsalgia. Today, many brands are incorporating air chambers in the soles or very soft materials such as memory foam, which allow many patients to function with tolerable pain. Rocker-soled shoes improve the transition from the first to the third rocker gait phase and can alleviate metatarsalgia symptoms. Those shoes may help as well in cases with reduced hallux range of motion [16].

It usually takes about 4–6 months for insoles and appropriate footwear to reach their maximum effect. If after that time the patient remains symptomatic and very limited in his or her daily activities, surgery may be indicated.

5.2   Surgical

The goal of metatarsalgia surgery is the achievement of a painless, plantigrade, functional foot.

Second rocker (non-propulsive metatarsalgia): Remembering the pathomechanics, a second rocker metatarsalgia can be due to two factors that can be found isolated or combined – a shortening of the gastrocnemius and an excessive inclination of a metatarsal – and solutions will go through modifying these two scenarios.

Lengthening of the gastrocnemius: With the Silfverskiöld test, we can confirm if the patient with second rocker metatarsalgia has a gastrocnemius-dependent

Fig. 6 Insoles. Test template with retrocapital bar for the treatment of third rocker metatarsalgia. Once its efficacy is confirmed, the lining is completed

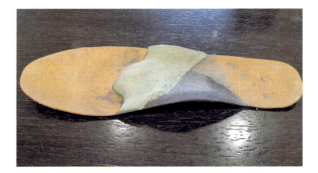

equinus. In these patients, tricep lengthening can be performed at different anatomical levels. The more distal (close to the calcaneus) is the release, more lengthening
is achieved, but also greater is the loss of muscle power in the gastrocnemius.
Numerous techniques – Baumann, Strayer, and Vulpius – have been described to
lengthen the triceps. Our experience indicates that it is not necessary to resort to
distal techniques and that most patients improve when the release of the gastrocnemius is limited to the medial gastrocnemius muscle head and is performed in the
most proximal region (popliteal zone of Silfverskiöld) [6]. Under local anesthesia
and through a small posterior and medial incision in the back of the knee, the surgeon easily accesses the superficial fascia in the popliteal region. After the fascia is
incised, the tendon of the medial gastrocnemius is individualized and cut. At this
level, the risk of excessive triceps surae elongation and neurovascular injury is
extremely low.

Figure 7 shows proximal gastrocnemius lengthening.

Proximal osteotomies: Traditionally, proximal osteotomies of the metatarsals
have been useful tools when it was necessary to elevate a metatarsal in the presence
of 2nd rocker metatarsalgia. A dorsal wedge osteotomy in the proximal metaphysis
of an excessively plantarized lesser metatarsal allowed relief of localized metatarsalgia. The two models of osteotomy that allow the controlled elevation of a metatarsal are the Goldfarb model and the BRT model (Barouk, Rippstein, Toullec) [17].
In the Goldfarb osteotomy, a dorsal closing wedge is performed in a chevron-shape.
Immediate weightbearing with a compliant patient is required to maintain the metatarsal elevation until consolidation. But it was frustrating at times, if the patient was
in pain or afraid to perform loading, that the osteotomy would not lift the operated
metatarsal as much as it should. For this reason, the BRT osteotomy incorporated
synthesis with a screw. The BRT osteotomy is an oblique dorsal closing wedge
osteotomy. But what happens in the Goldfarb osteotomy depends on the patient's
good work, in the BRT depends on the surgeon's good work. And it is very complicated to calculate (and execute) how much wedge to cut in order to raise the necessary amount.

Fig. 7 Proximal medial
gastrocnemius lengthening.
Proximal lengthening in
the popliteal zone of the
medial gastrocnemius:
semi-circumferential
incision of the fibers of the
aponeurosis

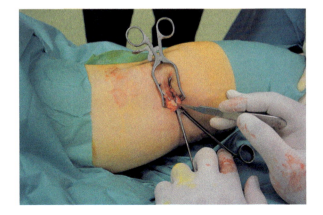

And, again, it was frustrating to perform a BRT and elevate a metatarsal with the clinical improvement of the metatarsalgia and the disappearance of the keratosis to, a few months later, find the same situation in the neighboring metatarsal. The appearance of transfer metatarsalgia is very common after a proximal elevation osteotomy [7].

Distal osteotomies: The highly variable results of proximal osteotomies led to the idea of a more reliable surgical procedure that would better control the elevation of the lesser metatarsal without causing transfer metatarsalgia. The more distal the osteotomy, the greater the control, but the lower the amount of elevation. The Suppan-type osteotomy ("tilt-up" in the Anglo-Saxon literature) [18] consists of an extra-articular cut preserving the cartilage, made in the neck of the metatarsal with extraction of a dorsal wedge that will allow (as in a Freiberg) [19] the restoration of the height of the metatarsal head and the relief of plantar pressure. If the collateral ligaments are maintained, the osteotomy does not require internal fixation and allows for immediate loading with very little discomfort to the patient, which usually makes them compliant with walking in postoperative shoes until the osteotomy is healed. The results are more predictable, and the potential risk of producing transfer metatarsalgia is much lower than with proximal osteotomies.

Figure 8 shows Suppan-type osteotomy.

There is no formula for deciding when to associate both surgeries – gastrocnemius lengthening and osteotomy – in the treatment of second rocker metatarsalgia, but our threshold for performing a gastrocnemius lengthening is low if the patient has a clear Silfverskiöld test or if he or she suffers or has suffered from other equine-related pathologies (non-insertional Achilles tendinopathy, proximal plantar fasciitis). Our most common treatment for second rocker metatarsalgia combines proximal lengthening of the medial gastrocnemius with a distal tilt-up osteotomy of the problem metatarsal without internal fixation.

Third rocker (propulsive metatarsalgia): As previously mentioned, in third rocker metatarsalgia, we can find two factors to be reconstructed in a surgery: a first radius with a deformity (hallux valgus) or dysfunction (hallux limitus or rigidus) and lesser metatarsals with a nonharmonic metatarsal parabola. The existence of an equinus has no role in the generation of third rocker metatarsalgia, so it will not make any sense to perform a gastrocnemius lengthening in these patients.

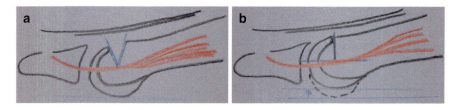

Fig. 8 Suppan-type osteotomy. (**a**) An extra-articular cut is designed, preserving the cartilage, performed on the metatarsal neck with extraction of a dorsal wedge. (**b**) The osteotomy allows elevation and restoration of the height of the metatarsal head and relief of plantar pressure

Hallux valgus treatment will not be treated in this chapter. This section will focus on what type of intervention can be performed to improve the metatarsal formula [5]. The controlled shortening of the lesser metatarsals, can be achieved through shortening osteotomies. It is very important to avoid metatarsal elevation or descent in order to avoid undesired a second rocker iatrogenic metatarsalgia. Although the most popular osteotomy for third rocker metatarsalgia is Weil's cervical-cephalic and its variants, mini-invasive techniques have increased in popularity in recent years.

Cervicocephalic Weil and triple Weil osteotomy: Distal metatarsal osteotomies, such as Weil and triple Weil osteotomies, are designed to produce a controlled shortening and allow the restoration of the ideal metatarsal parabola, with the secondary forefoot load redistribution. Weil described a simple technique to shorten the lesser metatarsals in a controlled manner [17]. In the distal area of the metatarsal, a single cut in the transverse plane allows the proximal sliding of the metatarsal head. The amount of shortening achieved can be calculated by measuring the length of the upper distal end of the proximal fragment. The osteotomy starts around 2 mm distal from the dorsal tip of the metatarsal head, and the inclination of the cut should be made almost parallel to the floor in the second metatarsal and progressively increasing the inclination of the cut as we progress toward the more lateral metatarsals. The surgeon must be familiar with the anatomy of the bone to achieve a proper tilt plane in each metatarsal. When planning shortening osteotomies, the surgeon should evaluate how many metatarsals should be shortened and how much shortening should be achieved in each one. A weightbearing anteroposterior X-ray is required for surgical planning. Barouk described the term "maximum shortening point" to assist in the preoperative planning [17]. This corresponds to the point of greatest deformity of the most affected metatarsal. This point is taken as a reference to calculate the amount of shortening required on that radius. The base of the phalanx is usually the location for the maximum shortening point. This spot is the reference point where the metatarsal should be after shortening it. In many occasions it is necessary to shorten more than one metatarsal. When we achieve a harmonic metatarsal parabola in the dorsal plane, without causing iatrogeny in the sagittal plane, we can be sure that the patient will achieve an improvement in pain and that the result will be very durable. The results of Weil's osteotomy have been well documented. Floating toes and joint stiffness are the most common complications after Weil's osteotomy [20]. These were especially evident in shortenings greater than 3 mm. In large shortenings, the center of rotation of the metatarsal head would be below the center of action of the interosseous muscles that would go from functioning as plantar flexors to functioning as dorsiflexors. To avoid these complications, Maceira [21] popularized the triple cut (triple Weil), achieving that the center of rotation of the metatarsal head would be above the working axis of the interosseous muscles, which would function as plantar flexors (avoiding floating toe). Furthermore, the postoperative bandages with plantar flexor effect during the first 4 weeks facilitate a good soft tissue healing and a better plantar motion of the lesser metatarsophalangeal joints. The bandage provides rotational stability in the transverse plane and helps prevent dorsal and distal displacement of the metatarsal head, which justifies that the Weil osteotomy without fixation can have similar results to the Weil with fixation, although assuming a greater risk of displacement according to the degree of compliance of the patient. Figure 9 shows triple Weil osteotomy.

When there is a degenerative metatarsophalangeal dislocation as a consequence of long-lasting propulsive metatarsalgia, a degenerative rupture of the plantar plate has occurred. In recent years, numerous techniques of reconstruction of the plantar plate have been described in association with Weil's osteotomy [22]. Most studies of plantar plate repair have shown favorable results in terms of patient satisfaction, pain, and AOFAS scores [23]. However, these results should be interpreted with caution because of the inherent limitations of the studies (mostly case series without

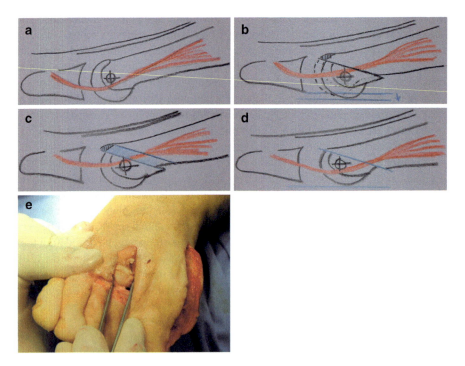

Fig. 9 Triple Weil osteotomy. Weil and triple Weil osteotomy design. (**a**) Diagram of the metatarsal head and interosseous musculature located at the center of rotation. (**b**) Weil's osteotomy with cut in the transverse plane and proximal and plantar sliding of the metatarsal head. The center of rotation remains plantar to the interosseous musculature. (**c**) Subtraction wedge design and double cut parallel to the first one. (**d**) Final result of the triple Weil osteotomy in which the metatarsal head is elevated and the center of rotation is restored. (**e**) Front view of the Weil metatarsal osteotomy ready to be fixed

a control group) and because most of the patients included had undergone several combined procedures (including Weil's osteotomy) that could have skewed the results [22, 23]. The authors are not in favor of the plantar plate repair in degenerative cases because of the most frequent complication of its reconstruction – joint stiffness. This complication is almost always symptomatic. In comparison, the most common Weil osteotomy complication is floating toe, which is rarely symptomatic and easy to repair. The Weil-type osteotomies and their variants are versatile and also allow displacements toward medial or lateral of the metatarsal heads in case of varus or valgus toe deviations. Figure 10 shows pre- and postoperative radiographs of a complete realignment of the forefoot.

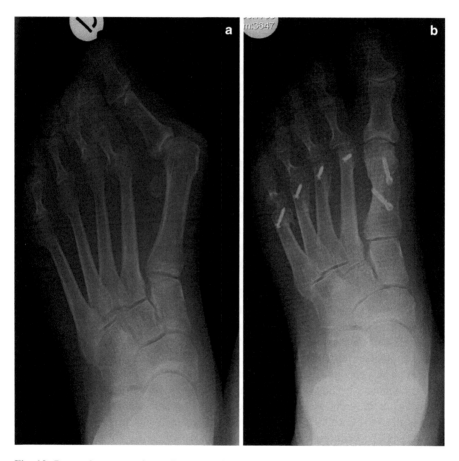

Fig. 10 Pre- and postoperative radiographs of a complete realignment of the forefoot. Surgical management of third rocker metatarsalgia. (Image **a**) Right foot with severe hallux valgus and complete dislocation of the second metatarsal. (Image **b**) Surgical correction of the first metatarsal with the head centered on the sesamoids and shortened to where the base of the proximal phalanx was. Shortening of the second metatarsal to where the base of the proximal phalanx was to reduce the dislocation. Shortening and regularization of the rest of the metatarsal parabola

Mini-invasive metatarsal osteotomies: Any surgical technique, open or mini-mally invasive (MIS), is valid as long as it achieves the final purpose previously indicated, to restore mechanical abnormalities and relieve pain. When a harmonic restoration of the metatarsal parabola is achieved under load, it is indifferent whether the result has been achieved with one or another osteotomy type or with an open or mini-invasive technique. The most popular type of osteotomy within MIS surgery of the forefoot is the distal metatarsal osteotomy ("distal metatarsal metaphyseal osteotomy," DMMO). This is a percutaneous extra-articular osteotomy of the metatarsal neck without any internal fixation. The amount of shortening in MIS osteotomies is influenced by multiple factors including the release of soft tissue and the geometric parameters of the osteotomy itself. Since no fixation is performed, the ground reaction forces together with the immediate shortening forces will determine the final position and orientation of the metatarsal heads. These mini-invasive techniques are usually associated with less joint stiffness, but their results are potentially more variable than open techniques because they depend on the patient's compliance so that the postoperative load is continuous and homogeneous and the osteotomies consolidate without movements in the sagittal plane [24]. Figure 11 shows metatarsal realignment by minimally invasive surgery.

The authors usually perform triple open Weil osteotomies in third rocker metatarsalgias. In the preoperative study, we calculate and draw on the radiography the ideal metatarsal parabola. During the surgery we check with radioscopy the new formula achieved. Once we reach the desired formula, we fix the osteotomies with self-breaking twist-off screws.

Iatrogenic (mixed metatarsalgia): The safer, more reliable, and faster the surgical procedures are, the more we increase the number of surgeries we do. The number of surgical procedures on the forefoot has increased continuously in the last decades, but with it the number of complications and new sequels has also increased. When the surgeon does not correctly identify the type of metatarsalgia, it is easy to end up creating sequelae in the patient. A metatarsal elevation osteotomy (second rocker solution) performed on a third rocker metatarsalgia will only succeed in creating a transfer metatarsalgia on the neighboring metatarsal. A shortening osteotomy (third rocker solution) performed on a patient with second rocker metatarsalgia will only change the location of the keratosis and pain. Many iatrogenic metatarsalgias are mixed and present a nonharmonic parabola in the dorsal and sagittal planes. These mixed patterns are a new challenge for the foot surgeon. These mixed metatarsals often require the combination, in the same operation, of shortening and elevation osteotomies in the same or different metatarsals. The physical examination and weightbearing X-rays allow to plan a "a la carte" treatment. When the joints are destroyed by previous surgical procedures, a frequently performed surgery for rheumatic forefeet is recommended, as it is the first metatarsophalangeal arthrodesis in addition to a lesser metatarsal heads resections (Hoffman procedure). The metatarsal head resection must also follow the formula of a harmonic parabola, with decreasing length from the second to the fifth. Thee neoformation of fibrous joints usually gives a great pain relief and a recovery of the plantar fat pad cushioning. Figure 12 shows iatrogenic metatarsalgia.

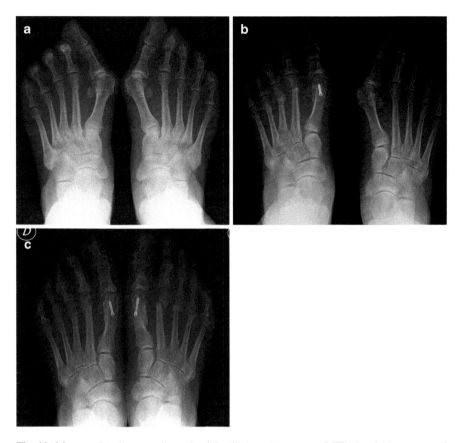

Fig. 11 Metatarsal realignment through minimally invasive surgery (MIS). Surgical treatment of third rocker metatarsalgia using minimally invasive techniques. (Image **a**) Severe bilateral hallux valgus and third rocker metatarsalgia. (Image **b**) Right foot: radiography 3 months after surgery with percutaneous correction of the first radius and percutaneous DMMO osteotomies without fixation of second, third, and fourth rays. (Image **c**) Radiological control 12 months after surgery of the right foot with healed osteotomies. Left foot with similar surgical management

Author's treatment of choice in metatarsalgia:

1. Clinical exploration:

   – Static: Standing
   – Dynamic: Gait cycle

2. Weight-bearing feet X-rays

   1 + 2: Provides 90% of the information needed to diagnose and discern between second or third rocker metatarsalgia

   Second rocker metatarsalgia: proximal medial gastrocnemius release in the popliteal fosa and/or distal tilt-up metatarsal osteotomy

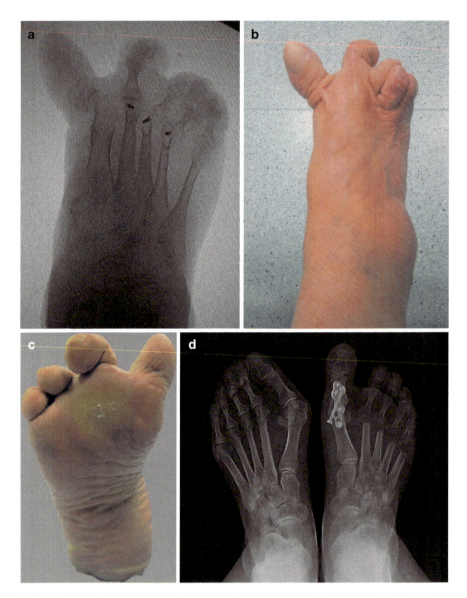

Fig. 12 Iatrogenic metatarsalgia. Case of a patient undergoing MIS surgery of the right foot. Images (**a**–**c**) show the sequelae of severe deformities, mixed metatarsalgia, and non-plantable and non-shoeable foot. Images (**d**, **e**) show surgical rescue using the Hoffmann technique. Figures (**f**, **g**) show the images of the plantigrade, aligned, and painless foot

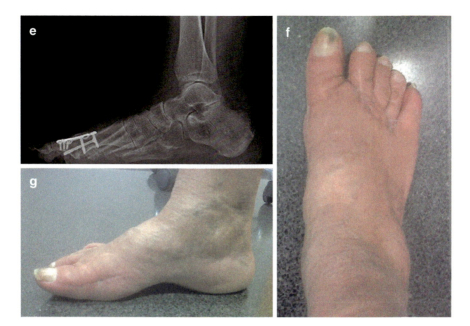

Fig. 12 (continued)

Third rocker metatarsalgia: approximately 90% of total cases of metatarsalgia. Weil's triple osteotomy used to shorten one or more metatarsals to achieve an ideal metatarsal parabola.

The postoperative protocol include bandages that keep toes in plantar flexion for 4 weeks.

6 Conclusions

Metatarsalgia can develop in any of the three walking cycles. Second rocker or non-propulsive metatarsalgia is less frequent than third rocker or propulsive metatarsalgia.

Physical examination, including gait analysis, and weightbearing X-rays will provide 90% of the most frequent metatarsalgia causes. That information will guide the treating surgeon to the most appropiate treatment.

Adequate insoles improve most metatarsalgias. If they fail, surgery is indicated. The surgical objective, regardless of the technique used, is to achieve a harmonic metatarsal parabola. The authors prefer distal elevation osteotomies in second rocker metatarsalgia assessing a proximal gastrocnemius lengthening if necessary and triple Weil osteotomies in third rocker metatarsalgia assessing a hallux correction if necessary.

Table 1 Management of second rocker –non-propulsive- metatarsalgia

Examination features		WB X-ray findings	Surgical options
Keratoses pattern	Isolated keratosis underneath the MT head Keratoses located strictly plantar to the MT head	Stress fracture located at the neck of the MT (Deutschländer fracture)	Goal: elevating the affected MT ray Procedures: Distal MT osteotomy: tilt-up Proximal MT osteotomy
Dislocations	Claw toes	Correct metatarsal formula in the dorsoplantar view	
Walking pattern	Extensor over recruitment		
Silfverskiöld test	Most patients positive (gastrocnemius tightness)		Proximal medial gastrocnemius release

MT metatarsal, *WB* weight-bearing

Table 2 Management of third rocker-propulsive-metatarsalgia

Examination features		WB X-ray findings	Surgical options
Keratoses pattern	Diffuse keratosis that may span several heads Keratosis located planto-distal to the MT head	Stress fracture at the head of the MT (Freiberg disease)	Goal: achieving a harmonic metatarsal formula. Procedure: realignment of the MT parabola
Dislocations	Rupture of the plantar plate MTPJ dislocations	Index minus MT formula Hallux valgus MTPJ dislocations	Correction of the HV Weil osteotomy Triple Weil osteotomy
Walking pattern	Worsen on heels		
Silfverskiöld test	Variable		No need to lengthen gastrocnemius in third rocker metatarsalgia

MT metatarsal, *WB* weight-bearing, *MTPJ* metatarsophalangeal joint, *HV* Hallux valgus

Table 1 explains management of second rocker metatarsalgia.
Table 2 explains management of third rocker metatarsalgia.

References

1. Perry J. Gait analysis: normal and pathological function. Thorofare: Slack; 1992.
2. Espinosa N, Brodsky JW, Maceira E. Metatarsalgia. J Am Acad Orthop Surg. 2010;18:474–85.
3. Amis J. The split second effect: the mechanism of how equinus can damage the human foot and ankle. Front Surg. 2016;27(3):38.

4. Espinosa N, Maceira E, Myerson MS. Current concept review: metatarsalgia. Foot Ankle Int. 2008;29:871–9.
5. Maestro M, Besse JL, Ragusa M, et al. Forefoot morphotype study and planning method for forefoot osteotomy. Foot Ankle Clin. 2003;8:695–710.
6. Barouk LS, Barouk P. Compte-rendu symposium gastrocnémien court. Toulouse Maitrise Orthopédique. 2006;159:21–8.
7. Maceira E, Monteagudo M. Transfer metatarsalgia post hallux valgus surgery. Foot Ankle Clin. 2014;19(2):285–307.
8. Viladot-Pericé A. Patología del antepié. Barcelona: Toray; 1974.
9. Maceira E, Monteagudo M. Mechanical basis of metatarsalgia. Foot Ankle Clin. 2019 Dec;24(4):571–84.
10. Ozonoff MB. Pediatric orthopedic radiology. Saunders; 1979. ISBN:0721670342.
11. David-West KS, Moir JS. Radiological assessment of tibial sesamoid position after scarf osteotomy for hallux valgus correction. Foot Ankle Surg. 2002;8:209–12.
12. Lintz F, de Cesar NC, Barg A, Burssens A, Richter M. Weight Bearing CT International Study Group. Weight-bearing cone beam CT scans in the foot and ankle. EFORT Open Rev. 2018 May;3(5):278–86.
13. Arias-Martín I, Reina-Bueno M, Munuera-Martínez PV. Effectiveness of custom-made foot orthoses for treating forefoot pain: a systematic review. Int Orthop. 2018;42(8):1865–75.
14. Park CH, Chang MC. Forefoot disorders and conservative treatment. Yeungnam Univ J Med. 2019;36(2):92–8.
15. Deshaies A, Roy P, Symeonidis PD, LaRue B, Murphy N, Anctil E. Metatarsal bars more effective than metatarsal pads in reducing impulse on the second metatarsal head. Foot (Edinb). 2011;21(4):172–5.
16. Hutchins S, Bowker P, Geary N, Richards J. The biomechanics and clinical efficacy of footwear adapted with rocker profiles--evidence in the literature. Foot (Edinb). 2009;19(3):165–70.
17. Barouk LS. Forefoot reconstruction. 2nd ed. Berlin: Springer; 2005.
18. Suppan RJ. The cartilaginous articulation preservation principle and its surgical implementation for hallux abducto valgus. J Am Podiatry Assoc. 1974;64:635.
19. Gauthier G. Maladie de Freiberg ou 2me maladie de Kholer, position d'un traitement de reconstruction au stade evolué de l'affection. 48e Réunion Annuelle de la SOFCOT. Rev Chir Orthop. 1974;60(11):337–42.
20. Migues A, Slullitel G, Bilbao F, Carrasco M, Solari G. Floating-toe deformity as a complication of the Weil osteotomy. Foot Ankle Int. 2004;25(9):609–13.
21. Espinosa N, Myerson M, Fernandez de Retana P, Maceira E. A new approach for the treatment of metatarsalgia: the triple Weil osteotomy. Tech. Foot Ankle Surg. 2007;6:254–63.
22. Elmajee M, Shen Z, A'Court J, Pillai A. A systematic review of plantar plate repair in the management of lesser metatarsophalangeal joint instability. J Foot Ankle Surg. 2017;56(6):1244–8.
23. Fleischer AE, Klein EE, Bowen M, McConn TP, Sorensen MD, Weil L Jr. Comparison of combination Weil metatarsal osteotomy and direct plantar plate repair versus Weil metatarsal osteotomy alone for forefoot metatarsalgia. J Foot Ankle Surg. 2020;59(2):303–6.
24. Biz C, Corradin M, Kuete Kanah WT, Dalmau-Pastor M, Zornetta A, Volpin A, Ruggieri P. Medium-long-term clinical and radiographic outcomes of minimally invasive distal metatarsal metaphyseal osteotomy (DMMO) for central primary metatarsalgia: do Maestro criteria have a predictive value in the preoperative planning for this percutaneous technique? Biomed Res Int. 2018;2018:1947024.

Deformity of the Lesser Toes

Pablo Sotelano and Daniel Sebastián Villena

1 Introduction

Pathology of the lesser toes is one of the most frequent reasons for consultation with the ankle and foot specialist [9, 15]. Problems with shoewear and walking have increased over the time. Patients seek quick and definitive solutions. The problem is that surgical treatment of lesser toes deformities have a long postoperative period. Another characteristic of these deformities is, that secondary to the muscle imbalance between the intrinsic and extrinsic toe muscles, the deformity is progressive.

Several nonsurgical treatments and toe devices have been described to reduce pain and improve digital position, but with poor results. Therefore, when the deformity is symptomatic and all the previous instances have been exhausted, surgical treatment is indicated.

Many articles have been published with varying levels of evidence, but even today, there is no consensus on the gold standard. With the development of percutaneous surgery or MIS (minimally invasive surgery), in the last decades it has been possible to achieve results similar to those of open surgery, with less soft tissue injury and better esthetic results.

In this chapter we are going to describe the different surgical options, both classic and MIS techniques.

P. Sotelano (✉) · D. S. Villena
Hospital Italiano de Buenos Aires, Buenos Aires, Argentina
e-mail: pablo.sotelano@hospitalitaliano.org.ar; daniel.villena@hospitalitaliano.org.ar

E. Wagner Hitschfeld, P. Wagner Hitschfeld (eds.), *Foot and Ankle Disorders*,
https://doi.org/10.1007/978-3-030-95738-4_21

467

2   Etiology

The deformity of the lesser toes frequently begins in the fourth decade of life and is slowly progressive, giving the greatest symptoms between the fifth and seventh decade [9]. But depending on the morphology of the foot, it may develop at an earlier age (Fig. 1). The toe most frequently affected is the second one [1, 30, 18]. The type of footwear is one of the most important external factors that generate deformity and discomfort.

From an anthropological point of view, the changes that were generated in the human species with respect to the lesser toes began three or four million years ago [19]. The modification through the years due to bipedestation was the increase of the MP dorsiflexion and morphological changes of the anatomical structures such as the plantar plate.

Due to human habits such as footwear, there is an altered foot biomechanics, with gastrosoleous and posterior tibial muscle hypotrophy. This limits the activation of the windlass mechanism, which is essential for a normal gait (Fig. 2).

Lesser toes deformities are underestimated by orthopedic surgeons and treated with poor interest. This leads to frequent patient complains and poor surgical solutions.

In the last two decades, MIS has gained prominence mainly in the treatment of forefoot pathology. Several surgical techniques have been developed for the lesser toes which will be described in this chapter.

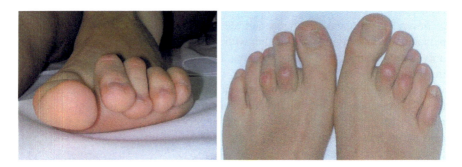

Fig. 1 Hammertoes in young patients

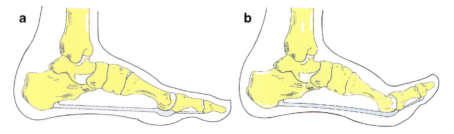

Fig. 2 Windlass mechanism of the plantar fascia. (**a**) At rest. (**b**) Tightening the base of the proximal phalanx to assist toe-off force

3 Anatomy and Pathophysiology

The lesser toes are named numerically (second to fifth) from medial to lateral. They are made up of three phalanges, with the exception of the fifth toe which in 15% of cases has only two phalanges.

The phalanges have three zones: the base, diaphysis and the head or epiphysis. The metatarsophalangeal (MP) and interphalangeal (IP) joints are joined by soft tissues through dynamic and static stabilizers.

Dynamic stabilization is generated by extrinsic muscles (muscles that originate in the leg) and intrinsic muscles (muscles that originate in the foot). The components of static stabilization are the joint capsule, the plantar plate, and the collateral ligaments.

3.1 Extrinsic Musculature

3.1.1 Extensor Digitorum Longus (EDL)

The EDL originates in the anterior compartment of the leg, passes under the inferior extensor retinaculum, and divides into four tendons for the second through the fifth toes; these are attached to the proximal phalanx dorsum by a fibro-aponeurotic structure known as the extensor hood. After leaving this structure distally, the tendon divides into three parts: one central that inserts dorsally at the base of the middle phalanx. The other two tendons continue on the sides towards the distal phalanx (one medial and one lateral). After receiving contributions from the intrinsic muscles, the two side components run distally inserting into the base of the distal phalanx through a single tendon known as the terminal tendon.

Although the proximal phalanx does not receive a direct tendinous extensor insertion, the extensor tendons generate an aponeurotic structure surrounding the MP called the extensor hood. This structure fuses with the plantar plate [12] (Fig. 3).

3.1.2 Flexor Digitorum Longus (FDL)

This muscle originates on the posterior aspect of the tibia. In the plantar region, the flexor hallucis longus provides a communicating tendinous fascicle; then at its lateral border, the quadratus plantar is inserted, followed by its division into four terminal tendons. At the level of the MP joint, it penetrates fibrous sheaths and inserts into the plantar base of the distal phalanx of the second, third, fourth, and fifth toes (Fig. 3).

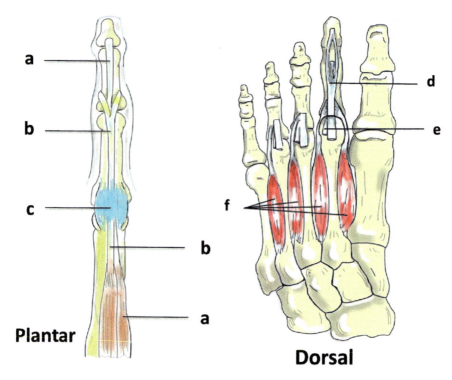

Fig. 3 Normal dorsal and plantar anatomy. (**a**) FDL, (**b**) FDB, (**c**) PP, (**d**) EDL, (**e**) EDB, (**f**) IO (interosseous). (*FDL* flexor digitorum longus; *FDB* flexor digitorum brevis; *PP* plantar plate; *EDL* extensor digitorum longus; *EDB* extensor digitorum brevis; *IO* interosseous)

3.2   *Intrinsic Musculature*

3.2.1   **Extensor Digitorum Brevis (EDB)**

The only muscle of the dorsum of the foot, also called the pedis muscle, originates from the anterosuperior process of the calcaneus. It runs obliquely medially and anteriorly before dividing into four fascicles, each of which ends in a flattened tendon. The tendons of the extensor digitorum brevis are generally thinner than those of the extensor digitorum longus and attach laterally to it at the level of the MP joint, contributing to the extensor apparatus from the first to the fourth toe.

3.2.2   **Flexor Digitorum Brevis (FDB)**

This muscle originates at the medial process of the calcaneal tuberosity. In the midfoot it divides into four fascicles that continue with four long flattened tendons on the plantar aspect of the FDL. Upon reaching the level of the MP joint, it divides into two portions to insert on the medial and lateral borders of the inferior aspect of the middle phalanx (Fig. 3).

3.2.3   Lumbricals (L)

They originate from the FDL tendons. From their point of origin, the lumbrical tendons run distally and diverge slightly to reach the medial side of the MP joints of the second through the fifth toes. They can also insert to the base of the proximal phalanx of the respective toe. Some authors report that the lumbrical muscles can also insert through tendon fibers, at the base of the proximal phalanx [36].

3.2.4   Interosseous (IO)

The seven interosseous muscles (three plantar and four dorsal) originate on the metatarsal shaft in the corresponding intermetatarsal space. The plantar muscles are located in the second, third, and fourth intermetatarsal spaces and arise on the medial and inferior aspect of these bones. The dorsal interosseous, which are thicker than the plantar interosseous, are found in all the intermetatarsal spaces. The tendons of the plantar and dorsal interosseous muscles run distally dorsal to the deep transverse metatarsal ligament. They are closely associated with the capsule, into which some fibers insert. The remaining fibers extend distally toward the base of the proximal phalanx (Fig. 3).

Given their location plantarly to the center of rotation of the MP joint, the interosseous muscles flex the proximal phalanx, opponent to the extensor function.

The second toe is anatomically different from the others because it has two dorsal interosseous muscles and no plantar interosseous muscles. This would explain the higher frequency of sagittal plane dislocation (MP dorsal dislocation).

3.3   Statics Stabilizers

3.3.1   Plantar Plate (PP)

The PP is a fibrocartilaginous structure, composed mainly of type I collagen (75%), and is the main stabilizer of the MP joint. It is a thick, square structure, originating proximally at the plantar fascia and metatarsal neck, inserting distally at the base of the proximal phalanx. The strongest insertion of the PP is found at the proximal phalanx base. The plate inserts into the bone through two bundles that derive directly from the plantar fascia. Between these two bundles, a synovial recess can be found and should not be confused with a tear. Proximally, the plantar plate attachment to the metatarsal neck is through a loose and fragile synovial sheath and does not participate in the joint stabilization. The plantar surface of the plate is covered with

Fig. 4 (**a**) Accessory
CL. (**b**) Phalangeal CL. (**c**)
FDB. (**d**) PP

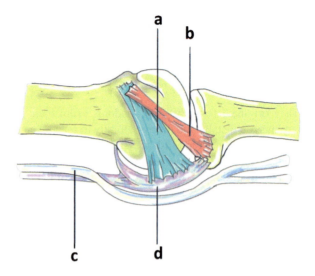

collagen fibers that attach to the deep transverse intermetatarsal ligament [32]
(Fig. 4).

3.3.2 Collateral Ligaments (CLs)

The lateral and medial collateral ligaments are composed of two structures: the phalangeal collateral ligament, which inserts at the base of the proximal phalanx, and the accessory collateral ligament, which sends an expansion toward the plantar plate.

These fan-shaped ligaments together with the plantar plate are the main stabilizers of the MP joint [8] (Fig. 4).

The pathophysiology of lesser toe deformities can occur gradually. Although they may be caused by trauma, mechanical or inflammatory processes (hallux valgus, systemic inflammatory diseases, diabetes, neuromuscular abnormalities, advanced age, improper footwear) [10]. During the toe-off phase, the forefoot may experience up to 120% of the total body load, predisposing to transverse plantar plate lesions at the MP joint. Some authors pointed out that these PP lesions are the first step to develop lesser toe deformities.

The major adult sagittal plane deformities consist of claw toes, hammertoes, and mallet toes. Axial plane deformities include crossover toes.

The position of the proximal phalanx in the MP joint is given by the powerful action of the EDL through the extensor hood mechanism. The antagonists are the intrinsic muscles (FDB, interosseous, and lumbrical) and the static stabilizers formed by the plantar plate collateral ligaments and plantar aponeurosis.

The position of the middle and distal phalanx is subject to the action of the FDL and FDB muscles, which are antagonized by the intrinsic extensor muscles (EDB).

In each of these joints, an imbalance between the intrinsic and extrinsic muscles can occur, causing different deformities.

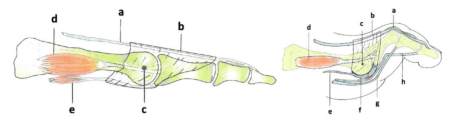

Fig. 5 Pathophysiology of the deformity. (**a**) EDL. (**b**) Extensor hood. (**c**) Center of rotation. (**d**) Interosseous. (**e**) Lumbricals. (**f**) PP. (**g**) FDB. (**h**) FDL

Chronic hyperextension of the proximal phalanx maintained during walking gradually weakens the static plantar structures until they become totally inefficient, thus keeping the proximal phalanx in an abnormal position in dorsal flexion. In addition, metatarsal overloads (originated in hallux valgus, pes cavus, flat foot, etc.) generate slowly progressive and degenerative lesions of the PP structures, which ends in its insufficiency to maintain the proximal phalanx flexion. The long and short flexors of the toes flex the proximal interphalangeal (PIP) joint. The EDL loses its tenodesis effect at the dorsum of the PIP joint, dislocating the two tendon bands laterally, thus contributing to the flexed position of the middle phalanx. As the proximal phalanx extends, the intrinsic flexors (interosseous and lumbrical) move dorsal to the center of rotation of the metatarsal head. In this position, they further worsen the MP extension deformity, not being mechanically able of flexing the proximal phalanx (Fig. 5). This explains the deformities mainly in the sagittal plane. When the imbalance between the extrinsic and intrinsic is combined with a lesion at the level of the plantar plate, there may be concomitant MP subluxation and axial plane misalignment.

The function of the plantar plate is to resist the dorsal displacement of the proximal phalanx during gait. The high functional demand on the plantar structures can ultimately lead to dorsal subluxation of the MP joint. As PP damage worsens, an imbalance between static and dynamic stabilizers leads to medial toe displacement and cross-over deformity (supraducted toe). Ford et al. [20] note that dorsal instability of the MP joint increases by 74% when the plantar plate is severed. Bhatia et al. [4] demonstrated in their biomechanical study a 48% reduction in the force required to dislocate the joint when both collateral ligaments were severed, compared to a reduction in force of only 29% when only the PP was severed. The same observation was made by Barg et al. [2] reporting that sectioning of both accessory collateral ligaments or both phalangeal collateral ligaments increased instability by 41.6% and 26.1% during dorsal subluxation of the MP joint, respectively. They conclude that the accessory collateral ligament is more important than the phalangeal collateral ligament for joint stability due to of its insertion into the PP. The deep transverse metatarsal ligament may also contribute to the dorsal stability of the MP joint. When this joint is in a plantigrade position, the lumbrical and interosseous muscles run plantar to the metatarsal head center of rotation. However, during the toe-off phase of gait, hyperextension of the proximal phalanx leads the interossei to run dorsal to the MP joint's center of rotation. As already stated, this hinders its toe flexion capabilities.

This dynamic imbalance can lead to a progressive MP dorsal displacement.

4   Diagnosis

Toe deformity can be congenital or acquired. The former is very rare, from 1% to 5% according to the literature (Fig. 6). And the acquired one can be primary, due to rheumatoid arthritis, iatrogenic, traumatic, or neurological [10].

Numerous names have been attributed to digital deformities: "mallet toe," "claw toe," "hammertoe," "supraducted toe," "infraducted toe," "rigid," and "flexible," but none of them define the complete deformity. The anatomy of the foot, and more specifically that of the lesser toes, allows us to evaluate by observing and quantifying the deformity in both the sagittal and axial planes without having to perform complementary studies to reach a diagnosis. That is why we are going to take the classification of Barbara Piclet-Legré, validated by the French Association of Foot and Ankle Surgeons, for the sagittal plane [25], which is based mainly on the simple visualization and morphology of the toes in the sagittal and axial planes, allowing us with the physical examination to define whether it is rigid or flexible and to make an accurate diagnosis and appropriate treatment for each pathology (Table 1).

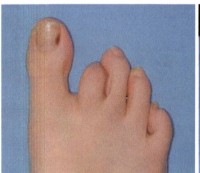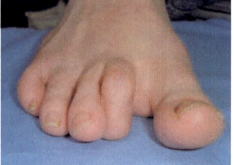

Fig. 6 Congenital second hammertoe

Table 1 French Association of Foot and Ankle Surgeons classification for toe deformities

Localization (proximal to distal)	Deformation	Reducibility	Cause
MP = metatarsophalangeal joint	f = flexion	f = flexible	rh = rheumatic
PIP = proximal interphalangeal	e = extension	sr = semi-rigid	pt = posttraumatic
DIP = distal interphalangeal	l = lateral deviation	r = rigid	nr = neurologic
	m = medial deviation		ic = iatrogenic

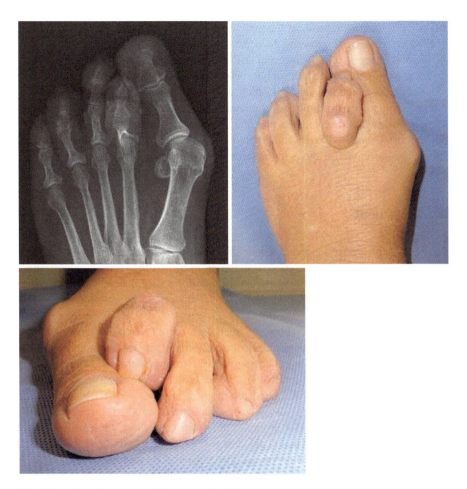

Fig. 7 Morphologic: second rigid claw and mallet

The cause of the deformity is placed after the toe number, while the deformity and the degree of stiffness are placed after the deformity. The most frequent MP deformity is in extension, so when it is in that position, the letter "e" is not added. The same happens when the PIP and distal (DIP) joints are in flexion – the letter "f" is not added. When any of the joints is dislocated, the sign "+" is added. The most important thing about this classification is that it is reproducible (inter- and intra-observer) and allows a treatment algorithm according to each subtype.

Example: a patient with rheumatoid arthritis (RA) and a subluxed or dislocated second toe supraducted medially (Fig. 7). From a morphological point of view, 2 MP + m PIP DIP, where the second toe presents a MP in extension and dislocated medially with the PIP and DIP in flexion. If we add the etiology (rheumatic [rh], posttraumatic [pt], Iatrogenic [ic], neurologic [nr]) and the criteria of reducible or not (rigid [r], semi-rigid [sr], flexible [f]), the above example would be 2 Ar MP + m

PIPsr DIPf, where 2 represents the second toe, "Ar" represents rheumatoid arthritis, "MP+" is the MP in flexion and dislocated, "m" is the medial toe deviation, "PIPsr" is the joint in semi-rigid flexion, and DIPf is the joint in flexible flexion (Fig. 7).

As complementary studies, weight-bearing AP and lateral view X-ray are sufficient for prior diagnosis and evaluation of postoperative evolution. In the case of having a diagnostic presumption of plantar plate lesion, it is suggested to complement with magnetic resonance imaging (MRI) or dynamic ultrasound (operator dependent). Computed axial tomography (CT scan) is only reserved for osteoarticular alterations and deformities in the three planes.

5 Treatment

To evaluate the type of treatment to be performed, we must mainly take into account the patient's age and expectations. The alteration of gait in elderly patients, where the lesser toes do not have an important role, will be very different from that of a 50-year-old patient, athlete, who needs the lesser toes to be able to perform his physical activity.

Consequently, the same pathology, such as a second supraducted toe, can be treated in an elderly patient and in an active patient in two different ways. The elderly patient, with rigid second crossover toe, chronic ulceration, needs to return quickly to his activity, and it is not advisable for him to rest for long periods of time. Therefore, amputation of the second toe might be the method of choice. On the other hand, the active patient, who needs the function of his second toe, is indicated a metatarsal osteotomy, a PIP arthrodesis, and a transfer the flexor longus toward the dorsal diaphysis of the proximal phalanx of the toe (Girdlestone-Taylor procedure), and in this way he will be able to perform his activity. The postoperative time in the latter case is much longer, but the functional result is better.

Another important point to make is the surgical result and the patient's expectations. Within the surgical treatment, osteotomies, tendon transfers, arthrodesis, and tendon elongation are performed. This implies that the operated toe will never have the functionality of a normal toe. We will greatly improve the position and symptoms but limiting the function. This information should be provided to the patient in a detailed and clear manner before surgery.

5.1 Nonsurgical

When the toe is reducible and flexible, the conservative treatment is based on strengthening the intrinsic and extrinsic muscles and windlass mechanism of the plantar fascia, which contributes to improve the MP plantar flexion. Strengthening and stretching of the Achilles and tibialis posterior tendons, help improve gait and decrease MP dorsiflexion deformity.

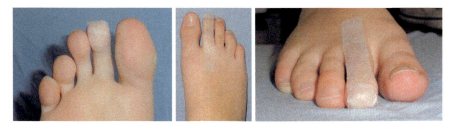

Fig. 8 Simple bandage. With correction in extension of the distal phalanx

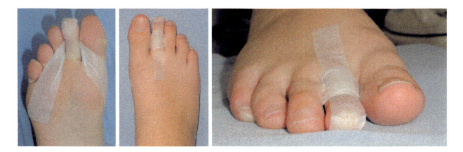

Fig. 9 Serpentine bandage. To the previous bandage, we add the descent of the proximal phalanx

Bandages aim to reduce the dorsiflexion position of the MP joint by bringing the toe into plantar flexion. They can be simple, in serpentine or in a tie shape (Figs. 8, 9, and 10).

Insoles is another good alternative. The insole can be partial size or full size (Fig. 11). They aim to elevate the lesser metatarsals with a retrocapital pad, located proximal to the metatarsal heads. This improves MP plantar flexion.

If the toe is rigid, conservative treatment will only be aimed at improving footwear with a wide and high toe box, insoles in the case of associated deformities to improve support, and biological silicone orthoses customized by specialists (Fig. 12).

5.2   Surgical Treatment

Numerous surgical techniques have been described for the various deformities. In our opinion, the clearest and most pedagogical way to list them is to evaluate each joint deformity, indicating the appropriate treatment for each one of them.

In a generic way, it is necessary to evaluate if the deformity is rigid or flexible. If it is flexible, the correction options are through tenotomies and osteotomies. On the other hand, if the deformity is rigid, the correction can be achieved through arthrodesis or joint arthroplasty.

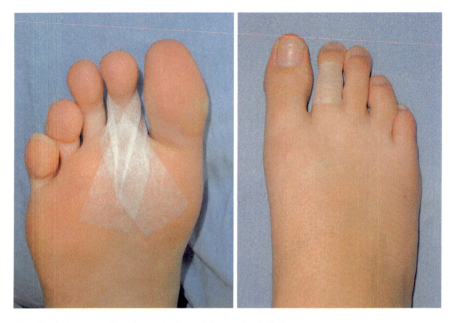

Fig. 10 Tie bandage. For plantar flexion of the proximal phalanx

Fig. 11 Shoe insoles

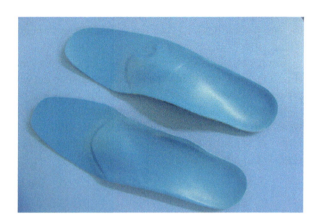

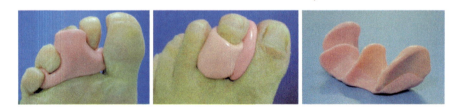

Fig. 12 Customized silicone orthoses

Due to the importance that MIS has taken in the last two decades, it should be noted that all the procedures mentioned have their adaptation to be performed with MIS. At the end of the description of the classical techniques, we will describe the MIS procedures and the author's preferred treatment method.

5.2.1 Open Surgery

Distal interphalangeal (DIP) joint deformity, also called mallet toe. In this pathology, the DIP joint is deformed in flexion and can be flexible or rigid.

Flexible DIP Flexion Deformity: Mallet Toe

The surgical objective is to release the FDL and perform a plantar DIP capsulotomy.

Through a longitudinal or transverse plantar incision at the distal skin fold, the tenotomy and capsulotomy are performed. Those procedures can also be performed through a dorsal transverse transarticular approach. The dorsal approach avoids soft tissue complications (dehiscence), common in transverse plantar incisions for toe flexion deformities.

Rigid DIP Flexion Deformity: Mallet Toe

The two gold standard open techniques are the DIP arthrodesis and the DuVries [16] technique.

DIP arthrodesis: Dorsal fishmouth approach, tenotomy, and dorsal capsulotomy releasing collateral ligaments. The joint is exposed, and the articular cartilage of both articular surfaces is resected using a rongeur. Then a closure is made with deep "U" or Donati skin stitches, which reach the articular capsule. If the deformity tends to recur after skin and capsule closure, a 1.25 mm ø intramedullary K-wire can be used across the DIP joint.

The DuVries [16] technique uses the same approach but only resects the articular cartilage of the middle phalanx epiphysis. In this way a fibrous union is obtained. The authors refer that the toe remains in a more anatomical position than with the arthrodesis.

If the deformity is in extension, tenotomy of the long extensor tendon is performed by a dorsal approach for flexible deformity or eventually arthrodesis for rigid deformity.

Flexible PIP flexion Deformity: Hammertoe or Claw Toe

The PIP flexion deformity, also called hammertoe or claw toe, occurs mainly in flexion and rarely in extension. This deformity, like the previous one, can be flexible or rigid.

Through a 2 cm longitudinal plantar approach at the level of the PIP toe crease, perform a PIP plantar capuslotomy and a FDB tenotomy at the base of the middle phalanx. If there is associated DIP joint deformity, perform a FDL and FDB tenotomy through the same approach. Use a postoperative K-wire for 3 weeks postoperative until soft tissues healing is achieved.

Rigid PIP flexion deformity: Hammertoe or Claw Toe

The PIP joint deformity is frequently associated with a metatarsophalangeal (MP) joint deformity. The joint deformity of PIP flexion and MP extension is called claw toe.

In case of a rigid PIP joint deformity, the surgical options are resection arthroplasty as described by DuVries [16], or PIP arthrodesis [11, 24]. Most used fixations are Kirschner wires or intramedullary devices (Fig. 13).

The surgical approach is similar for both techniques. Through a 20 mm dorsal and longitudinal approach over the PIP joint, an extensor tendon tenotomy, dorsal capsulotomy and collateral ligaments release are performed. If there is an associated mallet toe deformity, a transarticular flexor tendon tenotomy and plantar capsulotomy are performed.

DuVries arthroplasty includes resection of the proximal phalanx head cartilage and may or may not be fixed with a 1.5 Kirschner wire. PIP arthrodesis is performed by resecting both articular surfaces (proximal phalanx head and middle phalax base). It can be performed using a rongeur, oscillating microsaw, or burs [17, 37] (Fig. 14). It can be fixed with transient K-wires (kept in place for 6 weeks), resorbable wires, or intramedullary devices (Fig. 13).

These deformities may be associated with a dorsal MP dislocation. In these cases, metatarsal surgery is mandatory to reduce joint tension and thus reduce the MP joint. This deformity is mainly due to static stabilizers insufficiency, such as the PP and the collateral ligaments. In cases to acute PP or collateral ligaments injury, direct repair is recommended (plantar plate repair). If these lesions are chronic, indirect repair is recommended by performing a triple Weil osteotomy (discussed in other chapter of this book).

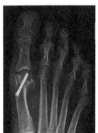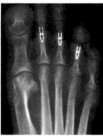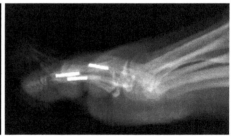

Fig. 13 Intramedullary devices. Pre- and postoperative

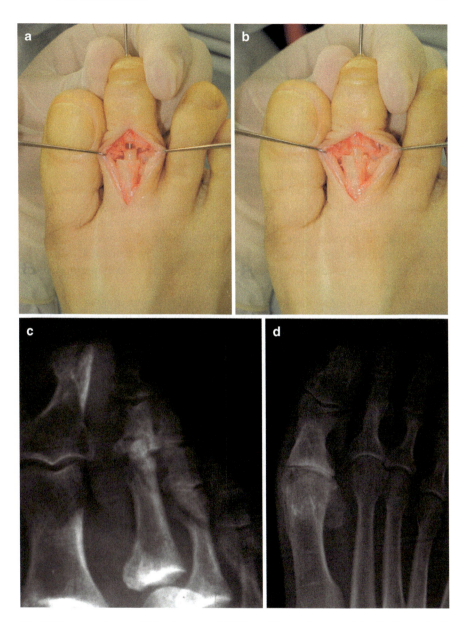

Fig. 14 Reciprocal socket PIP arthrodesis. (**a**) Joint milling and endomedular fixation with 1.5 mm ∅ K-wire. (**b**) Docking of proximal and middle phalanx. (**c**) Postoperative X-ray. (**d**) healed arthrodesis

MP Extension Deformity

This deformity is generally flexible and reducible as long as the joint is not dislocated or damaged by degenerative processes (such as Freiberg's disease). Keeping in mind that perfect reduction and position of this joint is not always achieved, many times we must perform extra-articular surgical procedures in order to achieve a good digital position, regardless of the joint reduction.

Through a 1 cm dorsal incision over the MP joint a "Z"- shaped tenotomy of the extensor digitorum longus tendon is performed. If the toe position does not improve, a dorsal capsulotomy is added. If further correction is needed, a Girdlestone-Taylor (GT) tendon transfer can be added. GT is technically demanding and often result in metatarsophalangeal stiffness. The objective of this technique is to change the insertion position of the FDL from the distal phalanx to the proximal phalanx. Most importantly, this transfer does not change the tendon traction vector; it is still a flexor agonist, therefore, it has a great correction power. The alternative to the GT is to perform a proximal phalanx tenotomy. This procedure is easily performed with MIS using a shannon burr.

Girdlestone-Taylor technique (Fig. 15): plantar DIP 3 mm approach. Perform a FDL tenotomy. Then perform a 5 mm plantar incision at the proximal phalanx diaphysis. The FDL is pulled and divided into two halfs. After that, a 15 mm dorsal proximal phalanx incision is performed. The FDL halfs are transferred dorsally, one on each side of the phalanx. Then, both ends are sutured together giving the necessary tension and balance to keep the proximal phalanx in neutral position [31].

PP ruptures evolve to a claw toe deformity or MP dislocation. Chronic ruptures progress to a PP degenerative lesion that ends in a rigid claw toe deformity. These lesions can be repaired; however, it is only recommended when there is an acute rupture in an athletic patient (to be discussed in the chapter on metatarsalgia). In patients with chronic PP injury, the authors recommend not repairing it, but to choose between the triple Weil and/or GT technique or proximal phalanx osteotomy MIS technique.

If the claw toe is associated with metatarsalgia, a Weil-Maceira-type osteotomy [28] or DMMO with MIS technique [13] (Fig. 16) will be recommended as metatarsalgia treatment. This will be discussed at length in the chapter on metatarsalgia.

5.2.2 MIS (Minimally Invasive Surgery)

The goal of MIS is to perform the same procedures as in open surgery but with less soft tissue injury, achieve a faster recovery of soft tissues, and reduce postoperative pain. The postoperative bandage should be kept in place for 3 weeks being fundamental in this technique, so that the osteotomies form a fibrous callus and heal in a good position [39].

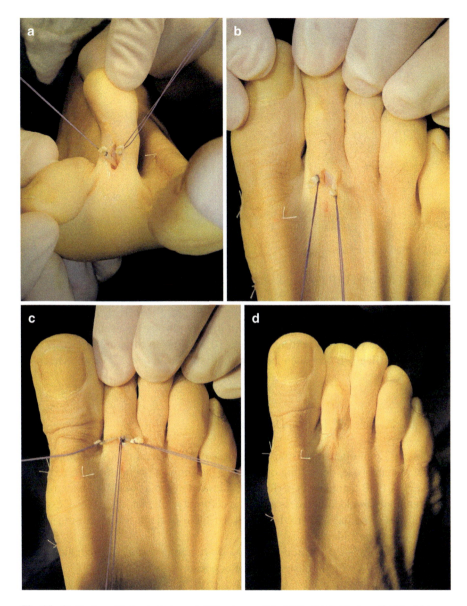

Fig. 15 Girdlestone-Taylor technique. (**a**) Tenotomy of the FDL divided in two. (**b**) Dorsal transfer. (**c**) Suture of the tendon to the dorsal. (**d**) Skin suture

For this surgery specific instruments are necessary such as a high-torque and low-revolution drill, cutting drills (15 and 10 mm long) and reaming drills depending on the brand (Shannon®, Arthrex®, Wright®, Vilex®), and Beaver 64, 64 MIS, and 67 blade scalpel for percutaneous surgery (Shannon®, Aesculap®).

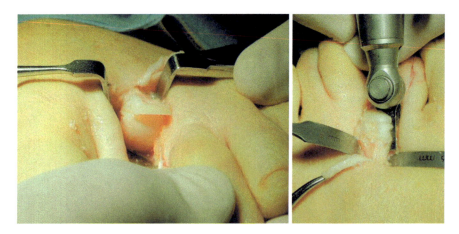

Fig. 16 Weil-Maceira osteotomy

Rigid and Flexible DIP Flexion Deformity

Perform a 2 mm plantar incision over the DIP joint. Proceed with a FDL tenotomy and plantar capsulotomy. If the joint is rigid, through the same plantar incision, introduce the short cutting reamer (10 mm) up to the joint and resect the articular cartilage. It can then be transiently fixed with a 1.25 mm Kirschner wire [27].

Rigid and Flexible PIP Flexion Deformity

Flexible: a 2 mm plantar incision is performed at the lateral or medial edge of the middle phalanx base, depending on whether the surgeon operates with the right or left hand. A FDB tenotomy is performed, followed by a plantar PIP capsulotomy. A FDL tenotomy is added if necessary. If the deformity still persists, a dorsal exostectomy of the proximal phalanx head and a middle phalanx dorsal closing wedge osteotomy can be added.

Rigid: Perform a PIP arthrodesis with a short cutting reamer through the a plantar incision. Fix it with a transient K-wire or a resorbable pin [3, 6].

Deformity in Extension of the MP Joint

Perform a 2mm dorsal incision at the level of the MP joint (Fig. 18). A EDL and EDB tenotomy in addition to a dorsal capsulotomy are performed. More than half of the MP deformities cannot be corrected with these procedures. In this case, we must act on the proximal phalanx, performing a plantar wedge base osteotomy if the deformity is only in the sagittal plane or a complete osteotomy if the deformity is in two or three planes (Fig. 17). Bandaging for 4 weeks is used to achieve osteotomy

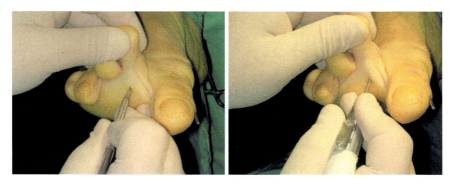

Fig. 17 MIS osteotomy at the base of the proximal phalanx

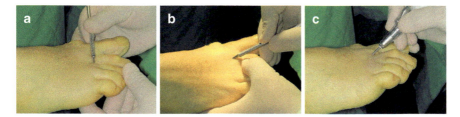

Fig. 18 (**a**) Extensor Tenotomy. (**b**, **c**) Minimally invasive distal metatarsal osteotomy (DMMO) [35]

healing and thus, deformity correction. If the deformity continues and metatarsalgia is present, a minimally invasive distal metatarsal osteotomy (DMMO) could be added (Fig. 18) [35].

5.2.3 Preferred Author's Treatment Method: PIP Arthrodesis with Resorbable Pin

For severe rigid hammertoe the author's preferred treatment method is a PIP arthrodesis with resorbable pins. The advantages of this technique are that it does not leave any implant outside the skin and it is minimally invasive. In addition, is a persistent deformity is evident after the PIP arthrodesis, a proximal phalanx osteotomy can be added.

As described, through a 2 mm plantar incision at the PIP, a FDB tenotomy and plantar capsulotomy are performed (Fig. 19). If there is distal deformity, tenotomy of the FDL is added as well. Through this approach, the articular surfaces are prepared with a 10 mm Shannon reamer. Under radioscopic control the intramedullary canal is prepared. A 1.5 resorbable intramedullary pin [5, 22] is introduced from the toe tip (Fig. 20).

If the toe is still extended after the PIP fixation, a minimally invasive proximal phalanx osteotomy or a Girdlestone-Taylor tendon transfer can be added.

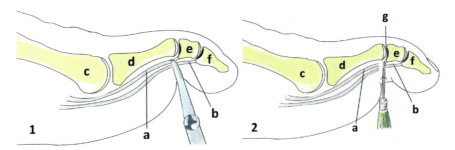

Fig. 19 (**1**) FDB tenotomy. (**2**) PIP arthrodesis. (**a**) FDB. (**b**) FDL. (**c**) Metatarsal. (**d**) Proximal phalanx. (**d, e**) Middle phalanx. (**f**) Distal phalanx. (**g**) PIP

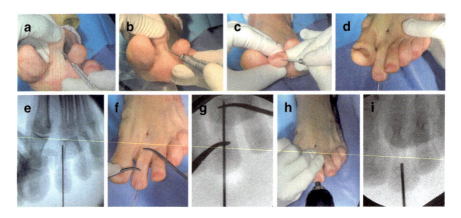

Fig. 20 (**a**) Plantar incision; (**b**) PIP arthrodesis with drill; (**c**) skin incision for guide passage; (**d**) guide placement; (**e**) fluoroscopy; (**f**) and (**g**) under fluoroscopy, measurement of the resorbable pin, avoiding to invade the MP joint; (**h**) insert the implant with drill; (**i**) progression of the implant with impactor leaving the DIP joint free

MIS techniques allow us to obtain similar results to open techniques with less soft tissue damage, low complication rate and early rehabilitation. It is important to note that when fixing the PIP joint, the FDL becomes a direct flexor of the MP joint and not of the PIP and DIP joints, developing a good and permanent toe plantar flexion moment.

6 Deformity of the Fifth Toe

Claw toes deformities of the fifth toe are treated the same way as mentioned above including arthrodesis, tenotomies and osteotomies. In cases of severe deformities associated with toe rotation, techniques that include EDL tendon transfer to the abductor tendon have been described (Lapidus technique). Often, skin elongation techniques must be added such as "V-Y" or "Z" plasty [14, 38].

7   Complications

The rate of complications range from 10% to 33% [7, 29, 33]. The complications that will be discussed include: malalignment, joint deformities, infection, ischemia and hardware related.

7.1 Malalignment: Many devices exist in the market that can maintain the position obtained in the immediate postoperative period, Nevertheless, they will probably fail in the long term if a DuVries resection arthroplasty (forms a fibrous union and not a bone fusion) was performed and not an arthrodesis. In addition, it is the author's advice to shorten the toe in severe deformities (at the proximal phalanx or metatarsal head). In this way soft tissue tension is reduced, and a better balance of the deforming forces is achieved.

Another common complication is floating toe. It is found in 36% of cases after the triple Weil - Maceira osteotomy is performed [21]. The incidence is even higher if a PIP arthrodesis is performed at the same time [26] (Fig. 21).

7.2 Extension contracture of the MP, either with or without joint subluxation, can be avoided by means of Girdlestone-Taylor tendon transfer and repair of the plantar plate and eventually the collateral ligaments. These static stabilizers are also responsible for deformities in the coronal plane. One way to avoid this deformity is to perform a complete or incomplete MIS osteotomy at the base of the proximal phalanx (to achieve flexion), as described in the MIS section.

7.3 Infection: The rate of superficial and deep infections does not exceed 11% (Fig. 22). Only 0.3% cause deep infections, often associated with the use of K-wires. Most infections evolve favorably with adequate antibiotic treatment [34].

Fig. 21 Floating toe after Weil-Maceira osteotomy and PIP arthrodesis

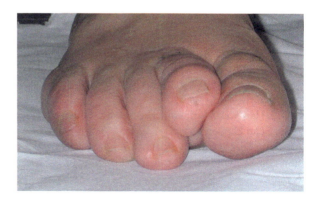

Fig. 22 Superficial infection after a DMMO of the second metatarsal

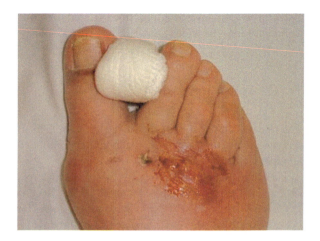

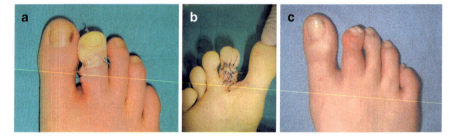

Fig. 23 Ischemic toe after correction of a complex deformity with Z-plantar skin advancement. (**a**) and (**b**) Immediate postoperative period. (**c**) Postoperative period at 1 year

7.4 Ischemia: Severe deformity corrections have a neurovascular risk. Kramer et al. reported 0.4% of severe ischemic complications [23]. After large deformity corrections, always evaluate the capillary filling at the end of the surgery. If any decrease in circulation occurs, there are a few options to perform: start by moving and partially removing the fixation wire. If this does not improve the ischemia, apply warm saline and nitro paste (nitroglycerin) to the toe. If none of the previous procedures improve the ischemia, remove the osteodesis regardless of the loss of correction (Fig. 23). Do not leave the operating room until ischemia is resolved.

7.5 Hardware Related: The most frequent problem is K-wire failure. Screw failure can happen as well if a screw or a metalic implant was used to stabilize the toe. This failure usually occurs after the patient starts to walk [40]. This complication can be avoided using resorbable pins or by keeping the toe immobilized for 6 weeks.

8   Summary

The pathology of the lesser toes is still a challenge for any orthopedic surgeon, due to its multiple deformities in a small segment of the anatomy. Many procedures are necessary to completely correct the deformities, which is the reason for its high recurrence rate. It is difficult after surgery to achieve normal function of the toe. This is something that the patient should be aware of before undergoing surgery.

Current percutaneous techniques have been able to correct deformities with less soft tissue damage. Classic MIS techniques solely depend on postoperative bandage. The evolution of some endomedullary devices help to achieve more predictable and reproducible results.

Although the lesser toes pathology is underestimated, surgical training and a detailed study of the anatomy and pathophysiology are necessary to obtain good results with a low complication rate.

References

1. Averous C, Leider F, Rocher H, Determe P, Guillo S, Cermolacce C, Diebold P. Interphalangeal arthrodesis of the toe with a new radiolucent intramedullary implant (toegrip). Foot Ankle Spec. 2015;8(6):520–4.
2. Barg A, Courville XF, Nickisch F, Bachus KN, Saltzman CL. Role of collateral ligaments in metatarsophalangeal stability: a cadaver study. Foot Ankle Int. 2012;33(10):877–82.
3. Basile A, Albo F, Via A. Intramedullary fixation system for the treatment of hammertoe deformity. J Foot Ankle Surg. 2015;54(5):910–6.
4. Bhatia D, Myerson MS, Curtis MJ, Cunningham BW, Jinnah RH. Anatomical restraints to dislocation of the second metatarsophalangeal joint and assessment of a repair technique. J Bone Joint Surg Am. 1994;76(9):1371–5.
5. Cicchinelli LD. Hammertoe surgery and the trim-it drill pin. Foot Ankle Spec. 2013;6(4):296–302. https://doi.org/10.1177/1938640013490123. Epub 2013 May 14. PMID: 23673417.
6. Coillard J, Petri G, van Damme G, et al. Stabilization of proximal interphalangeal joint in lesser toe deformities with an angulated intramedullary implant. Foot Ankle Int. 2014;35(4):401–7.
7. Cordier G, Nunes GA. Minimally invasive advances. Foot Ankle Clin 2020. 2020;25(3):461–78.
8. Coughlin MJ, Baumfeld DS, Nery C. Second MTP joint instability: grading of the deformity and description of surgical repair of capsular insufficiency. Phys Sportsmed. 2011;39(3):132–41.
9. Coughlin MJ, Saltzman CL, Mann RA. Mann's surgery of the foot and ankle E-book: expert consult – online. San Francisco, California: Elsevier Health Sciences; 2013.
10. Coughlin MJ. Lesser toe deformities. In: Coughlin MJSC, Anderson RB, editors. Mann's surgery of the foot and ankle. 9th ed. Elsevier; 2014. p. 322–424.
11. Coughlin MJ, Dorris J, Polk E. Operative repair of the fixed hammertoe deformity. Foot Ankle Int. 2000;21(2):94–104.
12. Dalmau-Pastor M, Fargues B, Alcolea E, Martínez-Franco N, Ruiz-Escobar P, Vega J, Golanó P. Extensor apparatus of the lesser toes: anatomy with clinical implications--topical review. Foot Ankle Int. 2014;35(10):957–69.

13. De Prado M, Ripoll PL, Metatarsalgias GP, editors. Cirugía percutánea del pie. Barcelona: Masson; 2003. p. 165–74.
14. Derhy Y, Binder JP, Mitrofanoff M, Haddad R, Pavy B. Quintus varus supraductus congénital: technique chirurgicale [Congenital quintus varus supraductus: surgical procedure]. Ann Chir Plast Esthet. 2004;49(4):373–7. French.
15. Doty JF, Coughlin MJ, Weil L, et al. Etiology and management of lesser toe metatarsophalangeal joint instability. Foot Ankle Clin. 2014;19(3):385–405.
16. DuVries HL. Dislocation of the toe. J Am Med Assoc. 1956;160:728.
17. Edwards WH, Beischer AD. Interphalangeal joint arthrodesis of the lesser toes. Foot Ankle Clin. 2002;7(1):43–8.
18. Femino JE, Mueller K. Complications of lesser toe surgery. Clin Orthop Relat Res. 2001;391:72–88.
19. Fernández PJ, Mongle CS, Leakey L, Proctor DJ, Orr CM, Patel BA, Almécija S, Tocheri MW, Jungers WL. Evolution and function of the hominin forefoot. Proc Natl Acad Sci U S A. 2018;115(35):8746–51.
20. Ford LA, Collins KB, Christensen JC. Stabilization of the subluxed second metatarsophalangeal joint: flexor tendon transfer versus primary repair of the plantar plate. J Foot Ankle Surg. 1998;37(3):217–22.
21. Highlander P, VonHerbulis E, Gonzalez A, et al. Complications of the Weil osteotomy. Foot Ankle Spec. 2011;4(3):165–70.
22. Konkel KF, Menger AG, Retzlaff SA. Hammer toe correction using an absorbable intramedullary pin. Foot Ankle Int. 2007;28(8):916–20.
23. Kramer W, Parman M, Marks R. Hammertoe correction with K-wire fixation. Foot Ankle Int. 2015;36(5):494–502.
24. Lehman D, Smith R. Treatment of symptomatic hammertoe with a proximal inter- phalangeal joint arthrodesis. Foot Ankle Int. 1995;16(9):535–41.
25. Lintz F, Beldame J, Kerhousse G, et al. Intra- and inter-observer reliability of the AFCP classification for sagittal plane deformities of the second toe. Foot Ankle Surg. 2020;26(6):650–6.
26. Migues A, Slullitel G, Bilbao F, et al. Floating-toe deformity as a complication of the Weil osteotomy. Foot Ankle Int. 2004;25(9):609–13.
27. Migues A, Campaner G, Slullitel G, Sotelano P, Carrasco M, Solari G. Minimally invasive surgery in hallux valgus and digital deformities. Orthopedics. 2007;30(7):523–6.
28. Monteagudo M, Maceira E. Evolution of the Weil osteotomy: the triple osteotomy. Foot Ankle Clin. 2019;24(4):599–614.
29. Mueller CM, Boden SA, Boden AL, Maidman SD, Cutler A, Mignemi D, Bariteau J. Complication rates and short-term outcomes after operative hammertoe correction in older patients. Foot Ankle Int. 2018;39(6):681–8.
30. Myerson MS, Shereff MJ. The pathological anatomy of claw and hammer toes. J Bone Joint Surg Am. 1989;71(1):45–9.
31. Nery C, Baumfeld D. Lesser metatarsophalangeal joint instability: treatment with tendon transfers. Foot Ankle Clin. 2018;23(1):103–26.
32. Nery C, Coughlin MJ, Baumfeld D, Raduan FC, Catena F, Macedo BD, de Andrade MA. Lesser metatarsal phalangeal joint arthroscopy: anatomic description and comparative dissection. Arthroscopy. 2014;30(8):971–9.
33. Nieto-García E, Ferrer-Torregrosa J, Ramírez-Andrés L, Nieto-González E, Martinez-Nova A, Barrios C. The impact of associated tenotomies on the outcome of incomplete phalangeal osteotomies for lesser toe deformities. J Orthop Surg Res. 2019;14(1):308.
34. Phisitkul P. Managing complications of lesser toe and metatarsophalangeal joint surgery. Foot Ankle Clin. 2018;23(1):145–56.
35. Redfern D, Vernois J. Percutaneous surgery for metatarsalgia and the lesser toes. Foot Ankle Clin. 2016;21(3):527–50.
36. Sarrafian SK, Topouzian LK. Anatomy and physiology of the extensor apparatus of the toes. J Bone Joint Surg Am. 1969;51(4):669–79.

37. Ferna S,ndez C, Wagner E, Ortiz C. Lesser toes proximal interphalangeal joint fusion in rigid claw toes. Foot Ankle Clin. 2012;17(3):473–80.
38. Tawil HJ, Pilliard D, Taussig G. Le quintus varus supraductus. Résultats du traitement chirurgical par plastie cutanée, capsulotomie interne et transfert externe de l'extenseur du 5e orteil [Quintus varus supraductus. Results of the surgical treatment by cutaneous graft, internal capsulotomy and external transfer of the extensor of the 5th toe]. Rev Chir Orthop Reparatrice Appar Mot. 1992;78(2):107–11. French.
39. Yassin M, Garti A, Heller E, et al. Hammertoe correction with K-wire fixation compared with percutaneous correction. Foot Ankle Spec. 2016;10(5):421–7.
40. Zingas C, Katcherian DA, Wu KK. Kirschner wire breakage after surgery of the lesser toes. Foot Ankle Int. 1995;16(8):504–9.

Morton's Neuroma

Rodrigo Melo Grollmus and Cristián Ortiz Mateluna

1 Introduction

Morton's neuroma (also called Morton's metatarsalgia, Morton's disease, plantar interdigital neuroma, interdigital neuritis, or plantar neuroma) is one of the common causes of metatarsalgia. It corresponds to a painful syndrome of the forefoot produced by the pathology of one of the interdigital plantar nerves, most commonly that of the third interosseous space and less frequently that of the second [1, 2].

The first anatomical report date back to 1835, in which Filippo Civinini, professor of anatomy at the University of Pisa (Italy), described an increase in volume of the plantar interdigital nerve in the third interosseous space [3, 4]. Ten years later, Lewis Durlacher [5] reported the first clinical case. But it was not until the clinical series published in 1876 by Thomas Morton [6] that the lesion between the third and fourth metatarsophalangeal joint was associated as a cause of metatarsalgia, which in turn produced a neuralgia due to the involvement of the plantar nerve [3].

In 1893, Hoadley [7] was the first to report the resection of a small neuroma in the area as a treatment of metatarsalgia, with good clinical results [8]. In 1940 Bett [9] described Morton's metatarsalgia as "neuritis of the fourth digital nerve," and Gauthier [10] in 1979 attributed it to nerve entrapment, supported by anatomical studies. In addition, he was the first to describe his successful clinical results with only release of the affected nerve.

R. Melo Grollmus (✉)
Department of Orthopedic Surgery, Foot and Ankle Unit, Clinica Las Condes, Santiago, Chile

Department of Orthopedic Surgery, Foot and Ankle Unit, Hospital Militar de Santiago, Santiago, Chile

C. Ortiz Mateluna
Department of Orthopedic Surgery, Foot and Ankle Unit, Clinica Universidad de los Andes, Santiago, Chile

© The Author(s), under exclusive license to Springer Nature Switzerland AG 2022
E. Wagner Hitschfeld, P. Wagner Hitschfeld (eds.), *Foot and Ankle Disorders*,
https://doi.org/10.1007/978-3-030-95738-4_22

493

2 Epidemiology

It is more frequent in the female sex (ratio 4:1) with an average age of presentation between 40 and 55 years [1, 2, 11, 12]. It is usually unilateral, but in up to 15–21% of cases, it is bilateral [11, 13, 14].

In the vast majority of patients, it affects the nerve in the third intermetatarsal space (66% of cases) and less frequently in the second interosseous space. Compromise of the first and fourth space is extremely rare and probably does not exist as a clinical entity [12–14]. On the other hand, the involvement of simultaneous adjacent spaces is unusual (< 3% of cases) [11, 15].

3 Anatomy

The medial plantar nerve is divided into four digital branches: the most medial to the hallux and the others to the first, second, and third interosseous spaces. The lateral plantar nerve gives two digital branches: one to the fifth toe and the other to the fourth interosseous space. This last branch, depending on the lateral plantar nerve, can give a communicating branch to the third space that joins the branch of the medial plantar nerve, which generates a thicker interdigital nerve (Fig. 1). Different cadaveric studies have demonstrated the existence of this branch in up to 66% of the population [11, 16–18].

The interdigital nerve is in a small osteofibrous space, limited laterally and medially by the adjacent metatarsals, distally by the metatarsal heads and their respective joints and periarticular structures (collateral ligaments, joint capsule, and flexor tendons), dorsally by the transverse intermetatarsal ligament which is inserted into the metatarsals slightly proximal to the heads, and plantarly by the plantar aponeurosis, fat, and thick plantar metatarsal skin. This space also contains the interdigital artery and veins [1]. The intermetatarsal bursa is located above the intermetatarsal transverse ligament (Fig. 2) [11, 19]. Each nerve at the level of the intermetatarsal transverse ligament normally measures about 1 mm in diameter. Distal to this and just proximal to the heads of the metatarsals, it is divided into the two digital nerves [1].

4 Etiopathogenesis

Although its etiology remains unclear, there are multiple theories described in the literature that attempt to explain its etiology, pathogenesis, and associated factors. Probably, as well as a large number of entities in orthopedics, it is a multifactorial condition in which each of the following factors collaborates to a greater or lesser degree [11, 20–23]:

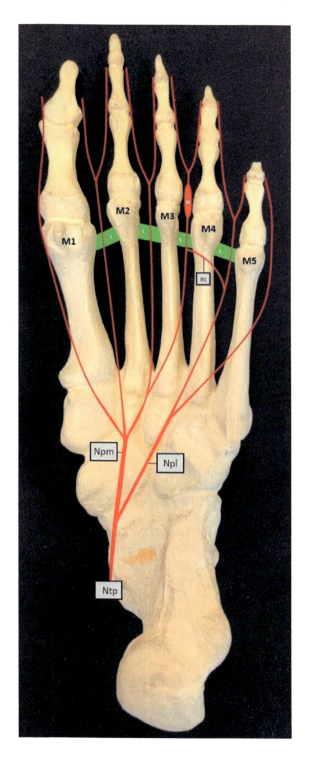

Fig. 1 Anatomical distribution of the plantar nerves (Ntp posterior tibial nerve, Npm medial plantar nerve, Npl lateral plantar nerve, Rc communicating branch of the third space, L transverse intermetatarsal ligament)

Fig. 2 Cross-section diagram of the intermetatarsal anatomical space. It is observed dorsal to the transverse intermetatarsal ligament (L) and the intermetatarsal bursa (B) and plantar to the ligament, the interdigital nerve (N), the artery (A), and the vein (V)

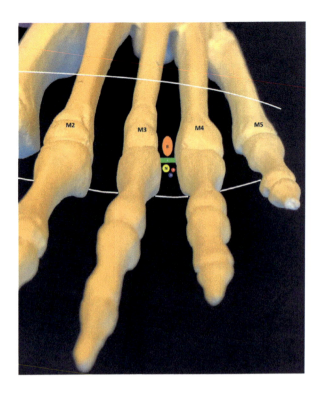

4.1 Anatomical Factors

Various anatomical conditions, especially the innervation of the forefoot, would be a fundamental etiopathogenic factor in the origin of Morton's neuroma. As mentioned in the anatomical description, in a high percentage of the population it has been demonstrated the existence of a communicating branch to the third space that joins the branch of the medial plantar nerve. This co-joined nerve generates a thicker interdigital nerve that it more exposed to trauma [16–18]. This branch can also pass under the head of the metatarsal or under the metatarsophalangeal joint, which increases its propensity for repetitive trauma [11, 16–18]. Another anatomical factor is referred to the anatomical space itself, since both the third and the second interosseous spaces would be smaller, compared to the first and the fourth [11, 16]. A widely discussed element is the difference in mobility and relative position of these metatarsals with respect to the ground, which occurs at the level of the midfoot joints between the medial and middle columns (rigid and inclined to the ground) and the lateral column (mobile and parallel to the ground). This difference explains that the third interosseous space is a more mobile transition area, which facilitates nerve and bursa friction and trauma, generating neuropathy and shear bursitis [11, 17, 24]. This factor would not be present in cases of second interosseous space neuroma. This is the reason, why some authors think that neuromas, other than in the third interosseous space, [25] do not exist and that symtoms are secondary to bursitis and metatarsophalangeal synovitis.

4.2   Mechanical Factors

Different orthopedic conditions can cause alterations in the biomechanics of plantar support, generating load transfer to the lesser metatarsals, which, added to some of the anatomical factors described above, would favor repetitive trauma on the interdigital nerve, generating neuropathy and symptomatology. These overload conditions can occur at different stages of gait. During the second rocker, for example, the shortening of the gastrocnemius favors a forefoot overload and the generation of an interdigital neuritis. In the third rocker, multiple alterations can generate load transfer to the lateral metatarsals, for example, hallux valgus, hallux rigidus, first ray insufficiency, long central metatarsals, etc. [26]. The previously mentioned alterations exacerbate the trauma on the plantar interdigital nerves during walking, especially when the metatarsophalangeal joints are in maximum dorsiflexion, which occurs, for example, with the use of high-heeled shoes. Anatomically, this exposes the interdigital nerves at the metatarsal level to trauma, which, associated with any of the anatomical predisposing factors described above, would increase the risk of traumatic neuropathy. This situation could explain the higher frequency of Morton's neuroma in the female population [11]. Likewise, in the context of a patient with plantar fat atrophy, repetitive loads can make the nerve more vulnerable to injury [8]. Watcher [27] and Franson [28] associate it to the pes cavus, through the increase of the tension of the plantar fascia on the transverse ligament, which would favor the microtrauma to the nerve. On the other hand, other authors associate it to the pronation present in flat foot, which would produce traction by neural stretching [29–33]. However, other authors [34] mention that there would be no evidence that Morton's neuroma is especially associated with any foot disorder.

4.3   Neural Compression Factor

The works of Lassman [21] and Graham [35] demonstrated a series of histological changes in the interdigital nerve, exclusively distal to the transverse intermetatarsal ligament. For this reason, Gautier in 1979 [10] and later other authors suggest that the most important factor in the etiopathogenesis of Morton's neuroma is a interdigital plantar nerve entrapment neuropathy at the level of the transverse intermetatarsal ligament, which would be predisposed by the anatomical characteristics of the osteofibrous space where the nerve is located [10, 11, 20, 21, 35–37].

4.4   Inflammatory Factor

Some authors have postulated that traumatic intermetatarsal bursitis, associated with any of the mechanical factors described above, could produce irritation due to nerve contiguity. Chronic perineural inflammation would secondarily produce neurofibrosis. Thus, intermetatarsal bursitis would not produce pathology by true compression, but secondarily by inflammation [11, 19, 38]. On the other hand, different pathologies of the metatarsophalangeal joints, especially those associated with metatarsphalangeal joint bursitis (e.g. deformity of the lesser toes or a metatarsophalangeal dislocation secondary to rupture of the plantar plate), could end up having neuropathy due to mechanical traction and inflammatory soft tissue changes [8, 11]. Thus, it has been described that 10–15% of the patients with metatarsophalangeal deformities have neurological symptoms [11].

4.4.1 Ischemic Factor

Nissen [39] and Ringertz [40] suggest that the decrease in blood supply as a result of degenerative changes in the lateral plantar artery would cause ischemia of the peripheral nerves, which in turn would increase perineural fibrosis and interdigital neuropathy. Although this etiopathogenic factor is not very considered today, multiple histopathological studies of Morton's neuromas show the presence of arteriolar vessels of diminished size [22, 23, 41].

4.4.2 Extrinsic Factors

The presence of extrinsic compressive and/or irritative lesions could also generate neurological symptoms, such as tumor lesions (e.g., synovial cyst of the metatarsophalangeal joint, hypertrophic pseudoarthrosis of the metatarsal, rheumatoid nodule, rupture of the plantar plate, etc.). The presence of a thickening of the intermetatarsal transverse ligament of the second space has been described in some patients, which would favor neural compression [11]. Also, direct trauma to the nerve, such as a fall from a heavy object, or a previous foot lesion could generate a traumatic neuropathy of the interdigital nerve [8].

5 Diagnosis

5.1 Clinical Presentation

The diagnosis of Morton's neuroma is eminently clinical, and many authors consider it the gold standard of diagnosis [1, 11, 41, 42]. The most common symptom is neuritic pain (present in more than 90% of cases), described by the patient as metatarsalgia in the third intermetatarsal space, usually radiated to one or both corresponding toes. Some patients refer to the sensation of "stepping on a foreign body" or "having a wrinkled sock" [8]. There can also be neurological symptoms with symptoms such as tingling, paresthesia, numbness or anesthesia of the corresponding toe(s) [1, 2, 11]. Symptoms in the second intermetatarsal space can also be present, frequently caused by bursitis secondary to a mechanical cause. This bursitis can secondarily generates neuritis.

Usually, the patients refer that their symptoms are exacerbated with the use of narrow anterior shoes and/or high heels and improve when retiring the footwear [11]. It is hypothesized that this phenomenon would be caused by nerve trapping between the metatarsal heads [11]. Less frequently, pain can migrate proximally to the foot, ankle, and leg [1, 11].

The physical examination should be complete, like that of any patient who consults for metatarsalgia. The whole affected extremity should be examined and compared with the healthy one. Special care must be taken with the morphological alterations of the forefoot, which favor the existence of mechanical factors or overloading of the lesser metatarsals, such as the presence of hallux valgus, rupture of the plantar plate, deformities of the lesser toes, etc. [11]. Thus, the inspection should focus on the areas of metatarsal support and the presence of hyperkeratosis [2, 26].

On palpation, the pain is usually located in the affected intermetatarsal space, mainly on plantar palpation. There is usually no dorsal or plantar pain of the metatarsal heads and metatarsophalangeal joints. Palpation of the interosseous space is initially performed locating the examiner's thumb plantarly and the index finger dorsally at the intermetatarsal space. This dorsal-plantar compressive maneuver of the interosseous space, also called intermetatarsal sensitivity test, reproduces the symptoms referred by the patient (pain, burning, paresthesia, which can radiate distally to the affected toes, etc.) [11]. Sometimes a slight increase in volume in the intermetatarsal space can be observed in the area of sensitivity.

Another maneuver to be performed during the physical examination is the lateral compression of the metatarsals or squeeze test (from the first and fifth metatarsals), which produces a decrease in the intermetatarsal space and thus generates a palpable click-type sensation. This can occur in association with pain, which is called "Mulder's sign or click" (Fig. 3). This sign is associated with the existence of Morton's neuroma with a sensitivity described by some authors of up to 94–98% [1, 43–45]. This sign is more usually seen in the third space than in the second one [11].

The neurological examination should include a sensory-motor evaluation of the entire limb, especially to rule out other proximal neurological etiologies with distal symptoms. Palpation and percussion of the posterior tibial nerve should be performed along its entire length. There is usually pain on percussion in the plantar intermetatarsal space (or plantar percussion test) [2, 8]. From the point of view of motor sensory evaluation, there are usually no specific alterations, except in some cases that digital hypoesthesia can be identified.

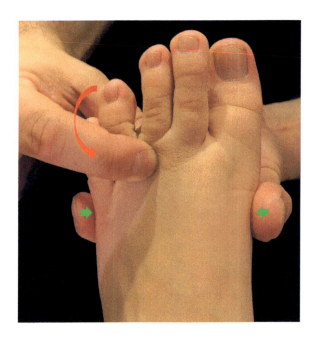

Fig. 3 Dorsal-plantar compression test of the interosseous space (red arrow) and lateral compression test of the metatarsals or squeeze test (green arrows). If this maneuver is associated with a palpable click-and-pain-type sensation, it is called "Mulder's sign or click"

5.2 Imaging Study

Because the diagnosis of Morton's neuroma is eminently clinical, many authors consider that the use of imaging tests is controversial, especially after reports such as Bencardino's [46] and Symeonidis' [47], where the presence of between 33% and 54% of Morton's neuromas in ultrasonography or magnetic resonance imaging in asymptomatic patients is observed. Likewise, Raouf [48] described a statistical correlation between clinical and histopathological findings. A sensitivity of 100%, a positive predictive value of 100%, and a false-positive rate of 0% was found. This calls into question the routine use of preoperative images, which in turn can represent a high economic cost.

For this reason, it is proposed that imaging studies should have the objective of supporting the etiological diagnosis, within the extensive differential diagnosis of metatarsalgia (see differential diagnosis of Morton's neuroma) [26]. Thus, the study begins with a weight-bearing X-ray of the affected foot (anteroposterior, oblique, and lateral projections), which collaborates in the evaluation of osteoarticular anatomy [11].

The most commonly used imaging studies that seek the presence of a thickening and/or increase in the size of the interdigital plantar nerve are ultrasonography (US) and magnetic resonance imaging (MRI). The US has the advantage of being dynamic, lower cost, being performed in less time, and presenting a high sensibility (90%) and specificity (88%). Some specialists consider it the test of choice [8, 49–52]. On the other hand, its limitations are that it is operator-dependent and does not show bone pathology (e.g., bone edema, stress fractures, etc.) that can be part of the

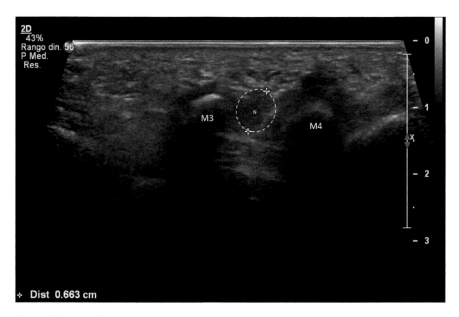

Fig. 4 Ultrasound image showing a 6 mm nodule (N) in the third interosseous space compatible with Morton's neuroma

differential diagnosis of metatarsalgia [8, 50]. Morton's neuroma is observed as an ovoidal mass in the short axis, and as a fusiform and elongated mass in the long axis, relatively hypoechogenic (Fig. 4). The lateral compression maneuver of the metatarsals helps to extrude the content of the space to improve the visualization of an eventual neuroma in the US [53].

Studies with MRI have shown a similarly high sensitivity as in the US (up to 93% in some series), however, with a lower specificity (reported as 68%) [49]. The advantages of this method are that it provides static images that are reproducible and not operator-dependent and can be interpreted by multiple clinicians. It allows an evaluation of all anatomical structures of the forefoot [52]. Its disadvantages are a lower specificity for Morton's neuroma with respect to US, its higher economic cost, and the longer time it requires to be performed [52].

In MRI, Morton's neuroma is usually observed as a well-demarcated ovoidal mass or a low-signal "dumbbell"- or "weight"-shaped mass in T1 and T2, which contrasts with the hyperintense liquid of the intermetatarsal bursa [51, 53]. Coronal cuts are usually the most useful (Fig. 5) [53]. With respect to the use of gadolinium, there are dissimilar reports in the literature, about whether its use allows improving the sensitivity of the exam with respect to the diagnosis of Morton's neuroma [51, 53].

The use of the lidocaine test (2 ml of lidocaine 2% in the affected intermetatarsal space, under the intermetatarsal ligament) with temporary cessation of pain can be useful for diagnostic support, especially if it is performed under US guidance [1].

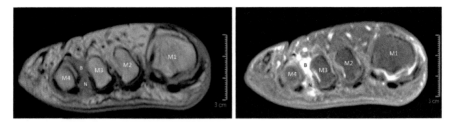

Fig. 5 Magnetic nuclear images showing a dorsal hyperintense area in the third interosseous space, compatible with bursitis (B), and plantar to it is a nodular image of about 7 mm compatible with Morton's neuroma (N)

Table 1 Differential diagnosis of Morton's neuroma

Bone	Mechanic metatarsalgia	First ray insufficiency
		Metatarsal length discrepancy
		Iatrogenic (hallux valgus failed surgery, etc.)
	Stress fracture	
	Freiberg disease	
Joint	Metatarsophalangeal synovitis	Metabolic (gout)
		Autoimmune (rheumatoid arthritis, psoriatic arthritis, etc.)
	Arthrosis/MTP osteochondral lesion	
	Plantar plate rupture	
Tumoral	Benign	Bone
	Malignant	Soft tissue
Neurologic	Peripheral neuropathy	
	Tarsal tunnel syndrome	
	Radiculopathy	
Others	Gastrocnemius tightness	
	Foreign body	

Electrodiagnostic studies are not useful, unless more proximal nerve compression or double crush syndrome is suspected [8, 11].

As already mentioned, because the diagnosis is eminently clinical and the problem to be solved with the imaging study is the differential diagnosis of metatarsalgia, we believe that the test that provides most information about the forefoot anatomy is MRI.

6   Differential Diagnosis

It is extensive, since it must include all the pathologies that cause metatarsalgia (see Table 1) [2, 26].

7 Pathological Anatomy

From the anatomopathological point of view, Morton's neuroma does not correspond to a true benign neoplasm and therefore does not correspond to a neuroma [21, 42]. Moreover, its histology is not very different from biopsies of asymptomatic interdigital nerves [2, 47, 54, 55].

Macroscopically, Morton's neuroma is observed as a whitish-yellowish fusiform volume increase, with a soft and smooth consistency in the nerve (Figs. 6 and 7),

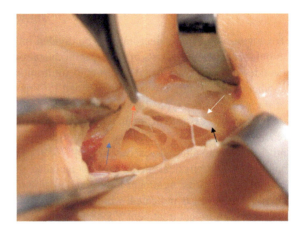

Fig. 6 Dorsal longitudinal approach, identifying the interdigital nerve (blue arrow), the thickened area of Morton's neuroma (red arrow), and both digital branches (white and black arrows)

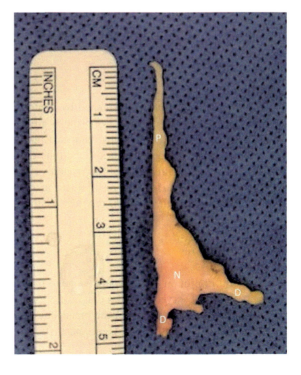

Fig. 7 Resected Morton's neuroma, with the neuroma as an area increased in volume (N), with its two distal branches (D) and its extensive proximal branch of at least 3 cm (P)

just distal to the intermetatarsal transverse ligament and before the digital nerve bifurcation [1].

Histologically, multiple reports characterize it by neural degeneration without signs of Wallerian degeneration, epineural degeneration, sclerohyalinosis of the interstitium, increase of elastic fibers in the stroma, endovascular hyalinization, and peri- and intraneural fibrosis [21, 35, 37, 54].

8 Treatment

Treatment of Morton's neuroma can be divided into conservative or surgical. The initial management consists of footwear modification associated with an insole (that includes a retrocapital insert). Corticoid infiltration at the site of the neuroma is another option. Using this scheme, Bennett [56] reports satisfactory results in 70% of the cases. Other types of infiltrations include the use of alcohol or botulinum toxin. The success rate of treatment using the different methods of infiltration has reached up to 85% [57]. The use of radiofrequency ablation and shock waves are other treatment alternatives described [57–59]. The use of anti-inflammatories, analgesics, and physical therapy is also included in the conservative treatment. In case of conservative treatment failure and symptom persistence after 3–6 months, surgical treatment is indicated, which consists of neuroma resection [56]. The success rate for surgical treatment is 89% [57].

8.1 Conservative Treatment

8.1.1 Orthotics

Initially Morton's neuroma is managed by placing a retrocapital insert associated with a wide shoe (wide toe box). The orthosis aligns the head of the metatarsals and relieves the pressure created by the neuroma on the forefoot, relieving the symptoms. There are retrocapital adhesive buttons that are options for narrower and smaller shoes and summertime shoes (sandals). With regard to the use of insoles, there is no difference in the final result by using alternatives for pronators or supinators [60]. The use of orthoses alone provides an improvement in 48% of patients [57].

8.1.2 Infiltrations

Corticoid infiltration of the neuroma is one of the most frequently used techniques. It is a method that serves both as a diagnostic and therapeutic alternative. There are multiple types of infiltrations for the management of Morton's neuroma, being the use of steroids associated with local anesthetic (usually lidocaine) the most used form in the treatment of the neuroma. A significant relief of symptoms is obtained after the infiltration in 60–80% of the patients, which lasts at least 3 months [61, 62]. The corticoid generates a decrease in the inflammation around the neuroma, which reduces the pressure of the anatomical space and therefore the pain. While Lizano-Díez's study [63] showed that for up to 6 months the isolated use of local anesthetic is as effective in improving pain and function as combining them with steroids, Thompson [61] found that the use of steroids was superior to the use of local anesthetic alone. In addition, other studies have shown favorable results in a wide spectrum of patients with the use of steroids [61, 64, 65]. When comparing corticosteroid infiltration with the use of orthotics, infiltration showed better results at 6 months [66]. The rate of recurrence of symptoms after steroid infiltration is 23% [57]. In addition, the greatest treatment success is achieved when the infiltration is carried out up to 1 year after the onset of symptoms [64]. Infiltration can be performed using ultrasound guidance. However, Mahadevan [14] presented a randomized double-blind study evaluating functional outcomes at 12 months after infiltration with and without ultrasound support, showing no statistically significant difference in functional outcomes between the two groups. Therefore, it is not recommended to routinely perform infiltration under ultrasound assistance. On the other hand, a maximum number of three infiltrations is recommended, separated by at least 3–4 weeks, with no other type of associated treatment. Caution should be exercised when performing the infiltration, due to possible damage to the joint capsule and collateral ligaments and/or atrophy of subcutaneous fat, when placing the medication outside the intermetatarsal space.

Infiltration using alcohol has shown promising results. Alcohol would induce chemical neurolysis, which helps with pain improvement. Studies with 1-year follow-up have shown improvement in functional scales and decrease in the size of the neuroma [67–69]. The treatment success rate is 71% [57], and it also generates a volume decrease of 30% of the neuroma [70, 71]. However, there is a wide range of alcohol concentrations used in the different studies. In Gurdezi's study [67], after 5 years of follow-up, 36% of patients required surgical resolution. Espinosa [72] reported improvement in only 20% of the patients. The use of alcohol generates an extensive fibrosis in the surrounding tissues because it is not specific for the nervous tissue. A secondary surgical resolution is more complex when required. That is why some authors do not recommend its use. This type of infiltration is not currently recommended as first-line treatment by this group of authors, being the infiltration with corticoids the recommendation with better evidence.

8.1.3 Other Conservative Treatments

The use of botulinum toxin A has shown an improvement of 71% of patients at 3 months after an application, without adverse effects. However, 29% showed no improvement [73]. The injection of hyaluronic acid by means of ultrasound support achieved a significant improvement in AOFAS scores (>50 points) at 1 year of follow-up [74]. Ultrasound-guided radiofrequency ablation is a method with promising short-term results, with a success rate of up to 85% [58, 59]. Brooks [75] demonstrated that performing three cycles of ablation obtained a high degree of satisfaction and a low rate of adverse effects. However, studies with a better level of evidence and greater follow-up and comparisons with different treatments are required to define the real efficacy of these treatments.

There is little evidence on the use of shock waves for the treatment of Morton's neuroma. Positive results have been obtained when comparing this treatment with a placebo control group [76]; however, it is not yet a recommended alternative, due to the lack of conclusive literature.

Other options include the use of high-dose vitamin B6 (200 mg daily for 3 months and then 100 mg daily) [77], anti-neuritic drugs, serotonin inhibitors, non-steroidal anti-inflammatory drugs, anti-epileptic drugs, and tricyclic antidepressants, which may reduce patient symptoms.

In general, the improvements achieved with conservative treatments can be permanent or transitory, total, or partial. Some patients decide to manage their symptoms with wide shoes combined with inserts and occasional infiltrations.

8.2   Surgical Treatment

If conservative measures fail, surgical treatment is recommended. Gaynor [78] determined that patients benefit from surgical resolution by obtaining a better success rate. In patients with symptoms lasting less than 6 months, conservative treatment was successful in 38% versus 62% with surgical treatment. In patients with symptoms lasting more than 6 months, 83% improved with surgical treatment. In order to achieve an adequate success rate of surgery, the etiological diagnosis must be adequately performed and the surgical technique carried out. Surgical resection of the thickened neural area (neurectomy) is the most frequently performed surgical treatment. Its success rate is between 51 and 85% in long-term follow-up studies [25, 38, 79, 80]. Fifty percent of patients report no pain after surgery; 30% report being better than before surgery, but with minimal residual pain; and only 10% report worse pain than before surgery [38, 81, 82].

It has also been proposed to associate other surgical gestures with neurectomy: intermuscular transposition to the intermetatarsal space, release of the transverse intermetatarsal ligament (open or endoscopic), neurolysis, transposition of the nerve, and/or osteotomy of the metatarsals. When comparing the results of patients with and without section of the intermetatarsal transverse ligament, a slight improvement was observed in the group where section was performed. In patients where no ligament section was performed, worse results were obtained [81]. Although 83% of good results were obtained with this technique, these were short term, and it remains to be seen whether the results will be maintained with greater follow-up [83].

Endoscopic decompression of the intermetatarsal transverse ligament has shown promising results with a considerable decrease in pain and a low rate of complications [84]. A variant of this technique without endoscopic support was described by Abdelaziz [85] obtaining complete resolution of pain at 26 months in 78% of the patients [85].

The role of metatarsal osteotomy is to increase the space available between the metatarsal heads, decreasing the compression and irritation of the surrounding tissue, specifically the nerve, thus achieving pain reduction. Park [86] compared the release of the transverse ligament versus osteotomies plus ligament release. The functional outcomes were improved in the combined group. However, the authors were unable to define the exact association between metatarsal shortening and neuroma decompression. Later Bauer [87] evaluated the efficacy of percutaneous distal metaphyseal osteotomy and transverse intermetatarsal ligament release when compared to neurectomy in the treatment of Morton's neuroma. After 2 years of follow-up, the patients with isolated neurectomy presented mechanical metatarsalgia, requiring plantar orthoses; however, the group that was also managed with distal metaphyseal osteotomies of the second, third, and fourth metatarsals did not require them. The authors of the study suggest that both treatments are effective, but the patients with osteotomy present better long-term evolution and a lower rate of residual metatarsalgia. The bias of this conclusion is that the study included patients with pain of mechanical origin (not only by the neuroma) and not only in the third intermetatarsal space. That is why it cannot be extrapolated for all Morton's neuroma patients. Therefore, there is currently not enough evidence to show that the outcome of the osteotomy is superior to neurectomy with release of the trans-metatarsal ligament.

There are two types of approaches to perform neurectomy: the dorsal approach and the plantar approach. The choice of approach depends on the surgeon's training and personal preference. No differences have been demonstrated in the functional results of patients operated on for neuroma in relation to the type of approach used [88]. However, the dorsal longitudinal approach would allow early loading and less pathological scarring (formation of hyperkeratosis or keloid) with respect to the plantar. Additionally, multiple authors have published successful results using the dorsal approach. The review carried out by Coughlin [38] with a follow-up of more than 5 years reported good and excellent results in 85% of the patients and pain-free in 65% of them with the same follow-up. For these reasons, the dorsal longitudinal approach is preferred by this group of authors.

In case there are two adjacent neuromas, it is advised the resection of the most symptomatic neuroma and the release of the intermetatarsal transverse ligament of the less symptomatic space, to avoid a significant hypoesthesia of the toe [15, 89]. The results are better when performing the resection of a single neuroma, compared to the resection of multiple neuromas. There is no difference in functional outcomes between patients who had resections of the second versus the third interdigital space [81].

8.2.1 Dorsal Approach

The patient is placed in a supine position by placing a tourniquet on the limb to be operated on. A longitudinal dorsal incision of 2–4 cm is made over the affected intermetatarsal space. Meticulous dissection is performed on the tissue of the inter-metatarsal space to find the intermetatarsal transverse ligament. The ligament is sectioned parallel to the metatarsals. A lamina spreader is placed between the meta-tarsals (to facilitate the vision of the content of the space), and pressure is applied from plantar to dorsal, allowing observation of the thickened region of the nerve. The common interdigital nerve will be observed proximal to the neuroma. A distal dissection is performed until the bifurcation is observed, which will continue dis-tally with two branches of the interdigital nerve (Fig. 6). The resection of the two distal branches of the nerve is performed. The trunk of the common interdigital nerve is identified, carrying out the resection at least 3 cm proximal to the bifurca-tion of the interdigital nerve, making sure not to leave communicating plantar branches. The sectioned plantar nerve is extracted, being bigger than 3 cm, and it is sent to biopsy for the corresponding anatomopathological evaluation (Fig. 7). The biopsy has to confirm that the nerve was resected and not only blood vessels that are anatomically located on the neuroma and can induce error in the surgical technique. Furthermore, it allows the occasional diagnosis of associated pathology such as vasculitis of rheumatological origin. The proximal end of the severed nerve is hid-den in the intrinsic musculature of the foot, reducing the possibility of recurrence by inhibiting the growth of the amputation neuroma [90]. At this point the tourniquet is released to perform hemostasis at the surgical site and to observe the vascular state of the affected toes. In addition, this reduces the possibility of adhesions and the formation of postoperative hematoma. The closure of the subcutaneous cellular tis-sue uses 3.0 resorbable suture. The skin is closed with 4.0 monocryl using the con-tinuous intradermal suture technique. The patient is placed in a compressive bandage and postoperative shoes being authorized to bear weight as tolerated.

8.2.2 Plantar Approach

The plantar longitudinal approach described by Betts [9] can be used for the resec-tion of Morton's neuroma presenting similar functional results in the long term as when performing the dorsal approach. The plantar approach presents better results in the treatment of relapses [90, 91], since a better visualization of the nerve and its residual plantar branches is obtained. The incomplete resection of the plantar branches in the primary surgery is one of the most frequent causes of recurrence.

This approach is done in a longitudinal way, 1 cm proximal to the metatarsal heads, to avoid the formation of scar that affects the load region of the forefoot. The incision is made through the plantar adipose tissue, avoiding the excision of this tissue. The plantar fascia is reached, and after separating the fascicles the neuroma is identi-fied, resecting it in the same way as when performing the dorsal approach. The inter-metatarsal ligament is preserved. The orientation of the incision could be transverse, proximal to the flexion crease of the forefoot. In this way the loading area is avoided, but it can lead to atrophy of the fatty tissue, and it is difficult to follow the interdigital nerve proximally [92]. As mentioned, we reserve the plantar approach mainly for relapses, since it is simpler to find the nerve amputation stump that is located closest to the plantar area (Fig. 8).

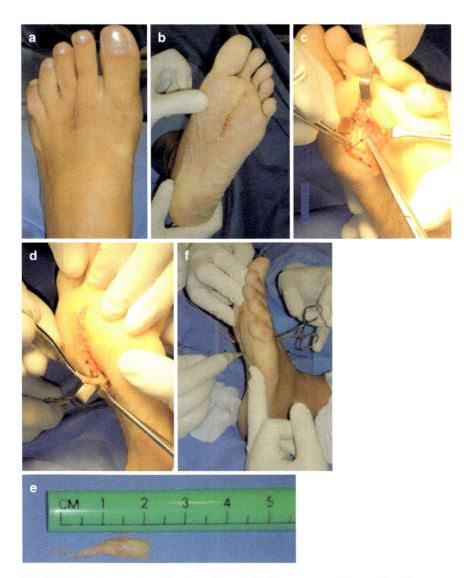

Fig. 8 (**a**) Dorsal approach previously performed. (**b**) Plantar approach for revision of recurrent Morton's neuroma. Longitudinal incision marking on the second plantar interdigital space, proximal to the metatarsal head. (**c**) Intraoperative picture using a plantar approach of recurrent Morton's neuroma with stump neuroma (red arrow). (**d**) Enlarged vision of neuroma in anatomical clamp. (e) Resected area of 2 cm of nerve with stump neuroma. (**f**) Relocation of nerve to a more proximal area, fixing it to the intermetatarsal muscles using fine suture (6-0)

8.2.3 Postoperative Management

Regardless of the approach used, the postoperative management consists of the placement of a compressive bandage, foot elevation, oral analgesics, and authorization to bear weight as tolerated using a postoperative shoe. Suture removal is after 14 days. The patient is warned that an area with hypoesthesia will be felt in the territory of the resected nerve. This hypoesthesia tends to progressively decrease in size, and finally the patient tends not to consciously perceive it despite its persistence. Due to the physiological growth of the amputation neuroma, patients usually experience an increase in local sensitivity around 10 weeks, which subsides after 2–3 weeks spontaneously. Physiotherapy can be prescribed to perform gait training and massage at the incision site to prevent adhesions, area desensitization, and edema management. High-impact activities such as jogging should be avoided until the tenth week.

9 Complications

Among the complications, we find surgical wound infection, residual hematoma, alterations in healing, or complex regional pain syndrome, among others. Akermark [88] conducted a prospective study comparing the plantar and dorsal approaches, obtaining good functional results in both groups. However, in spite of a low and comparable number of complications between both groups, each one of the types of approach has its own complications. The plantar approach presented hypertrophic scar formation. In contrast, the dorsal approach presented erroneous resection of the nerve (resected artery), operative wound dehiscence, operative wound infection, and deep vein thrombosis. Therefore, the patient should be educated about the complications according to the type of approach. It is important to note that the common digital artery is found next to the nerve and is resected in 39% of cases. However, this action does not generate major complications due to the presence of anastomotic communications, unless the arteries in adjacent spaces are resected as well [93]. As previously mentioned, what should not happen is to remove only the artery and leave the nerve in situ.

The failure rate for surgical treatment is 14–21% [94]. One of the usual causes of failure of surgical treatment is incorrect etiological diagnosis of metatarsalgia. To avoid this, it is essential to consider the entire differential diagnosis of Morton's neuroma (see Table 1). As it was already mentioned, the diagnosis is mainly clinical, and the imaging methods allow ruling out associated pathologies. Figure 9 shows a patient in whom an erroneous diagnosis of Morton's neuroma was made. Finally, the patient evolves with erythema nodosum in the lower left extremity being diagnosed with vasculitis. For this reason, the correct diagnosis is essentially with the clinical history and physical examination [95]. In addition, the patient's biomechanical alterations of the forefoot and comorbidities should also be considered.

Fig. 9 Erythema nodosum
of the lower left extremity,
consistent with the
diagnosis of vasculitis

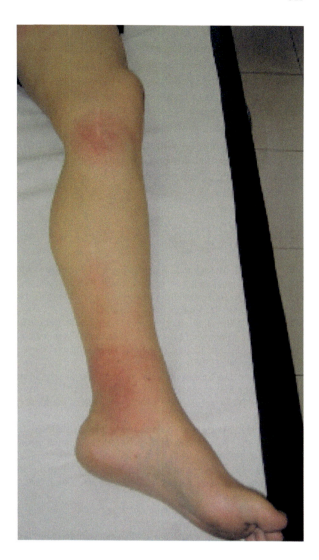

Fig. 9 Erythema nodosum of the lower left extremity, consistent with the diagnosis of vasculitis

9.1 Morton's Neuroma Revision Surgery

The main causes of failure of primary surgical treatment are the presence of an unidentified adjacent neuroma, incomplete resection of plantar branches, and recurrence of the neuroma, called amputation neuroma. The most common form of post-surgical residual pain treatment is the use of steroid infiltration. Using this method, adhesions and remaining scar tissue are released. If the symptoms persist, one option is revision surgery (Fig. 8a–f).

The resection of the proximal neuroma is performed through a plantar approach (Fig. 8b); after performing a dissection through the plantar fascia, the nerve is identified with its medial or lateral plantar branch (Fig. 8c and d). Afterwards, the neuroma is resected (Fig. 8e) with its plantar branches, and the remaining proximal nerve is redirected to a more proximal location, fixing it within the intermetatarsal muscles using a fine suture (6-0) (Fig. 8f). The nerve should be buried at least 1 cm away from the skin [96].

The success rate for eliminating pain from primary surgery is 80% [90]; however, the success rate for revision surgery is less than that of primary neurectomy, which should be discussed with the patient.

References

1. Di Caprio F, Meringolo R, Shehab Eddine M, Ponziani L. Morton's interdigital neuroma of the foot: a literature review. Foot Ankle Surg. 2018;24(2):92–8.
2. Gougoulias N, Lampridis V, Sakellariou A. Morton's interdigital neuroma: instructional review. EFORT Open Rev. 2019;4(1):14–24.
3. Larson EE, Barrett SL, Battiston B, Maloney CT Jr, Dellon AL. Accurate nomenclature for forefoot nerve entrapment: a historical perspective. J Am Podiatr Med Assoc. 2005;95(3):298–306.
4. Civinini F. Su di un gangliare rigonfiamento della pinata del plede. Mem Chir Archiespedale. 1835;4
5. Durlacher L. A treatise on corns, bunions, the diseases of nails, and the general management of the feet. Simpkin, Marshall, London, 1845, 52.
6. Morton TG. A peculiar and painful affection of the fourth metatarsophalangeal articulation. Am J Med Sci. 1876;71:37.
7. Hoadley A. Six cases of metatarsalgia. Chicago Med Rec. 1893;5:32–7.
8. Peters PG, Adams SB Jr, Schon LC. Interdigital neuralgia. Foot Ankle Clin N Am. 2011;16:305–15.
9. Betts L. Morton's metatarsalgia: neuritis of the fourth digital nerve. Med J Aust. 1940;1
10. Gauthier G. Thomas Morton's disease: a nerve entrapment syndrome. Clin Orthop Relat Res. 1979;142:90–2.
11. Schon LC, Mann RA. Disease of the nerves. In: Surgery of the foot and ankle surgery, vol. I. 8th ed. Mosby Elsevier. Philadelphia; 2007.
12. Bradley N, Miller WA, Evans JP. Plantar neuroma analysis of results following surgical excision in 145 patients. South Med J. 1976;69:853.
13. Mahadevan D, Salmasi M, Whybra N, Nanda A, Gaba S, Mangwani J. What factors predict the need for further intervention following corticosteroid injection of Morton's neuroma? Foot Ankle Surg. 2016;22:9–11.
14. Mahadevan D, Attwal M, Bhatt R, Bhatia M. Corticosteroid injection for Morton's neuroma with or without ultrasound guidance: a randomised controlled trial. J Bone Joint J. 2016;98-B:498–503.
15. Thompson FM, Deland JT. Occurrence of two interdigital neuromas in one foot. Foot Ankle. 1993;14:15–7.
16. Levitsky KA, Alman BA, Jesevar DS, Morehead J. Digital nerves of the foot: anatomic variations and implications regarding the pathogenesis of the interdigital neuroma. Foot Ankle. 1993;14:208–14.
17. Govsa F, Bilge O, Ozer MA. Anatomical study of the communicating branches between the medial and lateral plantar nerves. Surg Radiol Anat. 2005;27:377–81.

18. Frank PW, Bakkum BW, Darby SA. The communicating branch of the lateral plantar nerve: a descriptive anatomic study. Clin Anat. 1996;9(4):237–43.
19. Bossley CJ, Cairney PC. The intermetatarsophalangeal bursa: its significance in Morton's metatarsalgia. J Bone Joint Surg Br. 1980;62:184–7.
20. Valero J, Salcini JL, Gallart J, Gonzalez L. Revisión de las teorías acerca de la etiología del neuroma de morton. Revista Española de Podología. 2015;XXVI(2):42–9.
21. Lassmann G. Morton's toe: clinical, light, and electron microscopic investigations in 133 cases. Clin Orthop Relat Res. 1979;142:73–84.
22. Valero J, Gallart J, Gonzalez D, Deus J, Lahoz M. Multiple interdigital neuromas. A retrospective study of 279 feet with 462 neuromas. J Foot Ankle Surg. 2015;54(3):320–2.
23. Volpe A. La sindrome di Morton. Lo Scalpello. 2011;25:60–73.
24. Wu KK. Morton's interdigital neuroma: a clinical review of its etiology, treatment and results. J Foot Ankle Surg. 1996;35(2):112–9; discussion 187–8.
25. Mann RA, Reynolds JD. Interdigital neuroma: a critical clinical analysis. Foot Ankle. 1983;3:238.
26. Espinosa N, Brodsky JW, Maceira E. Metatarsalgia. J Am Acad Orthop Surg. 2010;18(8):474–85.
27. Wachter S, Nilson RZ, ThulJR. The relationship between foot structure and intermetatarsal neuromas. J Foot Surg. 1984;23(6):436–9.
28. Franson J, Baravarian B. Intermetatarsal compression neuritis. Clin Podiatr Med Surg. 2006;23:569–78.
29. Sgarlatto T. Compendium of podiatric biomechanics. San Francisco: California College of Podiatric Medicine; 1971. p. 31.
30. Levy M, Seelenfreund M, Maor P, Fried A. Post-traumatic Morton's neuroma. Harefuah. 1972;83(5):202–33.
31. Shephard E. Intermetatarsophalangeal bursitis in the causation of Morton's metatarsalgia. J Bone Joint Surg. 1975;57B:115–33.
32. Carrier PA, Janigan JD, Weil LS, Smith SD. Morton's neuroma: a possible contributing etiology. J Am Podiatry Assoc. 1975;65(4):315–21.
33. Silvermann LJ. Morton's toe or Morton's neuralgia. J Am Podiatry Assoc. 1976;66:749.
34. Tate RO, Rusin JJ. Morton's neuroma: its ultrastructural anatomy and biomechanical etiology. J Am Podiatry Assoc. 1978;68(12):797–807.
35. Graham CE, Graham DM. Morton's neuroma: a microscopic evaluation. Foot Ankle. 1984;5:150–3.
36. Dellon AL, Aszmann OC. Treatment of superficial and deep peroneal neuromas by resection and translocation of the nerves into the anterolateral compartment. Foot Ankle Int. 1998;19(5):300–3.
37. Weinfeld SB, Myerson MS. Interdigital neuritis: diagnosis and treatment. J Am Acad Orthop Surg. 1996;4(6):328–35.
38. Coughlin MJ, Pinsonneault T. Operative treatment of interdigital neuroma. A long-term follow-up study. J Bone Joint Surg Am. 2002;84:1276–7.
39. Nissen KI. Plantar digital neuritis. Morton's metatarsalgia. J Bone Joint Surg Br. 1948;30B(1):84–94.
40. Ringertz N, Unander-Scharin L. Morton's disease: a clinical and pathoanatomical study. Acta Orthop Scand. 1950;19:327.
41. Mulder JD. The causative mechanism in Morton's metatarsalgia. J Bone Joint Surg Br. 1951;33:94–5.
42. Giannini S, Bacchini P, Ceccarelli F, Vanini F. Interdigital neuroma: clinical examination and histopathologic results in 63 cases treated with excision. Foot Ankle Int. 2004;25(2):79–84.
43. Claassen L, Bock K, Ettinger M, Waizy H, Stukenborg-Colsman C, Plaass C. Role of MRI in detection of Morton's neuroma. Foot Ankle Int. 2014;35(10):1002–5.
44. Mahadevan D, Venkatesan M, Bhatt R, Bhatia M. Diagnostic accuracy of clinical tests for Morton's neuroma compared with ultrasonography. J Foot Ankle Surg. 2015;54(4):549–53.

45. Pastides P, El-Sallakh S, Charalambides C. Morton's neuroma: A clinical versus radiological diagnosis. Foot Ankle Surg. 2012;18(1):22–4.
46. Bencardino J, Rosenberg ZS, Beltran J, et al. Morton's neuroma: is it always symptomatic? AJR Am J Roentgenol. 2000;175(3):649–53.
47. Symeonidis PD, Iselin LD, Simmons N, Fowler S, Dracopoulos G, Stavrou P. Prevalence of interdigital nerve enlargements in an asymptomatic population. Foot Ankle Int. 2012;33(7):543–7.
48. Raouf T, Rogero R, McDonald E, Fuchs D, Shakked RJ, Winters BS, Daniel JS, Pedowitz DI, Raikin SM. Value of preoperative imaging and intraoperative histopathology in Morton's neuroma. Foot Ankle Int. 2019;40(9):1032–6.
49. Xu Z, Duan X, Yu X, Wang H, Dong X, Xiang Z. The accuracy of ultrasonography and magnetic resonance imaging for the diagnosis of Morton's neuroma: a systematic review. Clin Radiol. 2015;70(4):351–8.
50. Shapiro PP, Shapiro SL. Sonographic evaluation of interdigital neuromas. Foot Ankle Int. 1995;16(10):604–6.
51. Hulstaert T, Hulstaert T, Shahabpour M, Provyn S, Lenchik L, Simons P, Vanheste R, De Maeseneer M. Forefoot pain in the lesser toes: anatomical considerations and magnetic resonance imaging findings. Can Assoc Radiol J. 2019;70(4):408–15.
52. Bignotti B, Signori A, Sormani MP, Molfetta L, Martinoli C, Tagliafico A. Ultrasound versus magnetic resonance imaging for Morton neuroma: systematic review and meta-analysis. Eur Radiol. 2015;25(8):2254–62.
53. Ruiz F, Tomás P, Pryest P, Martínez A, Prados N. Role of imaging methods in diagnosis and treatment of Morton's neuroma. World J Radiol. 2018;10(9):91–9.
54. Morscher E, Ulrich J, Dick W. Morton's intermetatarsale neuroma: morphology and histological substrate. Foot Ankle Int. 2000;21(7):558–62.
55. Bourke G, Owen J, Machet D. Histological comparison of the third interdigital nerve in patients with Morton's metatarsalgia and control patients. Aust N Z J Surg. 1994;64(6):421–4.
56. Bennett GL, Graham CE, Mauldin DM. Morton's interdigital neuroma: a comprehensive treatment protocol. Foot Ankle Int. 1995;16(12):760–3.
57. Valisena S, Petri GJ, Ferrero A. Treatment of Morton's neuroma: a systematic review. Foot Ankle Surg. 2018;24(4):271–81.
58. Moore JI, Rosen R, Cohen J, Rosen B. Radiofrequency thermoneurolysis for the treatment of Morton's neuroma. J Foot Ankle Surg. 2012;51:20–2.
59. Chuter GS, Chua YP, Connell DA, Blackney MC. Ultrasound-guided radiofrequency ablation in the management of interdigital (Morton's) neuroma. Skelet Radiol. 2013;42:107–11.
60. Kilmartin TE, Wallace WA. Effect of pronation and supination orthosis on Morton's neuroma and lower extremity function. Foot Ankle Int. 1994;15(5):256–62.
61. Thomson CE, Beggs I, Martin DJ, McMillan D, Edwards RT, Russell D, Yeo ST, Russell IT, Gibson JN. Methylprednisolone injections for the treatment of Morton neuroma. J Bone J Surg Am. 2013;95(9):790–8.
62. Greenfield J, Rea J Jr, Ilfeld FW. Morton's interdigital neuroma. Indications for treatment by local injections versus surgery. Clin Orthop Relat Res. 1984;185:142–4.
63. Lizano-Díez X, Ginés-Cespedosa A, Alentorn-Geli E, Pérez-Prieto D, González-Lucena G, Gamba C, De Zabala S, Solano-López A, Rigol-Ramón P. Corticosteroid injection for the treatment of Morton's neuroma: a prospective, double-blinded, randomized, placebo-controlled trial. Foot Ankle Int. 2017;38:944–51.
64. Markovic M, Crichton K, Read JW, Lam P, Slater HK. Effectiveness of ultrasound-guided corticosteroid injection in the treatment of Morton's neuroma. Foot Ankle Int. 2008;29(5):483–7.
65. Thomson CE, Gibson JA, Martin D. Interventions for the treatment of Morton's neuroma. Cochrane Database Syst Rev. 2004; https://doi.org/10.1002/14651858.CD003118.pub2.
66. Saygi B, Yildirim Y, Saygi EK, Kara H, Esemenli T. Morton neuroma: compara- tive results of two conservative methods. Foot Ankle Int. 2005;26(7):556–9.

67. Gurdezi S, White T, Ramesh P. Alcohol injection for Morton's neuroma: a five- year follow-up. Foot Ankle Int. 2013;34(8):1064–7.
68. Dockery GL. The treatment of intermetatarsal neuromas with 4% alcohol sclerosing injections. J Foot Ankle Surg. 1999;38(6):403–8.
69. Pasquali C, Vulcano E, Novario R, Varotto D, Montoli C, Volpe A. Ultrasound- guided alcohol injection for Morton's neuroma. Foot Ankle Int. 2015;36(1):55–9.
70. Musson RE, Sawhney JS, Lamb L, Wilkinson A, Obaid H. Ultrasound guided alcohol ablation of Morton's neuroma. Foot Ankle Int. 2012;33(3):196–201.
71. Fanucci E, Masala S, Fabiano S, Perugia D, Squillaci E, Varrucciu V, Simonettiet G. Treatment of intermetatarsal Morton's neuroma with alcohol injection under US guide: 10-month follow-up. Eur Radiol. 2004;14(3):514–8.
72. Espinosa N, Seybold JD, Jankauskas L, Erschbamer M. Alcohol sclerosing therapy is not effective treatment for interdigital neuroma. Foot Ankle Int. 2011;32(6):576–80.
73. Climent JM, Mondéjar-Gómez F, Rodríguez-Ruiz C, Díaz-Llopis I, Gómez- Gallego D, Martín-Medina P. Treatment of Morton neuroma with botulinum toxin A: a pilot study. Clin Drug Investig. 2013;33(7):497–503.
74. Lee K, Hwang IY, Hyu Ryu C, Woo Lee J, Woo Kang S. Ultrasound guided hyaluronic acid injection for management of Morton's neuroma. Foot Ankle Int. 2018;39(2):201–4.
75. Brooks D, Parr A, Bryceson W. Three cycles of radiofrequency ablation are more efficacious than two in the management of Morton's neuroma. Foot Ankle Spec. 2018;11(2):107–11.
76. Fridman R, Cain JD, Weil L Jr. Extracorporeal shockwave therapy for interdigital neuroma: a randomized, placebo-controlled, double-blind trial. J Am Podiatr Med Assoc. 2009;99:191–3.
77. Bae SY, Jung EY, Oh SC. Pyridoxine in the treatment of peripheral nerve related foot pain. J Korean Foot Ankle Soc. 2013;17:203–8.
78. Gaynor R, Hake D, Spinner SM, Tomczak RL. A comparative analysis of conservative versus surgical treatment of Morton's neuroma. J Am Podiatr Med Assoc. 1989;79:27–30.
79. Womack JW, Richardson DR, Murphy GA, Richardson EG, Ishikawa SN. Long- term evaluation of interdigital neuroma treated by surgical excision. Foot Ankle Int. 2008;29:574–7.
80. Nery C, Raduan F, Del Buono A, Asaumi ID, Maffulli N. Plantar approach for excision of a Morton neuroma: a long-term follow-up study. J Bone Joint Surg Am. 2012;94(7):654–8.
81. Kasparek M, Schneider W. Surgical treatment of Morton's neuroma: clinical results after open excision. Int Orthop. 2013;37:1857–61.
82. Bucknall V, Rutherford D, Macdonald D, Shalaby H, McKinley J, Breusch SJ. Outcomes following excision of Morton's interdigital neuroma: a prospective study. Bone Joint J. 2016;98-B:1376–81.
83. Rosenberg G, Sferra J. Morton's neuroma, primary and recurrent and their treatment. Foot Ankle Clin. 1998;473–484
84. Shapiro SL. Endoscopic decompression of the inter-metatarsal nerve for Morton's neuroma. Foot Ankle Clin. 2004;9:397–407.
85. Abdelaziz M, Whitelaw K, Waryasz G, Guss D, Johnson A, Di Giovanni C. Isolated intermetatarsal ligament release as a primary surgical management for Morton neuroma: the carpal tunnel of the foot? Foot Ankle Orth. 2018;3(3):2473011418S0013.
86. Park EH, Kim YS, Lee HJ, Koh YG. Metatarsal shortening osteotomy for decompression of Morton's neuroma. Foot Ankle Int. 2013;34(12):1654–60.
87. Bauer T, Gaumetou E, Klouche S, Hardy P, Maffulli N. Metatarsalgia and Morton's disease: comparison of outcomes between open procedure and neurectomy versus percutaneous metatarsal osteotomies and ligament release with a minimum of 2 years of follow-up. J Foot Ankle Surg. 2015;54(3):373–7.
88. Akermark C, Crone H, Skoog A, Weidenhielm L. A prospective randomized controlled trial of plantar versus dorsal incisions for operative treatment of primary Morton's neuroma. Foot Ankle Int. 2013;34(9):1198–204.
89. Benedetti RS, Baxter DE, Davis PF. Clinical results of simultaneous adjacent interdigital neurectomy in the foot. Foot Ankle Int. 1996;17:264–8.

90. Wolfort SF, Dellon AL. Treatment of recurrent neuroma of the interdigital nerve by implantation of the proximal nerve into muscle in the arch of the foot. J Foot Ankle Surg. 2001;40(6):404–10.
91. Johnson JE, Johnson KA, Unni KK. Persistent pain after excision of an interdigital neuroma: results of reoperation. J Bone Joint Surg Am. 1988;70:651–7.
92. Alexander IJ, Johnson KA, Parr JW. Morton's neuroma: a review of recent concepts. Orthopedics. 1987;10(1):103–6.
93. Su E, Di Carlo E, O'Malley M, Bohne WH, Deland JT, Kennedy JG. The frequency of digital artery resection in Morton interdigital neurectomy. Foot Ankle Int. 2006;27(10):801–3.
94. Faraj AA, Hosur A. The outcome after using two different approaches for excision of Morton's neuroma. Chin Med J (Engl). 2010;123(16):2195–8.
95. Sharp RJ, Wade CM, Hennessy MS, Saxby TS. The role of MRI and ultrasound imaging in Morton's neuroma and the effect of size of lesion on symptoms. J Bone Joint Surg (Br). 2003;85-B:999–1005.
96. Wagner E, Ortiz C. The painful neuroma and the use of conduits. Foot Ankle Clin N Am. 2011;16:295–304.

Bunionette

Manuel Resende Sousa, Daniel Ribeiro Mendes, and João Vide

1 Introduction

The term "bunionette" refers to the lateral prominence of the fifth metatarsal (M5) head and the abnormality of its surrounding soft tissues. Such condition has been found frequently in tailors, due to the cross-legged position adopted at their work, thus being also commonly designated as "tailor's bunion" [1] (Fig. 1).

1.1 Epidemiology

Although the incidence and prevalence in the general population are not known, the bunionette deformity is three to ten times more common in women than men and has a peak incidence during the fourth and fifth decades of life [6, 7].

In one series 66% of the patients also had *pes planus* [15]. Other common associated forefoot abnormalities include adducted fifth toe, digital rotational component to the axial deformity, hammer fifth toe, and hallux valgus. When the latter occurs with a bunionette due to an increased angle between the fourth and the fifth

M. Resende Sousa (✉)
Foot and Ankle Unit at Hospital da Luz, Lisbon, Portugal

Department of Youth Football at Sport Lisboa e Benfica, Lisbon, Portugal
e-mail: manuelsousa@peetornozelo.pt

D. Ribeiro Mendes
Foot and Ankle Unit at Hospital Cuf Tejo, Lisbon, Portugal

J. Vide
Foot and Ankle Surgeon at Hospital da Luz, Lisbon, Portugal

Foot and Ankle Surgeon at Hospital Particular do Algarve, Faro, Portugal

E. Wagner Hitschfeld, P. Wagner Hitschfeld (eds.), *Foot and Ankle Disorders*,
https://doi.org/10.1007/978-3-030-95738-4_23

517

Fig. 1 Bunionette

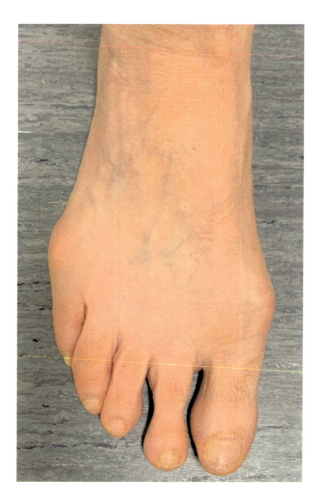

metatarsals (4–5 IM angle), a wide splayed foot deformity results [5, 12, 23, 32, 50]. A splayed foot is present in up to 7.4% of patients with hallux valgus, of which 60.7% meet surgical criteria and are sometimes overlooked [13]. The identification and appropriate treatment of this and other symptomatic foot pathology are paramount to success.

2 Anatomy and Etiology

Fifth metatarsal shape, rotation, and alignment, as well as exogenous factors, may predispose patients to a painful bunionette. These factors, adapted from Koti [30], are summarized in Table 1.

Table 1 Contributing factors for bunionette

Endogenous factors
A. M5 rotation

Abnormal foot position (lateral aspect of the foot resting on the ground)
Excessive pronation
  Fifth tarsometatarsal joint hypermobility
  Associated pronation of subtalar and midtarsal joints
  Pes planus

B. M5 alignment – varus/increased 4–5 IM angle
Incomplete insertion or development of the transverse metatarsal ligament Supernumerary ossicles attached to the lateral fourth metatarsal, pushing the fifth metatarsal laterally
C. M5 shape
Prominent lateral fifth metatarsal head "Dumbbell"-shaped fifth metatarsal head Lateral bending/deviation of the fifth metatarsal Congenital plantar or dorsiflexed fifth ray deformities
D. Hypertrophy of soft tissues overlying the lateral aspect of the M5 head
Exogenous factors   Tight footwear causing pressure around the M5 head

2.1 Clinical Symptoms and Signs

Bunionette is usually a static deformity. Repeated activities such as running or jogging cause friction between the bunionette and a constrictive footwear, leading to inflammation of soft tissues surrounding the fifth metatarsal head, including the overlying bursa [29, 53, 54]. Three main painful areas have been described in relation to the head of fifth metatarsal: the lateral, the dorsolateral, and plantar aspects.

Over time, continued friction and inflammation can evolve to an ulceration or keratosis. In patients with diabetes, advanced Charcot-Marie-Tooth disease, or spinal dysraphism with poor sensibility, can result in superinfection and loss of the entire fifth ray or even the foot [25].

Patients may present plantar keratosis (10–33%), lateral keratosis (50–70%), or a combination of the previous (17–20%) [11, 15, 20, 23, 26, 38]. This differentiation may affect the surgical procedure.

The clinical examination should include a thorough assessment of the patient's past and present medical history, with special emphasis placed on the chronicity of the symptoms, effect of the condition on the activities of daily living, employment responsibilities, and progression of the deformity.

A detailed evaluation of the fifth metatarsal cuboid joint and fifth metatarsal phalangeal joint range of motion, global forefoot posture, and palpation of the periarticular structures to determine areas of maximum signs and symptoms should be performed [44]. Assessment of the neurologic and vascular status is of paramount importance, as adequate peripheral circulation and protective sensation are necessary for postsurgical healing.

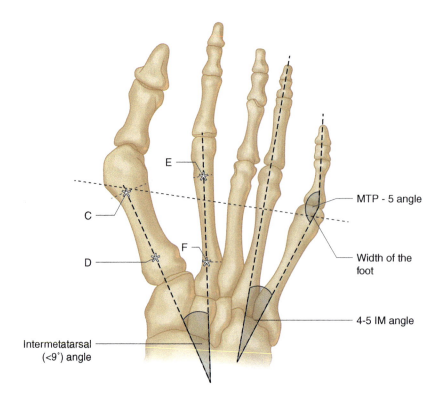

Fig. 2 Radiographic measurements

2.2 Diagnostic and Classification

The bunionette evaluation includes standing dorsoplantar (Fig. 2) and lateral radiographs. Occasionally, a medial oblique (MO) view is performed to assess lateral flare, metatarsal head, lateral tubercle, and lateral soft tissues.

Anatomic variations found in the fifth metatarsal define the classification and guide the treatment recommendations. Coughlin [9] described three types of bunionette deformities based on weight-bearing dorsoplantar radiographs.

Type I deformity (Fig. 3) is an enlargement of the lateral surface of the M5 head and occurs in 27% of cases, either due to an exostosis, a prominent lateral condyle, or a round, or dumbbell-shaped, metatarsal head. The normal width of the metatarsal head is 13 mm or less [17].

However, the radiographic shape of the fifth metatarsal head changes with the metatarsal pronation, just as does the shape of the first metatarsal head with increasing rotation in hallux valgus. With increasing pronation, the lateral plantar tubercle of the fifth metatarsal head becomes more prominent, creating the radiographic impression of an enlarged head [15, 54] and an increase of up to 3° in the 4–5 IM angle [17]; therefore, the radiographic technique may influence significantly the preoperative and postoperative assessment [4]. In fact, Nestor [40] defends that hypertrophy of the metatarsal head is not the cause of tailor's bunion. Diebold [15]

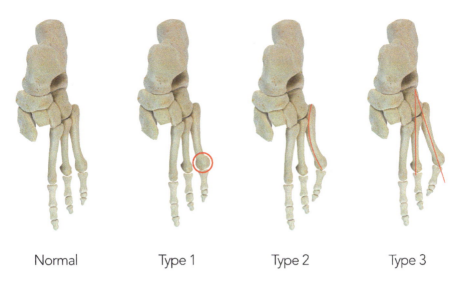

Normal   Type 1   Type 2   Type 3

Fig. 3 Classification

defends that the more or less bowed appearance of the fifth metatarsal is in fact due to its position when the X-ray is taken. Indeed, inversion and eversion of the foot modify this metatarsal appearance [17].

Type II deformity is secondary to abnormal lateral bowing of the distal fifth metatarsal and occurs in 23% of cases. The lateral bowing, or deviation, occurs at the distal third of the fifth metatarsal shaft and is measured between the line drawn from the center of the fifth metatarsal head to its neck and the line made along the medial cortex of the fifth metatarsal. The average lateral deviation angle is normally 2.6° (range, 0°–7°). Symptomatic patients with bunionette deformities have an average value of 8.05° (range, 0–16°) [10].

Type III deformity is an increased in the fourth to fifth intermetatarsal (4–5 IM) angle and occurs in 50% of cases. The 4–5 IMA is measured by bisecting the axis of both bone shafts. The average 4–5 IMA is 6.2° (range 3–11°). In symptomatic patients, the average IMA is 9.6° (range, 5–14°) [10, 13]. In general, a 4–5 IM angle greater than 8° is felt to be abnormal [36].

Differently from Coughlin, Kitaoka et al. [11] reported that fifth metatarsal bowing or an enlarged fifth metatarsal head was observed to be a cause in less than 10% of these cases, with most of the cases being caused by an increased 4–5 IMA (type III).

A *type IV deformity* suggested by Koty [30] consists of two or more components of the other three deformities. Although rare, it is most commonly seen in the rheumatoid patients [1, 8] and does not aid in selecting the appropriate treatment.

The fifth metatarsal-phalangeal (MTP-5) angle expresses the magnitude of the medial deviation of the fifth toe in relation to the axis of the fifth metatarsal. A normal MTP-5 angle is 14° or less [51], averaging 10.2 degrees [40].

The MTP-5 status should be assessed, as pain and swelling may be caused by inflammatory or degenerative pathology [14].

Sagittal plane deformities, although not so common, may also influence the surgical treatment.

3   Treatment

3.1   Conservative Treatment

No evidence-based guidelines exist for the conservative management of bunionette deformity; nevertheless, nonsurgical management should be considered initially.

This includes padding or shaving the keratotic lesion. Patients should wear altered shoes with wider toe box, to accommodate the lateral deformity. Nonsteroidal oral analgesics and corticosteroid injections can be used for the acutely inflamed bursa. Custom orthotics may be used to decrease pronation of the subtalar joint, hence decreasing pressure over the fifth metatarsal head [14].

3.2   Surgical Treatment

Surgery is indicated in the refractory patient (10–23% of all cases) [5]. Several surgical techniques have been described for deformity: lateral condylectomy, distal metatarsal osteotomy, diaphyseal osteotomy, and proximal fifth metatarsal osteotomy (Fig. 4). Other options, like metatarsal head resection, fifth metatarsal ray resection, and isolated soft tissue procedures, are of limited use.

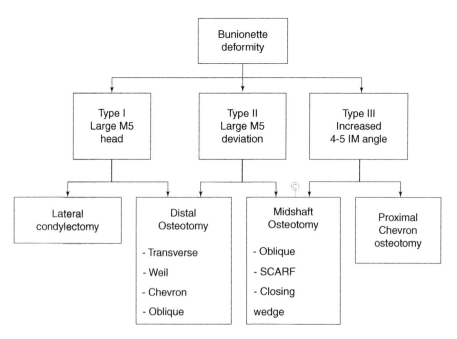

Fig. 4 Surgical treatment options

The goals of surgical intervention are resolution of the symptoms, decreased width of the forefoot as well as the prominence of the bunionette [14], and avoidance of complications [24].

3.2.1 Lateral Condylectomy

This technique was first presented by Davies in 1949 [12]. It is indicated in type I deformity and isolated or as part of other surgical techniques and can be done by either open or percutaneous approach. It is also indicated when more aggressive procedures are not tolerated, and the patient is allowed to immediately ambulate in a postoperative shoe for 3 weeks. A lateral condylectomy is often successful in relieving symptoms. Kitaoka and Holiday [27] reported that 71% of the patients were satisfied with their result.

In isolation, it is not effective in the presence of an intractable plantar keratosis. The presence of pes planus or forefoot pronation is considered a relative contraindication as the pressure will continue due to the position of the hindfoot and forefoot. The most common complications are recurrence of the deformity, MTP joint subluxation and poor weight bearing, the last due to excessive resection [31]. A tight capsule closure with excision of redundant soft tissue (or pant-over-vest suture) plus attention to repair the abductor digiti quinti muscle minimizes medial MTP joint subluxation [26, 29, 50]. Any angle correction is mostly due to associated soft tissue procedures, an effect that decreases over time. Therefore, to avoid deformity recurrence, this technique should be avoided if MTP5/4–5 IM angle is elevated [21, 23, 31, 33, 38, 50, 57].

3.2.2 Fifth Metatarsal Resections

Resection of the fifth metatarsal head, resection of the distal half of the metatarsal, and fifth ray resection have all been used to treat a bunionette deformity, but a high complications rate makes it inappropriate as an initial treatment. Common complications are transfer metatarsalgia to the fourth metatarsal head [16, 19, 31] (75%), malalignment (59%) [16], an average fifth toe retraction of 10 mm (36%) [16, 28, 31], continued symptoms (27%), stiffness (25%), toe subluxation [26, 28], and a flail fifth toe.

These procedures are used as a salvage procedure for infection, ulceration (excellent results in diabetic patients [2]), severe deformity, severe osteopenia, extensive degenerative joint changes, previous failed surgery, or poor medical health [14].

3.2.3 Osteotomy Procedures

Several fifth metatarsal osteotomies have been recommended for the treatment of symptomatic bunionettes. The choice depends on the case-specific anatomic variants and the surgeon's preference. Patients should weight-bear in a postoperative or Barouk shoe for 6 weeks (Fig. 5).

Distal Fifth Metatarsal Osteotomies

The main contraindication to a distal metatarsal osteotomy is a moderate or severe angular deformity.

In the *distal transverse medializing osteotomy*, a transverse vertical osteotomy, perpendicular to the long axis of the fifth metatarsal, is made from lateral to medial, completely transecting the metatarsal neck. The cut creates a shelf that tends to minimize dorsal translation of the capital fragment. A 1.8 mm Kirschner wire (K wire) is inserted into the soft tissue adjacent to the toe on the lateral aspect and driven distally out the tip of the fifth toe. With the capital fragment displaced as far

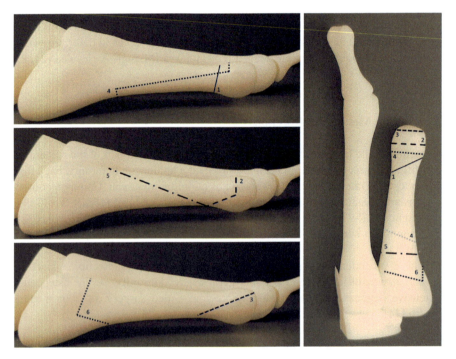

Fig. 5 M5 osteotomies. (1) Capital oblique; (2) chevron; (3) modified Weil; (4) scarfette – gray dots represent the dorsal projection of the plantar surface cut; (5) Ludloff; (6) proximal chevron

medialward as desired, the Kirschner wire is then driven proximal into the diaphyseal canal until it penetrates the proximal metaphyseal region. The K wire is removed 4–6 weeks after surgery. Weitzel et al. [56] reported on 21 patients (30 feet) who were noted to have 81% good and excellent results at an average follow-up of more than 7 years. Giannini et al. [21] reported on 32 patients (50 feet) at almost 5 years follow-up with 90% good and excellent results.

Smith and Weil [49] described a *distal oblique medializing osteotomy* without fixation, and later Steinke and Boll [52] added fixation. The osteotomy is oriented in a distal-lateral to proximal-medial direction at an angle of 70° and undercut by 15° (Fig. 5.1). The purpose of this angle is to have the bone slide medially and to avoid dorsal migration of the head. The osteotomy site is fixed with a K wire or with one or two mini-fragment screws.

The bone cut orientation of the *distal chevron osteotomy* is similar to the one performed in the first metatarsal (Fig. 5.2). The distal fragment is displaced medially and fixed according to the surgeon's preference. The remaining metaphyseal flare is shaved. In a case series by Kitaoka et al. [29] with a mean follow-up of 7.1 years, the authors reported improvement in pain control, IMA, forefoot width, and fifth MTP angle after distal chevron osteotomy. Satisfaction rate was 89.5% in 17 of 19 patients. Although the osteotomy is stable by design, fixation and a secure capsule closure are recommended to prevent malunion, nonunion, and recurrence.

Barouk [3] recommends the *capital oblique osteotomy (modified Weil osteotomy)* because of the inherent stability and ease of performance. However, like the chevron procedure, it has limitations in the narrow metatarsal head [55]. Similar to the Weil osteotomy of the lesser metatarsals, the bone cut is parallel to the plantar aspect of the foot (Fig. 5.3). The osteotomy is fixed with a dorsal-plantar mini-fragment screw. Radl et al. [43] reported an improvement in the AOFAS score from 42 to 87 points, no nonunions, and no transfer lesions.

The *percutaneous distal metatarsal osteotomy* is performed through the same incision as for the exostectomy, using a straight burr 2–15, following a 45° oblique angle from dorsal-distal to plantar-proximal. A lateral wedge osteotomy is performed, sparing the medial cortical. A valgus movement is performed on the fifth toe and metatarsal, thus completing the osteotomy with osteoclasis. The post-op bandage must be worn day and night for about 3 weeks [42].

Diaphyseal Fifth Metatarsal Osteotomies

In the presence of a type III deformity or a severe type II deformity, a diaphyseal osteotomy combined with a distal soft tissue procedure affords an excellent means of correction.

The *scarfette osteotomy* is similar to the SCARF osteotomy of the first ray (Fig. 5.4). The osteotomy is fixed with two vertical mini-fragment screws. The remaining lateral shelf of bone is resected with a sagittal saw. Seide and Petersen [46] reported successful results in a follow-up of 10 feet. Maher et al. [35] reported on 28 patients (36 feet) at a mean of 6.5 years. Eighty-six percent were completely satisfied. The mean AOFAS score improved from 44 to 92 points. The most reported complications are shaft fracture [34] and the need for hardware removal [22].

Ludloff first described an oblique osteotomy from the dorsal proximal to the plantar distal aspect of the first metatarsal in 1918 as a treatment option for hallux valgus. Coughlin [11] described a *diaphyseal oblique osteotomy* to correct an increased 4–5 IMA and/or an increased lateral bowing (Figs. 5.5 and 5.6). This oblique osteotomy is rotational rather than translational, which helps to maintain metatarsal length and avoid shortening. Two mini-fragment screws are used to fix the osteotomy site. The initial screw serves as the center of rotation for the osteotomy. Once the osteotomy has been aligned, a second screw is placed to further stabilize the osteotomy site (Fig. 6). Prominent bone at the osteotomy site is resected with a sagittal saw. The fifth MTP joint capsule is repaired, and the fifth toe is brought into proper alignment (Fig. 7). An unreliable patient may be treated with a below-knee walking cast for 6 weeks. Coughlin [11] reported on 30 feet (20 patients) with 31 months follow-up. Ninety-three percent had excellent or good clinical results; all osteotomies healed within 8 weeks, with only one case of a mild transfer lesion. In a report on 11 pediatric patients with a mean follow-up of 32 months, Masquijo et al. [37] noted all results were rated as excellent or good, and the final AOFAS score averaged 92 points (Fig. 6).

Several authors modified the oblique osteotomy to be more bio-mechanically stable with reverse Ludloff osteotomy. The theoretical benefit over the traditional Ludloff osteotomy is the force generated across the osteotomy with weight-bearing, which is a compression force rather than a distraction force across the osteotomy.

Mariano De Prado described the "DRP osteotomy" [42], a *percutaneous diaphyseal osteotomy* performed between the middle third and the distal third with the straight burr 2–15. The osteotomy starts at the medial cortical surface of the fifth metatarsal in a dorsal-distal to plantar-proximal direction at 45°, sparing the lateral cortical bone and creating a medial wedge. Once the desired size is reached, the

Fig. 6 Ludloff osteotomy

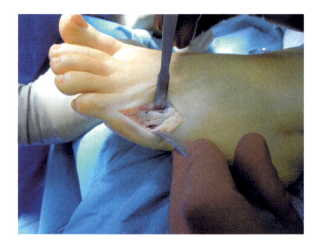

Fig. 7 Clinical result after bilateral Ludloff M5 osteotomies

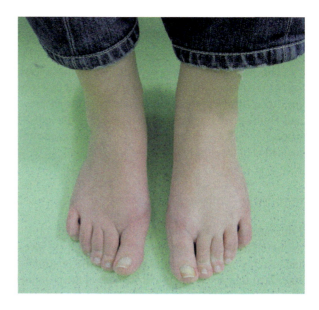

wedge is closed by pressing on the head of the fifth metatarsal to produce osteoclasis of the lateral cortical bone. The post-op bandage must be worn day and night for about 3 weeks (Fig. 7).

In 1972, Gerbert et al. [19] described a *long oblique closing wedge osteotomy* of the fifth metatarsal. The osteotomy runs from distal-medial to proximal-lateral ending at the junction of the lateral shaft and base of the fifth metatarsal and maintaining the proximal-lateral cortical-periosteal hinge. A small 2–3 mm medially based wedge of the bone is then resected from the proximal and medial portion of the fifth metatarsal. The osteotomy is closed with a small bone clamp, and fixation is done with a small, oblique screw, oriented from distal-lateral to proximal-medial. Patient is non-weight-bearing in either a short-leg cast or removable immobilization boot for 6–8 weeks.

Distal fifth metatarsal osteotomy complications are usually a result of either inappropriate soft tissue handling, fixation failure, or inappropriate end position of the M5 head.

After lateral capsulotomy, the remaining blood supply enters the metatarsal head from its medial aspect, so excessive dorsal and plantar soft tissue stripping should be avoided, as it increases the risk of AVN, instability, and fixation failure [41]. Excessive soft tissue tightening to compensate an insufficient bone procedure may result in recurrence of deformity due to progressive tissue attenuation.

The most common causes of fixation failure are no postsurgical protection, the choice of a lower stability osteotomy (transverse < oblique < modified Weill/chevron/scarfette) or the use of a weak implant (screws better the K wires). This may result in a delayed/nonunion with excessive callus formation and an inappropriate end position of the M5 head. Inappropriate surgical technique can also be the cause for failure. On the transverse plane, the M5 head can be located too medially (overcorrected – rare) or too laterally (undercorrection or deformity recurrence – common). On the sagittal plane, an excessive plantar displacement causes plantar keratosis, and a dorsal displacement may translate in transfer metatarsalgia.

Pontious et al. [41] compared distal fifth metatarsal osteotomies that were *internally fixed* to those not fixed. They concluded that osteotomies that were internally fixed healed more predictably and that fixation prevented displacement. Kitaoka and Holiday [29] and Frankel et al. [18] concluded that floating fifth metatarsal osteotomies that seek their own level in an uncontrolled manner have a significant incidence of transfer metatarsalgia.

Proximal Fifth Metatarsal Osteotomy

Fifth metatarsal base osteotomies may be used for severe type III deformities, but nonunion is a serious concern. Shereff et al. [47] investigated the extraosseous and intraosseous arterial vascular supply of the proximal fifth metatarsal. The authors suggested that an osteotomy or fracture in the proximal 2 cm of the fifth metatarsal can injure both the extraosseous and the intraosseous supply, leading to delayed union or nonunion.

A medial-to-lateral *proximal chevron osteotomy* performed with the apex 1 cm distal to the tip of the fifth metatarsal and its horizontal cut oriented distally (Fig. 5.6). The distal fragment is translated medially and stabilized to the fourth metatarsal with small Steinmann pins placed lateral to medial. The pins exit through the skin. Any prominent bone at the osteotomy site is beveled. A below-knee cast is applied for 6 weeks, when Steinmann pins are removed, and the patient is allowed to walk weight-bearing.

Diebold and Bejjani [15] reported excellent results in 90% of cases (12 patients with 1 year average follow-up). No nonunions were reported. Later, in a follow-up report, the same authors confirmed that 22 osteotomies had all successfully healed.

Minimal Incision Surgery

Techniques for minimally invasive osteotomy with or without fixation continue to emerge, with good to excellent results [48]. Postoperative dressings must keep the 4–5 IM angle closed and the fifth toe in the correct position in the first 3 weeks. The first dressing change occurs 7–10 days postoperatively. A postoperative shoe is used for 4 weeks [39].

Delayed bone healing is a well-known phenomenon after percutaneous surgery on the lateral metatarsals. Clinical healing usually precedes radiographic evidence of bone healing by several weeks. In most patients, the osteotomy site was pain free at 6 weeks postoperatively, despite only limited callus formation on X-ray [39].

Concerns of inferior outcomes after minimally invasive correction of type II and III deformities are possibly the result of the inability to address the underlying pathology.

The great majority of cases yielded an acceptable cosmetic result with no scarring or dorsal contracture, but because of the limited outcomes studies available and the tendency toward dorsal malunion, it is difficult to recommend this technique routinely until more extensive data are reported.

Intractable Plantar Keratosis

In the presence of a plantar keratosis (Fig. 8), the chosen osteotomy should allow a controlled elevation of the metatarsal head. This is possible in most osteotomies, as in the distal chevron osteotomy, the modified Weil osteotomy, the scarfette osteotomy, the diaphyseal oblique osteotomy, or the proximal chevron osteotomy. Instead of a horizontal cut, the saw blade is oriented from lateral-plantar to medial-dorsal, so that the capital fragment elevates as it is translated in a medial direction (Fig. 9b).

The amount of sagittal plane M5 head translation increases with the inclination of the osteotomy cut and with the osteotomy site: more proximal osteotomies allow a larger translation. One should be mindful about excessive dorsal translation as transfer metatarsalgia may occur.

Deformity Correction Power

The ability to correct the deformity varies with the type and site of the osteotomy. Proximal procedures are reported to have a larger 4–5 IM angle and MTP5 angle correction power (Table 2).

Surgical Pearls
1. Soft tissue:

    (a) Avoid excessive soft tissue stripping
    (b) Avoid additional correction with soft tissue tightening

2. Use internal fixation device
3. Select correct procedure

    (a) Enough correction power – adequate site
    (b) Address sagittal plane
    (c) Stable enough and low risk of delayed or nonunion

Fig. 8 Intractable plantar
keratosis

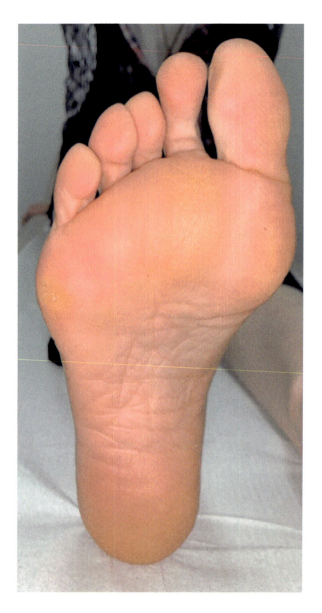

4   Summary

Most painful bunionette deformities respond to nonsurgical management. When
intractable symptoms are refractory to nonsurgical treatment, operative intervention
may be necessary. Lateral eminence resection is reserved for patients with a focal
prominence and no angular deformity of the metatarsal. Metatarsal osteotomies narrow the forefoot, maintain the length of the metatarsal, and preserve function of the

Fig. 9 M5 head translation with medialization (**a**) none; (**b**) dorsal translation; (**c**) plantar translation

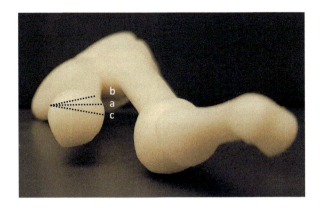

Table 2 Deformity correction power

Bone procedure		4–5 IM A	MTP5 A	Power
Lateral condyle resection		None	Low	Very low[a]
Distal osteotomy		4–5°	8° (55b, 71b)	Low
Percutaneous		4,5°	12°	Low to average
Mid-diaphyseal osteotomy	Scarfette	5–10° (14, 47, 62)	15° (62)	Average
	Oblique	10° [9, 45]	15–17°	Average
Proximal osteotomy		Highest	N/A	High

[a]Correction due to soft-tissue procedure

MTP joint. When appropriate correction can be achieved with the chevron osteotomy, it should be the procedure of choice, because it has the greatest strength and fails in the same manner as the intact fifth metatarsal. Diaphyseal oblique osteotomy and scarfette osteotomy are indicated to treat mild to moderate transverse and sagittal plane deformities and have inherent stability that allow early weight-bearing. Proximal osteotomies allow for larger correction of the IMA compared with distal osteotomies but carry a risk of potential injury to the already tenuous proximal fifth metatarsal blood supply. Newer minimally invasive techniques with expanded corrective power have been reported, with promising results; however, sufficiently powered, prospective, randomized, controlled trials related to surgical bunionette correction are not available.

References

1. Addante JB, Chin M, Makower BL, Lescosky FA, Nowick AR. Surgical correction of tailor's bunion with resection of fifth metatarsal head and silastic sphere implant: an 8-year follow-up study. J Foot Surg. 1986;25:315–20.
2. Armstrong DG, Rosales MA, Gashi A. Efficacy of fifth metatarsal head resection for treatment of chronic diabetic foot ulceration. J Am Podiatr Med Assoc. 2005;95:353–6.

3. Barouk LS. Some pathologies of the fifth ray: tailor's bunion. In: Barouk LS, editor. Forefoot reconstruction. Paris: Springer-Verlag; 2002. p. 276–83.
4. Baumhauer JF, Benedict FD. Osteotomies of the fifth metatarsal. Foot Ankle Clin. 2001;6:3.
5. Bishop J, Kahn A 3rd, Turba JE. Surgical correction of the splayfoot: the Giannestras procedure. Clin Orthop Relat Res. 1980;146:234–8.
6. Boyer ML, Deorio JK. Bunionette deformity correction with distal chevron osteotomy and single absorbable pin fixation. Foot Ankle Int. 2003;24:834–7.
7. Buchbinder IJ. DRATO procedure for tailor's bunion. J Foot Surg. 1982;21:177–80.
8. Catanzariti AR, Friedman C, DiStazio J. Oblique osteotomy of the fifth metatarsal: a five-year review. J Foot Surg. 1988;27:316–20.
9. Cohen BE, Nicholson CW. Bunionette deformity. J Am Acad Orthop Surg. 2007;15:300–7.
10. Coughlin MJ. Etiology and treatment of the bunionette deformity. Instr Course Lect. 1990;39:37–48.
11. Coughlin MJ. Treatment of bunionette deformity with longitudinal diaphyseal osteotomy with distal soft tissue repair. Foot Ankle. 1991;11:195–203.
12. Davies H. Metatarsus quintus valgus. Br Med J. 1949;1:664.
13. Deveci, et al. An overlooked deformity in patients with hallux valgus: Tailor's bunion. JAPMA. 2015;15(3):233–7.
14. Didomenico, et al. Revisiting the Tailor's bunion and adductovarus deformity of the fifth digit. Clin Podiatr Med Surg. 2013;30:397–422.
15. Diebold PF, Bejjani FJ. Basal osteotomy of the fifth metatarsal with intermetatarsal pinning: a new approach to tailor's bunion. Foot Ankle. 1987;8:40–5.
16. Dorris MF, Mandel LM. Fifth metatarsal head resection for correction of tailor's bunions and sub-fifth metatarsal head keratoma: a retrospective analysis. J Foot Surg. 1991;30(269):275.
17. Fallat LM, Buckholz J. An analysis of the tailor's bunion by radiographic and anatomical display. J Am Podiatry Assoc. 1980;70:597–603.
18. Frankel JP, Turf RM, King BA. Tailor's bunion: clinical evaluation and correction by distal metaphyseal osteotomy with cortical screw fixation. J Foot Surg. 1989;28:237–43.
19. Gerbert J, Sgarlato TE, Subotnick SI. Preliminary study of a closing wedge osteotomy of the fifth metatarsal for correction of a Tailor's bunion deformity. J Am Podiatry Assoc. 1972;62:212–8.
20. Giannestras NJ. Other problems of the foot. In: Giannestras NJ, editor. Foot disorders: medical and surgical management. Philadelphia: Lea and Febiger; 1973. p. 420–1.
21. Giannini S, Faldini C, Vannini F, et al. The minimally invasive osteotomy "S.E.R.I." (simple, effective, rapid, inexpensive) for correction of bunionette deformity. Foot Ankle Int. 2008;29:282–6.
22. Glover JP, Weil L Jr, Weil LS Sr. Scarfette osteotomy for surgical treatment of bunionette deformity. Foot Ankle Spec. 2009;2:73–8.
23. Haber JH, Kraft J. Crescentic osteotomy for fifth metatarsal head lesions. J Foot Surg. 1980;19:66–7.
24. Haddon TB, SJ LP. Relative strength of Tailor's bunion osteotomies and fixation techniques. J Foot Ankle Surg. 2013;52:16–23.
25. Ishikawa SN, Murphy GA. Lesser toe abnormalities. In: Canale ST, editor. Campbell's operative orthopaedics. 10th ed. Philadelphia: Mosby; 2003. p. 4652–60.
26. Kaplan EG, Kaplan G, Jacobs AM. Management of fifth metatarsal head lesions by biplane osteotomy. J Foot Surg. 1976;15:1–8.
27. Kitaoka HB, Holiday AD Jr. Lateral condylar resection for bunionette. Clin Orthop Relat Res. 1992;278:183–92.
28. Kitaoka HB, Holiday AD Jr. Metatarsal head resection for bunionette: long-term follow-up. Foot Ankle. 1991;11:345–9.
29. Kitaoka HB, Holiday AD Jr, Campbell DC 2nd. Distal chevron metatarsal osteotomy for bunionette. Foot Ankle. 1991;12:80–5.
30. Koti M, Maffulli N. Bunionette. J Bone Joint Surg Am. 2001;83-A:1076–82.

31. Leach RE, Igou R. Metatarsal osteotomy for bunionette deformity. Clin Orthop. 1974;100:171–5.
32. Legenstein R, Bonomo J, Huber W, Boesch P. Correction of tailor's bunion with the Boesch technique: a retrospective study. Foot Ankle Int. 2007;28:799–803.
33. Lelièvre J: [Exostosis of the head of the fifth metatarsal bone; tailor's bunion].*Concours Med.* 1956;78:4815–16.
34. Magnan B, Samaila E, Merlini M, Bondi M, Mezzari S, Bartolozzi P. Percutaneous distal osteotomy of the fifth metatarsal for correction of bunionette. J Bone Joint Surg Am. 2011;93:2116–22.
35. Maher AJ, Kilmartin TE. Scarf osteotomy for correction of Tailor's bunion: mid- to long-term followup. Foot Ankle Int. 2010;31:676–82.
36. Mann RA. Keratotic disorders of the plantar skin. In: Mann RA, editor. Surgery of the foot. St Louis: Mosby; 1986. p. 194–8.
37. Masquijo JJ, Willis BR, Kontio K, Dobbs MB. Symptomatic bunionette deformity in adolescents: surgical treatment with metatarsal sliding osteotomy. J Pediatr Orthop. 2010;30:904–9.
38. McKeever DC. Excision of the fifth metatarsal head. Clin Orthop. 1992;278:183–92.
39. Michels F, Bauwhede J, Guillo S, Oosterlinck D, Lavigne C. Percutaneous bunionette correction. Foot Ankle Surg. 2013;19:9–14.
40. Nestor BJ, Kitaoka HB, Ilstrup DM, Berquist TH, Bergmann AD. Radiologic anatomy of the painful bunionette. Foot Ankle. 1990;11:6–11.
41. Pontious J, Brook JW, Hillstrom HJ. Tailor's bunion. Is fixation necessary? J Am Podiatr Med Assoc. 1996;86:63–73.
42. Prado M, Ripoll PL, Golanó P. Cirurgía percutánea del pie 2003.
43. Radl R, Leithner A, Koehler W, Scheipl S, Windhager R. The modified distal horizontal metatarsal osteotomy for correction of bunionette deformity. Foot Ankle Int. 2005;26:454–7.
44. Roukis TS. The tailor's bunionette deformity: a field guide to surgical correction. Clin Podiatr Med Surg. 2005;22:223–45.
45. Schabler JA, Toney M, Hanft JR, Kashuk KB. Oblique metaphyseal osteotomy for the correction of Tailor's bunions: a 3-year review. J Foot Surg. 1992;31:79–84.
46. Seide HW, Petersen W. Tailor's bunion: results of a scarf osteotomy for the correction of an increased intermetatarsal IV/V angle. A report on ten cases with a 1-year follow-up. Arch Orthop Trauma Surg. 2001;121:166–9.
47. Shereff MJ, Yang QM, Kummer FJ, Frey CC, Greenidge N. Vascular anatomy of the fifth metatarsal. Foot Ankle. 1991;11:350–3.
48. Shi GG. Management of Bunionette Deformity. J Am Acad Orthop Surg. 2018;26:e396–404.
49. Smith SD, Weil LS. Fifth metatarsal osteotomy for tailor's bunion deformity: minor surgery of the foot. Mt. Kiscoe: Futura; 1971.
50. Sponsel KH. Bunionette correction by metatarsal osteotomy: preliminary report. Orthop Clin North Am. 1976;7:809–19.
51. Steel MW 3rd, Johnson KA, DeWitz MA, Ilstrup DM. Radiographic measurements of the normal adult foot. Foot Ankle. 1980;1:151–8.
52. Steinke MS, Boll KL. Hohmann-Thomasen metatarsal osteotomy for tailor's bunion (bunionette). J Bone Joint Surg Am. 1989;71:423–6.
53. Stewart M. Miscellaneous affections of the foot. In: Edmonson SA, Crenshaw AH, editors. Campbell's operative orthopaedics. St Louis: Mosby; 1980. p. 1733.
54. Throckmorton JK, Bradlee N. Transverse V sliding osteotomy: a new surgical procedure for the correction of tailor's bunion deformity. J Foot Surg. 1978;18:117–21.
55. Weil L, Consul D. Fifth metatarsal osteotomies. Clin Podiatr Med Surg. 2015;32:333–53.
56. Weitzel S, Trnka HJ, Petroutsas J. Transverse medial slide osteotomy for bunionette deformity: long-term results. Foot Ankle Int. 2007;28:794–8.
57. Yancey HA Jr. Congenital lateral bowing of the fifth metatarsal. Report of 2 cases and operative treatment. Clin Orthop Relat Res. 1969;62:203–5.

Part IV
Adult Orthopaedics: Midfoot, Rearfoot and Ankle

Progressive Collapsing Foot Deformity – Flatfoot

Jaeyoung Kim and Jonathan T. Deland

1 Introduction

The flatfoot deformity in adults comprises a wide spectrum of ligament and posterior tibial tendon (PTT) failure that results in significant deformity and disability. Because dysfunction of the PTT has been considered the culprit of flatfoot deformity in adults, this condition was initially termed posterior tibialis tendon dysfunction (PTTD) and later renamed adult-acquired flatfoot deformity (AAFD). However, the dysfunction of the PTT has not been proven to be the cause of the condition. Results from new imaging modalities have revealed that the shape of the tarsal bones and slope of the posterior facet may be an important predisposing factor contributing to why certain flatfeet get this condition and others do not. Also, because the most debilitating problem is the collapse of the foot secondary to the ligament failure and the tendon can be graded separately, there is now a proposal to rename this condition in order to emphasize the progressive collapse of the foot appropriately. In 2020, an expert consensus group proposed progressive collapsing foot deformity (PCFD) as the better name for the condition with the tendon failure graded separately [1]. Therefore, this book chapter will use the term PCFD when referring to this condition. Paralleling the changes in terminology, the treatment for PCFD has also evolved to shift the focus away from the tendon to increased emphasis on how to treat the collapsing foot deformity. The collapse of the foot and its treatment are the most important determinants of a patient's outcome.

J. Kim · J. T. Deland (✉)
Hospital for Special Surgery, New York, NY, USA
e-mail: delandj@hss.edu

© The Author(s), under exclusive license to Springer Nature
Switzerland AG 2022
E. Wagner Hitschfeld, P. Wagner Hitschfeld (eds.), *Foot and Ankle Disorders*,
https://doi.org/10.1007/978-3-030-95738-4_24

2   Etiology and Pathophysiology

As this condition has long been thought to be associated with the PTT problem, much of the previous description of its etiology has primarily focused on factors that cause attenuation, tear, or dysfunction of the PTT [2]. However, this does not describe the failure of the ligamentous structures in the medial longitudinal arch, such as the spring and deltoid ligaments. Although degeneration of the PTT is a common finding and is often a presenting symptom, the timing of the failure of the ligaments is not necessarily in parallel with that of the tendon. The failure of the ligaments that support the medial longitudinal arch of the foot can occur before, during, or after tendon failure. Multiple factors have been described as associated with the PTT abnormality, which can be fallen into two categories: extrinsic or intrinsic. The extrinsic factors exert more physical force on the tendon, and these include preexisting flatfoot deformity [3], accessory navicular [4, 5], obesity [6, 7], and acute traumatic injury [8]. The intrinsic factors make the tendon more susceptible to degeneration, and these include inflammatory disorders (rheumatoid arthritis or seronegative spondyloarthropathy) [9–11], vascular insufficiency (steroid use), diabetes mellitus, hypertension [7], and polymorphisms at genes involved in collagen degeneration (matrix metalloproteinases 13 & 18) [12, 13]. Also the morphology of the talus with its effect on the valgus angulation of the subtalar joint may be an important predisposing factor.

There are several underlying etiologies in which patients with a normal PTT can develop PCFD. Failure of the spring ligament has been identified as a potential cause of PCFD in patients in which the PTT is normal based on imaging and intra-operative exploration [14, 15]. Some researchers have proposed that medial column instability can be a primary driving force rather than the result of PTT dysfunction in the development of the flatfoot deformity [16, 17]. Certainly, that could contribute as well as a more valgus subtalar joint axis.

Once the PTT becomes insufficient, the foot is subject to the unopposed pull of the peroneus brevis, which is the primary antagonist of the posterior tibial muscle. This results in increased abduction through the talonavicular joint, leading to increased stress on the medial ligaments and abduction deformity seen in PCFD [18, 19]. A tight Achilles tendon or gastrocnemius muscle may be causally related, a result of the deformity or both. The force vector of the Achilles becomes lateral relative to the center of the subtalar joint. This contributes to stress on medial ligaments and the resultant peritalar subluxation mentioned above. Thordarson et al. demonstrated that the triceps surae has the most significant arch flattening effect in the sagittal plane [20]. Tight triceps surae is also associated with abduction deformity of the forefoot in the transverse plane. In later stages, the deltoid ligament may fail, causing ankle instability and talar tilt.

3   Anatomy

Through its medial course to the subtalar axis and multiple insertions in the midfoot, the posterior tibialis functions as plantarflexor and inverter of the hindfoot and adductor and supinator of the forefoot [21]. There are several proposed anatomical theories why the PTT is prone to develop degenerative or inflammatory changes. First, the PTT courses directly behind the medial malleolus at a relatively acute angle [22]. This creates excessive frictional forces with physical activity. Second, the PTT courses underneath the tight overlying flexor retinaculum which can cause compression and constriction of the tendon through synovial enlargement [23]. This can affect the circulation of the tendon, leading to degenerative changes. Finally, a cadaveric study demonstrated a hypovascular zone in the retromalleolar region, with fibrocartilaginous changes in tendon structure identified in this region [24].

The spring ligament complex (SLC) is one of the static ligamentous structures frequently involved in PCFD. The primary function of the SLC is to support the head of the talus, an essential part of the articular surface of the talocalcaneonavicular joint. Alterations of the spring ligament are commonly seen with PTT degeneration or tears, making them the most common secondary abnormality seen in PCFD [25]. While acute tears of the spring ligament are uncommon, degeneration, plastic deformation, and/or tears occur. The SLC has been known to be composed of two distinct bands: a stronger superior medial calcaneonavicular (SMCN) ligament and an inferior calcaneonavicular (ICN) ligament just lateral to it. Recently, a third additional component (third ligament) or midplantar oblique ligament has been described as a distinct structure within the SLC. It runs from the notch between the anterior and middle calcaneal facets to the tubercle of the navicular in the lower layer of the SLC, lying beneath the cartilaginous surface of the complex [26].

The interosseous ligament also functions to maintain the alignment of the calcaneus relative to the talus. In a magnetic resonance imaging (MRI) study, the talocalcaneal interosseous ligament was the third most commonly involved ligament in patients with PCFD, after the SMCN and ICN ligaments of the SLC [25]. Unlike the SLC, it is located near the center of the subtalar joint and therefore likely has an important role in resisting anterior/posterior and medial/lateral displacement rather than inversion/eversion rotatory displacement. In advanced cases, subtalar subluxation with both eversion rotation presumably from SLC failure and lateral calcaneal drift from interosseous failure becomes apparent.

4   Diagnosis

4.1   Clinical

The typical patient with PCFD is an overweight, middle-aged woman. Patients may describe the insidious onset of vague, activity-induced pain on the medial side of the foot due to posterior tibial tendon degeneration and failure. In later stages, symptoms may include lateral-sided pain, which may be attributed to talocalcaneal or calcaneofibular impingement. At advanced stages of the disease, patients may have little to no pain along the PTT course due to elongation or rupture of the tendon. Therefore, the absence of medial pain does not preclude the diagnosis of PCFD.

Physical examination is especially important in evaluating the degree of actual deformity, as radiographs may not fully reflect the deformity. The examination begins with the patient standing barefoot and allowing the foot to fully pronate. Asymmetrical swelling and fullness about the medial ankle and hindfoot may be present. In advanced stages, abduction of the forefoot is evident, resulting in a characteristic "too many toes" sign. The function and strength of the posterior tibialis muscle can be tested in a standing position by performing the heel-rise test. On bilateral heel rise, the examiner looks for symmetric hindfoot inversion. Lack of symmetry indicates that the affected PTT is incompetent in inverting the subtalar joint, locking the transverse tarsal joint, and allowing heel rise through the gastrocnemius-soleus complex power. A more sensitive and specific finding is the inability to perform a single heel-rise test, but it can still be a false positive with other causes of midfoot pain. A sensation of weakness or medial pain along the course of the PTT may also be appreciated. At the earlier stages of disease progression, a repetitive single heel-rise test with comparison to the contralateral uninvolved side may be helpful.

Patients with chronic deformity may have enlarged tendon size upon palpation, especially at the retromalleolar region. The motor strength of the PTT can be assessed by asking the seated patient to invert the foot against resistance. The foot should be fully plantarflexed to ensure that the anterior tibial tendon is not substituting for the PTT. Tenderness over the joint line may be identified when there is a valgus tilt of the talus within the tibiotalar joint. Heel cord tightness should be checked, most commonly with the Silfverskiöld test. This test is considered positive when ankle dorsiflexion increases with the knee in flexion, and the foot and ankle cannot go into any dorsiflexion with the knee straight. The rigidity of the midfoot and hindfoot should be checked under a range of motion assessment. A fixed forefoot varus should be checked with the heel in the neutral position. Dorsal instability of the first tarsometatarsal (TMT) joint should also be evaluated.

4.2   Radiographic

When taking radiographs, it is especially important to educate patients to fully load their weight on the involved foot and let it pronate completely; otherwise the deformity can be underestimated. Four studies are commonly recommended for radiographic assessment: weight-bearing anteroposterior (AP) and lateral views of the foot, hindfoot alignment view, and weight-bearing AP view of the ankle. The abduction deformity of the foot is best visualized on the AP view of the foot. Talonavicular coverage angle, talo-first metatarsal angle, and talar incongruency angle are radiographic parameters that represent the amount of abduction deformity of the forefoot [27–29]. Collapse of the medial longitudinal arch is best evaluated on the lateral view of the foot. The talo-first metatarsal angle (Meary's angle; flatfoot >20 degrees) is an angle between the longitudinal axis of the talus and the first metatarsal bone [27, 30]. The calcaneal pitch angle is formed by the line parallel to the ground and the line along the inferior inclination axis of the calcaneus [27, 30]. When evaluating the lateral view, the location of collapse within the medial column should be carefully inspected. Failure to fully address the apex of the instability may lead to persistent postoperative deformity and poor patient outcomes. Instability at the first TMT joint often presents as plantar gapping. However, there may be dorsal displacement of the metatarsal bone in relation to the medial cuneiform without angulation of the joint. Bony impingement at the sinus tarsi can also often be identified at the angle of Gissane in the sinus tarsi in patients with advanced hindfoot valgus deformity on the weight-bearing lateral X-ray. Hindfoot alignment view, frequently called the Saltzman view, can quantify hindfoot valgus and guide operative planning on how much medial slide of the calcaneus will be needed [31]. The hindfoot moment arm is measured by the shortest orthogonal distance between the axis of the tibia and the most inferior point of the calcaneus. Hindfoot alignment angle is formed by the intersection of the longitudinal axis of the tibial shaft and the axis of the calcaneal tuberosity. On the AP view of the ankle, the height of the tibiotalar joint line of the involved side may be lower than the uninvolved contralateral side due to collapse of the medial arch and eversion of the calcaneus. Valgus talar tilt and evidence of ankle arthritis can be observed in the later stages of PCFD. Calcaneofibular bony impingement can sometimes be identified in the case where there is severe subluxation at the subtalar joint but may not be able to be seen on plain X-rays and is best seen on a weight-bearing computed tomography (WBCT) scan. In addition, a whole limb radiograph can be beneficial to rule out other causes of the deformity that might be associated with malalignment of the lower limb.

Although not universally available, MRI and WBCT are increasingly being used to understand the extent of PCFD. MRI can be used as an adjunctive diagnostic test in identifying soft tissue involvement, such as the PTT, deltoid ligament, SLC, and interosseous ligaments. The information obtained from MRI can aid in determining surgical treatment. WBCT is an emerging technique that has been proven to more precisely measure bone position than conventional weight-bearing radiographs due to its ability to evaluate multiplanar deformity with the patient weight-bearing [32]. When compared to conventional radiographs, WBCT is free from superimposition and can minimize rotational errors. WBCT helps identify subluxation of joints within the medial column as well as findings of hindfoot deformity such as sinus tarsi impingement and calcaneofibular impingement (Fig. 1) [33].

4.3   Clinical Staging

The classification system is helpful because it aids in describing the deformity and therefore directs the method of surgical treatment. There have been several classification systems previously described, depending on the etiology and the location of the deformity. A four-stage classification system popularized by Johnson and Strom and later modified by Myerson is commonly cited [34, 35].

Stage I refers to the mildest form of the deformity within this classification system, with an absence of abnormal alignment. It is the alignment of the flatfoot they have had all their adult life without any progressive deformity. Tenosynovitis or tendinosis with pain over the PTT tendon is the most important finding in this stage.

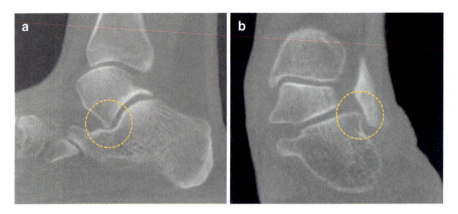

Fig. 1 Weight-bearing computed tomography analysis reveals sinus tarsi impingement (**a**) and calcaneofibular impingement (**b**), potentially explaining the presence of lateral hindfoot symptoms

However, in actual practice, the patients who truly fit into Stage I are relatively rare. Radiographs are of a normal flatfoot, although MRI may show inflammation or early signs of degeneration of the PTT. Stage II, with its different amounts and types of deformity, is the most controversial part of this classification system. Stage II is associated with an elongated or torn PTT and ligament failure, the latter of which results in structural deformity. The deformity in Stage II is still flexible, which makes it different from Stage III, and favors joint-preserving surgical methods rather than joint arthrodesis. Depending on the amount of forefoot abduction, Stage II is further divided into IIA and IIB. Stage IIA deformity is characterized by minimal abduction at the midfoot with less than 40% talonavicular uncoverage on the standing AP radiograph. In Stage IIB, there is greater forefoot abduction, 40% or more talonavicular uncoverage. This division is useful in the determination of the type of osteotomy, as lateral column lengthening is known to be more effective in addressing abduction deformity than the medial displacement calcaneal osteotomy. Stage III signifies a more rigid or fixed deformity, in which the malalignment at the triple joint complex cannot be corrected past neutral with passive inversion. The stiffness of each joint is not objectively measurable, and it is unclear exactly how much stiffness defines a Stage III presentation. However, if the talonavicular joint cannot be placed in neutral and the talonavicular joint is passively incapable of inversion, a tendon transfer will not be of benefit, and deformity should be considered Stage III. Finally, Stage IV is a deformity of the ankle joint with talar tilt due to the attenuation of the deltoid ligament. The foot deformity in Stage IV can be either fixed or flexible.

Despite its wide use, this classification system has significant limitations. A limitation of this classification system is that Stage I is a misnomer and is not typically encountered in the outpatient clinic. Another is that PCFD is a progressive disorder, and, interestingly, the deformity described in the current classification system is not on a continuum. For example, Stage III refers to rigid flatfoot, which frequently requires double or triple arthrodesis, whereas Stage IV includes deformities that are still flexible which can be treated with osteotomy and ligament reconstruction.

Table 1 Consensus group classification of progressive collapsing foot deformity (2020)

Stage of the deformity		
Stage I (flexible)	Stage II (rigid)	
Types of deformity (classes – isolated or combined)		
	Deformity type/location	Consistent clinical/radiographic findings
Class A	Hindfoot valgus deformity	Hindfoot valgus alignment Increased hindfoot moment arm, hindfoot alignment angle, foot and ankle offset
Class B	Midfoot/forefoot abduction deformity	Decreased talar head coverage Increased talonavicular coverage angle Presence of sinus tarsi impingement
Class C	Forefoot varus deformity/ medial column instability	Increased talus-first metatarsal angle Plantar gapping first TMT joint/NC joints Clinical forefoot varus
Class D	Peritalar subluxation/ dislocation	Significant subtalar joint subluxation/ subfibular impingement
Class E	Ankle instability	Valgus tilting of the ankle joint

Reprinted from Myerson et al. [1]
Abbreviations: *NC* naviculocuneiform; *TMT* tarsometatarsal

In light of these limitations, in 2020, the expert consensus group proposed a new classification system based on the flexibility and the type and location of the deformity. In this new classification system, the deformity is designated into Stage I (flexible) or Stage II (rigid) depending on the flexibility stage of the deformity [1]. In addition, depending on the type and location of the deformity, this is further classified into A through E (Table 1).

5 Conservative Treatment

In most circumstances, initial treatment should start with nonoperative measures. However, as the majority of symptomatic patients present with a deformity that will progress, conservative treatment, in general, has a limited role. The goal for conservative treatments would be to decrease the force exerted through the posteromedial soft tissues theoretically. This can be done by encouraging weight loss, using orthosis, and reducing repetitive loading by activity modifications. Often, this is usually supplemented with nonsteroidal anti-inflammatory drugs. For patients with acute symptoms, a short period of immobilization may be indicated in a removable boot or, in severe cases, a cast. After immobilization, patients may be transitioned to a custom brace or orthosis and begin a rehabilitation program. A variety of orthotic options are available. These options include off-the-shelf orthoses, customized arch supports, customized UCBL (University of California Biomechanics Laboratory), Arizona brace, and Ritchie brace. Although braces may slow down deformity progression, none of them have been shown to stop it. In our opinion, they do not stop the progression of deformity, and patients should be made aware of this. However, it is also true that the rate of progression is variable. Physical therapy and rehabilitation protocols can be helpful after initial inflammation dissipates. Goals for rehabilitation center around mechanically strengthening ankle inversion power, stretching the Achilles and gastrocnemius, and minimizing further tendon lengthening and foot deformity.

6 Surgical Management

Surgical treatment is recommended for patients who have failed conservative management. In reality, many patients who present with symptoms already have a deformity from PCFD and therefore will highly likely need surgery. A wide breadth of surgical treatment options for PCFD has been reported in the literature. In general, a combination of procedures is preferred to address the complex multiplanar deformity. The two most important things to check when determining the surgical plan are (1) whether the deformity is still flexible or rigid and (2) the location of the deformity. When the deformity is rigid and cannot be corrected back to neutral, this favors arthrodesis of the involved joint. Joint instability or sagging within the medial column is not always appreciable preoperatively. Therefore, this should be carefully examined intraoperatively, and an effort should be made to address deformities within the medial column. An exception is a naviculocuneiform joint, which in the case of a mild to moderate sag in our experience is not necessary to fuse. The choice of procedures must depend on the specific deformity to be addressed. Therefore, it is essential to understand the strengths and weaknesses of each procedure.

6.1 Hindfoot Valgus Deformity

6.1.1 Medial Displacement Calcaneal Osteotomy

Medial displacement calcaneal osteotomy (MDCO) is a commonly employed technique to correct hindfoot valgus. By translating the posterior tuber of the calcaneus medially, this repositions the axis of the Achilles and subsequently decreases strain on the medial column. In one study investigating the factors associated with postoperative hindfoot alignment, MDCO was the only significant predictor. This can be performed as an isolated bony procedure when there is an isolated hindfoot valgus in the setting of mild talonavicular joint uncoverage (less than 40% uncovered) and a lack of significant forefoot supination, varus, or abduction. Since some patients can hold up their arch or lean back and do not let their arch fully sag, the X-ray can be an underestimation of the true deformity. If no WBCT is available and no subtalar impingement seen on plain X-rays, use the preoperative standing clinical exam as a possible alert to significant talonavicular abduction or plantar sag to suggest a lateral column lengthening or subtalar arthrodesis may be necessary. A 7–15 mm of medial slide osteotomy is recommended, and clinically straight heel (hindfoot moment arm 0–5 mm by X-ray) is known to be associated with better clinical outcomes. A lateral oblique incision along the suspected line of osteotomy is most

Fig. 2 Clinically straight heel alignment should be obtained after osteotomy fixation for better patient outcomes

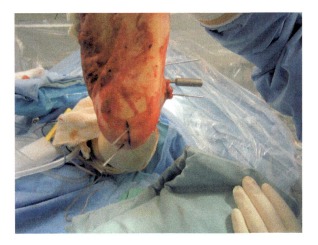

commonly employed, but some endorse an L-shaped incision. Various types of fixation can be utilized, such as compression screws, step plates, or blade plate. Regardless of the method, union rates are high. Lateral column lengthening (LCL) can also correct the hindfoot valgus deformity but to a much smaller degree. The key is achieving a clinically straight heel (Fig. 2).

6.2 Midfoot/Forefoot Abduction Deformity

6.2.1 Lateral Column Lengthening

LCL is a powerful procedure to correct forefoot abduction deformity as well as restore the medial arch. Lengthening of the lateral column can be performed through either an arthrodesis of the calcaneocuboid joint or an osteotomy of the anterior calcaneus. However, the former can lead to nonunion, stiffness, and lateral foot overload, causing residual discomfort, and has largely been abandoned. Theoretically, lengthening through the anterior process preserves motion at the calcaneocuboid joint, but overlengthening can lead to stiffness of the lateral column when an adequate amount of eversion is not preserved. Therefore, performing the correct amount of lengthening is a critical portion of the operation. The amount will vary depending on the individual deformity, but the range of ideal graft size is recommended to be 5–7 mm. Hintermann pin distractor can be placed across the osteotomy and opened gradually to allow for correction of forefoot abduction. The ideal amount of correction is assessed both visually and with a simulated anteroposterior weight-bearing fluoroscopic view (Fig. 3). A moderate amount of eversion motion from neutral should be maintained in the subtalar joint, approximately 15 degrees. If necessary, give less correction to the alignment in the arch to allow this critical motion to remain, or the patient will complain of excessive stiffness or lateral overload of the foot.

Once an ideal amount of correction has been achieved, passive hindfoot motion, particularly eversion, should be assessed. When an adequate degree (usually 10 degrees)

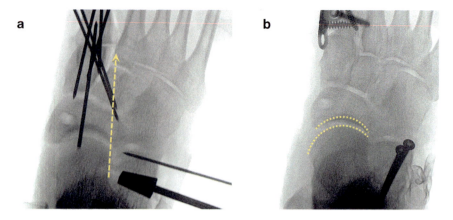

Fig. 3 A metal trial wedge is especially helpful in titrating the amount of correction. Any possibility of overcorrection should be checked and avoided to obtain better patient outcomes. There is a high probability of overcorrection in our clinical experience when the lateral talar neck aims lateral to the proximal-medial corner of the second metatarsal base (arrow, **a**). Some residual amount of talonavicular uncoverage is allowed when the complete correction leads to stiffness in eversion (**b**)

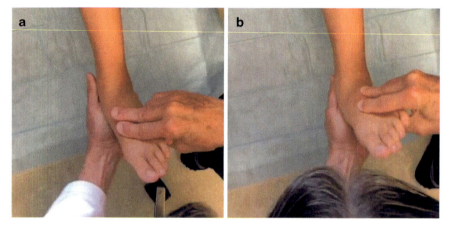

Fig. 4 Physical examination on the passive motion of the subtalar joint (**a, b**). Passive hindfoot motion, at least 10 degrees of eversion (**b**), should be preserved; otherwise the patient will complain of stiffness and possibly excessive lateral weight-bearing and pain

of eversion is not obtained, the graft size should be decreased to prevent overcorrection. We aim to avoid adduction at the talonavicular joint, and avoidance of this adduction has been shown to lead to better clinical results [36]. To get the most accurate size measurement of the actual wedge to be implanted, the use of trial wedges is helpful. While an Evans-type osteotomy is performed parallel and 1 cm posterior to the calcaneocuboid joint, other osteotomies such as the central Hintermann-type or step-cut lengthening osteotomies have been described with comparable outcomes. Regardless, subtalar/talonavicular eversion motion should be maintained, or the patient will complain of stiffness and possibly excessive lateral weight-bearing and pain (Fig. 4).

In the senior author's experience, a difference of 1–2 mm of lengthening can make the difference between a happy patient with good eversion motion remaining and an unhappy patient with stiffness and possible lateral excessive weight-bearing. Unfortunately, it is a very sensitive procedure. Either an autograft or allograft can be used, while the use of trabecular metal wedges has also been described with low nonunion rates. Metal wedges make the revision of LCL procedures very problematic and should be avoided. The fixation of the osteotomy can be achieved in the form of screws or plates.

6.3 Forefoot Varus or Supination Deformity/Medial Column Instability

6.3.1 Cotton Osteotomy and Tarsometatarsal Joint Fusion

Forefoot varus or supination refers to the condition in which there is an elevation of the first ray and/or rotation of forefoot in the coronal plane. Generally, it is considered as a correction for an elevated first ray but does not correct or counteract hindfoot stiffness from excessive stiffness from LCL. Through a dorsal approach, the medial cuneiform is osteotomized from dorsal to plantar, and the plantar hinge of the cortex is left intact. The typical amount of correction ranges from 5 to 7 mm, and an allograft, autograft, or metal implant can be inserted [37]. This is usually indicated for patients with stable first TMT joints to correct both forefoot varus deformity. However, when the TMT joint is unstable with excessive motion (plantar gapping or dorsal instability in lateral radiographs), arthrodesis of the TMT joint is needed. In cases when there is concomitant instability at other joints in the medial column, an additional arthrodesis may be required, although this may not be necessary. Mild to moderate naviculocuneiform plantar sag can be tolerated. More recently, a technique which Recent study has established a technique for successfully transferring the flexor hallucis longus tendon to the first metatarsal base. This method has been shown to successfully correct the entire medial arch, with the added benefit of correcting medial arch instability even in the presence of gapping or arthritic changes without undergoing joint arthrodesis.

6.3.2 Flexor Hallucis Longus Tendon Transfer and LapiCotton Procedure

Kim et al. described a procedure called dynamic medial column stabilization in which the flexor hallucis longus tendon is transferred to the first metatarsal base [38]. This method has been shown to successfully correct the entire medial arch as well as three-dimensional deformities associated with PCFD, with the added benefit of correcting medial arch instability even in the presence of plantar gapping or arthritic changes in the first TMT joint. More recently, de Cesar Netto et al. described another technique called LapiCotton as a surgical technique that combines the mechanical advantages of a Cotton osteotomy with a modified Lapidus procedure to treat medial column collapse by fusing the first TMT with a dorsal opening wedge distraction allograft [39]. The procedure has the potential benefit of maintaining/increasing the length of the first ray and plantarflexing the medial column, as well as restoring the first ray's mechanical competence in the foot tripod. Although their outcomes are limited to short-term follow-up or reporting on surgical technique, these two procedures have the potential to treat PCFD without or with a smaller amount of LCL, thereby reducing the risk of complications such as foot stiffness.

6.4 Peritalar Subluxation/Dislocation (Rigid Deformity)

6.4.1 Double or Triple Arthrodesis

Subtalar joint arthrodesis is indicated when there are severe arthritic changes or peritalar instability characterized by subtalar coronal subluxation or subfibular impingement. This may be caused by laxity or failure of the interosseous talocalcaneal ligament. In patients of older age, lower physical demand, or excessive weight, arthrodesis may be an acceptable surgical option than LCL as fusing the subtalar joint in neutral/mildly everted position makes lateral column overcorrection less likely. When performing subtalar arthrodesis, it is imperative to correct the joint to neutral as the deltoid ligament may otherwise fail in a poorly positioned fusion (Fig. 5).

An MDCO should be added to obtain an ideal heel position, a clinically straight heel. Talonavicular joint arthrodesis can be added when there is a severe arthritic change at the joint or excessive abduction after hindfoot correction. If more than 50% of the abduction is corrected, spring ligament reconstruction is an option to avoid talonavicular joint fusion. Whether or not the talonavicular joint is fused, the calcaneocuboid joint can usually be spared. Unfortunately, even in the setting of a double arthrodesis, patients are still at an increased risk for adjacent joint arthritis.

6.5 Ankle Instability

6.5.1 Deltoid Ligament Reconstruction

When there is valgus talar tilt in the tibiotalar joint in PCFD, there is likely to be an insufficiency of the deltoid ligament as long as there is not lateral tibial bone defect. When used as a supplement to complete the correction of the flatfoot deformity, deltoid reconstruction has been shown to result in good clinical outcomes as well as correction of valgus talar tilt (Fig. 6) [40, 41].

Reconstruction can be achieved using either peroneus longus autograft or Achilles tendon allograft. It is imperative to address all deformities in the foot when performing deltoid reconstruction in order to minimize the risk of failure from

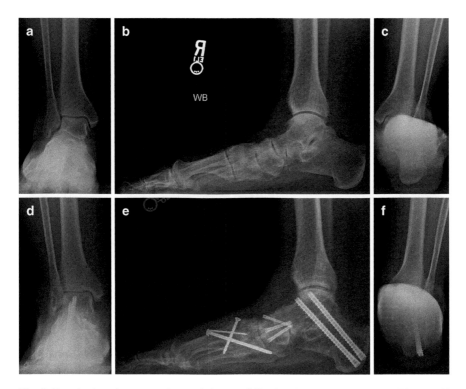

Fig. 5 Pre- (**a–c**) and postoperative (**d–f**) images following double arthrodesis in a 74-year-old male patient. Heel alignment should be in the right position (straight) to make deltoid ligament failure less likely

increased strain on the medial soft tissues in the longer term. Before proceeding with deltoid reconstruction either at the same operation or as a staged procedure if necessary, there must be a clinically straight heel in relation to the tibial and a moderately plantarflexed first ray with moderate prominence of the first metatarsal head in relation to the lesser metatarsal heads.

6.6   Soft Tissue Procedures

6.6.1   Flexor Tendon Transfer

The purpose of flexor tendon (flexor digitorum longus [FDL] or flexor hallucis longus [FHL]) transfer is to substitute or augment the function of the impaired PTT and to balance the force of the peroneus muscle. The FDL is usually utilized due to its proximity to the PTT and because there are fewer comorbidities associated with harvesting the FDL tendon compared to the FHL. Although tendon transfer is a widely performed technique in PCFD treatment, it alone fails to correct the

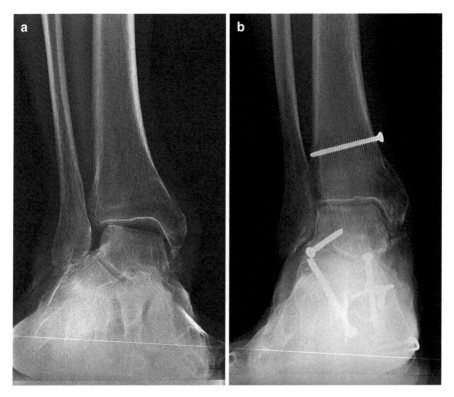

Fig. 6 Pre- (**a**) and 7-year postoperative (**b**) ankle standing radiographs show a successful outcome of deltoid ligament reconstruction in an 81-year-old female patient

deformity, and the correction would deteriorate over time. Therefore, it is combined with bony realignment procedures such as LCL or MDCO. The optimal location of tendon transfer has also been discussed, with options including the navicular, medial cuneiform, or PTT. These locations have been shown to be biomechanically similar in a cadaveric study. FHL transfer?

6.6.2 Gastrocnemius Recession/Achilles Tendon Lengthening

Heel cord tightness or equinus contracture is a common pathology observed in PCFD and may lead to worsening hindfoot valgus deformity if heel alignment is not fully corrected to a clinically straight heel. During PCFD correction, gastrocnemius recession is usually performed first before performing other bony or tendinous procedures, while percutaneous tri-cut lengthening is most often performed at the end of the procedure. The former is performed when the Silfverskiöld test is positive (isolated gastrocnemius tightness), and the latter is performed to address both gastrocnemius and soleus tightness.

6.6.3   Spring Ligament Reconstruction

Spring ligament reconstruction is indicated when non-fusion bony procedures such as LCL or subtalar fusion most often combined with medial heel slide correct at least 50% of the abduction/plantarflexion deformity, but adequate correction is not achieved. In cadaveric and clinical studies, spring ligament reconstruction resulted in the correction of talonavicular deformity and talonavicular arthrodesis avoided [42–44]. Multiple techniques have been described for spring ligament reconstruction, including allograft, autograft, and synthetic materials. However, this is technically demanding, and the data supporting this procedure is not yet sufficient. A long-term study of spring ligament reconstruction is underway by the senior author of this chapter.

7   Complication of Treatment

There are numerous surgical options in the treatment of PCFD, and all of these procedures have the potential for a range of complications. Complications may be due to poor presurgical planning, intraoperative errors, and inherent complications of each procedure, such as delayed union, nonunion, over- or undercorrection, or neurovascular injury.

7.1   Medial Displacement Calcaneal Osteotomy

While this procedure yields a high rate of osseous union, lateral incision risks injury to the sural nerve. Several studies have described alternative incisions to minimize the risk of sural nerve injury. In addition, the medial neurovascular bundle can also be compromised when performing the osteotomy. A safe zone for the osteotomy has been described as being within 11.2 ± 2.7 mm anterior to the line connecting the posterosuperior apex of the calcaneal tuberosity to the origin of the plantar fascia [45]. However, there is still some debate on whether a safe zone truly exists due to inherent variation in anatomy. Finally, irritation from prominent hardware is also a frequently described complication following MDCO.

7.2   Lateral Column Lengthening

Much of the concern for complications following PCFD reconstruction is associated with the LCL procedure. Due to the nature of non-anatomical lengthening, this procedure can result in stiffness of the adjacent joints. Subsequently, lateral column overload, fifth metatarsal stress fracture, and calcaneocuboid joint arthritis have all been reported following this procedure. It is known that overcorrection leads to a higher rate of lateral column pain and increased lateral foot pressures with a higher rate of patient dissatisfaction. Therefore, as mentioned above, slight undercorrection of the abduction deformity and maintaining an adequate amount of eversion after lengthening are paramount. Adequate eversion motion remaining is much more important than arch height. Given the choice between an X-ray with a fully restored Meary's angle with stiffness and adequate eversion motion with a mild talonavicular sag remaining, the latter is preferable and will usually result in a happier patient.

7.3   Arthrodesis

When an arthrodesis is chosen, the potential for adjacent joint overload and subsequent arthritis or secondary collapse should be explained to patients, and this should be carefully assessed during the follow-up period. For example, triple arthrodesis will limit the motion of the foot through arthrodesis of the talonavicular and calcaneonavicular joints, resulting in more stress placed on the midfoot joints. One should always be aware of possible arthritis as a source of patient's recurrent symptoms in the long term. Preservation of talonavicular motion is particularly important as it is not only a key motion to the foot but is associated with the development of ankle arthritis over the long term. Triple arthrodesis, of which talonavicular fusion is a key part, has been shown to cause ankle arthritis over the long term. Talonavicular motion is also a motion that most patients in one way or another will miss. Preservation of even some of this motion, whether by early correction of PCFD or the use of spring ligament reconstruction when needed, will preserve important motion and probably lessen the chance of adjacent joint arthritis.

8   Summary

In treating patients with PCFD, prompt early nonsurgical or surgical management is essential to avoid deformity progression. The location and the severity of the deformity may vary between the patients; therefore, an individualized approach is required. Generally, the goal of treatment is to achieve good correction of the deformity while maintaining as much as normal motion as possible both in the medial and the lateral column of the foot. Poor alignment of joints, particularly the talonavicular, subtalar, or first metatarsal joints, or over- or undercorrection of heel alignment or lateral column lengthening correction leads to a dissatisfied patient.

References

1. Myerson MS, Thordarson D, Johnson JE, Hintermann B, Sangeorzan BJ, Deland JT, et al. Classification and nomenclature: progressive collapsing foot deformity. Foot Ankle Int. 2020;1071100720950722.
2. Beals TC, Pomeroy GC, Arthur MI. Posterior tibial tendon insufficiency: diagnosis and treatment. JAAOS-J Am Acad OrthopSurg. 1999;7(2):112–8.
3. Cody EA, Williamson ER, Burket JC, Deland JT, Ellis SJ. Correlation of talar anatomy and subtalar joint alignment on weightbearing computed tomography with radiographic flatfoot parameters. Foot Ankle Int. 2016;37(8):874–81.
4. KIDNER FC. The prehallux (accessory scaphoid) in its relation to flat-foot. JBJS. 1929;11(4):831–7.
5. Kim J, Day J, Seilern, Aspang J. Outcomes following revision surgery after failed kidner procedure for painful accessory navicular. Foot Ankle Int. 2020:1071100720943843.
6. Fuhrmann R, Trommer T, Venbrocks R. The acquired buckling-flatfoot. A foot deformity due to obesity? Der Orthopade. 2005;34(7):682–9.
7. Holmes GB, Mann RA. Possible epidemiological factors associated with rupture of the posterior tibial tendon. Foot Ankle. 1992;13(2):70–9.
8. Giblin MM. Ruptured tibialis posterior tendon associated with a closed medial malleolar fracture. Aust N Z J Surg. 1980;50(1):59–60.
9. Myerson M, Solomon G, Shereff M. Posterior tibial tendon dysfunction: its association with seronegative inflammatory disease. Foot Ankle. 1989;9(5):219–25.
10. Downey DJ, Simkin PA, Mack LA, Richardson ML, Kilcoyne RF, Hansen ST. Tibialis posterior tendon rupture: a cause of rheumatoid flat foot. Arthritis Rheum. 1988;31(3):441–6.
11. Michelson J, Easley M, Wigley FM, Hellmann D. Posterior tibial tendon dysfunction in rheumatoid arthritis. Foot Ankle Int. 1995;16(3):156–61.
12. Godoy-Santos A, Ortiz R, Junior RM, Fernandes TD, Santos M. MMP-8 polymorphism is genetic marker to tendinopathy primary posterior tibial tendon. Scand J Med Sci Sports. 2014;24(1):220–3.
13. de Araujo Munhoz FB, Baroneza JE, Godoy-Santos A, Fernandes TD, Branco FP, Alle LF, et al. Posterior tibial tendinopathy associated with matrix metalloproteinase 13 promoter genotype and haplotype. J Gene Med. 2016;18(11–12):325–30.
14. Orr JD, Nunley JA. Isolated spring ligament failure as a cause of adult-acquired flatfoot deformity. Foot Ankle Int. 2013;34(6):818–23.
15. Tryfonidis M, Jackson W, Mansour R, Cooke P, Teh J, Ostlere S, et al. Acquired adult flat foot due to isolated plantar calcaneonavicular (spring) ligament insufficiency with a normal tibialis posterior tendon. Foot Ankle Surg. 2008;14(2):89–95.
16. Greisberg J, Assal M, Hansen ST Jr, Sangeorzan BJ. Isolated medial column stabilization improves alignment in adult-acquired flatfoot. Clin Orthop Relat Res®. 2005;435:197–202.
17. Cohen BE, Ogden F. Medial column procedures in the acquired flatfoot deformity. Foot Ankle Clin. 2007;12(2):287–99.
18. Funk DA, Cass J, Johnson K. Acquired adult flat foot secondary to posterior tibial-tendon pathology. J Bone Joint Surg Am. 1986;68(1):95–102.
19. Imhauser CW, Siegler S, Abidi NA, Frankel DZ. The effect of posterior tibialis tendon dysfunction on the plantar pressure characteristics and the kinematics of the arch and the hindfoot. Clin Biomech. 2004;19(2):161–9.
20. Thordarson DB, Schmotzer H, Chon J, Peters J. Dynamic support of the human longitudinal arch: a biomechanical evaluation. Clin Orthop Relat Res (1976–2007). 1995;316:165–72.
21. Kelikian AS, Sarrafian SK. Sarrafian's anatomy of the foot and ankle: descriptive, topographic, functional. Lippincott Williams & Wilkins; 2011.
22. Supple KM, Hanft JR, Murphy BJ, Janecki CJ, Kogler GF. Posterior tibial tendon dysfunction. Semin Arthritis Rheum: Elsevier. 1992:106–13.

23. Jahss MH. Spontaneous rupture of the tibialis posterior tendon: clinical findings, tenographic studies, and a new technique of repair. Foot Ankle. 1982;3(3):158–66.
24. Frey C, Shereff M, Greenidge N. Vascularity of the posterior tibial tendon. J Bone Joint Surg Am. 1990;72(6):884–8.
25. Deland JT, de Asla RJ, Sung I-H, Ernberg LA, Potter HG. Posterior tibial tendon insufficiency: which ligaments are involved? Foot Ankle Int. 2005;26(6):427–35.
26. Taniguchi A, Tanaka Y, Takakura Y, Kadono K, Maeda M, Yamamoto H. Anatomy of the spring ligament. JBJS. 2003;85(11):2174–8.
27. Ellis SJ, Yu JC, Williams BR, Lee C. Chiu Y-l, Deland JT. New radiographic parameters assessing forefoot abduction in the adult acquired flatfoot deformity. Foot Ankle Int. 2009;30(12):1168–76.
28. Williamson ER, Chan JY, Burket JC, Deland JT, Ellis SJ. New radiographic parameter assessing hindfoot alignment in stage II adult-acquired flatfoot deformity. Foot Ankle Int. 2015;36(4):417–23.
29. Sangeorzan BJ, Mosca V, Hansen ST Jr. Effect of calcaneal lengthening on relationships among the hindfoot, midfoot, and forefoot. Foot Ankle. 1993;14(3):136–41.
30. Younger AS, Sawatzky B, Dryden P. Radiographic assessment of adult flatfoot. Foot Ankle Int. 2005;26(10):820–5.
31. Saltzman CL, El-Khoury GY. The hindfoot alignment view. Foot Ankle Int. 1995;16(9):572–6.
32. Conti MS, Ellis SJ. Weight-bearing CT scans in foot and ankle surgery. JAAOS-J Am Acad Orthop Surg. 2020;28(14):e595–603.
33. de Cesar NC, Myerson MS, Day J, Ellis SJ, Hintermann B, Johnson JE, et al. Consensus for the use of weightbearing CT in the assessment of progressive collapsing foot deformity. Foot Ankle Int. 2020;1071100720950734.
34. Johnson KA, Strom DE. Tibialis posterior tendon dysfunction. Clin Orthop Relat Res. 1989;239:196–206.
35. Bluman EM, Myerson MS. Stage IV posterior tibial tendon rupture. Foot Ankle Clin. 2007;12(2):341–62.
36. Conti MS, Chan JY, Do HT, Ellis SJ, Deland JT. Correlation of postoperative midfoot position with outcome following reconstruction of the stage II adult acquired flatfoot deformity. Foot Ankle Int. 2015;36(3):239–47.
37. Ellis SJ, Johnson JE, Day J, de Cesar NC, Deland JT, Hintermann B, et al. Titrating the amount of bony correction in progressive collapsing foot deformity. Foot Ankle Int. 2020;41(10):1292–5.
38. Kim J, Kim J-B, Lee W-C. Dynamic medial column stabilization using flexor hallucis longus tendon transfer in the surgical reconstruction of flatfoot deformity in adults. Foot Ankle Surg. 2021;27(8):920–7.
39. de Cesar Netto C, Ahrenholz S, Iehl C, Vivtcharenko V, Schmidt E, Lee H, et al. Lapicotton technique in the treatment of progressive collapsing foot deformity. J Foot Ankle. 2020;14(3):301–8.
40. Deland JT, de Asla RJ, Segal A. Reconstruction of the chronically failed deltoid ligament: a new technique. Foot Ankle Int. 2004;25(11):795–9.
41. Ellis SJ, Williams BR, Wagshul AD, Pavlov H, Deland JT. Deltoid ligament reconstruction with peroneus longus autograft in flatfoot deformity. Foot Ankle Int. 2010;31(9):781–9.
42. Deland JT, Arnoczky SP, Thompson FM. Adult acquired flatfoot deformity at the talonavicular joint: reconstruction of the spring ligament in an in vitro model. Foot Ankle. 1992;13(6):327–32.
43. Choi K, Lee S, Otis JC, Deland JT. Anatomical reconstruction of the spring ligament using peroneus longus tendon graft. Foot Ankle Int. 2003;24(5):430–6.
44. Williams BR, Ellis SJ, Deyer TW, Pavlov H, Deland JT. Reconstruction of the spring ligament using a peroneus longus autograft tendon transfer. Foot Ankle Int. 2010;31(7):567–77.
45. Talusan PG, Cata E, Tan EW, Parks BG, Guyton GP. Safe zone for neural structures in medial displacement calcaneal osteotomy: a cadaveric and radiographic investigation. Foot Ankle Int. 2015;36(12):1493–8.

Latest Trends in Flatfoot Management: Contributions of the Spring Ligament Complex and the Deltoid Ligament

Brian T. Sleasman and Anish R. Kadakia

1 Introduction

Flatfoot deformity is a common complaint of patients presenting to a foot and ankle surgeon. It has long been accepted as a source of pain and disability and affects upwards of five million Americans [1]. Originally, flatfoot was described as posterior tibial tendon dysfunction (PTTD) due to the contribution of posterior tibial tendon (PTT) insufficiency to the deformity. This idea was conceptualized in the original flatfoot classification in 1989 by Johnson and Strom [2] and later refined by Bluman [3] in 2007 to include a broader spectrum of pathologies. Despite the breadth of this classification, it still failed to incorporate some components of the deformity, specifically the spring and deltoid ligaments. Regardless, this classification is well known and frequently referenced when discussing treatment algorithms.

Recently, a group of experts on flatfoot advocated for the use of the term progressive collapsing foot deformity (PCFD) to include adults and children and to state the progressive nature of this condition [4]. With continued research it has become evident that the medial stabilizers of the ankle provide essential support to the arch and are critical in the prevention of this deformity. Several authors have noted that in patients who have progressed to this deformity, the spring ligament is almost universally compromised [5–7]. The deltoid ligament, which was included in the late stage disease in Bluman's classification, may have implications in the earlier diseased states. For these reasons, understanding and treatment of PCFD must include an evaluation of these two medial soft tissue structures, and they should be addressed at the time of correction.

B. T. Sleasman (✉) · A. R. Kadakia
Northwestern University – Feinberg School of Medicine, Northwestern Memorial Hospital, Department of Orthopedic Surgery, Chicago, IL, USA

© The Author(s), under exclusive license to Springer Nature Switzerland AG 2022
E. Wagner Hitschfeld, P. Wagner Hitschfeld (eds.), *Foot and Ankle Disorders*,
https://doi.org/10.1007/978-3-030-95738-4_25

555

In this chapter we will focus on how to address the medial soft tissue structure damage in PCFD. Please refer to the previous chapter for a more detailed analysis of the clinical history, physical examination findings, and bone deformity correction.

2 Etiology: Pathophysiology

PCFD is a complex problem which results in the compromise of the soft tissue and osseous structures in the foot. This compromise ultimately leads to the classic progressive collapse of the medial longitudinal arch.

Historically, the PTT has been implicated in the development of PCFD. This tendon is a powerful plantar flexor and inverter of the hindfoot. It originates in the posterior aspect of the intermuscular septum, and its tendon passes posterior to the axis of rotation of the ankle and medial to the subtalar axis. Thus, it acts as a strong plantarflexor and inverter of the hindfoot. Through the stages of gait, this tendon is responsible for locking the transfer tarsal joints during gait which allows for efficient propulsion. In patients without this tendon, the hindfoot is not effectively inverted, and thus medial ligaments can be attenuated [8]. However, several authors noted that it is not uncommon for patients with a normal PTT to have a planovalgus deformity of the hindfoot [9, 10]. Additionally, we do not see PCFD in patients in which the PTT is transferred for foot drop.

In an MRI study, evidence of spring ligament dysfunction was strongly associated with the planovalgus deformity, alongside with multiple other soft tissue insufficiencies like the deltoid ligament and subtalar interosseous ligament [7]. The spring ligament has a crucial role as the soft tissue hammock in which the talar head rests. The structure provides static stability to the talar head, and thus, when intact, the foot cannot abduct nor the talus plantar flex at the TN joint. Therefore, it is not without failure or attenuation of the spring ligament that the classic flatfoot deformity should occur.

2.1 Relevant Anatomy

The medial soft tissue stabilizers of the ankle and talus include the spring ligament complex (SLC) and the deltoid ligament, which are intimately related. The SLC is comprised of a group of ligaments that connect the sustentaculum tali of the calcaneus to the navicular bone. Together these ligaments support the head of the talus and form part of the articular cavity of the talocalcaneonavicular joint, which is referred to as the acetabulum or coxa pedis [11]. The SLC is comprised of three main components. The most important of which is the superomedial band (SMCN). This band is the longest and most medial of the components originating on the medial sustentaculum tali and projecting anteromedially to attach over a broad spectrum to the navicular. Its deep surface is covered in fibrocartilage and is the specific portion of the SLC primarily responsible for articulating with the talar head. The inferoplantar (ICN) band is the shortest and most lateral part of the SLC. It is slightly thicker than the SMCN, and biomechanical analysis shows that it does play a minor role in stabilizing the talocalcaneonavicular joint as well as the medial arch of the foot [12]. The medioplantar oblique band (MPO) is a distinct band that lies between the SMCN and the ICN.

The deltoid ligament is composed of two main components, namely, the superficial and deep components. The deep deltoid originates on the distal aspect of the medial malleolus and inserts over a wide non-articular portion of the medial and posteromedial aspect of the talus. Its main function is to prevent lateral displacement and external rotation of the talus. The superficial deltoid ligament is broad and sends distinct bands to the navicular, the spring ligament, the calcaneus, and the talus. The tibiospring and tibionavicular portions of the superficial deltoid ligament highlight the intimate relationship between these two medial soft tissue structures [13]. The tibionavicular band helps to suspend the spring ligament and works in conjunction with the SLC to prevent inward displacement of the talus. The talocalcaneal portion helps to prevent valgus.

3   Conservative Management

As with most conditions of the foot and ankle, flatfoot treatment begins with nonoperative management. These options typically focus on alleviating pain and symptoms by attempting to off-load the medial foot and arch. This can be done with a combination of weight loss, activity modification, and improving footwear. Orthoses are often incorporated into early treatment algorithms to improve symptoms. Typically, these included a medial post to support the medial arch. The University of California Biomechanics Laboratory (UCBL) semirigid orthosis was created to control the valgus of the hindfoot as well as support the medial arch. In biomechanical studies the UCBL was effective in partially correcting these deformities [14].

In patients who are inflamed, or who have severe pain, a period of rest in a cast or CAM boot immobilization combined with NSAIDs may be helpful. It is important to note however that in most instances, in patients with true flatfoot deformity, rather than PTT tendinitis, these treatments will not affect the long-term position of the foot. Nonoperative treatment is most effective for patients with Stage I disease.

4   Surgical Management

Surgical treatment of PCFD is determined by the level of deformity and the radiographic and clinical findings. While there are many described treatments for PCFD, we will focus on the medial ligamentous structures, specifically the SLC and the deltoid.

4.1   Isolated Spring Ligament Injury

While it is much more common that the spring ligament is injured in conjunction with the PTT, there have been several case reports which suggest that an isolated injury to the SLC is enough to cause PCFD. In these cases, patients often present with pain anterior to the medial malleolus and deep in the medial arch as opposed to along the PTT. Patients often typically maintain their ability to perform a single heel raise [15]. Due to the paucity of literature, there is no well-established recommendation on how to treat these patients. Despite the literature on these isolated injuries being very limited, good results have been published with surgical treatment.

In a case series of nine patients with PCFD with normal PTT function, Tryfonidis et al. reported on three patients who went on to have surgery. One patient with an acute spring ligament injury underwent direct repair of the torn spring and deltoid ligaments, while the remaining two patients underwent a spring ligament repair in conjunction with a flexor digitorum longus (FDL) transfer and medializing calcaneal osteotomy (MCO). He noted good results with both techniques [15]. In two separate case reports of high-level athletes with isolated spring ligament injury with no evidence of PTT dysfunction, the patients returned to their prior level of competition after undergoing a repair of the sprained ligament. In one case the spring ligament repair was supplemented with an FDL transfer [16, 17]. In 2013, Orr and Nunley reported on six patients with PCFD with isolated spring ligament dysfunction [18]. In their cohort ligament repair was done in conjunction with LCL, MCO, or cuneiform osteotomy as determined by pre-op deformity.

4.2   Spring Ligament Repair in Flexible PFCD

Stage II of PCFD is characterized by a valgus deformity of the hindfoot, flattening on the medial arch of the foot, and a variable degree of abduction of the forefoot. The amount of forefoot abduction differentiates between IIA and IIB deformities and is based on the amount of talonavicular uncoverage. Historically, this stage is treated with a FDL transfer, MCO, and/or LCL. However, in order for the forefoot to abduct, and the talus to plantarflex, we know there has to be an attenuation of the SLC. Therefore, in the flexible Stage II-A/B of PCFD, the ligament complex should be addressed to correct abduction deformity directly. LCL has traditionally been done for this deformity and, while effective [19, 20], can lead to lateral column overload, pain, and a rigid hindfoot [21, 22]. In 2015, Conti et al. [23] showed that excess abduction correction, by LCL, can lead to worse patient outcome, and this should be avoided. Additionally, we know that the lateral column is not necessarily short in patients with PCFD.

Studies have looked at SLC repair and reconstruction in the acute and chronic setting and concluded that it can be an effective treatment for forefoot abduction. In some cases, the spring ligament repair with or without augmentation can reduce the need to perform a LCL [24]. There are many different approaches to repair and reconstruct the SLC. In a cadaver model, Tan et al. [25] performed augmentation from the talar head to the navicular and found correction of the AP talo-first metatarsal angle, lateral talo-first metatarsal angle, and medial cuneiform height. Aynardi et al. in 2019 [26] compared SLC repair vs repair plus augmentation in eight cadaveric models. In their group, all of the ligament repairs failed, while only one of the augmented repairs failed. Several other authors have had success in vivo with various reconstruction techniques [26–30]. Most recently, Haye et al. [31] in 2020 compared SLC reconstruction with hamstring allograft with synthetic ligament augmentation and found patient outcomes were better with synthetic reconstruction. Historically, a LCL is performed in patients with greater than 30% uncoverage of the talar head. With new SLC reconstruction techniques with improved outcomes and a better understanding of the consequences of over lengthening the lateral column, we feel that SLC reconstruction should be the preferred technique and LCL only reserved for greater deformities of greater than 50% uncovering, given the power of modern medial soft tissue reconstruction.

4.2.1 Author's Recommended Technique

When performing this reconstruction, we developed a technique to reconstruct both the calcaneonavicular and tibiospring components due to the intimate relationship of the spring and deltoid ligaments. We chose to use the internal brace for our reconstruction technique due to the superior radiographic results with synthetic ligament reconstruction. A standard medial approach over the PTT is assessed for disease. If there is disease or attenuation, a FDL transfer is first performed in the standard fashion. If the PTT is found to be intact and in good condition, it can be left alone. After addressing the PTT, attention is turned to the SLC. The SLC is incised, and the sustentaculum of the calcaneus is identified. Utilizing the cannulated InternalBrace System (Arthrex®), a guide wire is placed into the sustentaculum and confirmed using fluoroscopy (Fig. 1). The sustentaculum is then further prepared with a drill and tap in a standard fashion, and a 3.5 mm SwiveLock®, loaded with a single long FiberTape®, is inserted. A wire is then placed from plantar to dorsal through the navicular and again confirmed with fluoroscopy (Fig. 2). A 2.7 mm drill is passed over the wire to create a passage for the FiberTape® (from the sustentaculum) which is routed from plantar to dorsal through the navicular (Fig. 3). The spring ligament component is then tensioned with the foot held in neutral dorsiflexion and neutral adduction by pulling on both limbs of the FiberTape® as it exits the dorsal navicular. After obtaining appropriate tension, the FiberTape® is secured by placing a SwiveLock® in the navicular tunnel. Attention is then turned to the deltoid component of our reconstruction. A guide wire is first placed into the tip of the medial malleolus and confirmed with fluoroscopy (Fig. 4). The bone is then prepped with a drill and tap for a 4.75 SwiveLock®. Again, the foot is held in neutral dorsiflexion and neutral adduction, and both limbs of the FiberTape® are appropriately tensioned and inserted into the medial malleolar tunnel (Fig. 5). We then imbricate the native spring ligament in a pants-over-vest fashion using 0 Vicryl suture to complete the reconstruction.

Fig. 1 An axial view of
the calcaneus demonstrates
appropriate fluoroscopy
image to confirm
placement of the guide
wire into the sustentaculum
tali. Care must be taken to
place the wire from
proximal to distal to avoid
violation of the subtalar
joint

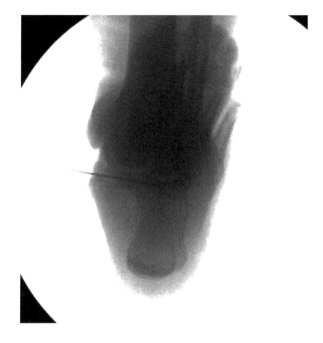

Fig. 2 An AP view of the
foot demonstrates wire
placement within the
navicular for creation of
the navicular tunnel

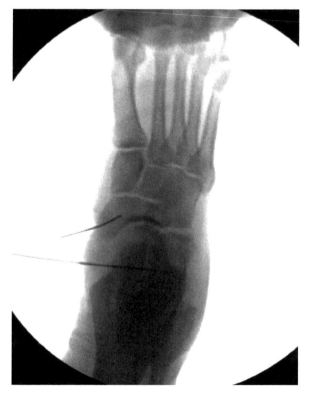

Fig. 3 Intraoperative photograph demonstrating the passage of the FiberTape® from the sustentaculum tali, plantar to the stump of the posterior tibial tendon, and routed from plantar to dorsal through the navicular tunnel. The sustentaculum tali are marked with a white dotted line and the letters "ST." The navicular bone is marked with a white dotted line and the letter "N"

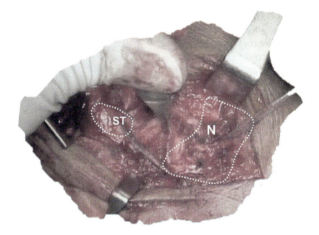

Fig. 4 A mortise view of the ankle demonstrating appropriate drilling position within the medial malleolus for insertion of the tibiospring component of the reconstruction

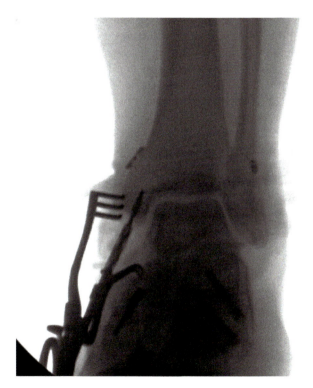

4.3 Medial Ligament Reconstruction in Rigid PCFD

As the progression of flatfoot deformity continues, the medial arch collapses, there is increased forefoot abduction, the hindfoot becomes rigid with subtalar arthritis (Stage III), and ultimately the deltoid will fail leading to asymmetry of the ankle

Fig. 5 Intraoperative photograph demonstrating the tibiospring component of the reconstruction with the FiberTape® now anchored into the medial malleolus. The medial malleolus is marked with a white dotted line and the letters "MM." The navicular is marked with a white dotted line and the letter "N"

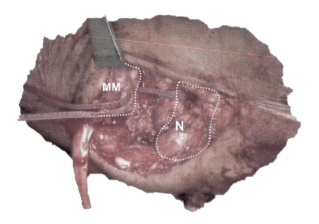

mortise with increased talar tilt. This ankle asymmetry is the hallmark of Stage IV of PCFD and was further subdivided by Bluman in 2007 into IV-A and IV-B, based on the presence or absence of ankle arthritis [3]. Historically, IV-A deformity is treated with deltoid reconstruction in conjunction with bony procedures, often a triple arthrodesis. When the ankle becomes arthritic, the tibiotalar joint is involved, and thus patients are historically treated with a pantalar arthrodesis. While this may be required to effectively correct deformity, extensive hindfoot fusions have a high morbidity, and when possible, joint sparing procedures should be attempted [32].

During surgical decision-making for patients with III and IV-A disease, there are several factors that must be considered. These include the ability to fully correct the hindfoot valgus and to realign and restore the ankle mortise and the identification and treatment of concomitant lateral ankle instability. We know through cadaveric studies that flatfoot deformity causes a shift and reduction in tibiotalar contact areas which can lead to point loading and development of arthritis [33]. In Stage III disease, the subtalar and talonavicular arthrodesis procedure or triple arthrodesis has had good results as the deformity has not progressed to include the tibiotalar joint. However, the increased rigidity of the construct will place increased stress on the deltoid ligament and medial-sided structures which may ultimately lead to failure and progression of deformity [34, 35]. Therefore, it is critical that the hindfoot deformity is completely corrected to decrease the risk of progression to Stage IV of disease despite arthrodesis. In patients with existing deltoid function and ankle asymmetry, but with intact cartilage (Stage IV-A) successful alignment of the mortise must be obtained. This can be obtained through reconstruction of deltoid ligament. Several procures have been described and have had good success [29, 30, 36–38]. In general, these procedures involve a reconstruction of some or all of the components of the tibiocalcaneonavicular ligament, term given to the functional ligament comprising the superficial and deep deltoid and spring ligament complex [39] which spans the tibiotalar, tibiocalcaneal, tibionavicular, and calcaneonavicular segments. This triangularly shaped complex reconstruction has been described using autograft, allograft, with or without augmentation due to the attenuation of the native ligament [30]. While often not considered a hallmark of early PCFD, Presaud et al. showed that there is MRI evidence of lateral ligament injury in approximately 63% of patients with Stage II or III disease [40]. When present this should be addressed.

Stage IV-B deformity, which is defined by the presence of ankle arthritis is a unique situation. In these patients joint-sparing procedures are often limited. Typically, when patients reach this stage, we surgeons are limited to ankle fusion vs total ankle replacement (TAR). Although TAR has been contraindicated in patients with deformity, as our understanding of deformity correction has improved, and our techniques have evolved, indications have expanded. In this instance most authors would recommend staged procedures that initially address the deformity and stability of the ankle and hindfoot, followed by TAR after complete recovery, to address the coexisting ankle arthritis [41].

4.3.1   Author's Recommended Technique

In our practice we attempt to avoid hindfoot fusion when possible in the early Stage IV disease. This can only be accomplished when there is not significant subtalar arthrosis. In these instances, both the superficial and deep deltoid ligaments must be reconstructed to provide stability. We prefer a technique that was described by Nery et al. in which the deep and superficial deltoid ligaments are reconstructed along with the spring ligament. This procedure involves anchoring a FiberTape® into the medial malleolus. One of the limbs is then anchored to the talus to reconstruct the deep deltoid, while the other is anchored, with a second FiberTape®, into the sustentaculum to reconstruct the superficial limb. This second FiberTape® is then routed through the navicular (in a similar fashion as described in detail above) to reconstruct the SLC. In all cases this reconstruction must be combined with a MCO. Alternatively, a double-loaded 3.5 mm SwiveLock® can be placed into the sustentaculum, and the use of the longer FiberTape® is recommended. Two limbs are taken into the navicular as described previously, tensioned with foot in neutral adduction, and secured with a 3.5 mm SwiveLock®. The superficial deltoid and tibiospring components are then reconstructed by taking the two limbs from the sustentaculum and the two limbs from the navicular and securing them into the medial malleolus with a 4.75 SwiveLock® with the foot held in slight inversion. The deep deltoid is then reconstructed immediately anterior to the MM with a 3.5 SwiveLock® with two of the four limbs that were anchored into the medial malleolus.

In cases in which the arthrosis of the hindfoot progresses to end-stage disease and a hindfoot fusion is required, a MCO is also performed to further medialize the forces on the ankle. In these cases, the deltoid ligament should also be reconstructed as we know this ligament must be attenuated or torn for this deformity to occur and repair is not sufficient. For this technique a medial incision is made, and the native deltoid ligament is elevated of the medial malleolus. Augmentation is completed by placing a 4.75 mm double loaded SwiveLock® into the medial malleolus. One of the limbs is anchored into the talus 5 mm distal and 5 mm anterior to the tip of the medial malleolus, and the second is inserted into the sustentaculum, reconstructing the deep and superficial deltoid ligaments, respectively. In these instances, fusion of the subtalar and talonavicular joints obviates the need for SLC reconstruction. It is imperative that the ankle is held in neutral dorsiflexion with a reduced mortise, while each limb of the reconstruction is separately tensioned. This reconstruction is then imbricated with the native deltoid ligament using anchors and additional 0 Vicryl.

In instances of Stage IV-B deformity where the ankle has progressed to end-stage arthritis, we feel that this should be treated in a staged fashion using the techniques described above to correct deformity and provide stability during the index procedure. When the patient has a stable and aligned foot, a TAR can be performed, understanding that there is still persistent risk of recurrent valgus in this case. In all cases, it is our protocol to utilize an ASO and an arch support for 3–6 months to protect the soft tissue repair.

References

1. Coughlin M, Mann R. Surgery of the foot and ankle. 7th ed. St. Louis: Mosby; 1999.
2. Johnson KA, Strom DE. Tibialis posterior tendon dysfunction. Clin Orthop Relat Res. 1989;239:196–206.
3. Bluman EM, Title CI, Myerson MS. Posterior tibial tendon rupture: a refined classification system. Foot Ankle Clin. 2007;12(2):233–49, v. https://doi.org/10.1016/j.fcl.2007.03.003.
4. de Cesar NC, Deland JT, Ellis SJ. Guest editorial: expert consensus on adult-acquired flatfoot deformity. Foot Ankle Int. 2020;41(10):1269–71. https://doi.org/10.1177/1071100720950715.
5. Deland JT. The adult acquired flatfoot and spring ligament complex. Pathology and implications for treatment. Foot Ankle Clin. 2001;6(1):129–35, vii. https://doi.org/10.1016/s1083-7515(03)00086-x.
6. Deland JT, de Asla RJ, Sung IH, Ernberg LA, Potter HG. Posterior tibial tendon insufficiency: which ligaments are involved? Foot Ankle Int. 2005;26(6):427–35. https://doi.org/10.1177/107110070502600601.
7. Williams G, Widnall J, Evans P, Platt S. Could failure of the spring ligament complex be the driving force behind the development of the adult flatfoot deformity? J Foot Ankle Surg. 2014;53(2):152–5. https://doi.org/10.1053/j.jfas.2013.12.011.
8. Funk DA, Cass JR, Johnson KA. Acquired adult flat foot secondary to posterior tibial-tendon pathology. J Bone Joint Surg Am. 1986;68(1):95–102.
9. Oburu E, Myerson MS. Deltoid ligament repair in flatfoot deformity. Foot Ankle Clin. 2017;22(3):503–14. https://doi.org/10.1016/j.fcl.2017.04.001.
10. Hintermann B, Knupp M, Pagenstert GI. Deltoid ligament injuries: diagnosis and management. Foot Ankle Clin. 2006;11(3):625–37. https://doi.org/10.1016/j.fcl.2006.08.001.
11. Omar H, Saini V, Wadhwa V, Liu G, Chhabra A. Spring ligament complex: illustrated normal anatomy and spectrum of pathologies on 3T MR imaging. Eur J Radiol. 2016;85(11):2133–43. https://doi.org/10.1016/j.ejrad.2016.09.023.
12. Davis WH, Sobel M, DiCarlo EF, Torzilli PA, Deng X, Geppert MJ, et al. Gross, histological, and microvascular anatomy and biomechanical testing of the spring ligament complex. Foot Ankle Int. 1996;17(2):95–102. https://doi.org/10.1177/107110079601700207.

13. Campbell KJ, Michalski MP, Wilson KJ, Goldsmith MT, Wijdicks CA, LaPrade RF, et al. The ligament anatomy of the deltoid complex of the ankle: a qualitative and quantitative anatomical study. J Bone Joint Surg Am. 2014;96(8):e62. https://doi.org/10.2106/JBJS.M.00870.

14. Havenhill TG, Toolan BC, Draganich LF. Effects of a UCBL orthosis and a calcaneal osteotomy on tibiotalar contact characteristics in a cadaver flatfoot model. Foot Ankle Int. 2005;26(8):607–13. https://doi.org/10.1177/107110070502600806.

15. Tryfonidis M, Jackson W, Mansour R, Cooke PH, Teh J, Ostlere S, et al. Acquired adult flat foot due to isolated plantar calcaneonavicular (spring) ligament insufficiency with a normal tibialis posterior tendon. Foot Ankle Surg. 2008;14(2):89–95. https://doi.org/10.1016/j.fas.2007.11.005.

16. Borton DC, Saxby TS. Tear of the plantar calcaneonavicular (spring) ligament causing flatfoot. A case report. J Bone Joint Surg Br. 1997;79(4):641–3. https://doi.org/10.1302/0301-620 x.79b4.7396.

17. Chen JP, Allen AM. MR diagnosis of traumatic tear of the spring ligament in a pole vaulter. Skelet Radiol. 1997;26(5):310–2. https://doi.org/10.1007/s002560050242.

18. Orr JD, Nunley JA. Isolated spring ligament failure as a cause of adult-acquired flatfoot deformity. Foot Ankle Int. 2013;34(6):818–23. https://doi.org/10.1177/1071100713483099.

19. Dumontier TA, Falicov A, Mosca V, Sangeorzan B. Calcaneal lengthening: investigation of deformity correction in a cadaver flatfoot model. Foot Ankle Int. 2005;26(2):166–70. https://doi.org/10.1177/107110070502600209.

20. Sangeorzan BJ, Mosca V, Hansen ST. Effect of calcaneal lengthening on relationships among the hindfoot, midfoot, and forefoot. Foot Ankle. 1993;14(3):136–41. https://doi.org/10.1177/107110079301400305.

21. Oh I, Imhauser C, Choi D, Williams B, Ellis S, Deland J. Sensitivity of plantar pressure and talonavicular alignment to lateral column lengthening in flatfoot reconstruction. J Bone Joint Surg Am. 2013;95(12):1094–100. https://doi.org/10.2106/JBJS.K.01032.

22. Benthien RA, Parks BG, Guyton GP, Schon LC. Lateral column calcaneal lengthening, flexor digitorum longus transfer, and opening wedge medial cuneiform osteotomy for flexible flatfoot: a biomechanical study. Foot Ankle Int. 2007;28(1):70–7. https://doi.org/10.3113/FAI.2007.0013.

23. Conti MS, Chan JY, Do HT, Ellis SJ, Deland JT. Correlation of postoperative midfoot position with outcome following reconstruction of the stage II adult acquired flatfoot deformity. Foot Ankle Int. 2015;36(3):239–47. https://doi.org/10.1177/1071100714564217.

24. Acevedo J, Vora A. Anatomical reconstruction of the spring ligament complex: "internal brace" augmentation. Foot Ankle Spec. 2013;6(6):441–5. https://doi.org/10.1177/1938640013499404.

25. Tan GJ, Kadakia AR, Ruberte Thiele RA, Hughes RE. Novel reconstruction of a static medial ligamentous complex in a flatfoot model. Foot Ankle Int. 2010;31(8):695–700. https://doi.org/10.3113/FAI.2010.0695.

26. Aynardi MC, Saloky K, Roush EP, Juliano P, Lewis GS. Biomechanical evaluation of spring ligament augmentation with the fiber tape device in a cadaveric flatfoot model. Foot Ankle Int. 2019;40(5):596–602. https://doi.org/10.1177/1071100719828373.

27. Baxter JR, LaMothe JM, Walls RJ, Prado MP, Gilbert SL, Deland JT. Reconstruction of the medial talonavicular joint in simulated flatfoot deformity. Foot Ankle Int. 2015;36(4):424–9. https://doi.org/10.1177/1071100714558512.

28. Pasapula C, Devany A, Fischer NC, Wijdicks CA, Hübner T, Reifenscneider F, et al. The resistance to failure of spring ligament reconstruction. Foot (Edinb). 2017;33:29–34. https://doi.org/10.1016/j.foot.2017.05.006.

29. Nery C, Lemos AVKC, Raduan F, Mansur NSB, Baumfeld D. Combined spring and deltoid ligament repair in adult-acquired flatfoot. Foot Ankle Int. 2018;39(8):903–7. https://doi.org/10.1177/1071100718770132.

30. Brodell JD, MacDonald A, Perkins JA, Deland JT, Oh I. Deltoid-spring ligament reconstruction in adult acquired flatfoot deformity with medial peritalar instability. Foot Ankle Int. 2019;40(7):753–61. https://doi.org/10.1177/1071100719839176.

31. Heyes G, Swanton E, Vosoughi AR, Mason LW, Molloy AP. Comparative study of spring liga-ment reconstructions using either hamstring allograft or synthetic ligament augmentation. Foot Ankle Int. 2020;41(7):803–10. https://doi.org/10.1177/1071100720917375.
32. Taylor R, Sammarco VJ. Minimizing the role of fusion in the rigid flatfoot. Foot Ankle Clin. 2012;17(2):337–49. https://doi.org/10.1016/j.fcl.2012.03.010.
33. Friedman MA, Draganich LF, Toolan B, Brage ME. The effects of adult acquired flatfoot deformity on tibiotalar joint contact characteristics. Foot Ankle Int. 2001;22(3):241–6. https://doi.org/10.1177/107110070102200312.
34. Miniaci-Coxhead SL, Weisenthal B, Ketz JP, Flemister AS. Incidence and radiographic predic-tors of valgus tibiotalar tilt after hindfoot fusion. Foot Ankle Int. 2017;38(5):519–25. https://doi.org/10.1177/1071100717690439.
35. Song SJ, Lee S, O'Malley MJ, Otis JC, Sung IH, Deland JT. Deltoid ligament strain after cor-rection of acquired flatfoot deformity by triple arthrodesis. Foot Ankle Int. 2000;21(7):573–7. https://doi.org/10.1177/107110070002100708.
36. Deland JT, de Asla RJ, Segal A. Reconstruction of the chronically failed deltoid ligament: a new technique. Foot Ankle Int. 2004;25(11):795–9. https://doi.org/10.1177/107110070402501107.
37. Haddad SL, Dedhia S, Ren Y, Rotstein J, Zhang LQ. Deltoid ligament reconstruction: a novel technique with biomechanical analysis. Foot Ankle Int. 2010;31(7):639–51. https://doi.org/10.3113/FAI.2010.0639.
38. Jeng CL, Bluman EM, Myerson MS. Minimally invasive deltoid ligament reconstruction for stage IV flatfoot deformity. Foot Ankle Int. 2011;32(1):21–30. https://doi.org/10.3113/FAI.2011.0021.
39. Cromeens BP, Kirchhoff CA, Patterson RM, et al. An attachment-based description of the medial collateral and spring ligament complexes. Foot Ankle Int. 2015;36(6):710–21. https://doi.org/10.1177/1071100715572221.
40. Persaud S, Hentges MJ, Catanzariti AR. Occurrence of lateral ankle ligament disease with stage 2 to 3 adult-acquired flatfoot deformity confirmed via magnetic resonance imag-ing: a retrospective study. J Foot Ankle Surg. 2019;58(2):243–7. https://doi.org/10.1053/j.jfas.2018.08.030.
41. Dodd A, Daniels TR. Total ankle replacement in the presence of talar varus or valgus deformi-ties. Foot Ankle Clin. 2017;22(2):277–300. https://doi.org/10.1016/j.fcl.2017.01.002.

Cavus Foot

Mark S. Myerson and Shuyuan Li

1   Introduction

The cavus foot represents an incredibly complex spectrum of deformities all caused by muscle imbalance leading to structural changes in the foot. There is no classic presentation of the cavus foot, since cavus, cavovarus, cavoadductovarus, and cavo-equinovarus are all different types of structural deformity associated with muscle imbalance and soft tissue contracture [1–5]. To add to this, there is a very wide and varied spectrum of the severity of deformity even within each of the above subtypes. There are references to the mild or subtle cavus foot in the literature, those which appear to be idiopathic [6–12] and those which we easily recognize as being quite severe. The keys to understanding *all of these deformities* are based on some very straightforward principles, since treatment is determined by recognition of the flexibility or rigidity of the hindfoot, midfoot, and forefoot, the structural changes of the foot, the apex of each of these separate deformities, and the inherent muscle imbalance which is the cause of every neurological cavus foot deformity [13–15]. The management of the cavus foot does not have to be complicated provided one understands this muscle imbalance and the role of correction in multiple planes at the apex of each structural deformity. One should not rely on correction of deformity with osteotomy or arthrodesis alone since balancing the muscle forces with tendon transfer(s) should be considered fundamental for many procedures and in all cases of neuromuscular cavus deformity [5].

This chapter will focus on the neurological cavus foot deformities, and the principles of deformity correction can be summarized here:

M. S. Myerson (✉) · S. Li
Department of Orthopaedics, University of Colorado Anschutz Medical Campus,
Aurora, CO, USA

Steps2Walk, Greenwood Village, CO, USA
https://www.steps2walk.org

E. Wagner Hitschfeld, P. Wagner Hitschfeld (eds.), *Foot and Ankle Disorders*,
https://doi.org/10.1007/978-3-030-95738-4_26

- Tendon transfer(s) must be performed to improve muscle imbalance in neurological cavus foot.
- A tenotomy of the posterior tibial tendon may be necessary if there is severe scarring of the foot and ankle.
- A plantar fascia release is routinely performed.
- Osteotomies or arthrodesis must be performed at the apex of deformity.
- A triplanar calcaneal osteotomy may be necessary in addition to hindfoot arthrodesis.
- Resection of the base of the fifth metatarsal combined with triple or pantalar arthrodesis is useful to correct fixed midfoot varus deformity.

2   Examination of the Foot

Is the deformity rigid or flexible? How will one use this information? The classic clinical test of rigidity is the Coleman "block test" where the lateral forefoot and heel rest on a block of wood, while the plantarflexed first ray is allowed to drop off the edge of the block [16–18]. If the hindfoot varus remains uncorrected after removing the plantarflexed first ray as a deforming force, then the hindfoot varus is considered to be rigid. The challenge to effectively and predictably use this test is that there is a spectrum to flexibility and rigidity, and it is difficult to know what to do when the hindfoot *partially* corrects. While the Coleman block test can tell you if there is *some* flexibility, its downfall is that it does not give the examiner a "feel" for how correctable the hindfoot really is [5]. The Coleman block is not the only way to assess hindfoot rigidity, and others have suggested maneuvers for evaluating hindfoot flexibility while the patient is non-weight-bearing. One described method is performed by placing the patient in a prone position with the knee flexed 90° [19]. In this position, the foot is allowed to move freely without the influence of the first ray, and hindfoot manipulation is easily performed allowing for determination of rigidity. We agree that while a test of rigidity while weight-bearing is relevant, it is not nearly as useful as the "feel" that one obtains when examining the foot in the seated position. We therefore always perform the examination of the foot by manipulating the heel with the patient in a seated position and the foot dangling from the exam table. With the foot in equinus, it takes out the effect of any Achilles or gastrocnemius contracture as well as the position of the first metatarsal. We believe that this method gives the examiner a better sense for the amount of retained hindfoot motion and is easier to perform than the Coleman block test or by having the patient lie prone [20]. With this method, if the heel is correctable to a valgus position, then, regardless of what happens to the forefoot, there is still the likelihood that an arthrodesis can be avoided. If the hindfoot is only partially correctible, then it is our practice to lean toward arthrodesis rather than trying to "push the limits" of a joint-sparing procedure. One should also realize that final decision-making regarding flexibility of the foot can sometimes only be made intraoperatively following medial soft tissue release. Some surgeons use the Coleman block test to determine whether a single dorsal closing wedge osteotomy at the base of the first metatarsal can correct the varus deformity of the heel, based on a concept that this is a "forefoot-driven hindfoot varus deformity." However, there are very no neurologic cavovarus deformities which are caused by a fixed equinus of the first metatarsal in the absence of muscle imbalance. Secondly, in order to correct a "forefoot-driven hindfoot varus" deformity with a single first metatarsal osteotomy, the midfoot and hindfoot must be flexible to allow sufficient derotation, which is very difficult to achieve due secondary medial and plantar soft tissue contracture. It is a general principle of deformity correction to commence with the most proximal deformity, and heel varus is no different where an osteotomy of the calcaneus may be the ideal way to start. We suggest that if one wants to start by correcting the first metatarsal plantar flexion, always check intraoperatively under simulated weight-bearing if the hindfoot is corrected. If the foot is not able to be reduced under anesthesia during the surgery, then it is unlikely to do so after surgery.

Standard anteroposterior, oblique, and lateral weight-bearing radiographs of the foot and ankle should be taken, and often forgotten, but most important, are weight-bearing radiographs of the ankle [21]. We know that the foot is deformed, but if deformity, instability, or arthritis of the ankle persists, this will significantly affect the outcome of treatment. Weight-bearing computerized tomography (WBCT) scan can give us three-dimensional detailed information of the alignment, structure, biomechanics, and condition of the joints. It is always helpful to quantify the amount of deformity. For example, on weight-bearing radiographic images, using the calcaneal pitch angle, Meary's angle, Hibbs angle, to evaluate pes cavus; using hindfoot alignment, talonavicular coverage, metatarsus adductus, and Kite's angle to assess varus deformities, and on three-dimensional WBCT scan images using foot and ankle offset (FAO), parameters of peritalar subluxation and the arch index to assess the general cavovarus deformity [22, 23].

The apex of the deformity, which is nearly always multiplanar, will be very useful to decide where and which procedure(s) need to be performed [24]. The location of the apex in the sagittal plane will determine whether the deformity is an anterior (midfoot) or posterior (hindfoot) cavus (or both since there can be more than one apex). One must plan for correction in the coronal plane as well in particular adduction and rotational malalignment. The hindfoot alignment view is a very useful adjunct in radiographic evaluation. It is helpful in measuring the amount of deformity present and can provide an objective gauge of the amount of correction of hindfoot varus achieved after surgical intervention. When one chooses to use WBCT scans in helping surgical planning, it is critical to realize that the foot and ankle offset (FAO) which was developed based on the tripod theory of the foot should not be used to substitute for the hindfoot alignment view. The FAO is a three-dimensional parameter which gives the reader a general idea of how well the foot is balanced as a tripod, but one cannot say that a patient with a higher negative FAO value has a more severe cavus or varus deformity than another patient with a lower negative FAO value. Several recent publications [25–27] were designed by grouping patients using FAO as a direct substitution for the assessment of hindfoot alignment which is misleading. In treating a cavus deformity, one must see the whole picture, that is, you cannot see the forest for the trees, since one should address each individual problem by taking the whole picture apart and then reassembling it. One can use the peritalar subluxation assessment in the subtalar, talonavicular, calcaneocuboid, and ankle joints and the relationship between the first and the fifth metatarsal and the floor to help with preoperative planning [23]. Ideally, after derotation around those joints, the declination of the first metatarsal and the height of the medial cuneiform to the floor should decrease postoperatively, and the position and height of the fifth metatarsal from the floor should increase postoperatively.

3   Approach to Correction

As the heel moves into varus, the first metatarsal has to compensate for the hindfoot position by dropping into equinus, in order to maintain the forefoot in a plantigrade position. This equinus position of the first metatarsal is perpetuated and aggravated by contracture of the plantar fascia, and in cases where there is weakness of the anterior tibial muscle as in Charcot-Marie-Tooth (CMT) disease, the equinus of the first metatarsal is worsened. With increasing contracture of the plantar fascia, and in particular as a result of atrophy of the intrinsic muscles of the foot when associated with CMT, the forefoot deformity worsens. In neurological cavus deformity, there is frequently an imbalance between the peroneus longus and the anterior tibial muscles, and the posterior tibial muscle is always stronger than the peroneus brevis muscle in more severe deformities, with a variable degree of contracture of the gastrocnemius and soleus muscles present. Understanding this will be very useful for planning the structural changes in the foot [28]. In order to successfully correct structural deformity, it is useful to perform a release of any contracted soft tissue, including the plantar fascia release, which can be the initial procedure followed by preparation of the posterior tibial tendon for transfer, since the calcaneus is difficult to move with osteotomy if the plantar fascia remains contracted. The sagittal apex is either in the midfoot or the hindfoot or both and will determine the location as well as the type of the procedure. Recognize that whatever is done to correct one plane of deformity will have an impact on the rest of the foot. For example, as the hindfoot varus is corrected through eversion and pronation, the medial forefoot equinus worsens. The medial column of the foot is always more plantarflexed than the lateral column, but the lateral column tends to be more fixed, rotated, and slightly adducted. Thus, when correcting the plantarflexion of the first ray, rotational malalignment must also be addressed or else the midfoot will be left in a supinated position with continued overload of the lateral column. The assessment of muscle strength is important to plan the tendon balancing which will be a necessary part of the correction. While this is understood in the setting of the joint-sparing procedures for a flexible deformity, it has often been overlooked when treating a rigid deformity. It has been our observation that without proper soft tissue balancing, bony procedures alone are likely to fail in the long run [4].

One can simplistically approach deformity correction based on the flexibility of the foot and the severity of the deformity [29]. Although it is difficult to quantify flexibility, it implies that the subtalar joint is easily correctable to neutral, there is mild forefoot equinus deformity, and no fixed adductovarus. For a flexible foot associated with a mild deformity, we perform a combination of a plantar fascia release, a calcaneal osteotomy, a transfer of the peroneus longus to brevis, and then whatever else is necessary to complete the correction, which may have to include a dorsal closing wedge osteotomy of the first metatarsal, an arthrodesis or the first TMT joint, or a dorsal closing wedge osteotomy of the medial cuneiform. There is often an associated equinus deformity, and the correction is performed with either a percutaneous Achilles lengthening or a gastrocnemius recession depending on the nature of the contracture. For a moderate deformity, we perform the same sequence of procedures above but recognize that the midfoot deformity is greater with an increased cavus of the medial part of the midfoot as well as increased rotation of the lateral foot which creates a much greater load along the entire length of the fifth metatarsal. If present, adductovarus is mild, and a transfer of the posterior tibial tendon is unusual in these cases unless the cavus is caused by CMT disease associated with a drop foot, in which case the posterior tibial tendon is transferred through the interosseous membrane to the midfoot. The most important aspect of correcting a moderate deformity is a midfoot osteotomy-arthrodesis. For severe deformity correction, the sequence of steps includes the same approach as outlined above but performed with one or another modification of a triple arthrodesis and additional procedures which are necessary including peroneus brevis repair and a lateral ankle ligament reconstruction. It is easy to distinguish between a mild and a severe deformity, but the difficulty lies in the approach to correct a moderate deformity where the foot appears to be correctible on a Coleman block test, the hindfoot is flexible on examination, and one tries to avoid an arthrodesis leading to less-than-ideal results.

3.1 The Plantar Fascia Release

Correcting the malposition of the calcaneus is difficult without first releasing the plantar fascia, and this is part of the overall soft tissue releases medially which include the posterior tibial tendon transfer. This simplest fasciotomy is done percutaneously through a 1 cm medial longitudinal incision adjacent to the heel, at the junction of the dorsal and plantar skin (Fig. 1). Although uncommon, this may lead to a small area of numbness on the medial aspect of the heel pad but of no clinical relevance. Following the skin incision, a pair of scissors is inserted to bluntly push above and below the fascia to separate and to locate the fascia which will also avoid any injury to the branch of the lateral plantar nerve. The fascia is then cut with scissors by advancing the scissors without a cutting motion, but simply allowing the scissors to split the fascia until both the medial and lateral bands are completely released. For severe adductovarus deformity, the fascia of the abductor hallucis

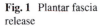
Fig. 1 Plantar fascia release

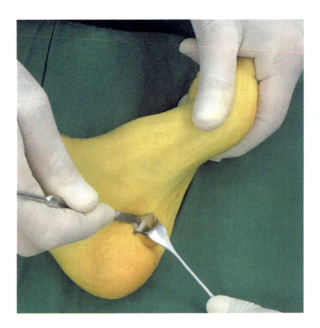

tendon also must be completely released. This release must be very carefully planned because multiple incisions cannot be used for the posterior tibial tendon transfer, the plantar fascia release, the abductor hallucis tendon release, and the talonavicular joint capsule and the spring ligament release. By carefully planning, these procedures can be completed through the same medial approach.

3.2 Calcaneus Osteotomy

The calcaneus osteotomy is a very utilitarian procedure to correct a cavus foot and, depending on the magnitude of the deformity, is always required in one form or another. When correcting a very severe hindfoot varus deformity, in addition to a subtalar or triple arthrodesis, a triplanar calcaneus osteotomy can be added. This triplane osteotomy corrects the varus with a laterally based wedge and then moves the tuberosity laterally as well as cephalad [30]. One has to be careful with the extent of the lateral shift of the calcaneus, since this can cause tarsal tunnel syndrome [31]. If the varus is severe, we think that a prophylactic release of the tarsal tunnel is useful and can be performed by extending the medial incision for the exposure of the posterior tibial tendon. At times one can perform the osteotomy and then palpate the skin on the medial side of the foot to determine if it remains soft, and if so a release may not be necessary.

The incision for the calcaneal osteotomy varies according to the type of procedure performed (Fig. 2a). If an osteotomy alone is performed, then a shorter incision is made directly inferior to the peroneal tendons. Invariably however, the calcaneal osteotomy often needs to be performed with additional lateral procedures, including repair of the peroneal tendon(s), reconstruction of lateral ankle instability, a peroneus longus-to-brevis tendon transfer, and a cuboid osteotomy. For these cases, the incision is simply extended posteriorly along the axis of the peroneal tendons behind the fibula.

The incision is deepened through subcutaneous tissue in the plane between the peroneal tendon and the sural nerve. The peroneal tendon repair or transfer is performed before the osteotomy (Fig. 2b). The nerve can be retracted either superiorly or inferiorly, depending on its position. The periosteum needs to be elevated over a broad area, because a wedge of bone is going to be removed. Two small, curved retractors are used on either side of the incision to expose the entire lateral tuberosity. A saw should be used to make the wedge cuts, with the first cut perpendicular to the axis of the calcaneus at a 45-degree angle to the tuberosity and the second at an angle of approximately 20 degrees, but this depends on the size of the wedge. It is far easier to start out with a smaller wedge and then remove more bone if the correction is not sufficient. The osteotomy rarely closes down perfectly at this time, so additional perforation of the calcaneus typically is necessary to permit it to close down smoothly. Depending on the deformity, the calcaneus is moved in two or three planes as described above (Fig. 2c-e). The valgus closing wedge osteotomy constitutes the first plane. The tuberosity is then shifted laterally by 8–10 mm, and cephalad movement is the third plane which is added according to the pitch angle of the calcaneus. We use two guide pins to hold the calcaneus in the corrected position. The first guide pin is inserted centrally into the body of the posterior tuberosity, which can then be manipulated into the corrected position. While the guide pin is being held and the heel held in the desired position, a second guide pin is introduced for screw fixation. It is best to insert the screw from slightly posterior lateral to slightly anterior and medial to gain maximal compression. Tamping the overhanging inferior ledge of the bone is unnecessary.

3.3   Tendon Transfers

Cavovarus deformities tend to be both dynamic and progressive, and only a well-balanced foot will be stable over time. Soft tissue balancing contributes to the long-term success of the bony structural correction, as it will remove the major deforming forces going forward [32]. In cavovarus deformities the deforming forces are the posterior tibial and the peroneus longus tendons, which overpower the peroneus brevis and anterior tibial tendon, respectively. This imbalance leads to a varus hindfoot and a pronated and plantarflexed medial column. However, this muscle imbalance is always a little different in each patient, and variations in muscle strength will always be encountered, and therefore, evaluation of their *relative* differences is important. The peroneus longus-to-brevis transfer is an important part of correction, and without release of the force of the peroneus longus, recurrence of first metatarsal plantarflexion will occur even if a midfoot or triple arthrodesis is performed. We transfer the peroneus longus to the weakened peroneus brevis to increase eversion

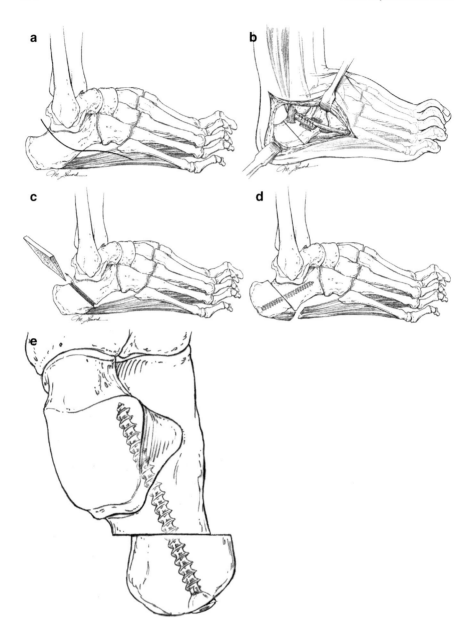

Fig. 2 (**a**) An extensile incision is used laterally to approach the calcaneus, the peroneal tendon transfer, and also expose the cuboid for osteotomy. (**b**) The peroneus longus-to-brevis tendon transfer is performed and the calcaneal osteotomy marked out with electrocautery. (**c**) The calcaneus osteotomy is performed as a triplane shift. A wedge is removed laterally, (**d**) and the calcaneus shifted cephalad and fixed with a fully threaded screw. (**e**) Note the lateral shift of the tuberosity

strength. Ideally, this procedure is done in younger patients and even in children to achieve maximal advantage or when the foot is more flexible. One must be careful using this transfer to augment the eversion strength when a posterior tibial tendon transfer is performed simultaneously in the absence of a hindfoot arthrodesis. In this situation, one can cause an irreversible flatfoot deformity. If the peroneus brevis tendon is scarred, torn, or absent, the longus tendon can still be transferred to the stump of the base of the brevis tendon into the fifth metatarsal. This is the first tendon transfer to be performed, and we usually do it before commencing with the calcaneus osteotomy. The technique for this transfer involves pulling the longus tendon distally while suturing both tendons together before cutting the longus to achieve the appropriate tension. If the longus is cut before suture, it is more difficult to find the correct resting tension for the transfer. Additional tendons to consider for transfer are the anterior tibial tendon, the extensor hallucis longus, and extensor digitorum longus. Even though the anterior tibial tendon is overpowered by the peroneus longus, it still has some strength and contributes to the deformity by creating a dorsal apex in the midfoot. In certain deformities, without release and transfer of the tendon, it may be impossible to unwind the foot adequately for correction.

A typical tendon transfer for the cavus foot is to use the posterior tibial tendon (PTT) and place it in a position that is beneficial for function and stability of both the foot and the ankle. There are two reasons to perform a tendon transfer: the first is to remove a deforming force, and the second is to gain power in a direction that is missing. Muscle power of any commonly transferred tendon in the cavus foot, particularly the posterior tibial, is variable, and when the posterior tibial muscle is weak, surgeons commonly do not perform a transfer judging it to lack sufficient power for transfer. However, there is always *some* power left in the muscle that will overcome its antagonist and gradually lead to recurrence of deformity, and we perform a posterior tibial tendon transfer routinely, regardless of the type of bony surgery chosen. If not transferred, an arthrodesis will eventually fail since overpull by the posterior tibial tendon will cause adduction at the level of the talonavicular joint if a midfoot arthrodesis is planned or at the naviculo-cuneiform joint if a triple is done. In either setting, a new apex of deformity is created by the intact insertion of the tendon. We try to use whatever tendon is available and, in particular, whichever muscle is a deforming force on the foot or ankle. This applies to the extensor hallux longus, the extensor digital longus, the posterior tibial tendon, the peroneus longus, and any other tendon that may be used to correct deformity. The principles of tendon transfer are similar to those performed for paralytic deformities; however, the incisions must be planned more carefully when calcaneal and midfoot osteotomies are performed simultaneously. We prefer not to use an interference screw or bone suture anchor to secure the posterior tibial tendon to the midfoot, but use a broad rubber button which is used over a gauze pad. We use the syringe top from a 20 or 30 syringe and then take off the rubber cap and perforate it with two clamps to make a hole and then pass sutures attached to the posterior tibial tendon transfer through the rubber cap which are then tied over a gauze pad on the under surface of the foot.

3.4   Midfoot Osteotomy-Arthrodesis

Midfoot osteotomy and arthrodesis are ideally suited for a deformity where the apex is located distal to the transverse tarsal joint. A triple arthrodesis will not correct the forefoot and midfoot present in this deformity and is therefore the incorrect procedure in this situation. For so many moderate to severe deformities, rigid or flexible, one can perform correction with soft tissue procedures, a triplanar osteotomy of the calcaneus, an osteotomy through the cuneiforms and cuboid, or an arthrodesis of the naviculocuneiform joints and an osteotomy of the cuboid (Fig. 3). Concerns about wound healing, nonunion, and technical difficulty of the operation have led surgeons away from midfoot arthrodesis, but one cannot correct the forefoot only with an osteotomy of the first metatarsal since this is at a point distal to the apex and will only create a banana shape to the medial forefoot.

Several techniques for dorsal wedge osteotomy have been described including Jahss [33] who performed the procedure at the level of the tarsometatarsal (TMT) joints and Cole [34] and Jappas [35] who performed correction at the naviculocuneiform/cuboid joints [36]. Our preferred technique is similar to that proposed by Cole, since this provides correction at the apex of the deformity, and it allows for multiplanar correction including the plantarflexion and adductus. The midfoot arthrodesis must be performed with a release of the plantar fascia. An extensile dorsal midline incision from the ankle to the mid-metatarsal is made. One should not compromise wound healing by limiting the length of the incision, because skin retraction and wound dehiscence are potential risks with a shorter incision. The superficial peroneal nerve is retracted laterally, and the deep peroneal nerve and dorsalis pedis artery are elevated via a subperiosteal plane and retracted medially followed by tenotomy of the extensor hallucis brevis tendon if necessary, to visualize the midfoot. The apex of the deformity is identified under fluoroscopy, and an electrocautery is used to mark out the wedge of bone which is removed with a saw (Fig. 4). Predicting the size of the wedge is not easy, so we always begin with a small amount of bone resection and then gradually increase this as necessary for correction. The entire osteotomy-arthrodesis of the midfoot and cuboid can be performed through one dorsal incision, but this requires a lot of retraction laterally to visualize the cuboid. We will frequently use two incisions to approach correction, the first one dorsally and the second by extending the incision used for the calcaneus osteotomy distally to the fifth metatarsal. In this way the cuboid can be very easily visualized and cut. It is rare that the wedge correction can be obtained with a single bone cut, because the first metatarsal declination is always more depressed than the fifth, and the wedge is biplanar, with more bone removed from the dorsal than from the lateral midfoot. It is very important to understand that one cannot remove a medially based wedge which will cause or worsen any adductus deformity. The wedge is therefore based dorsally toward the middle and medial cuneiform but tapered laterally into the cuboid where no wedge is removed. However, more of a *dorsal wedge* will need to be removed medially than laterally – the medial correction is achieved mostly by dorsiflexion through the wedge resection, whereas the lateral correction through the cuboid is achieved more by dorsal translation and rotation. A very useful technique

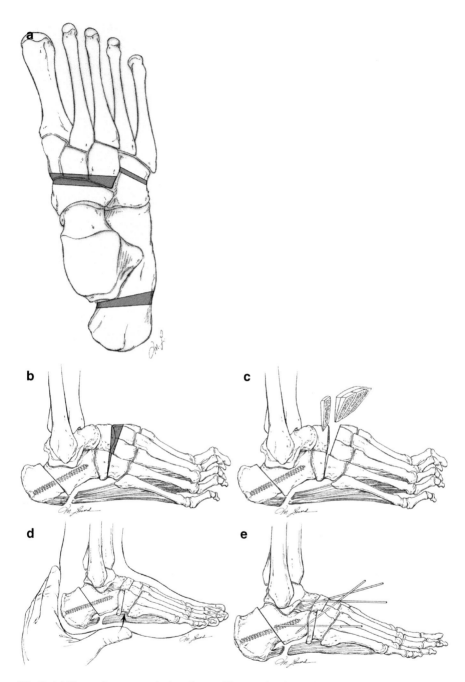

Fig. 3 (**a**) The wedges are marked out here to illustrate the size and orientation from the navicular cuneiform joint, the cuboid, and calcaneus. It is not always necessary to remove a wedge from the cuboid, and a vertical osteotomy in the center of the cuboid with dorsal translation may be sufficient. (**b**, **c**) The location and extent of the wedge from the naviculocuneiform joints and the cuboid is illustrated. Note the plantar fasciotomy and the position of the calcaneus tuberosity. (**d**) A key part of the correction of the midfoot deformity is to push up under the base of the fifth metatarsal and cuboid in order to derotate the supination of the midfoot. (**e**) Final fixation is demonstrated

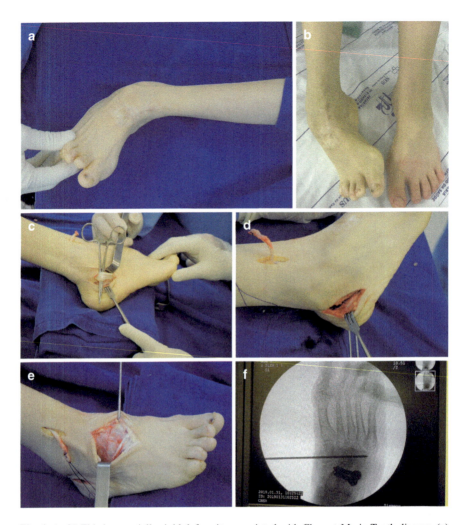

Fig. 4 (**a, b**) This is a partially rigid deformity associated with Charcot-Marie-Tooth disease. (**c**) Following the plantar fascia release and the harvest of the posterior tibial tendon for transfer, the lateral incision is made for calcaneal osteotomy and peroneus longus-to-brevis transfer. (**d**). The triplane calcaneal osteotomy is performed and shifted laterally and cephalad. (**e, f**) The midfoot is exposed, and a guide pin is inserted across marking out the osteotomy both clinically and under fluoroscopy to ensure that the osteotomy is performed in the center of the naviculocuneiform joint and across into the cuboid at the correct level. (**g**) Following the osteotomy and fixation with 3 mm pins, a drill hole is made to pass the posterior tibial tendon from dorsal to plantar, in this case through the medial edge of the cuboid. (**h, i**) The posterior tibial tendon is secured on the plantar surface of the foot over soft tissue bolster and a rubber stopper from a 30 mL syringe. (**j**) Note the correction obtained with the naviculocuneiform arthrodesis, the dorsal translation of the cuneiform on the navicular, and the triplanar calcaneal osteotomy

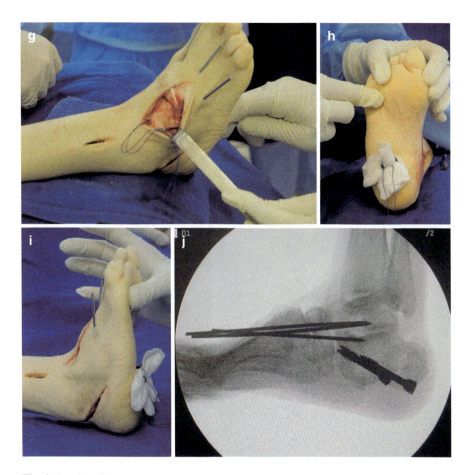

Fig. 4 (continued)

now is to close the wedge but add additional dorsal translation of the forefoot. This can usually be done, but depends on the plantar soft tissue contracture, and the size of the wedge resected. More dorsal translation should be obtained medially, but this depends on the severity and location of the equinus. This step will significantly reduce the residual forefoot deformity and decrease the likelihood of metatarsalgia (Fig. 5). Because the first metatarsal declination is always more depressed than the fifth, the wedge is biplanar, with more bone removed from the dorsal than from the lateral midfoot. Also note that one should not try to remove a huge wedge medially in order to elevate the first metatarsal since this will unnecessarily shorten the foot, and it is easier to perform a double osteotomy, one in the midfoot and an additional osteotomy of the first metatarsal. If the latter is performed with a long oblique wedge instead of a vertical wedge, the length of the metatarsal can also be preserved. Be careful of the location of the anterior tibial tendon which must be retracted out of the way of the excursion of the saw blade. If adductus needs to be corrected in addition to the cavus, a biplanar correction is achieved by resecting more bone laterally, in

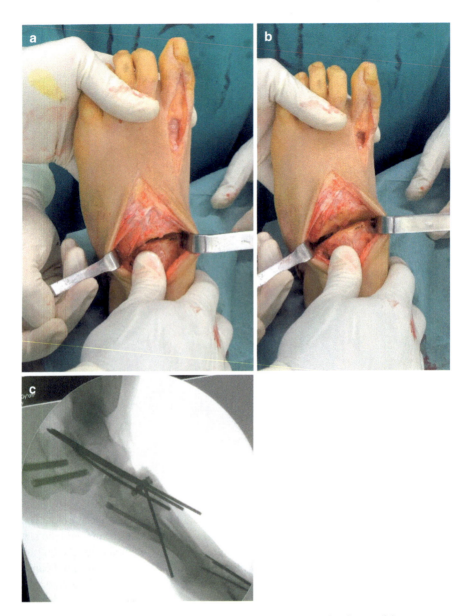

Fig. 5 (**a**) Following the biplanar osteotomy, an alternative technique for closure of the osteotomy is to adjust the distal aspect of the midfoot which is pushed dorsally. (**b**) The thumb on the right hand is pushing down on the navicular, while the forefoot and midfoot are elevated. Bone contact with this elevation is quite adequate. (**c**) Following fixation, one can appreciate the dorsal translation of the cuneiforms on the navicular which simultaneously elevates the forefoot to correct the equinus

particular through the cuboid. The osteotomy cut is shaped such that the medial limb forms one aspect of a wedge that is 8 mm in diameter and at a 15–20-degree angle to the dorsal plane of the midfoot. The first lateral osteotomy cut is made extending the saw cut toward the cuboid from the middle or lateral cuneiform, and then the second osteotomy cut is made at a much smaller angle so that the apex is in the cuboid without removing much of the cuboid at all. It is far easier to perform the lateral correction by dorsally translating the cuboid and then rotating it slightly to elevate the base of the fifth metatarsal.

Once the midfoot has been corrected through dorsiflexion, elevation, and translation as well as lateral column rotation, good bony apposition can be achieved with any available fixation (Fig. 6). Typically, we use multiple 3 mm Steinmann pins. Using pins in

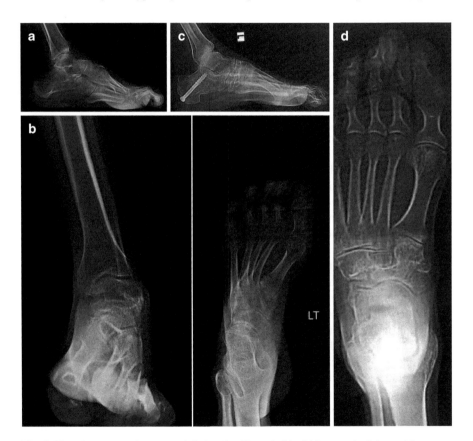

Fig. 6 Note the preoperative non-weight-bearing X-ray (**a**, **b**) of this severely deformed foot associated with Charcot-Marie-Tooth disease. The hindfoot and the midfoot were quite rigid. Note the severely supinated midfoot with a dorsal apex at the naviculocuneiform joint. The subtalar joint is open, and in varus, and the fifth metatarsal is close to the floor with a marked change in the arch height index. (**c**, **d**) Even though these are not weight-bearing X-rays, it is easy to see the marked change in appearance of all of the features of the cavus foot in the postoperative X-ray. The subtalar joint is no longer in varus, and the arch height index (the ratio between the height of the medial cuneiform and fifth metatarsal to the floor) has been completely restored. On the anteroposterior review, the talus-first metatarsal angle, the adductus, and supination have all been corrected

this location is easier than plates, staples or screws because of the plane of the osteotomy and the small bone segments between each articulation. The pins are inserted from the medial and lateral portion of the foot, from distal to proximal, and then removed at 4–6 weeks in children and 8 weeks in adults, once ambulation begins. Once the osteotomy has been stabilized, the tendon transfer(s) can be completed. We typically place the posterior tibial tendon into the lateral cuneiform, although if severe adductus is present and some anterior tibial muscle power is present, we will insert it into the cuboid.

3.5   Correction of Forefoot Equinus

As the heel is brought into valgus, increased pronation of the forefoot occurs, with an increased plantar flexion of the first metatarsal which is counterproductive in a cavus foot. For a flexible deformity, the worsening of the first metatarsal equinus occurs commonly but may also be required following a midfoot osteotomy-arthrodesis or even a triple arthrodesis. One must understand that the apex of the cavus deformity is never in the first metatarsal and is either at the first TMT joint, the cuneiform, the naviculocuneiform (NC), or the talonavicular (TN) joint. Why then is a dorsiflexion osteotomy of the first metatarsal so frequently performed? Although this is an easy procedure to perform, and intentionally elevates the first metatarsal to correct the distal overload, it is technically incorrect. It is our preference therefore to perform the osteotomy or arthrodesis directly at the apex of the deformity which will either be the first TMT joint, the medial cuneiform, or the NC joint, and a first metatarsal osteotomy will be used for convenience purposes only for minor deformities or after hindfoot correction. One should consider the balance of the foot with the combination of a calcaneal osteotomy, a peroneus longus-to-brevis tendon transfer, and a first metatarsal osteotomy. With the peroneus longus tendon transfer, the plantar flexion of the first ray is clearly weakened, and this weakening has to be considered when the osteotomy is performed to prevent overcorrection with ultimate shift of weight to the second metatarsal. Another issue is whether the forefoot cavus deformity is global or limited to one or two metatarsals. More frequently, the first metatarsal alone is in equinus, so this single forefoot osteotomy is most commonly used.

An incision is made on the dorsal medial aspect of the first metatarsal extending to the metatarsal cuneiform joint. The periosteum is stripped, and the extensor hallucis longus tendon is retracted laterally. The osteotomy cut is made 1 cm distal to the articulation in the metaphyseal bone with an oblique saw cut on the metatarsal from distal and dorsal to proximal and plantar. It is useful to preserve the plantar cortex to maintain stability, although one can even gain some length by allowing the metatarsal to shift distally before fixation. Once the bone wedge has been resected, the first metatarsal is pushed up dorsally, and the plantar surface of the forefoot is palpated with the foot in maximal dorsiflexion. More bone can be shaved through the osteotomy itself until an appropriate amount of the wedge has been resected. The easiest way to secure this osteotomy is with a vertically inserted screw which is why one uses a long oblique osteotomy cut. If the bone fractures with insertion of the screw, a two-hole plate is used. Frequently, the first metatarsal osteotomy is performed in conjunction with an arthrodesis of the hallux interphalangeal joint and transfer of the extensor hallux longus tendon for correction of a claw hallux. In this situation, the extensor hallux longus should be cut first, the dorsal capsule of the hallux metatarsophalangeal joint released, and then the first metatarsal osteotomy performed. At the completion of the osteotomy, the extensor hallux longus can be transferred into the first metatarsal or the midfoot (which is our preference).

3.6   Triple Arthrodesis

The triple arthrodesis is a safe and reliable option for the management of severe and rigid cavus regardless of the subtype of deformity. Triple arthrodesis has not had enough focus in the recent literature. Older reports [37, 38] demonstrated poor long-term outcomes associated with degenerative changes of the ankle and joints of the midfoot. These deformities were caused by muscle imbalance since many feet that initially had had satisfactory alignment and deformity developed as a result of inadequate muscle balance at the time of the triple arthrodesis. The posterior tibial tendon inserts distal to the talonavicular joint, and unless it is transferred, the medial foot deformity will gradually recur, with onset of adductovarus. Therefore, if a triple arthrodesis is thought to be the procedure of choice, it should be performed with appropriate transfer of the posterior tibial tendon, as well as additional tendon transfers as required. We have previously reported that one cannot rely on a triple arthrodesis to correct as well as *maintain correction* of deformity secondary to a neuromuscular disease process [4]. As noted above, if performed in isolation, a triple arthrodesis may fail since the arthrodesis must be accompanied by additional procedures to address the muscle imbalance and soft tissue contractures. There are several techniques of triple arthrodesis described in the literature. The original description by Hoke utilized a lateral incision and fused only the subtalar and talonavicular joints. He described making a cut through the neck of the talus and removing the head and neck for preparation for arthrodesis. The neck portion had to be shortened because when the equinus deformity was corrected with dorsiflexion, the head and neck piece was too long to go back in [39]. Ryerson's technique involves taking a wedge from the transverse tarsal joint for correction of transverse or sagittal plane deformity [40]. Lambrinudi's technique [41] creates a notch in the posteroinferior portion of the navicular and then an oblique cut through the talar head. The cut surface of the neck of the talus is then plantarflexed down to the anterior process of the calcaneus and wedged under the notch that was made in the navicular. The angle produced posteriorly by the flexed talus on the calcaneus is filled with the bone graft piece obtained from the talar head and neck [41].

The Siffert "beak" triple arthrodesis [42] was described specifically for correction of the cavus deformity. In this technique, the dorsal cortex of the navicular is removed. An osteotomy of the anterior calcaneus and talar head and neck are performed in order to create the talar "beak." The forefoot is then displaced downward, and the navicular is locked under the talar "beak" for correction of the deformity. Despite its appearance, this arthrodesis actually gains length of the foot. It works extremely well when the apex is dorsal, directly at the talonavicular joint.

Our method of triple arthrodesis for the cavus foot is to utilize a single lateral incision to the three joints, although one can use the medial incision used for the posterior tibial tendon transfer for more visualization of the talonavicular joint. Furthermore, there is frequently a separate dorsal incision used for the posterior tibial tendon transfer, and the dorsal surface of the talonavicular joint is visible and can be approached under more direct vision. The lateral incision is begun at the tip of the fibula and extended distally toward the base of the fifth metatarsal long enough to expose the calcaneocuboid (CC) joint. It is important to watch for the sural nerve during the dissection, and it should be retracted plantarward along with the peroneal tendons. The extensor digitorum brevis is retracted dorsally, and the soft tissues are elevated sharply from the floor of the sinus tarsi. The sinus tarsi is then distracted with a toothed laminar spreader allowing visualization of the interosseous ligament, which can be sharply divided and removed with a rongeur. This allows access to the posterior and middle facets of the subtalar joint. Preparation of the subtalar joint is begun by removing the cartilage, and then a curved osteotome is used to rigorously "fish-scale" the surfaces of the middle and posterior facets. Next, a large periosteal elevator is used to strip the lateral surfaces of the calcaneus and cuboid at the level of the calcaneocuboid joint. The peroneal retinaculum is retracted inferiorly, and a knife is swept vertically through the calcaneocuboid joint and rotated dorsally through the bifurcate ligament. Preparation of the joint is performed in the same manner as for the subtalar joint. For most severe deformities, the talonavicular joint is easy to visualize from the lateral approach, and a separate incision medially is not necessary. After the cartilage is denuded with a chisel, we will often use a burr in order to break through the subchondral plate while still maintaining the overall shape of the joint. Once all the joints have been prepared, one must plan the deformity correction which will include a wedge resection of the lateral subtalar and calcaneocuboid joints and a lateral rotation of the talonavicular joint (Fig. 7). In more severe cases, a saw can be used to remove a wedge from the

---

Fig. 7 (**a**) This is an extremely rigid deformity fixed in equinovarus. The posterior tibial tendon has been transferred through the interosseous membrane to the anterolateral compartment. (**b**) With the foot in adductovarus, it is easy to see the subluxation of Chopart's joint with both the talonavicular and calcaneocuboid joint easily visible. (**c**) The correction is begun with a wedge cut through the calcaneocuboid joint using a saw. (**d**) The size of the wedge is approximately 8–10 mm, which should start on the smaller size and then more bone taken out as needed once the correction has been done. (**e**) A wedge has now been removed from the posterior facet of the subtalar joint as the second step in the sequence of correction. This too is between 8 and 10 mm in diameter at the base of the wedge. (**f**) The wedge across the talonavicular joint begins with an angled cut across the talar head. All of the head is removed as part of this wedge. (**g**) Following wedge resection of all three joints, it is easy to see that the forefoot has been corrected and well aligned but the heel remains in varus. (**h**) The hindfoot alignment also demonstrates the persistent varus indicating that more needs to be done to correct this persistent heel deformity. (**i**) A wedge has now been repeated, this time by adding a calcaneal osteotomy to the resection of the subtalar joint. Although further bone removal from the subtalar joint could have been attempted, the joint was coming together very well, and it was felt to be easier to correct the remaining varus through calcaneal osteotomy. (**j**, **k**) The final appearance of the foot is shown here from the plantar and lateral surface after the completion of internal fixation for the triple arthrodesis and the posterior tibial tendon transfer to the dorsocentral aspect of the foot.

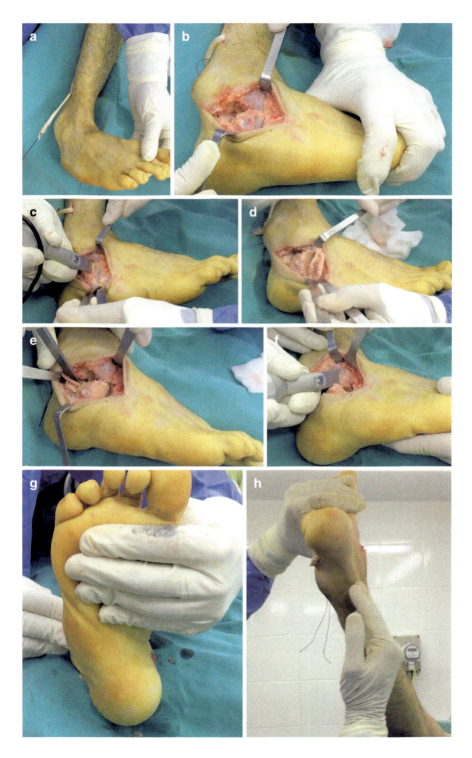

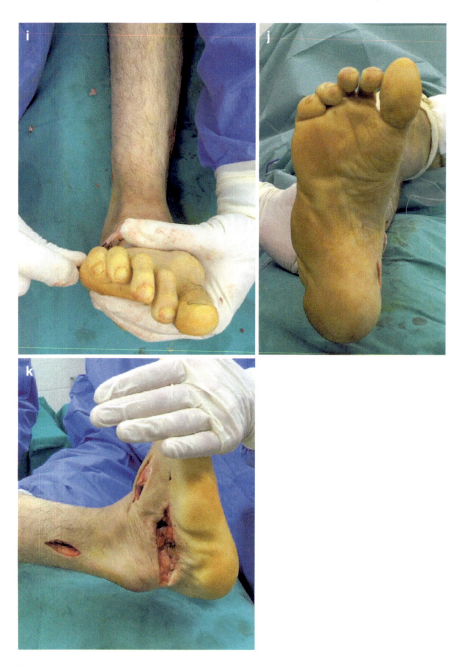

Fig. 7 (continued)

calcaneocuboid joint across to the talonavicular joint. The position of the heel is then assessed and corrected at the subtalar joint to approximately 5 degrees of valgus. Fixation of the subtalar joint is then performed with a partially threaded large cannulated screw inserted from the heel but off the weight-bearing surface of the calcaneus into the body of the talus. The talonavicular joint is not easy to palpate nor visualize for screw insertion, but one should use two cannulated partially threaded screws or a single screw and dorsal two-hole plate depending on the quality of the bone and the purchase and compression achieved by the first screw. The compression screws are inserted from distal to proximal beginning at the medial tuberosity of the navicular. It is important to make sure that the screw head sits flush with the margin of the joint so as not to protrude into the naviculocuneiform joint. Finally, fixation of the calcaneocuboid joint is performed. The cuboid has a tendency to subluxate plantarward and if fixed in this position, it will tend to cause lateral column overload with weight-bearing. It is therefore vital to elevate the lateral forefoot to make sure that the plantar surface of the cuboid is even with that of the calcaneus on the lateral fluoroscopic view prior to fixation. The calcaneocuboid joint can be fixed in an antegrade or retrograde fashion, and we generally use screw(s) placed across the joint from proximal to distal after creating a lateral notch in the calcaneus approximately 1 cm proximal to the calcaneocuboid joint in order to recess the screw head. If screw purchase or compression across the joint is poor, a four-hole plate can be applied to the dorsolateral surface of the joint for added stability and compression.

Sometimes, even though the calcaneocuboid joint has been reduced completely, the rotation of the forefoot is such that the base of the fifth metatarsal is still very plantar, and in this situation resection of the base of the fifth metatarsal will be required [43]. In these cases, there is typically a large hard callus under the base of the fifth metatarsal, and the ostectomy can be done in conjunction with any additional necessary procedure (Fig. 8). The incision that is used for the calcaneal osteotomy, peroneal tendon procedure, or triple arthrodesis is extended, or an additional incision is made from the base of the fifth metatarsal distally along the course of the dorsal shaft of the metatarsal. A saw cut is made obliquely in the shaft of the fifth metatarsal in two planes so that the starting point of the osteotomy is dorsal and slightly lateral. With this orientation of the osteotomy, no bone prominence remains on the plantar lateral weight-bearing surface. The metatarsal base is grasped with a clamp, rotated on its pedicle, and then cut sharply by detaching the short plantar ligament and the remnant of the attachment of the peroneus brevis tendon. The peroneus brevis tendon can be detached from the fifth metatarsal and can be left with its attachment to the adjacent soft tissues, because it is generally nonfunctional with these more severe deformities. If a peroneus longus-to-brevis tendon transfer is performed, however, then the longus tendon needs to be securely attached to the cuboid using a suture anchor for fixation. At the completion of the ostectomy, the hypertrophic callus needs to be shaved, and it is helpful to soften the hard callus with a moist sponge before it is cut. Finally, always assess the stability of the ankle, and if the posterior tibial tendon transfer does not hold the foot stable, then it may be necessary to add lateral ligament stabilization.

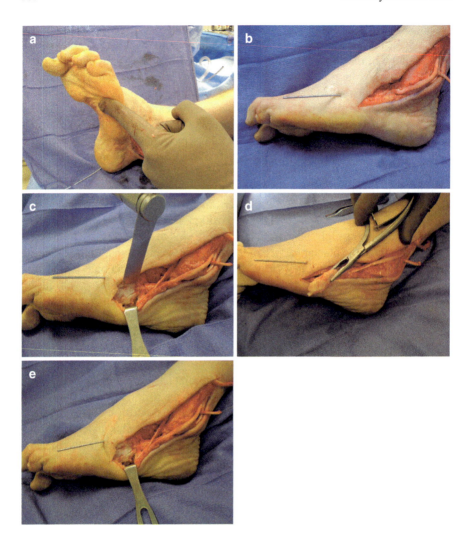

Fig. 8 (**a–c**) Following fixation of the triple, one should get a sense of the alignment of the foot. Note here that there's a large prominence at the base of the fifth metatarsal. This needs to be addressed since a maximum supination has already been obtained through rotation of the calcaneocuboid joint. Note also the severely torn peroneus brevis tendon, which was split and routed through the fibula as part of a non-anatomic ankle ligament reconstruction which was necessary in this case for severe ankle instability. (**d, e**) The ostectomy is made obliquely at the base of the metatarsal removing as much as is necessary to address the bone prominence. Note also the split half of the peroneus brevis tendon attached to the insertion point of the tendon distally. This is not a problem, since the tendon is easily reattached to the soft tissues adjacent to the base of the metatarsal

4   Conclusions

- Rigid deformity is usually treated with a triple arthrodesis although a midfoot correction in combination with a triplanar calcaneus osteotomy may be sufficient.
- A triple arthrodesis is a good procedure, provided that the foot is correctly balanced with additional osteotomy and tendon transfers.
- Be careful of causing a tarsal tunnel syndrome with correction of the hindfoot varus.
- Even with a large wedge resection in the midfoot, the foot will usually be longer and not shorter.
- Persistent and recurrent deformity will occur if soft tissue and muscle balance is not achieved.
- Posterior tibial tendon transfer and peroneus longus transfer are nearly always required for correction.
- Soft tissue procedures (such as anterior tibial tendon transfer, plantar fascia release, Achilles tendon lengthening, gastrocnemius recession) may be necessary.

References

1. Barg A. The cavus foot. Foot Ankle Clin. 2019;24(2):xiii–xiv.
2. Younger AS, Hansen ST Jr. Adult cavovarus foot. J Am Acad Orthop Surg. 2005;13(5):302–15.
3. Chesler SM, Grumbine NA. An examination procedure for cavo-adducto-varus. J Foot Surg. 1979;18(1):1–6.
4. Li S, Myerson MS. Failure of surgical treatment in patients with cavovarus deformity: why does this happen and how do we approach treatment? Foot Ankle Clin. 2019;24(2):361–70.
5. Li S, Myerson MS. Managing severe foot and ankle deformities in global humanitarian programs. Foot Ankle Clin. 2020;25(2):183–203.
6. Brewerton DA, Sandifer PH, Sweetnam DR. Idiopathic. Pes Cavus Br Med J. 1963;2(5358):659–61.
7. Harris N, Stevens M. A cavovarus foot is a predisposing factor for rather than a result of peroneus longus tendinopathy. Foot Ankle Int. 2001;22(6):525.
8. Larsen E, Angerman P. Association of ankle instability and foot deformity. Acta Orthop Scand. 1990;61:136–9.
9. Vienne P, Schöniger R, Helmy N, et al. Hindfoot instability in cavovarus deformity: static and dynamic balancing. Foot Ankle Int. 2007;28:96–102.
10. Fortin PT, Guettler J, Manoli A. 2nd idiopathic cavovarus and lateral ankle instability: recognition and treatment implications relating to ankle arthritis. Foot Ankle Int. 2002;23:1031–7.
11. Manoli A 2nd, Graham B. The subtle cavus foot, "the underpronator". Foot Ankle Int. 2005;26:256–63.
12. Di Fabio R, Lispi L, Santorelli FM, et al. Idiopathic pes cavus in adults is not associated with neurophysiological impairment in the lower limbs. Neurol Sci. 2015;36(12):2287–90. https://doi.org/10.1007/s10072-015-2334-7.
13. Heron JR. Neurological syndromes associated with pes cavus. Proc R Soc Med. 1969 Mar;62(3):270–1.
14. Nagai MK, Chan G, Guille JT, Kumar SJ, Scavina M, Mackenzie WG. Prevalence of Charcot-Marie-Tooth disease in patients who have bilateral cavovarus feet. J Pediatr Orthop. 2006;26(4):438–43.

15. Krause FG, Wing KJ, Younger AS. Neuromuscular issues in cavovarus foot. Foot Ankle Clin. 2008;13(2):243–vi.
16. Coleman SS, Chesnut W. A simple test for hindfoot flexibility in the cavovarus foot. Clin Orthop Relat Res. 1977;123:60–2.
17. Deben SE, Pomeroy GC. Subtle cavus foot: diagnosis and management. J Am Acad Orthop Surg. 2014;22(8):512–20.
18. Dreher T, Beckmann NA, Wenz W. Surgical treatment of severe cavovarus foot deformity in Charcot-Marie-Tooth disease. JBJS Essent Surg Tech. 2015;5(2):e11.
19. Price BD, Price CT. A simple demonstration of hindfoot flexibility in the cavovarus foot. J Pediatr Orthop. 1997;17(1):18–9.
20. Myerson MS. Cavus foot correction. In: Myerson MS, editor. Reconstructive foot and ankle surgery: management of complications. 2nd ed. Philadelphia: Elsevier; 2010. p. 155–73.
21. Perera A, Guha A. Clinical and radiographic evaluation of the cavus foot: surgical implications. Foot Ankle Clin. 2013;18(4):619–28.
22. Lintz F, Welck M, Bernasconi A, et al. 3D biometrics for hindfoot alignment using weightbearing CT. Foot Ankle Int. 2017;38(6):684–9.
23. Li S, Myerson MS, Netto CC. Peritalar Subluxation: A Key Finding for Both Cavovarus and Flatfoot Deformities. Foot Ankle Orthop. 2022;7(1):2473011421S00316.
24. Joseph TN, Myerson MS. Correction of multiplanar hindfoot deformity with osteotomy, arthrodesis, and internal fixation. Instr Course Lect. 2005;54:269–76.
25. Lintz F, Bernasconi A, Baschet L, et al. Relationship between chronic lateral ankle instability and hindfoot varus using weight-bearing cone beam computed tomography. Foot Ankle Int. 2019;40(10):1175–81.
26. Lintz F, Mast J, Bernasconi A, et al. 3D, weightbearing topographical study of periprosthetic cysts and alignment in total ankle replacement. Foot Ankle Int. 2020;41(1):1–9.
27. Zhang JZ, Lintz F, Bernasconi A; Weight Bearing CT International Study Group, Zhang S. 3D biometrics for hindfoot alignment using weightbearing computed tomography. Foot Ankle Int. 2019;40(6):720–6.
28. Aminian A, Sangeorzan BJ. The anatomy of cavus foot deformity. Foot Ankle Clin. 2008;13(2):191-v.
29. Myerson MS, Myerson CL. Cavus foot: deciding between osteotomy and arthrodesis. Foot Ankle Clin. 2019;24(2):347–60.
30. Myerson M, editor. Current therapy in foot and ankle surgery. St Louis: Mosby Year Book; 1993.
31. VanValkenburg S, Hsu RY, Palmer DS, Blankenhorn B, Den Hartog BD, DiGiovanni CW. Neurologic deficit associated with lateralizing calcaneal osteotomy for cavovarus foot correction. Foot Ankle Int. 2016;37(10):1106–12.
32. Huber M. What is the role of tendon transfer in the cavus foot? Foot Ankle Clin. 2013;18(4):689–95.
33. Jahss MH. Tarsometatarsal truncated-wedge arthrodesis for pes cavus and equinovarus deformity of the fore part of the foot. J Bone Joint Surg Am. 1980;62(5):713–22.
34. Cole WH. The classic. The treatment of claw-foot. By Wallace H. Cole. 1940. Clin Orthop Relat Res. 1983;181:3–6.
35. Japas LM. Surgical treatment of pes cavus by tarsal V-osteotomy. Preliminary report. J Bone Joint Surg Am. 1968;50(5):927–44.
36. Sullivan RJ, Aronow MS. Different faces of the triple arthrodesis. Foot Ankle Clin. 2002;7(1):95–106.
37. Wetmore RS, Drennan JC. Long-term results of triple arthrodesis in Charcot-Marie-Tooth disease. J Bone Joint Surg Am. 1989;71(3):417–22.
38. Wukich DK, Bowen JR. A long-term study of triple arthrodesis for correction of pes cavovarus in Charcot-Marie-Tooth disease. J Pediatr Orthop. 1989;9(4):433–7.
39. Hoke M. An operation for stabilizing paralytic feet. J Orthop Surg. 1921;3:494–507.
40. Ryerson EW. Arthrodesing operations on the feet. J Bone Joint Surg. 1923;5:453–71.

41. Lambrinudi C. New operation on drop-foot. British J Surg. 1927;15:193–200.
42. Siffert RS, Forster RI, Nachamie B. "Beak" triple arthrodesis for correction of severe cavus deformity. Clin Orthop Relat Res. 1966;45:101–6.
43. Shariff R, Myerson MS, Palmanovich E. Resection of the fifth metatarsal base in the severe rigid cavovarus foot. Foot Ankle Int. 2014;35(6):558–65.

"Management of Severe Untreated and Recurrent Clubfoot Deformity in the Child and Adult"

Mark S. Myerson and Shuyuan Li

1 Introduction

The approach to treatment of severe untreated or recurrent clubfoot deformities is very different in the world where patients are mobile and have access to repeated return visits for follow-up treatment and where more sophisticated options for gradual correction with external fixation are available [1–4]. While the Ponseti treatment can be applied to untreated deformity even in older children and young adults [5], many of these patients do not have the ability to return from rural regions for repeated casting and bracing following this treatment [1, 6]. The spectrum of these deformities in children and adults is tremendous, ranging from minor procedures such as an anterior tibial tendon transfer, tendon transfers with or without osteotomy, to arthrodesis or even talectomy. The goal of treatment for these severe deformities is to obtain a plantigrade foot with no likelihood for recurrent deformity. Our extensive experience with these deformities has been on global humanitarian programs where we have very limited resources and a lack of availability of implants and where the needs of patients are quite different from those we as surgeons are accustomed to in the Western world. This setting will affect decision-making since resorting to a Ponseti treatment is invariably not possible and prolonged treatments with external fixation is not practical for these patients. These deformities are so variable that a simplistic algorithm for surgical treatment is not possible (Fig. 1a, b). There are those with a fixed equinus and no dorsiflexion of the ankle due to a flat-top talus. Addressing the foot alone will not correct the deformity and where an anterior closing wedge osteotomy of the tibia is required in addition to tri-planar correction of

M. S. Myerson (✉) · S. Li
Department of Orthopaedics, University of Colorado Anschutz Medical Campus, Aurora, CO, USA

Steps2Walk, Greenwood Village, CO, USA
https://www.steps2walk.org

© The Author(s), under exclusive license to Springer Nature
Switzerland AG 2022
E. Wagner Hitschfeld, P. Wagner Hitschfeld (eds.), *Foot and Ankle Disorders*,
https://doi.org/10.1007/978-3-030-95738-4_27

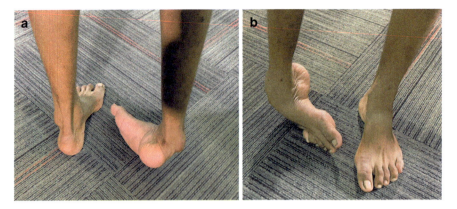

Fig. 1 (**a, b**) These are multiplanar deformities, and this untreated clubfoot in an adolescent typifies how challenging correction can be. The ankle is in equinus, the heel in varus, and the midfoot is adducted as well as in cavus. This would correctly be termed an equino-cavo-adductovarus deformity, and each component of this deformity must be corrected

the foot. In patients with some range of motion of the ankle but an equinus deformity, it may be very difficult to regain dorsiflexion because of severe scarring of the Achilles tendon which may even be adherent to the skin. Provided that some ankle range of motion is present, most deformities of the foot no matter how severe can be corrected with a combination of osteotomies and tendon transfers or arthrodesis, and a triple arthrodesis would be the procedure of choice. For rigid severe deformities of the foot and ankle where no motion whatsoever is present, talectomy is preferable. The indications for talectomy in the setting of an untreated or recurrent club foot deformity are nowadays uncommon and rarely necessary with the use of modern external fixation techniques [7, 8]. As noted however, this is not a treatment option for our patients in rural settings where continuous monitoring of fixation is necessary.

2 Patient Evaluation

Decision-making is based on the mobility of the foot and ankle, the presence of scarring from prior surgeries, the presence of bilateral deformity, and the overall needs of the patient. These feet are already small; therefore, anything other than gradual correction with external fixation will further reduce the foot size, since lateral shortening is always safer and easier than medial lengthening. One has to anticipate a significant leg length discrepancy following talectomy which averages 2.5 cm and approximately 3 cm if a tibiocalcaneal (TC) arthrodesis is performed. For this reason, a unilateral talectomy must be a last resort. If bilateral deformities are present, this decision-making is easier since both limbs will be shorter, and leg length discrepancy will not be a concern [9, 10]. If some albeit limited ankle range of motion is present and the foot can be passively corrected into neutral, a talectomy is not indicated since a triple arthrodesis combined with tendon transfers and additional osteotomies can be performed regardless of the magnitude of deformity. If a flat-top talus is present in the child associated with a fixed equinus deformity and limited dorsiflexion, it is quite reasonable to perform an anterior closing wedge osteotomy of the distal tibia to regain dorsiflexion which is similar to the procedure of anterior distal tibial epiphysiodesis performed in children with residual or recurrent equinus deformity [11]. Therefore, it is the magnitude of the equinus deformity, the associated soft tissue scarring or contracture, and the possibility of ischemia with an attempt of correction with alternative methods that will determine the need for a talectomy. Scarring can be quite daunting and will limit the ability to perform a revision with additional soft tissue release procedures, and if so, one may need to be versatile with the use of skin Z-plasty due to the medial contracture (Fig. 2).

Bear in mind that active dorsiflexion will rarely be present in these very severe equinovarus deformities. It is rare that any of the extensor muscles of the foot are functional, and following any procedure whether arthrodesis (triple, tibiotalocalcaneal (TTC), or pantalar), although the hindfoot position may be recovered from equinus to neutral, no active dorsiflexor is present, and a static and dynamic equinus of the midfoot or forefoot may persist. Equinus of the forefoot is usually not fixed, but dynamic following correction of the ankle and hindfoot, and generally the foot, can be passively pushed up into a neutral position. However, the forefoot will drop back down into equinus. In such cases, a tendon transfer can be used as a dynamic or static force to help correcting the mid- and forefoot equinus [12].

The same philosophy of muscle rebalancing will apply to correcting the deformity in the midfoot. This is difficult to determine preoperatively due to rigidity of the contracture, but an effort should be made to try to carefully examine the foot for function of various muscles since these will determine the need for a tendon transfer.

Transfer of the posterior tibial tendon is indicated if one can demonstrate that some posterior tibial muscle function remains, in which case the tendon can be transferred through the interosseous membrane to the dorsum of the foot to provide

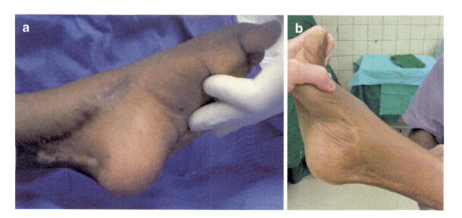

Fig. 2 Note the severe fixed equinus deformity in both these feet associated with significant scarring along the posteromedial foot and the length of the Achilles tendon. The scars are thick, hypertrophic, and in the skin completely adherent to the Achilles tendon (**a**, **b**)

some degree of active dorsiflexion or at least to change its deforming force into a static dorsiflexion power. Tendon transfer is very difficult to perform in the feet which have undergone a few prior surgeries. If there is little identifiable posterior tibial tendon, a tenotomy is more useful. If there is no functioning muscle (either the anterior or posterior tibial or the peroneus brevis and/or longus) to consider for a tendon transfer to increase dorsiflexion, then a tenodesis should be considered using one of the extensor tendons, generally the extensor digitorum longus.

3   Anterior Tibia Closing Wedge Osteotomy

If the equinus deformity cannot be fully corrected due to a flat-top talus but range of motion in the ankle is however present, one can consider a closing wedge anterior distal tibial osteotomy. Most of the time, this procedure will be performed in older adolescents or adults, in which case a combination of screw and plate fixation will be ideal. The bone cut is made in the metaphysis, leaving enough room in the distal metaphysis for application of a T-shaped or L-shaped plate. We begin with a small wedge, approximately 4 mm in diameter, and see how much dorsiflexion is obtained since dorsiflexion to 10° is preferable. It is important to translate the distal tibia posteriorly following the wedge resection in order to center the ankle under the tibia (Fig. 3). If not, the foot will move forward after the wedge resection, which is not ideal biomechanically. An osteotomy of the fibula is also required, and generally we will make a small oblique cut on the distal fibula almost at the same level as the tibial osteotomy. The fibula osteotomy does not require fixation.

A lengthening of the Achilles tendon should be performed before the tibial osteotomy which is made through an anterior incision centered over the distal tibia. In many of these feet, the equinus is difficult to manage because of scarring around the Achilles tendon posteromedially, which limits the ability to perform a further lengthening. The Achilles tendon can be scarred, ropelike, and adherent to the skin, and one has to be careful with the lengthening procedure chosen. Tenotomy is not a good choice here, since one wants to preserve whatever push-off strength remains in the Achilles.

Fig. 3 Note the severe equinovarus in this 8-year-old child following three failed attempts at Ponseti treatment. There was no dorsiflexion associated with a flat-top talus and severe scarring posteriorly (**a–c**). A closing wedge osteotomy including both distal tibia and fibula was performed. Note the size of the wedge (**d**), and with dorsiflexion of the foot, the distal tibia translated anteriorly (**e**), and the foot and distal tibia needed to be translated posteriorly in order to center the foot under the tibia (**f**). The final appearance of the foot is shown following a lateral transfer of the anterior tibial tendon, the tibia and fibula osteotomy, and a closing wedge osteotomy of the cuboid (**g, h**)

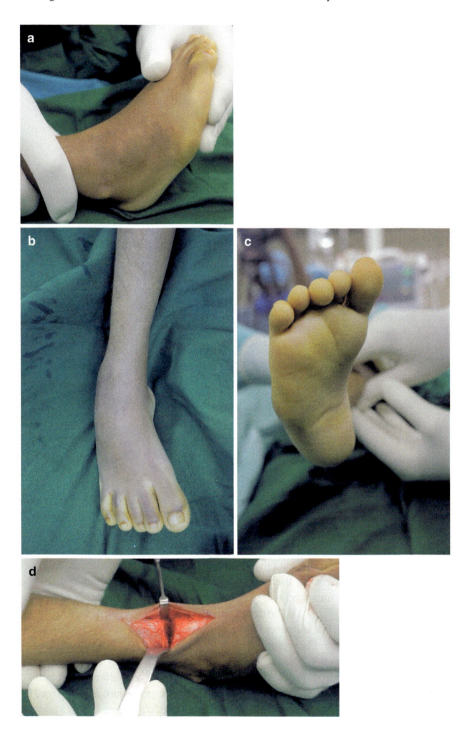

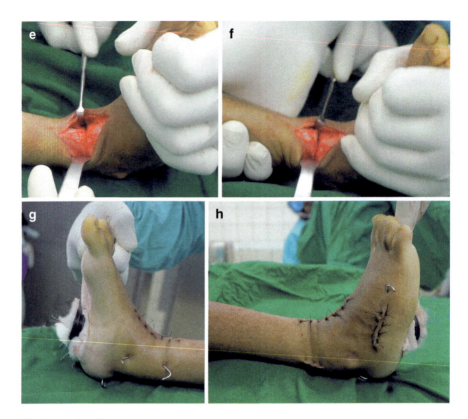

Fig. 3 (continued)

4 Triple Arthrodesis

This topic is discussed elsewhere in the book (Chap. 26), as well as a brief overview in the section on the cavus foot (Chap. 26). A triple arthrodesis is an option for correction of severe equinovarus deformity, but only when range of motion is present in the ankle. Ideally, one would want the ankle to reach at least a neutral position, even in the presence of a flat-top talus. Because of the adductovarus of the Chopart joint and the fixed varus of the subtalar joint, much larger wedges need to be removed from these joints than one may be accustomed to doing with a more routine triple arthrodesis (Fig. 4a). The deformities that are amenable to a triple arthrodesis vary significantly, but are generally fixed in equinovarus, but with some passive range of motion of the ankle present (Fig. 4b–e).

Other than a tenotomy of the posterior tibial tendon which may be necessary, no medial incision is required, and if a tenotomy is performed, we prefer to do it behind the medial malleolus and not over the medial foot. The procedure is performed in conjunction with a plantar fascia release and tendon transfers or tenotomies as necessary. The steps for the triple arthrodesis are illustrated here in sequence (Fig. 5). The

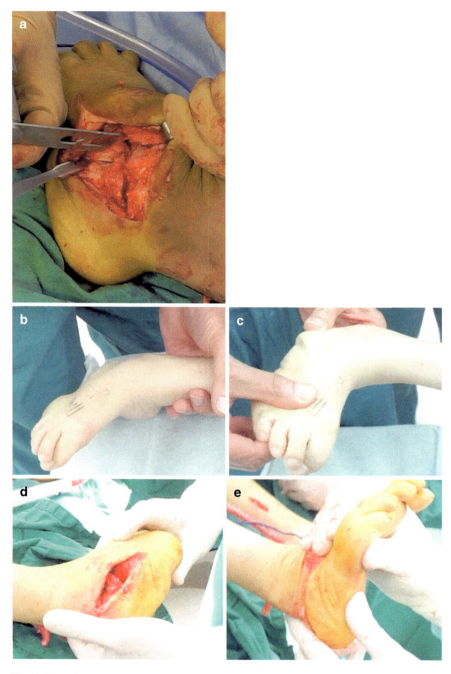

Fig. 4 The triple arthrodesis was performed through an extensile lateral incision. Note the large wedge that was first taken out of the calcaneocuboid and talonavicular joints (**a**). This patient had bilateral equinovarus deformities which were treated simultaneously with a plantar fascia release, a posterior tibial tendon transfer, Achilles lengthening, and a triple arthrodesis (**b, c**) and the wedge removed from the calcaneocuboid joint (**d**). The final plantigrade position of the hindfoot was accomplished by pushing up under the base of the fifth metatarsal and cuboid in order to elevate through translation the lateral column of the foot (**e**)

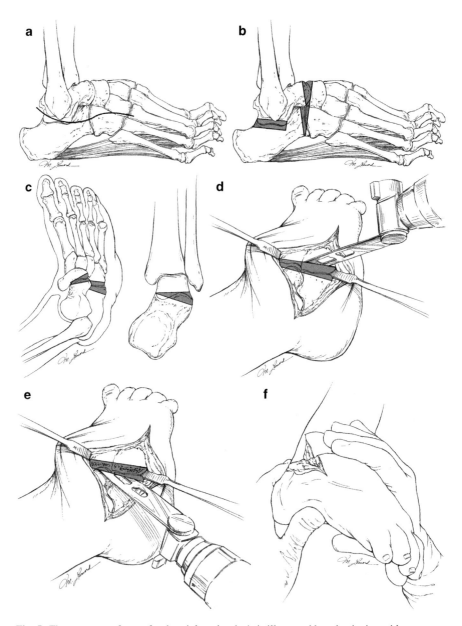

Fig. 5 The sequence of steps for the triple arthrodesis is illustrated here beginning with an extensile incision (**a**). Planning for the wedge resection is illustrated noting a large wedge removed from the subtalar joint and a biplanar wedge removed from the calcaneocuboid and talonavicular joints with more bone resected laterally and dorsally across the Chopart joints (**b–e**). Prior to commencing with fixation, it is important to manipulate the foot into the correct position maintaining hindfoot valgus and pressure underneath the lateral column of the foot, generally directly under the cuboid. This dorsal translation of the lateral column is important (**f**). Note that a calcaneal osteotomy may be required in addition to the subtalar arthrodesis. One may have to translate the calcaneus slightly cephalad to improve the pitch angle as well as laterally if any persistent valgus is present (**g**). The options for fixation are presented (**h, i**)

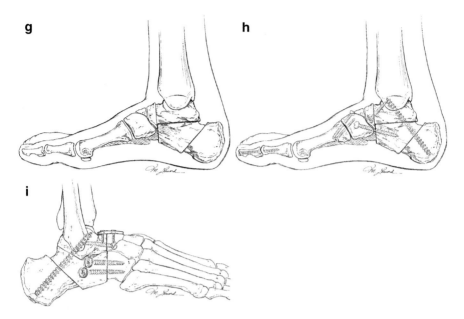

Fig. 5 (continued)

entire triple arthrodesis procedure should be performed through an extensile lateral approach beginning at the distal fibula and ending at the base of the fourth metatarsal. Beginning with the calcaneocuboid joint, a wedge of approximately 8 mm is resected, followed by debridement of the subtalar joint and then the talonavicular joint. It is often possible to extend the saw cut on the calcaneocuboid joint directly across the navicular and the head of the talus, but this may have to be cut separately depending on the size of the wedge required for correction. Once these wedges have been removed, it should be quite easy to shift the foot into the correct position. The heel should be placed in a few degrees of valgus, and there should be no residual pressure under the lateral border of the foot. The adduction should be completely corrected with the wedge resection of Chopart joint. A useful tip is to push up under the fifth metatarsal and cuboid in order to correct the supination deformity across the midfoot. Screw fixation is preferable, and the size, type, and number of screws are surgeon preference. Since the medial screw(s) are inserted percutaneously, depending on access to the navicular, it is sometimes necessary to add a two-hole plate dorsally to the talonavicular joint to improve stability of fixation of the talonavicular fusion.

5 Talectomy

Talectomy is not by any means a physiologic procedure, but because of the ankylosis that it creates between the tibia and calcaneus and the ability to accept full body weight, it is a very reasonable procedure despite the limb shortening [7–10, 13].

Most patients are free of pain and fairly functional and ambulate satisfactorily. Another option is to correct the deformity gradually with an external fixator, which does maintain limb length; however, the foot is no more functional following correction of the deformity since rigidity persists (Fig. 6).

A talectomy should only be performed with very specific indications, and although always associated with severe foot deformity, a rigid ankle often associated with a flat-top talus is invariably present [10]. Talectomy is rarely performed as an isolated procedure, since this will only correct a severe equinus deformity of the ankle and hindfoot and to a lesser extent the changes in the transverse tarsal joint. Frequently, the adduction deformity of the Chopart joints is too severe to permit correction without an additional procedure which abducts the foot at the apex of the deformity, usually the calcaneocuboid joint. In addition to the talectomy and

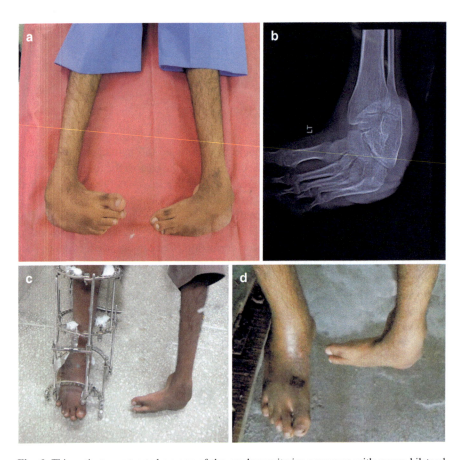

Fig. 6 This patient was treated on one of the our humanitarian programs with severe bilateral deformities, a flat-top talus, and no range of motion in either the foot or ankle (**a**, **b**). In this case an Ilizarov fixator was used to gradually correct the deformity with a well-aligned plantigrade foot at the completion of treatment (**c**, **d**). (Case courtesy of Dr. Saad Ilyas, on Steps2Walk humanitarian programming, Lahore Pakistan)

calcaneocuboid wedge arthrodesis, there are further procedures which must be considered to correct any residual adduction or equinus deformity of the midfoot and forefoot, as well as balance the soft tissue contracture. These could involve a transfer of the posterior tibial tendon, the anterior tibial tendon, or the peroneus longus to the peroneus brevis. Rarely, the deformity is in the ankle *and* hindfoot, and there is no severe midfoot deformity. In these cases, correction of the equinus deformity and the hindfoot varus can be addressed with a tibiotalocalcaneal (TTC) arthrodesis.

A decision will need to be made preoperatively and then again intraoperatively as to whether or not an isolated talectomy will be performed or whether this will be done in conjunction with a TC or a TC and tibionavicular (TN) arthrodesis [14, 15]. In general, a talectomy without arthrodesis is preferred since the residual motion is generally painless and functional. The decision is based on stability of the hindfoot following temporary pin fixation and the age of the patient, since it is very rare that an arthrodesis is necessary in childhood or even in adolescence. The range of motion after a talectomy is generally not significant, but it does improve function.

We have found that the anterolateral approach for performing an isolated talectomy is the most versatile, since one has the opportunity to obtain a complete lateral exposure, extending the incision distally to include the calcaneocuboid joint and the peroneal tendons as necessary. This extensile approach permits a complete removal of the talus successfully (Fig. 7). One has to always consider the potential for skin complications with any approach to correction of these very severe deformities, but a laterally based incision is not likely to lead to problems as a result of decompression of the soft tissue contracture following the talectomy. The extensile lateral approach has to be long, commencing behind the fibula towards the fifth metatarsal. One can either leave the fibula intact or remove the distal 2 cm for visualization. The main advantage of the transfibular approach is easy visualization and removal of the talus and molding of the tibia and calcaneus for an arthrodesis. It is also easy to mold the anterior tibia and the navicular to include a tibionavicular arthrodesis. Most importantly, access to the lateral foot for a wedge resection of the calcaneocuboid joint can be done with an extensile approach (Fig. 8). When considering a talectomy without arthrodesis, one can consider an anterior approach to the ankle. This is more useful for deformities which are predominantly locked in equinus, without midfoot adductus caused by a rigid contracture medially and which does not necessitate many additional procedures. By removing the talus from the anterior approach, both malleoli can be left intact, which may serve to provide some stability to the periarticular tissues as the calcaneus gradually scars into position. Occasionally, the anterior approach may lead to impingement between the margins of the malleolus and either the calcaneus or navicular medially and less laterally. If this is the case, a subsequent secondary procedure may need to be performed with an ostectomy of the offending bone causing the impingement. The one disadvantage of approaching a talectomy anteriorly is that it is not as easy to remove the talus as through a lateral approach since the talus has to be cut into pieces with an osteotome and then gradually removed.

Thick skin flaps should be maintained. If one is certain that a TC arthrodesis will be performed, then the distal fibula can be resected to gain access to the talectomy

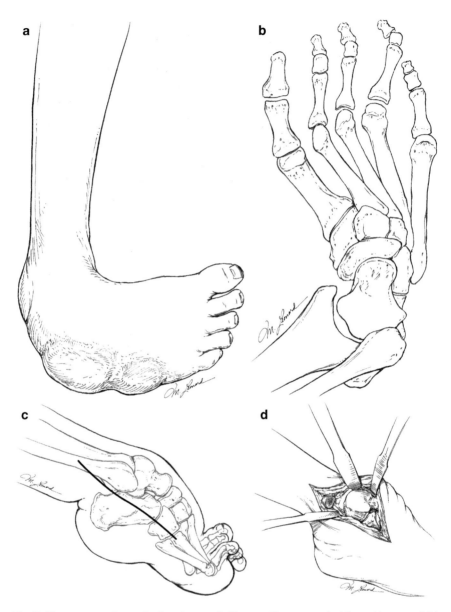

Fig. 7 The sequence of steps for the talectomy is illustrated in a very typical foot with severe rigid equinovarus, weight-bearing on the dorsal surface of the foot noted by hypertrophy of the dorso-lateral skin (**a**). It is not just the magnitude of the deformity of the foot that determines the need for talectomy but the fixed rigid deformity of the ankle in equinus (**b**). Following an extensile lateral approach, the talus is exposed with or without removing the distal 2 cm of the fibula (**c–e**). Often, additional wedges need to be removed, one from the calcaneocuboid joint and the other from the anterior tibia and dorsal surface of the navicular (**f**). Provisional fixation is performed with can-nulated guide pins if available (**g**) and the screw fixation demonstrated after molding the tibia to the calcaneus and inserting bone graft as noted between the tibia and calcaneus (**h**)

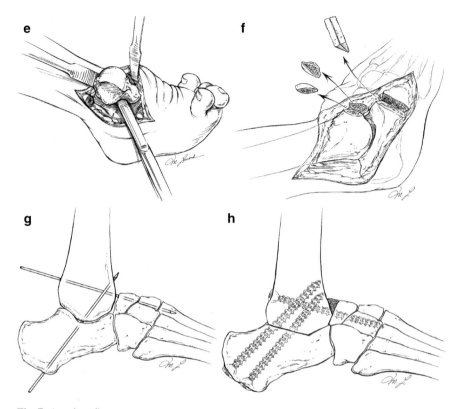

Fig. 7 (continued)

and preparation of the joint surfaces. All of the ligaments and capsules connecting the talus to the adjoining bones are divided, trying to avoid any injury to the articular surfaces, particularly in children. The anterior talofibular ligament is first cut followed by the calcaneofibular ligament which should be detached as much as possible off the fibula so as to reattach it at the completion of the procedure if there is any coronal plane instability. It is generally not possible to maximally invert the foot and expose the talus without cutting the calcaneofibular ligament. The main ligament that anchors the talus is the talocalcaneal interosseous ligament which is easier to cut from the lateral approach, thereby freeing up lateral attachments and subsequently dislocating the foot to remove the talus. This is not as easy if an anterior approach is used. After freeing up the lateral ligaments, the foot can be manipulated into more equinus and varus, and by holding the talus with a large towel clamp, the medial capsule of the subtalar joint and the deep portion of the deltoid ligament as well as the posterior ankle and posteromedial calcaneal capsule are cut. A posterior capsulotomy is easier to perform under direct vision noting however the position of the flexor hallucis longus and the neurovascular bundle posteromedially. It is important to remove the entire talus and not leave any small bone fragments behind, which can lead to secondary deformity.

The foot should now be quite mobile and can easily reach a neutral position without any residual equinus or adductovarus. By manipulation the foot is positioned under the tibia ensuring that there's no residual equinus nor any tension

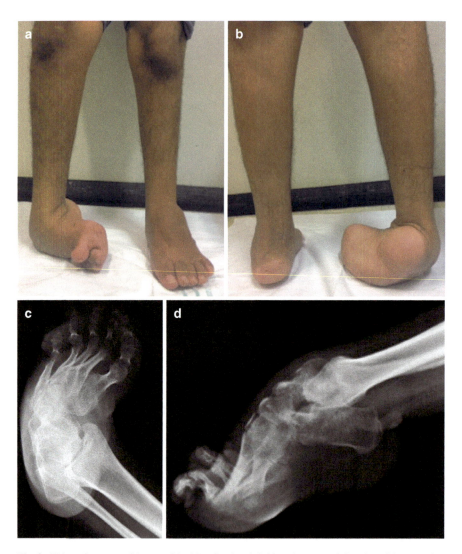

Fig. 8 This patient was a 26-year-old with a fixed and rigid equinovarus deformity with no motion in either the ankle or foot (**a**–**d**). Note the ostectomy of the terminal fibula (**e**,1) and the articular surface of the distal tibia (**e**, 2), with the osteotome perforating through the interosseous ligament to lever out the talus (**e**). Saw cuts were made on the articular surface of the calcaneus, the tibia across to and including the medial malleolus, and then finally the anterior aspect of the tibia where it would articulate with the navicular (**f**–**h**). A wedge was removed from the calcaneocuboid joint followed by provisional fixation of the foot (**i, j**). The final clinical and radiographic appearance of the foot 5 months following surgery is demonstrated. Note that there is very little limb length inequality as a result of prior surgery on the contralateral foot (**k**–**n**)

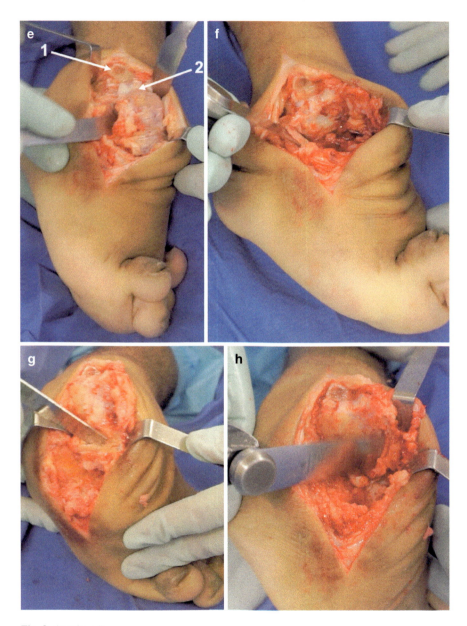

Fig. 8 (continued)

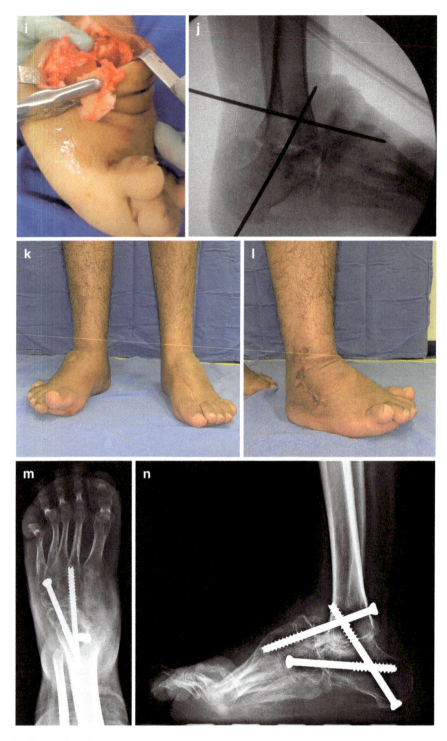

Fig. 8 (continued)

in the posterior ankle capsule. Division of the anterior inferior tibiofibular ligament in the syndesmosis has been described to widen the ankle mortise and more easily fit the calcaneus underneath the tibia, but we do not have experience with this step [16]. It is essential that the foot is positioned correctly, and it should be translated slightly posteriorly under the tibia. Adequate posterior capsular release needs to be performed in order to move the foot posteriorly. At times this requires additional release as well as tenotomy of the Achilles tendon if contracture still presents. As the foot is moved posteriorly, the tip of the medial malleolus will be immediately adjacent to the navicular and the tip of the fibula just posterior to the calcaneocuboid joint. The goal is to provide a long lever to the foot by shifting the foot posteriorly to give mechanical advantage to the gastrocnemius-soleus [17]. Once positioned, the foot is fixed to the tibia with two 3 mm Steinman pins. If any impingement occurs between the calcaneus and the fibula and prevents correction, one can remove the tip of the fibula or the medial malleolus to decrease the jamming. Occasionally, the tibia will abut against the navicular with the posterior shift of the calcaneus, but in a child an arthrodesis should be avoided, and to regain a neutral position, the anterior tibia can be shaved with an ostectomy in order to permit slightly more posterior translation. Slight dorsiflexion and plantarflexion may be possible despite the ankylosis and can provide some function.

Dorsiflexion may not be possible because the anterior tibia is impinging against the navicular. The same may occur because of a medially rotated navicular where it is impinging against the medial malleolus. In either of these situations one has to trim the anterior distal tibia or the dorsal and medial navicular. Both of these procedures are necessary if one is performing a tibionavicular arthrodesis. The latter procedure is only occasionally necessary in conjunction with a tibiocalcaneal arthrodesis and never with an isolated talectomy. The incision is then extended more distally to the base of the fifth metatarsal and a large wedge removed from the calcaneocuboid joint. The distal cut can be extended medially to include the navicular as one cut if a tibionavicular arthrodesis is going to be considered. Once the calcaneocuboid wedge has been removed, the foot should now assume a perfectly neutral position. Prior to completing the tendon transfer dorsally, the hindfoot is fixed to the tibia using two or three 3 mm pins. The one is introduced from the posterior and inferior calcaneus passing through the anterior cortex of the distal tibia, and the second is inserted vertically through the calcaneus into the tibia (Fig. 9).

6   Additional Procedures

An equinus deformity of the forefoot may still persist following the talectomy, and if present, it is helpful to stabilize the deformity with a tenodesis using the extensor tendons. A 2 cm incision is made over the midfoot, and the longus extensor tendons to the second, third, and fourth toes are cut, sutured together, and inserted into the midfoot using either an interference screw, a suture anchor, or a soft tissue bolster on the plantar surface of the foot. In children, we prefer to use a padded bolster and not a suture button, which can cause necrosis of the skin. A 4 mm drill through the lateral cuneiform is made, and the tendons are passed through to the plantar surface. A useful technique to pass the tendon is to insert a guide pin through the cuneiform, hold the guide pin with a clamp below the foot, and then drill through the bone. Using a #15 blade, a small skin incision is made over the guide pin; then, a metallic

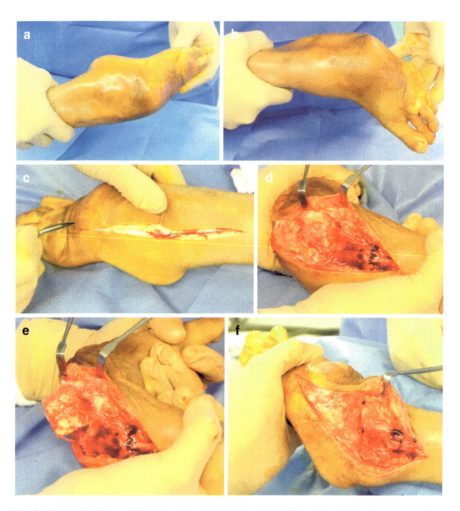

Fig. 9 The surgical steps of talectomy are demonstrated in this 26-year-old female who was walking on the dorsolateral surface of the foot (**a**, **b**). An anterolateral extensile incision was made followed by manipulation of the foot into varus. With further manipulation the talus can be extruded laterally (**c–e**). Note that at completion of the talectomy and articular surface resection, the foot remains in adduction and equinus (**f**). Large wedges were then removed from the calcaneocuboid joint as well as the anterior distal tibia in order to bring the foot into a neutral plantigrade position (**g**, **h**). When the tourniquet was deflated, severe ischemia of the foot was present. Nitroglycerin paste was applied to the foot as shown (**i**) which resulted in reperfusion (**j**)

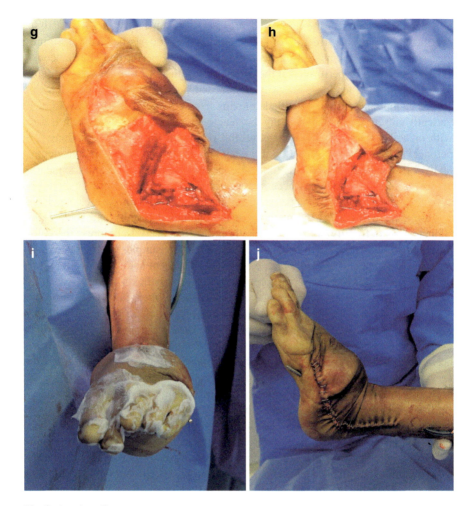

Fig. 9 (continued)

suction tip is passed over the guide pin from plantar to dorsal and pushed out dorsally [18]. The suture attaching the tendons is then inserted into the suction which is then pulled out into the drill hole through to the plantar surface. The foot is then positioned in neutral and the sutures tied over a soft tissue bolster. We use the rubber stopper from a 30 mL syringe which is perforated twice with a small clamp, and the sutures are passed through the rubber stopper, and a soft tissue bolster is inserted between the stopper and the skin and then again over the stopper to prevent the suture from cutting through the rubber, thereby losing tension. In children, it is useful to reinforce this with a 2.0 absorbable suture through the dorsal bone and into the tendon. The bone may be too hard to accomplish this in the adult, in which case small holes are made with a 1.6 mm K wire, or a suture anchor can be inserted into the cuneiform directly. If a suture anchor is used, one should ensure that this does not pull out with very vigorous tension on the suture.

Talectomy without arthrodesis will provide sufficient laxity of the soft tissue contracture to permit correction of the equinus and various associated deformities. Occasionally however, an Achilles tenotomy needs to be performed simultaneously and only needs to be performed at the completion of the talectomy if equinus deformity persists. The tendon can easily be reached posterolaterally, grasped with a curved clamp, and cut with the blade moving from outside to inside to avoid inadvertently cutting the skin. Following the talectomy, regardless of whether it is done with or without an arthrodesis, it is useful to shorten the peroneal tendons. The peroneal muscles will not function if the tendons are left alone due to considerable laxity following reduction of the foot, and one may want to restore muscle balance by shortening the tendons as necessary. Certainly, the peroneus brevis should be tightened, and a transfer of the peroneus longus to the brevis can also be considered.

Talectomy will correct the majority of the equinus deformity and some of the adductovarus deformity but is occasionally not sufficient to decompress the deformity, and additional procedures must be considered. The simplest would be to transfer the posterior tibial tendon which ensures that recurrent adductovarus deformity does not occur and also may help provide an active dorsiflexor albeit weak to the foot. It is rare that the extensor muscles are functional. If one is not able to perform a transfer of the posterior tibial tendon, a tenotomy of the tendon will need to be performed. Harvesting the tendon may not be easy because of prior scarring if a posteromedial incision has been used in early childhood. Since it is never clear what has been previously performed, we initiate the incision at the level of the medial malleolus and try to find the posterior tibial tendon in its sheath which is opened. The tendon is usually firmly adherent to the posterior aspect of the medial malleolus, and a smooth small clamp is inserted underneath the tendon to visualize it. From here, one can work distally by opening the sheath as far as possible distally. Because of scarring, one may not be able to harvest the entire tendon, but it is essential to attempt to obtain as long a piece of tendon possible for the interosseous transfer. If so, the distal 2 or 3 cm may have to be shaped and narrowed knowing that this is predominantly a scar tissue. Once the tendon has been dissected free and sutured, one should take note of any persistent adduction contracture. In cases where on examination one is certain that either the anterior tibial or extensor tendon function is present, then these can be considered for use as an active transfer in combination with the talectomy. Essentially, the foot must be balanced so that recurrent deformity of the midfoot and forefoot is less likely to occur. Bear in mind that the peroneal tendons are also not likely to be functioning in these advanced cases, but one can perform a longus-to-brevis transfer in an effort to aid eversion and balance the hindfoot. This transfer should not be considered however if the peroneal muscles are functioning strongly and the posterior and anterior tibial tendons are scarred or the muscles dysfunctional.

At this stage one should check the alignment of the toes since a flexion contracture may now be present. To some extent this will always occur because of the pre-existing equinus deformity, and as the foot is dorsiflexed, the long flexor tendons are contracted. Since passive dorsiflexion of the toes of 45° is desirable, the contracture may be decompressed by virtue of the talectomy in which case nothing needs to be done. Since these muscles may still be functional, if there are residual flexion contractures after the talectomy, one can consider a lengthening at the musculotendinous junction or through the tendon depending on the magnitude of the contracture. If severe scarring is present posteromedially, then lengthening is not necessary, and tenotomies can be performed. If so, we find it easier to perform the tenotomy of the flexor hallucis longus looking through the ankle from posterior to anterior under direct vision. Needless to state, make sure that one is grasping the flexor tendon and not the tibial nerve.

At the completion of the above procedures, the tourniquet must be left down to ensure adequate circulation to the foot. This is frequently compromised because of the magnitude of the deformity, the inevitable traction on the neurovascular bundle, hypoplasia of the dorsalis pedis artery, or prior scarring around the posteromedial ankle from prior surgeries. If perfusion does not return immediately, apply warm moist cloths to the foot and ankle, and wait for 10 minutes. It is also useful to drop the foot down slightly off the side of the table to a dependent position. If circulation does not improve following 10 minutes, we recommend applying nitroglycerin paste (Nitro-Bid) (Fig. 9h–j). This promotes vasodilatation and may sufficiently improve venous return such that the ischemia is resolved. If not, use a Doppler to mark out the tibial artery, and if there is an appreciable change at the level of the ankle, open posteromedially and perform a complete tarsal tunnel release. When releasing the tibial nerve and artery, it is important to trace the bundle distally beyond its bifurcation to the medial and lateral branches since the flexor retinaculum may be constricting either or both vessels.

7   Conclusions

The spectrum of severe untreated or recurrent clubfoot deformities that one encounters makes it impossible to provide a clear algorithm for treatment. We have highlighted a few of the more common approaches that are used on our global humanitarian programs including tendon transfer, tibial osteotomy, triple arthrodesis, and talectomy. By no means are these the only options for treatment, since combinations of procedures and additional osteotomies of the cuboid and calcaneus and other soft tissue procedures must be considered on a case-by-case basis. As we noted above, the approach to treatment of these deformities may be quite different where patients have access to regular return visits for follow-up treatment and where more sophisticated options for gradual correction with external fixation are available.

References

1. Li S, Myerson MS. Managing severe foot and ankle deformities in global humanitarian programs. Foot Ankle Clin. 2020;25(2):183–203.
2. Dobbs MB, Morcuende JA, Gurnett CA, Ponseti IV. Treatment of idiopathic clubfoot: an historical review. Iowa Orthop J. 2000;20:59–64.

3. Radler C, Mindler GT. Treatment of severe recurrent clubfoot. Foot Ankle Clin. 2015;20(4):563–86.
4. Thomas HM, Sangiorgio SN, Ebramzadeh E, Zionts LE. Relapse rates in patients with clubfoot treated using the Ponseti method increase with time: a systematic review. JBJS Rev. 2019;7(5):e6.
5. Dragoni M, Farsetti P, Vena G, Bellini D, Maglione P, Ippolito E. Ponseti treatment of rigid residual deformity in congenital clubfoot after walking age. J Bone Joint Surg Am. 2016;98(20):1706–12.
6. Eidelman M, Kotlarsky P, Herzenberg JE. Treatment of relapsed, residual and neglected clubfoot: adjunctive surgery. J Child Orthop. 2019;13(3):293–303.
7. Holmdahl HC. Astragalectomy as a stabilising operation for foot paralysis following poliomyelitis; results of a follow-up investigation of 153 cases. Acta Orthop Scand. 1956;25(3):207–27.
8. Joseph TN, Myerson MS. Use of talectomy in modern foot and ankle surgery. Foot Ankle Clin. 2004;9(4):775–85.
9. Letts M, Davidson D. The role of bilateral talectomy in the management of bilateral rigid clubfeet. Am J Orthop (Belle Mead NJ). 1999;28(2):106–10.
10. El-Sherbini MH, Omran AA. Midterm follow-up of talectomy for severe rigid equinovarus feet. J Foot Ankle Surg. 2015;54(6):1093–811.
11. Ebert N, Ballhause TM, Babin K, Schelling K, Stiel N, Stuecker R, Spiro AS. Correction of recurrent equinus deformity in surgically treated clubfeet by anterior distal tibial hemiepiphysiodesis. J Pediatr Orthop. 2020;40(9):520–5.
12. Malik SS, Knight R, Ahmed U, Prem H. Role of a tendon transfer as a dynamic checkrein reducing recurrence of equinus following distal tibial dorsiflexion osteotomy. J Pediatr Orthop B. 2018;27(5):419–24.
13. Cooper RR, Talectomy CW. A long-term follow-up evaluation. Clin Orthop Relat Res. 1985;201:32–5.
14. Mirzayan R, Early SD, Matthys GA, Thordarson DB. Single-stage talectomy and tibiocalcaneal arthrodesis as a salvage of severe, rigid equinovarus deformity. Foot Ankle Int. 2001;22(3):209–13.
15. Mann RA, Chou LB. Tibiocalcaneal arthrodesis. Foot Ankle Int. 1995;16(7):401–5.
16. Arthrogryposis. In: McCarthy JJ, Drennan JC, editors. Drennan's the child's foot and ankle. Vol. 2. Philadelphia: Lippincott Williams & Wilkins; 2009. p. 252–253.
17. Hsu LC, Jaffray D, Leong JC. Talectomy for club foot in arthrogryposis. J Bone Joint Surg Br. 1984;66(5):694–6.
18. Melamed EA, Myerson MS, Schon LC. A review of tendon passing techniques and introduction of a new method using a suction tip. Foot Ankle Int. 2000;21(8):693–6.

Muller Weiss Disease

Manuel Monteagudo and Ernesto Maceira

1 Introduction

Müller-Weiss disease (MWD) is defined as a dysplasia of the navicular bone, a consequence of abnormal development during its ossification in childhood, the pathomechanical consequences of which are experienced in adulthood. There are several possible origins for MWD, but all combine an environmental factor (e.g., malnutrition) with a predisposing mechanical factor (e.g., a short first metatarsal), during the ossification stage of the navicular. The progressive thinning of the lateral region of the bone produces a progressive lateral translation of the head of the talus until it is positioned over the calcaneus, thus generating a subtalar varus. This subtalar varus, together with the medial prominence of the medial navicular tuberosity, creates a "paradoxical varus flatfoot" pathognomonic of MWD. Dysplastic changes and altered talonavicular coverage are evident on plain weightbearing radiographs. There is no direct correlation between radiological and clinical involvement. The patient usually complains of pain in the dorsal talonavicular region, over the anterior chamber of the ankle, lateral instability due to subtalar varus effect, and pain in the tarsal sinus and peroneal tendons. Some patients with MWD do not have much pain or dysfunction and do not require treatment. When pain and functional limitation are present, the most effective conservative treatment is the use of insoles with a varus/pronator wedge in the hindfoot and internal longitudinal arch support. The varus/pronator wedge promotes passive medial displacement of the talar head to take advantage of healthy ("virgin") cartilage in the medial

M. Monteagudo (✉)
Quironsalud University Hospital Madrid, Madrid, Spain

E. Maceira
Orthopaedic Foot and Ankle Unit, Complejo Hospitalario La Mancha Centro,
Alcázar de San Juan, Ciudad Real, Spain

© The Author(s), under exclusive license to Springer Nature
Switzerland AG 2022
E. Wagner Hitschfeld, P. Wagner Hitschfeld (eds.), *Foot and Ankle Disorders*,
https://doi.org/10.1007/978-3-030-95738-4_28

region of the navicular. Most patients improve with orthotic treatment. Patients who show limiting pain, despite insoles, may require surgery. Since this is an asymmetric talonavicular joint osteoarthritis, surgery should provide the necessary mechanical change to take advantage of the medial region of healthy joint cartilage. Performing a calcaneal valgus osteotomy allows translation of the talar head medially to achieve good talonavicular coverage. In most patients, clinical improvement allows us to avoid arthrodesis. In patients with no clinical response to calcaneal valgus osteotomy, we can perform an arthrodesis which, depending on the location and extent of osteoarthritic involvement, can be talonavicular, talonaviculocuneiform, or double/triple tarsal.

2   Epidemiology

Understanding the epidemiology and historical development of MWD is very important in order to understand the origin, pathogenesis, and diagnosis of the disease. In 1925, Schmidt reported a compressed and flattened tarsal navicular in a patient with a multiple endocrine deficiency syndrome but did not publish any x-ray images [1]. In 1927, Walther Müller a German surgeon did publish the first images of a fragmented, compressed, and condensed tarsal navicular [2]. Konrad Weiss, an Austrian radiologist, studied the radiological signs of the fragmented, compressed, and condensed tarsal navicular to conclude that it was osteonecrosis [3]. This was a logical deduction because the radiological details pointed to poor bone vitality but also because of professional bias since Weiss was a disciple of Kiemböck who had described a similar condition in the lunate bone of the wrist (lunatomalacia). However, in later studies no necrotic changes were found in histological analysis of biopsies of navicular bones affected by this pathology [4, 5]. MWD was named after the findings of these two physicians. Since then, numerous etiopathogenic theories have been suggested to explain its development (congenital malformation, anomalous evolution of Köhler's disease, posttraumatic migration of an accessory cuboid, etc.) [6].

Brailsford proposed that a history of previous trauma was an important factor for the development of MWD and named it "listhesis navicularis" because of the crushing and sliding of the fragments after their separation from the bone [7]. This author had a large series of cases for the time (5 patients in 1935, 17 in 1945, and 20 in 1953). He also reported that it was predominantly bilateral and asymmetric between the feet, and 88% of the patients were women. Interestingly, he commented that the disease was more prevalent than previously thought and that many cases were not correctly diagnosed. This is something we fully subscribe to in our experience to date. MWD is largely unknown in many parts of the world. Understanding its epidemiology explains to a large extent why it is underdiagnosed.

In 1948, Fontaine et al. coined the term "adult tarsal scaphoiditis," and it became the most popular non-eponymic name in Europe [8]. In 1981, Willey and Brown published the longest series in North America (Ottawa) and suggested that it was not an osteonecrosis but the result of heterogeneous ossification centers inducing dysplasia [9].

In a seminar paper (2004) for MWD, Maceira and Rochera described the types of radiological presentation and also analyzed epidemiological data that pointed to environmental factors, interacting with a mechanical predisposition of the foot, for the development of the disease [10]. The authors studied the clinical records of 191 cases of MWD registered at the Hospital de San Rafael in Barcelona, and from the analysis of the data, they realized several very interesting facts. Eighty-five percent of the patients were born outside Barcelona and had migrated from different rural areas of southern Spain to Barcelona in the 1950s, with a homogeneous distribution of birth dates. Most were born around 1932, about 4 years before the outbreak of the Spanish Civil War. However, 70% of the controls seen for other foot and ankle reasons in the same hospital and the same time period were born in Barcelona. Most of the patients with MWD were immigrants whose families had escaped from conditions of extreme poverty and hunger in southern Spain after the Spanish Civil War (1936–1939). Southern Spain (Andalusia, Extremadura, Castilla-La Mancha) suffered devastating war and postwar conditions of extreme poverty and hunger. Environmental and nutritional stress in children with a growing navicular may have played a fundamental role in the later development of a navicular that, for a time until complete ossification, may have been subjected to abnormal loads that eventually deformed it. Poverty and lack of food were also due to the disappearance of traditional agriculture in Spain, due to the progressive mechanization of agricultural techniques that required less labor. For all these reasons, in the 1950s, there were massive migratory movements from the most disadvantaged areas of southern Spain to the big capitals – Madrid, Barcelona, and Valencia – and the new inhabitants occupied the lower-skilled jobs. Some 73% of the patients with MWD in Maceira and Rochera's study were women, housewives, or housekeeping staff [10]. Müller and Weiss's patients had also suffered a very similar situation with the First World War, which raged in Europe between 1914 and 1918 [1–3]. Their published cases had the same temporal pattern with respect to a war as those in Barcelona. The low incidence of MWD in some countries such as the United States can be explained by the absence of the predisposing environmental factors already explained. They have not suffered wars (on their territory) in the last century, and they have not suffered poverty or hunger, so cases of MWD in the United States are usually "imported" in immigrants who did suffer hardships during their childhood in their countries of origin [10]. It is interesting how archeological studies have been able to identify cases of MWD and how the stigmata of malnutrition coincided in our ancestors and in our epidemic patients [11]. Anthropologists believe that the presence of Harris lines (radiological striations indicating tortuous bone growth due to malnutrition), dental enamel hypoplasia (which will cause severe dental problems at early ages), and cribra orbitalia (porotic hyperostosis of the orbital roof due to childhood stress) represents episodes of nutritional stress among populations of children in different civilizations throughout history [12]. Most patients with MWD show these signs of nutritional stress.

The authors, after studying more than 600 cases of MWD over the last 20 years (including those in the study by Maceira and Rochera), can explain that there are different types of MWD, which are due to different etiological factors, although all of them share the fundamental characteristics of navicular dysplasia and subtalar varus [10, 13]:

1. Cases of unknown origin
2. Epidemic environmental stress during childhood
3. Individual environmental stress during childhood
4. Obvious or less obvious anatomical deformities, such as metatarsus adductus or varus hindfoot
5. Athletes with intensive training during childhood
6. A special type of adult-onset MWD known as "Müllerweissoid foot"

These different types of MWD will be discussed in the following section in order to understand their pathomechanics and development.

3   Pathomechanics

Once the epidemiology of MWD is understood, the most important question to understand its pathomechanics would be: Is delayed navicular ossification a sufficient condition to develop MWD? The answer would be no. There must also be an abnormal ("nonideal") mechanical factor that irregularly compresses a maturing (ossifying) navicular. Children who, subjected to severe nutritional environmental stress, did not develop MWD underwent compressive forces that were homogeneously distributed along the entire length and width of the navicular, whereby the ossifying cartilage structure could accommodate these loads and not deform, except if we occasionally consider a symmetrical flattening in its antero-posterior width. This scenario is found in Köhler's disease, a benign, self-limiting condition also known as naviculare pedis retardatum.

Environmental factors alone are not a sufficient condition for developing MWD; otherwise, the prevalence would be higher and more homogeneous in risk groups. It is necessary for a mechanical factor to act on the slowly maturing navicular to cause asymmetric load distribution and consequent dysplasia. The most frequent predisposing mechanical factor (almost 100% of cases) is the presence of a short first metatarsals (metatarsal index minus formula) [8, 10, 14]. When the first ray of the foot is not able to transmit the loads to the ground due to the short length of the first metatarsal, the compressive moments are transferred to the second-third-fourth metatarsal producing a "nutcracker" effect on the immature navicular to eventually cause dysplasia with crushing in the lateral region. A more or less marked metatarsus adductus (metatarsus adductus) or the sequel of a clubfoot can also cause the same effect on the navicular (Fig. 1).

At this stage of bony stress, during ossification of the navicular, it is common for some orthopedic surgeons unfamiliar with MWD to diagnose as a navicular stress

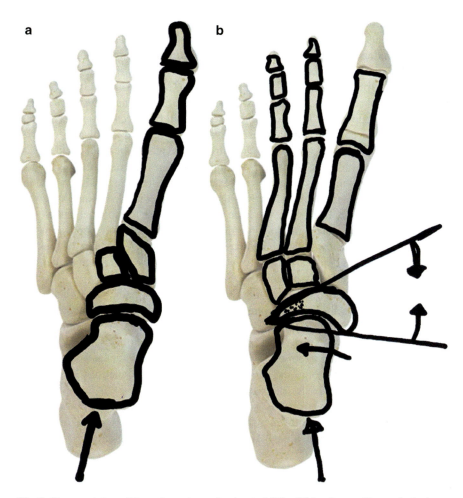

Fig. 1 Representation of the pathogenic mechanism in Müller-Weiss disease. The navicular bone is compressed between the head of the talus and the central cuneiforms producing a "nutcracker" effect. (**a**) In a foot with a non-dysplastic navicular, compressive forces during gait act between the head of the talus and the first metatarsal through the medial cuneiform, maintaining the shape of the coxa pedis. (**b**) In a dysplastic navicular due to Müller-Weiss disease, with a short first metatarsal, compressive forces act between the head of the talus and the medial cuneiforms producing bony stress in the lateral region of the navicular

fracture what is actually the natural evolutionary process of the disease [15]. The progressive compression, condensation, and crushing of the lateral region of the navicular cause the head of the talus to progressively migrate laterally and plantarly, progressively overlapping the calcaneus (decreased kite angle). The overlapping of the talus and calcaneus is physiological during the third rocker of gait ("propulsive calcaneal foot"), but is not physiological when maintained throughout the gait cycle. The superimposition of the talus over the calcaneus results in subtalar varus. The forces transmitted by the triceps and those of ground reaction are transformed into varus moments that end up damaging the lateral structures of the ankle and foot. Peroneal tendon pathology and calcaneocuboid pain are common among patients with MWD [13]. Subtalar varus also leads to the loss of the shock-absorbing "talar foot" during the first and second rocker gait. The shock-absorbing work during the first and second rocker gait must be then performed by an upper segment, the knee extensor apparatus. This extensor apparatus will be forced to work with rotation and greater compression than usual against the femoral trochlea in order to compensate for subtalar varus. This load transfer explains the high incidence of patellofemoral problems and patellar tendinopathies in patients with MWD [13]. When an insole is modified to achieve a greater valgus effect, the foot improves, and the knee worsens. Conversely, when the valgus effect is reduced, the knee improves, and the foot worsens. If for years the knee has to compensate and assume the cushioning that the midtarsal joint does not do, not only the patellofemoral joint will suffer but also the femorotibial joint will eventually be damaged, which justifies that the incidence of total knee arthroplasty in patients with MWD is much higher than in the general population (without MWD) (Fig. 2) [10].

Talonavicular osteoarthritis may also be responsible for pain, but in many cases it is also due to the mechanical compression causing damage to the deteriorated bone and soft tissue [16]. Today we know the beneficial effects on pain and function of joint preservation surgeries in cases of asymmetric osteoarthritis. Similarly, with conservative or surgical treatment, when we manage to transfer loads to the most preserved region of the joint, the patient improves pain and function. With a common pathomechanical basis, the asymmetric compression of a navicular with delayed ossification due to various predisposing factors, we can differentiate some special pathomechanical pathways that would justify that not all patients with MWD are the same, although they all share common clinical findings:

1. Cases of unknown origin.

   In very few patients, we do not find a clear cause for the development of MWD. Surely there was some subtle mechanical problem that acted in childhood (but later disappeared by development) on the growing navicular and caused dysplasia.

2. Epidemic environmental stress during infancy.

   This group includes the cases of the so-called "epidemic group" described by Müller, Weiss, Brailsford, Maceira, and other authors in which the "children of war" were unable to ossify their naviculars normally [1–3, 7, 10]. Nowadays wars are far from the Western world in which many of us live, but there are continents with millions of children in a situation of famine and nutritional stress silently generating new cases of MWD. In malnourished children, the fragility of the navicular during its maturation (last tarsal bone to ossify) makes it sensitive to any mechanical factor, banal in any other stage of life, to end up developing dysplasia. Nutritional stress in children is also associated with Harris lines, enamel hypoplasia, and cribra orbitalia, and these findings are very frequent in adult patients with MWD and very rare in the general population [10, 13].

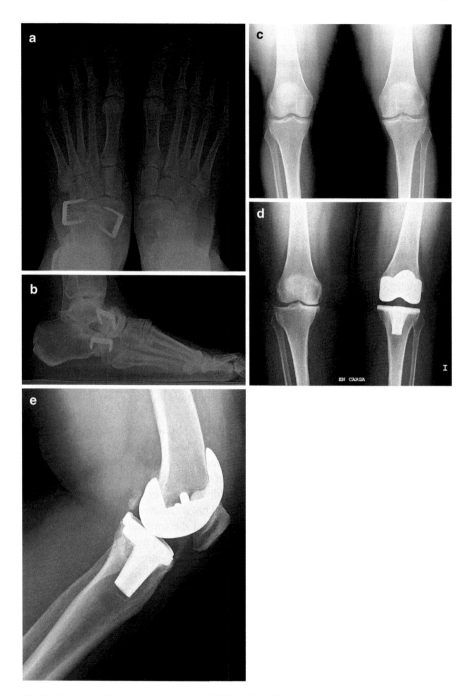

Fig. 2 Lack of cushioning of the foot with Müller-Weiss disease leads to load transfer to the knee. (**a**) Dorsoplantar view of weightbearing radiograph of a patient showing bilateral involvement, already operated with an unsuccessful attempt at arthrodesis and without varus correction. (**b**) X-ray in lateral weightbearing view of the same case. (**c**) Anteroposterior view of weightbearing radiographs of both knees showing gonarthrosis. (**d**) The patient required a total knee replacement. (**e**) Total knee replacement is a common and an early event in patients with Müller-Weiss disease

3. Individual environmental stress during childhood.

   There are non-epidemic cases in which a child may suffer malnutrition or malabsorption and produce altered navicular ossification. Some diseases, such as inflammatory bowel disease and chronic kidney disease, which can occur in childhood, produce a decreased appetite and increased energy expenditure, with consequent alteration of navicular ossification [17]. Some of these children may later, as adults, have good control of the underlying disease, and the pathomechanical correlation described above may be difficult.

4. Obvious or less obvious anatomical deformities such as metatarsus adductus or varus hindfoot.

   Sometimes the mechanical causes are obvious and sufficient to "take advantage" of any slight delay in navicular ossification and cause dysplastic development. A very short first metatarsal (brachymetatarsia of the first metatarsal), a marked metatarsus adductus, a cavovarus foot, can cause a great imbalance of compressive and shearing forces on a navicular with "normal" development to end up deforming it (Delpech's law).

5. Athletes with intensive training during childhood.

   Another scenario in which the pathomechanics have more to do with non-epidemic factors is found in high-level athletes who, during childhood with their developing naviculars, were subjected to intensive training. These "non-epidemic" cases show no Harris lines, no dental problems, and no orbital cribra [10, 13]. The vast majority of these child athletes, some of them later elite professionals, have a short first ray, and their naviculars were subjected to "too much work, too soon." The short first ray can be explained by the existence of a short first metatarsal or by the secondary relative shortening of the medial column of the foot as a result of the internal rotation of the navicular in the transverse plane and the relative retroposition of the first cuneometatarsal joint with respect to the second. Kidner and Muro already indicated to us that children with metatarsal palette adduction had delayed ossification of their naviculars [18]. Spontaneous correction of the adductus in some children involves external rotation of the cuboid and of the "en bloc" cuneiforms. This rotation is possible if the medial region of the navicular acts as a fulcrum and the rotation is at the expense of compression of the lateral region of the navicular and a medial subluxation of the cuboid. It would simulate the "nutcracker effect" already outlined, the arms being the talus and cuneiforms, the fulcrum the medial region of the navicular, and the nut the lateral region of the navicular. The lack of cushioning of the foot means that, during the "adult" phase of their sporting career (between 25 and 35 years of age), many suffer from patellofemoral problems and tendinopathies of the extensor apparatus of the knee. It is not easy for some of these patients, many of them professional athletes and some of them elite athletes, to find a balance for the correct functioning of the foot-knee pair with adequate insoles. Some of them have several insoles with pronator wedges of different heights, which they change during the competition or the season to increase the work of the foot or knee according to their symptoms. Some of these athletes compete in environments with a low historical prevalence of MWD, and their pain is mistaken for navicular stress fractures, when radiological studies leave no doubt about their problems [19]. Sometimes, misdiagnosed athletes are treated by fixation (osteosynthesis) with grafting, and many of these surgeries fail because they do not heal, and the athlete maintains pain and functional limitation. The subtalar varus and the "nutcracker effect" will cause distraction forces on the focus of injury and with the result of a nonunion in many of these athletes. The newspaper archives (see the American professional basketball league players with navicular stress fractures on the Internet) have plenty of examples of failures of supposed navicular stress fractures in elite athletes, which are a "career-ending" injury because of treating the consequence and not the cause of their problem.

6. A special type of adult-onset MWD known as "Müllerweissoid foot".

A less obvious scenario of MWD development can be observed in adult life on the basis of a healthy navicular. The combined existence of a constitutional subtalar varus and a short first metatarsal stimulates repeated pronation of the forefoot during gait and results in subtle osteoarthritis of the Lisfranc joint. Lisfranc arthrosis and midfoot abduction and pronation create a dorsomedial prominence in the midfoot and a false valgus flatfoot appearance. Lisfranc arthropathy may divert our attention away from subtalar varus and direct damage to the lateral region of the acetabulum pedis. These "Müllerweissoid" feet do not show lateral navicular fragmentation, and the bone dysplasia is very subtle, but they share the pathomechanics and clinical and treatment strategy of a patient with "conventional" MWD (Fig. 3). If MWD goes undiagnosed in many cases, the "Müllerweissoid" foot is even more complicated to diagnose. Many cases are

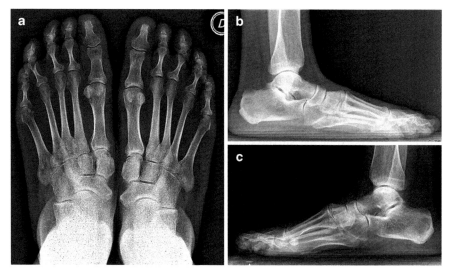

Fig. 3 The "Müllerweissoid" foot is the result of a combination of constitutional subtalar varus and a short first metatarsal. There is no obvious navicular dysplasia, but it shares the pathogenetic mechanisms of Müller-Weiss disease. The radiological signs are identifiable on a weightbearing radiograph. (**a**) In a dorsoplantar view we can appreciate the existence of a short first metatarsal and a subtle varus of the hindfoot. (**b**) In the lateral view, we can see the dorsal prominence in the midfoot. (**c**) And an associated arthropathy at the Lisfranc joint that almost always accompanies the "Müllerweissoid" foot

treated as flat feet instead of subtalar varus feet. When the type of treatment is changed, the response is often comparable to that of classic MWD.

4 Diagnosis

As in any other mechanical pathology of the foot, the combination of a good physical examination with the reading of radiographs of both feet should allow us to make a diagnosis of MWD.

5 Clinical Examination

The examination should begin by observing the patient walking in the office, barefoot and with the ankles free. In many patients we observe what we call a "paradoxical varus flatfoot," because it is usual for the flatfoot to be valgus and the pes cavus to be varus. However, in MWD, the flatfoot appearance is conferred by the protrusion of the medial tuberosity of the navicular that simulates a collapse of the medial arch, unlike true flatfoot in which the medial protrusion is due to the head of the talus. The varus may be obvious or subtle. When the varus is subtle, a good examination maneuver for diagnosis is to grasp the patient's heel while asking the patient to do a bipodal toe-off. The "palpable" varus is maintained throughout the entire length of the toe-off and up to the plantigrade position of the foot, unlike valgus flatfoot in which (when the subtalar is mobile) a change into valgus position of the heel is noticed with the bipodal or monopodal toe-off. Pain in the dorsal region of the talonavicular joint is frequent, as well as pain attributable to lateral overload due to subtalar varus, such as pain in the peroneal tendons, in the sinus tarsi, and in the calcaneocuboid region. Often the patient reports a sensation of ankle instability, also related to subtalar varus. The existence of an associated equinus can be assessed by the Silfverskiöld maneuver. The presence of a third rocker metatarsalgia in the context of an index minus is also common in patients with MWD.

6 Imaging Studies

It is essential to obtain a reliable weightbearing radiograph of both feet. The "mechanical reading" of the radiographs gives us almost all the information necessary to complete the diagnosis and to know the existence of other typical changes of MWD [20, 21]. After analyzing the radiological variants of MWD, Maceira formulated a radiological classification that allows us to identify the different evolutionary changes of navicular dysplasia [10]. The radiological classification has no direct correlation with clinical findings or with pain, but it is very useful to identify different evolutionary stages of the same problem. The degree of asymmetry and fragmentation of the navicular is more visible in the dorsoplantar view of the feet weightbearing. In this projection we can see the existence of an index minus, with a first metatarsal much shorter than the second, in the great majority of patients with MWD. The overlapping of the talus and calcaneus reduces the visible surface of the calcaneocuboid joint and exposes most of the medial tuberosity of the navicular which is "uncovered" without articulating with the talus. The head of the talus faces the heads of the second-third (and even fourth) metatarsals instead of facing the first metatarsal, as in a mechanically normal foot (Fig. 4). CT can help quantify arthropathy and fragmentation of the lateral region of the navicular and check for the absence of osteoarthritis in neighboring joints, including the subtalar. MRI often reveals bone edema in the lateral talonavicular region and the lateral region of the subtalar joint [22]. MRI is also useful to assess for tendinopathy or longitudinal tears in the peroneals and to assess the status of the lateral collateral ligament of the ankle. Talonavicular joint asymmetry usually preserves the medial region of the joint with healthy cartilage that will be the basis for improving patient's symptoms using a joint preservation surgery (calcaneal osteotomy). Other tests such as SPECT-CT scintigraphy or weightbearing CT scan (WBCT) can help to assess subtalar joint congruency and associated injuries in neighboring joints but are not necessary for diagnosis [23].

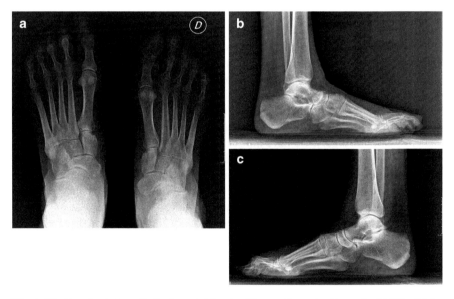

Fig. 4 The "mechanical reading" of a weightbearing X-rays allows the diagnosis of Müller-Weiss disease. (**a**) Weightbearing dorsoplantar view of a patient showing greater radiological involvement of the right foot. It is important to see that the head of the talus "faces" the second metatarsal and the presence of a bilateral short first metatarsal. (**b** and **c**) Lateral view of a weightbearing radiograph of the same case

7   Treatment

Regardless of the evolutionary stage or the patient's pain at the first consultation, we should always try to exhaust the resources of conservative treatment before considering surgery. There is no minimum time of effect of conservative therapies to consider surgery. The surgical decision will depend above all on the limitation of quality of life and poor pain control experienced by the patient during the evolution of MWD.

7.1   *Conservative*

As with any mechanical pathology of the foot, conservative treatment should always precede any surgical indication. Physical means of rehabilitation and anti-inflammatory medication generally have little effect in the treatment of MWD. When there is a lot of bone edema, some patients improve with magnetotherapy [13].

Conservative treatment in mechanical foot disorders has as a fundamental element the use of insoles. When we were aware of the importance of hindfoot varus, our indication of the type of insoles focused on using pronator/valgus wedges of about 10–12 mm of lateral base in the hindfoot, to try to counteract the subtalar varus moments during the first rocker of gait, and the use of a medial longitudinal arch support to stop the collapse of the medial tuberosity of the navicular. With the correct insoles, most patients experience marked improvement in their symptoms and improve their function (Fig. 5) [13]. With a mobile and healthy subtalar joint, the pronator wedge forces subtalar pronation and the head of the talus to move toward the more medial region of the joint. Loading on a region of the bone with healthy cartilage allowed patients' pain and function to improve. Many patients with MWD present with incorrect insoles, with the heel wedge being supinator/varus rather than pronator/valgus. Switching to the correct wedge improves most patients. Although it would be logical to think that patient response to insole use might anticipate response to surgery, we have not seen a direct correlation in our patients [13]. Some did not respond adequately to insoles but were much improved by surgically correcting the hindfoot varus. The same situation applies to the degree of radiological compromise. We have not found a direct relationship between the degree of osteoarthritic involvement and deformity and the response to the use of insoles, which leads us to indicate them in any evolutionary situation of the disease before surgery is considered. In a short series with ten patients, Ruiz-Escobar et al. report a significant improvement in seven of the patients, with the remaining three requiring surgery [24].

Footwear may also be important in some cases of MWD. Rocker-bottom shoes allow a smoother transition from the first to the third rocker of the gait, with less energy expenditure and reduced joint work [25]. Some patients improve with rocker-bottom shoes. Some of our patients have also improved with the use of ankle braces to limit anterolateral instability associated with MWD.

Fig. 5 Insoles used in Müller-Weiss disease with pronator/valgus wedges for the hindfoot and with internal longitudinal arch support

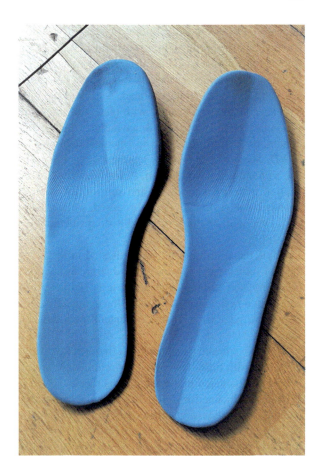

7.2 Surgical

When the patient is unable to perform basic activities of daily living because of pain and functional limitation, and conservative treatments have been reasonably exhausted, surgery can functionally improve patients with MWD. About 20 years ago, the gold standard of treatment was to perform arthrodesis of the painful arthritic segments. We associated then (about 25 years ago) osteoarthrosis and arthrodesis as an appropriate diagnosis-treatment pair in MWD.

7.2.1 Arthrodesis

The most common arthrodesis in our past treatments was talonavicular. This selective arthrodesis could be considered in cases of isolated talonavicular involvement and with a healthy naviculocuneiform joint, but it is associated with a high risk of nonunion. From a technical point of view, it was not easy to perform an isolated talonavicular arthrodesis in a foot with MWD. The most common approach was the medial approach. To achieve an adequate valgus, the talar head had to be "pushed" from lateral to medial to achieve a favorable alignment between the talar head and the first metatarsal head. And then the talus had to be held in position with adequate stable fixation with plate and screws. But the varus moments were still acting on a dysplastic talonavicular, which explained the high percentage of nonunions and malunions in medial column arthrodesis in patients with MWD. Some of our patients required salvage surgery after attempted arthrodesis due to nonunion or malunion. A few years ago, Hintermann et al. added lateral fixation with a tension band and screws that neutralized the varus forces in the talonavicular region to be arthrodesed, obtaining homogeneously good results [26]. Other authors have reported good results in this type of arthrodesis in MWD [27, 28].

Triple tarsal arthrodesis was indicated in the few patients with added involvement of subtalar and calcaneocuboid arthrosis and, occasionally, to avoid nonunion of the isolated talonavicular arthrodesis. Triple arthrodesis can have good results both with an open approach and arthroscopically in patients with MWD, although there were patients with residual lateral pain attributable to residual uncorrected varus [29–31].

With a dysplastic navicular, with frequent involvement of the naviculocuneiform joint, and with little bone stock for arthrodesis, we often expanded the number of joints to be included in the arthrodesis block and frequently resorted to performing a talonaviculocuneiform (medial column) arthrodesis. Watson-Jones described internal longitudinal arch arthrodesis for the treatment of navicular fracture sequelae [32]. Restoration of medial column length of the foot is desirable in a posttraumatic setting but is challenging to achieve in MWD. Improved length in the medial column has been associated with a better clinical outcome in this type of arthrodesis [33]. Several authors have achieved good results with talonaviculocuneiform arthrodesis in MWD, most using a tricortical iliac crest graft to connect the segments to be arthrodesed [34–37]. Some authors opted for complete removal of the navicular and replacement with a femoral head allograft to cover the defect and fixation with an eight-hole plate with solid union [38]. The poor vitality of the navicular has led some authors to try using a vascularized femoral condyle graft to successfully perform a medial column arthrodesis, replacing the nonviable part of the navicular [39].

Our overall experience with arthrodeses in MWD was variable. We learned from the technical difficulty of fusion and used a talonaviculocuneiform arthrodesis with "Watson-Jones" grafting in most of our cases. But objectively, the arthrodesis required long postoperative unloading times, slow recovery, the need for grafting, a non-negligible percentage of nonunions, and some malunions with residual subtalar varus (Fig. 6). By 2003, our perception of pathomechanics in MWD changed from considering osteoarthritis as the problem causing the pain to hindfoot varus as the true culprit. Asymmetric talonavicular osteoarthritis led us to believe that, if we

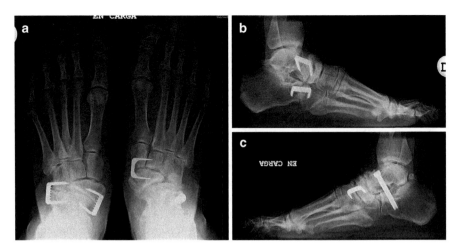

Fig. 6 In tarsal arthrodesis for the treatment of Müller-Weiss disease, it is common to find non-union and malposition without hindfoot varus correction. (**a**) In the dorsoplantar view we can appreciate the presence of nonunion. In one of the feet, a screw ("talus-stop") was used to stop the lateral displacement of the talus. (**b** and **c**) Lateral weightbearing view of the same case

could modify the moments acting on the lateral region of the joint toward the medial region, the existing "virgin" cartilage in the medial region of the navicular could allow an improvement in joint conditions and pain relief. The same was true for other asymmetric osteoarthritis such as the knee in genu varum after valgus osteotomy of the proximal tibia. The use of pronator wedge inserts achieved this goal in most patients [13]. We went from operating on 10–15 cases per year to only 2–4. The next question was then logical: could we achieve the same effect of the insoles with surgery?

7.2.2   Joint Preservation Osteotomies/Surgery

The response was to perform a calcaneal valgus osteotomy to allow the triceps to function by generating valgus moments rather than favoring varus moments. The Dwyer-type calcaneal valgus osteotomy was a simple technique and allowed early loading in patients with MWD. And it worked, in most cases with mild varus, but not to the same extent when the varus was significant. We then made two modifications that allowed improvement in cases of more accentuated varus. The first modification in our surgical technique to achieve greater valgus with the Dwyer-type osteotomy was to perform it in the most anterior region of the calcaneus. When we perform a varus osteotomy of the calcaneus, the translation has the same effect if it is performed on the posterior tuberosity as if it is placed closer to the sinus of the tarsus. The triceps will act in the same way, generating the same varus moments.

However, in a Dwyer-type osteotomy, the location of the osteotomy does matter. The same lateral base wedge of about 8–10 mm will produce a greater varus effect the further forward the osteotomy cut is placed. The lever arm from the osteotomy to the insertion of the Achilles at the posterior calcaneal tuberosity will be greater the further the distance from the Achilles insertion in the calcaneus and the greater the valgus effect. The second modification was to add a lateral displacement (reverse Koutsogiannis effect) to the Dwyer osteotomy to achieve an even greater valgus effect. When attempting to shift the posterior region of the calcaneus laterally, it is necessary to stretch/weaken the medial soft tissues. In our experience it is not necessary to section the plantar fascia to achieve a "valguizating" osteotomy. Sectioning the plantar fascia can also have unpredictable consequences, such as medial arch collapse and lateral column overload syndrome of the foot. It is sufficient to spend about 2 minutes during surgery, using a laminar spreader, to open and close the osteotomy several times, resulting in a controlled fractional elongation of the medial soft tissues including the plantar fascia. When this effect is achieved, it is easy to gain about 8–10 mm of lateral translation in the osteotomy, achieving the desired valguizating effect that has given us considerably better results than those obtained with the Dwyer osteotomy alone [13]. Fixation of the osteotomy is performed with two 6.5 or 7.0 millimeter cannulated screws (Fig. 7). The immediate postoperative period includes non-weightbearing for 2 weeks until the wounds and soft tissues are healed. At 2 weeks, weightbearing is started with an orthopedic boot and crutches according to the patient's tolerance. The boot is abandoned between the second and third month. In recent years, and in view of our results, this "supervalgus" osteotomy – very anterior lateral closing wedge and lateral translational calcaneal osteotomy – has become our surgery of choice for patients with MWD, regardless of the radiological stage at the time of surgery [13]. Any modification to the calcaneus-triceps loading axis requires a minimum of 6 months of "brain habituation" so that our cortex receives reliable mechanical stimuli and can develop an effective and homogeneous motor plan for the patient to gain gait fluidity and reflex speed with the operated foot. Most of the patients operated on with an isolated calcaneal osteotomy improved without the need for secondary surgery [40]. But, as is obvious and as we explain to our surgical patients, some patients may require secondary arthrodesis after an osteotomy that did not produce the desired effect or that produced it for a time only to worsen later. When talonavicular coverage improves, arthrodesis over a previous osteotomy is quicker and easier and possibly more likely to be successful than primary arthrodesis over the original deformity.

The first series in our case series with an isolated "supervalgus" osteotomy was the subject of a joint study with Myerson's group series with 13 patients in total (14 feet) treated with a calcaneal valgus osteotomy [40]. The mean age at the time of surgery was 56 years, with a mean of 10.6 years of previous symptomatology. With a mean follow-up of 3.7 years (1–8.5 years), the visual analog pain scale improved from 8 (7–9) preoperatively to 2 (0–4), and the hindfoot AOFAS scale improved from 29 (20–44) to 79 (70–88). Most patients were very satisfied with the

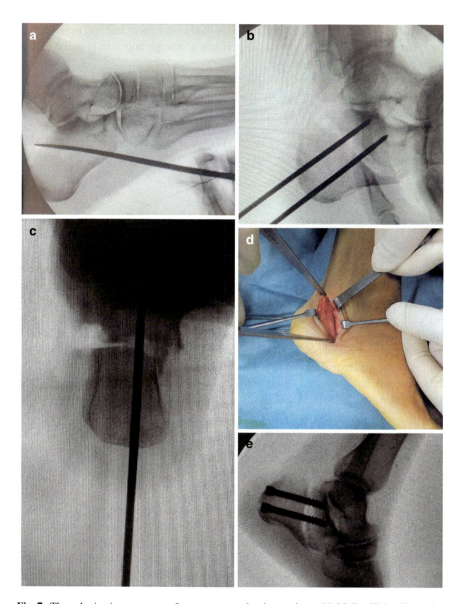

Fig. 7 The valguizating osteotomy for varus correction in a patient with Müller-Weiss disease has several key steps. (**a**) Radioscopy image showing the optimal location of the osteotomy, as anterior as possible, to achieve the greatest valgus effect. (**b**) The osteotomy already performed and provisional fixation with k-wires can be seen. (**c**) Axial view of the intraoperative fluoroscopy shows the lateralizing effect of the osteotomy. (**d**) Intraoperative image showing the lateral step after displacement of the osteotomy and provisional fixation with k-wires. E: Radioscopy showing fixation of the osteotomy with two cannulated 6.5 mm screws

outcome of surgery. When we published this study, no patient had had to be reoperated, but we have subsequently had to perform a salvage arthrodesis in the patient who showed a worse outcome.

We have recently reviewed our series of joint preservation surgeries in 17 cases with very satisfactory results and comparable to those obtained in the bi-center study discussed above, with one patient reintervened with an arthrodesis 4 years after osteotomy (Fig. 8) [41]. With these results, supervalgus calcaneal osteotomy has become our surgery of choice in MWD regardless of radiological and clinical involvement, although it is clear that some patient will need a salvage arthrodesis some time after the osteotomy.

7.2.3   Other Surgeries

Some authors have proposed joint preservation surgery for MWD, consisting of performing a calcaneal osteotomy to lengthen the lateral column [42]. In their work they confuse MWD with a valgus flatfoot and adopt a solution contrary to the pathomechanics of the disease. It is clear that an Evans-type lengthening of the lateral column can only increase lateral translation of the talar head and increase subtalar varus and the clinical problems of MWD. The work was challenged shortly thereafter, and the authors of this chapter believe that the starting error was the confusion of a paradoxical varus flatfoot with a conventional valgus flatfoot [43]. Other authors have reported a good outcome after decompression with biopsy/forages of the navicular with MWD [44].

8   Conclusions

MWD is a dysplasia of the navicular that develops during childhood and is suffered in adulthood. Epidemiologic study of many cases over the past 25 years has allowed us to understand that not all patients have the same origin of their deformity, but they all share common pathomechanics that includes translation of the talar head laterally to lie over the calcaneus, inducing subtalar varus. Confusion in the clinical diagnosis of a paradoxical varus flatfoot instead of a conventional valgus flatfoot will lead to inadequate treatment and failure to respond to conservative and surgical treatment. Plain weightbearing radiographs are the most cost-effective diagnostic tool in MWD. Conservative treatment consists primarily of the use of pronator/valgus wedge insoles in the rearfoot to reduce subtalar varus effects and internal longitudinal arch support. Joint preservation surgery in asymmetric osteoarthritis of MWD, by means of a supervalgus osteotomy of the calcaneus, allows in most cases a good clinical and radiological result and thus avoids the need for arthrodesis. Arthrodesis could be reserved for cases that do not improve with osteotomy.

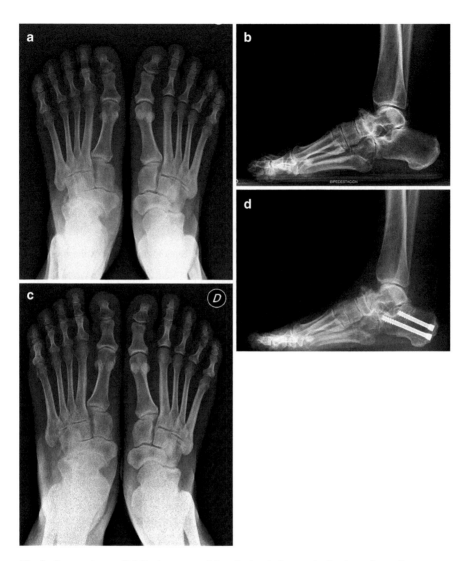

Fig. 8 Progressive medial displacement of the talar head after a valguizating calcaneal osteotomy is evident by comparing the radiographs shown. (**a**) Preoperative dorsoplantar weightbearing view showing significant involvement of the left foot. (**b**) Lateral view of the same foot where the talonavicular degenerative changes can be seen, and it is not possible to visualize the joint. (**c**) One year after surgery, the improvement in the talonavicular coverage can be seen after the medial displacement of the talus produced by the osteotomy. (**d**) Lateral view 1 year after surgery where the talonavicular joint is already visible

References

1. Müller W. On a typical deformity of the tarsal navicular and its clinical presentation [in German]. ROEFO. 1928;37:38–42.
2. Müller W. On an odd double-sided change of the tarsal navicular [in German]. Deutsche Zeitschrift für Chirurgie Leipzig. 1927;201:84–7.
3. Weiss K. On the malacia of the tarsal navicular [in German]. Fortschr Geb Rontgenstr. 1927;45:63–7.
4. Maceira E. Clinical and biomechanical aspects of Müller Weiss disease [in Spanish]. Revista de Medicina y Cirugía del Pie. 1996;10:53–65.
5. Zimmer EA. Diseases, injuries and varieties of the tarsal navicular [in German]. Arch Orthop Trauma Surg. 1937;38:396–411.
6. Viladot A, Rochera R, Viladot A Jr. Necrosis of the navicular bone. Bull Hosp Jt Dis Orthop Inst. 1987;47(2):285–93.
7. Brailsford JF. Osteochondritis of the adult tarsal navicular. J Bone Joint Surg Am. 1939;26(1):111–20.
8. Fontaine R, Warter P, de Lange CH. The adult tarsal scaphoiditis (Müller-Weiss disease) [in French]. J Radiol Électrol. 1948;29:540–1.
9. Wiley JJ, Brown DE. The bipartite tarsal scaphoid. J Bone Joint Surg. 1981;63B(4):583–6.
10. Maceira E, Rochera R. Müller-Weiss disease: clinical and biomechanical features. Foot Ankle Clin. 2004;9(1):105–25.
11. Chiavegatti R, Canales P, Saldias E, Isidro A. Earliest probable case of Mueller-Weiss disease from ancient Egypt. J Foot Ankle Surg. 2018;57(5):1034–6.
12. Nowak O. The influence of conditions of life on the formation of morphological features of human long bones in historical populations. Variabil Evol. 2000;8:129–34.
13. Monteagudo M, Maceira E. Management of Müller-Weiss disease. Foot Ankle Clin. 2019;24(1):89–105.
14. Vilaseca JM, Casademunt M. Escafoidopatı'a tarsiana del adulto [Adult tarsal scaphoidopathy]. Anales de Medicina Sección Médica Barcelona. 1957;43:157–72. [In Spanish]
15. Frosch L. The pathologic fracture of the tarsal navicular [in German]. Deutsche Z für Chirurgie. 1931;232:487–92.
16. Doyle T, Napier RJ, Wong-Chung J. Recognition and management of Müller-Weiss disease. Foot Ankle Int. 2012;33(4):275–81.
17. Sylvester FA, Wyzga N, Hyams JS, Davis PM, Lerer T, Vance K, Hawker G, Griffiths AM. Natural history of bone metabolism and bone mineral density in children with inflammatory bowel disease. Inflamm Bowel Dis. 2007;13(1):42–50.
18. Kidner FC, Muro F. Köhler's disease of the tarsal scaphoid or os naviculare pedis retardatum. JAMA. 1924;83(21):1650–4.
19. Khan M, Madden K, Burrus MT, Rogowski JP, Stotts J, Samani MJ, Sikka R, Bedi A. Epidemiology and impact on performance of lower extremity stress injuries in professional basketball players. Sports Health. 2018;10(2):169–74.
20. Wong-Chung J, McKenna R, Tucker A, Gibson D, Datta P. Radiographic analysis of Müller-Weiss disease. Foot Ankle Surg. 2020:S1268–7731(20)30119–3. https://doi.org/10.1016/j.fas.2020.06.009. Online ahead of print.
21. Samim M, Moukaddam HA, Smitaman E. Imaging of Mueller-Weiss syndrome: a review of clinical presentations and imaging spectrum. Am J Roentgenol. 2016;207(2):W8–W18.
22. Nguyen AS, Tagoylo GH, Mote GA. Diagnostic imaging of the mueller-weiss syndrome: findings of a rare condition of the foot. J Am Podiatr Med Assoc. 2014;104(1):110–4.
23. Welck MJ, Kaplan J, Myerson MS. Müller-Weiss syndrome: radiological features and the role of weightbearing computed tomography scan. Foot Ankle Spec. 2016;9(3):245–51.
24. Ruiz-Escobar J, Viladot-Pericé R, Álvarez-Goenaga F, Ruiz-Escobar P, Rodríguez-Boronat E. Tratamiento con soportes plantares en la enfermedad de Müller-Weiss. Reporte preliminar Acta Ortopédica Mexicana. 2020;34(2):112–8.

25. Myers KA, Long JT, Klein JP, et al. Biomechanical implications of the negative heel rocker sole shoe: gait kinematics and kinetics. Gait Posture. 2006;24(3):323–30.
26. Fornaciari P, Gilgen A, Zwicky L, Horn Lang T, Hintermann B. Isolated talonavicular fusion with tension band for Müller-Weiss syndrome. Foot Ankle Int. 2014;35(12):1316–22.
27. Cao HH, Lu WZ, Tang KL. Isolated talonavicular arthrodesis and talonavicular-cuneiform arthrodesis for the Müller-Weiss disease. J Orthop Surg Res. 2017;12:83. https://doi.org/10.1186/s13018-017-0581-4.
28. Harnroongroj T, Chuckpaiwong B. Müller-Weiss disease: three- to eight-year follow-up outcomes of isolated talonavicular arthrodesis. J Foot Ankle Surg. 2018;57(5):1014–9.
29. Cao HH, Tang KL, Xu JZ. Peri-navicular arthrodesis for the stage III Müller-Weiss disease. Foot Ankle Int. 2012;33(6):475–8.
30. Hetsroni I, Nyska M, Ayalon M. Plantar pressure distribution in patients with Müller-Weiss disease. Foot Ankle Int. 2007;28(2):237–41.
31. Lui TH. Arthroscopic triple arthrodesis in patients with Müller Weiss disease. Foot Ankle Surg. 2009;15(3):119–22.
32. Watson-Jones R. Fractures of the tarsal navicular bone. In: Watson-Jones R, editor. Fractures and joint injuries, vol. 2. 4th ed. Edinburgh: E & S Livingstone; 1955. p. 900.
33. Fernández de Retana P, Maceira E, Fernández-Valencia JA, Suso S. Arthrodesis of the talonavicular-cuneiform joints in Müller-Weiss disease. Foot Ankle Clin. 2004;9(1):65–72.
34. Mohiuddin T, Jennison T, Damany D. Müller-Weiss disease - review of current knowledge. Foot Ankle Surg. 2014;20(2):79–84.
35. Yu G, Zhao Y, Zhou J, Zhang M. Fusion of talonavicular and naviculocuneiform joints for the treatment of Müller-Weiss disease. J Foot Ankle Surg. 2012;51(4):415–9.
36. Yuan C, Wang C, Zhang C, Huang J, Wang X, Ma X. Derotation of the talus and arthrodesis treatment of stages II-V Müller-Weiss disease: midterm results of 36 cases. Foot Ankle Int. 2019;40(5):506–14.
37. Zhang H, Li J, Qiao Y, Yu J, Cheng Y, Liu Y, Gao C, Li J. Open triple fusion versus TNC arthrodesis in the treatment of Mueller-Weiss disease. J Orthop Surg Res. 2017;12(1):13.
38. Tan A, Smulders YC, Zöphel OT. Use of remodeled femoral head allograft for tarsal reconstruction in the treatment of Müller-Weiss disease. J Foot Ankle Surg. 2011;50(6):721–6.
39. Levinson H, Miller KJ, Adams SB Jr, Parekh SG. Treatment of spontaneous osteonecrosis of the tarsal navicular with a free medial femoral condyle vascularized bone graft: a new approach to managing a difficult problem. Foot Ankle Spec. 2014;7(4):332–7.
40. Li S, Myerson M, Monteagudo M, Maceira E. Efficacy of calcaneus osteotomy for treatment of symptomatic Müller-Weiss disease. Foot Ankle Int. 2016;38(3):261–9.
41. Buendía I, Gaviria ME, Monteagudo M, Maceira E, Martínez de Albornoz P. Enfermedad de Müller–Weiss, ¿cómo hemos cambiado? Rev Pie Tobillo. 2020;34(2):125–32. in press.
42. Ahmed AA, Kandil MI, Tabl EA. Preliminary outcomes of calcaneal lengthening in adolescent flatfoot in Müller-Weiss disease. Foot Ankle Int. 2019;40(7):803–7.
43. Myerson MS. Letter regarding: preliminary outcomes of calcaneal lengthening in adolescent flatfoot in Muller-Weiss disease. Foot Ankle Int. 2019;40(7):808.
44. Janositz G, Sisák K, Tóth K. Percutaneous decompression for the treatment of Mueller-Weiss syndrome. Knee Surg Sports Traumatol Arthrosc. 2011;19(4):688–90.

Surgical Techniques for Peritalar Osteoarthrosis: Talonavicular, Subtalar, Calcaneocuboid, and Midfoot

José Antônio Veiga Sanhudo and Marco Túlio Costa

1 Introduction

Osteoarthrosis of the peritalar joints is usually post-traumatic, secondary to pre-existing deformities and/or systemic inflammatory diseases. Calcaneus fracture is undoubtedly one of the major causes of arthrosis of the subtalar joint and, less frequently, of the calcaneocuboid joint. The overload and alignment changes observed in the cavus varus foot or flatfoot are often associated with degenerative changes of the peritalar joints, especially the subtalar joint.

2 Anatomy and Biomechanics of the Subtalar Joint

The subtalar is a complex joint, with an important role in impact absorption, propulsion and adaptation to irregular surfaces during walking. Separated by a medially cylindrical bone tunnel, called the tarsal canal, and laterally conical, called the sinus tarsi, it can be divided into anterior, composed of the talocalcaneonavicular joint, and posterior, composed of the talocalcaneal joint.

During walking, the joint is responsible for impact absorption in the heel contact phase, when it is in valgus and with the transverse tarsal joints unlocked and flexible. As it progresses to the propulsion phase, the subtalar joint inverts, the transverse tarsal joints lock to transform the hindfoot into a lever arm for impulse and

J. A. V. Sanhudo (✉)
Hospital Moinhos de Vento de Porto Alegre, Porto Alegre, RS, Brazil

M. T. Costa
Hospital Santa Casa de Misericórdia de São Paulo, São Paulo, Brazil

locomotion. During walking, a complex triplane movement involving eversion/inversion, abduction/adduction, supination/pronation of the middle and the hindfoot alternate successively, involving mainly the talonavicular joint, but also the calcaneocuboid and subtalar joints [1].

3 Diagnosis

3.1 Clinical

The typical history of subtalar osteoarthrosis is pain in the lateral subfibular region and sinus of the tarsus, associated with difficulty in walking on uneven surfaces. The diagnostic investigation begins with the clinical examination, observing the alignment of the lower limb as a whole, especially the alignment of the knee, ankle and hindfoot, the medial longitudinal arch and the presence of increased volume, common in more advanced cases. Valgus or varus deviations of the hindfoot are often associated with subtalar degeneration and it is important to remember that the varus deviation of the hindfoot is often associated with fibular tendinopathy, which can simulate subtalar arthropathy.

Dynamic inspection is of paramount importance in the identification of gait changes, often associated with pain, muscle imbalance and neurological disorders.

In the physical examination, the palpation of the pain site, as well as the evaluation of the active and passive ankle, subtalar and midfoot joints range of motion allows the identification of joint degeneration, among other causes. The pain in subtalar osteoarthrosis usually worsens with active and passive eversion/inversion of the hindfoot. Silfverskiöld test, comparing the degree of ankle dorsiflexion with the flexed and extended knee, should be routinely performed in these patients, since the shortening of the calf muscle is often associated with hindfoot misalignment, especially in valgus [2].

4 Imaging

The initial image evaluation involves an anteroposterior, oblique and lateral foot weight bearing radiographs. Narrowing of the joint space, sclerosis and/or subchondral cysts and formation of osteophytes are the most frequent findings in degenerative changes of the hindfoot. Additional incidences, such as the axial calcaneus or the long leg view, are requested in selected cases for evaluation of the mechanical axis. An anteroposterior ankle x-ray with 40° internal rotation allows an excellent visualization of the subtalar joint. Nuclear magnetic resonance is extremely useful for demonstrating incipient degenerative changes and in evaluating soft tissues, especially tendons and ligaments of the hindfoot. The emerging weight bearing computed tomography (WBCT) has been proving extremely useful in the evaluation of hindfoot disorders, especially regarding functional alignment and joint incongruity. The demonstration of changes in subtalar joint orientation in flatfoot was possible with the advent of WBCT [3–6].

5   Conservative Treatment

Infiltration of the subtalar joint with anesthetic (xylocaine or ropivacaine 2%) guided or not by radioscopy or another imaging method may be useful in confirming the source of pain. The association of anesthetic with steroid can also be used aiming at a combined therapeutic effect [7]. The intra-articular injection of hyaluronic acid at weekly intervals for 21 days was shown to be beneficial, with pain improvement, AOFAS score and greater tolerance for walking, in 18 of 20 patients aged between 22 and 72 years with subtalar ostheoarthritis. The benefit of the treatment lasted more than six months [8]. The association of hyaluronic acid and intra-articular chondroitin sulfate was beneficial in patients with knee and hip osteoarthrosis, but there are no studies demonstrating the same benefits in other joints of the lower limb [9, 10].

The conservative treatment is the first choice for osteoarthrosis of the foot and involves the modification of the activity and the footwear, as well as the use of orthoses aiming at a better load distribution. Decreasing high demand physical activities and losing weight help with symptoms relief as well. The treatment of osteoarthrosis involves the use of painkillers, anti-inflammatory drugs and chondroprotectors, but the efficacy of the latter in the treatment of degenerative foot disorders has not yet been proven.

6   Subtalar Joint Osteoarthrosis

Few options exist between conservative treatment and arthrodesis in the management of subtalar joint osteoarthritis. Thus, after conservative treatment failure, the most performed surgical procedure is arthrodesis, which can be in situ or modelling, depending on the existence or not of associated deformity. The use of bone block grafting is indicated for correction of malunion with flattening of the calcaneus and loss of height on the hindfoot [11].

Although less invasive procedures, such as arthroscopy, are procedures performed in many centers, few cases present in a phase of osteoarthrosis that would benefit from this less invasive approach that does not involve subtalar arthrodesis.

6.1 Biomechanics

Although widely used in the treatment of flatfoot, subtalar arthrodesis alone has been shown, in a cadaveric study, to be less effective in promoting support for the medial and lateral longitudinal arch than combined calcaneocuboid and talonavicular arthrodesis. However, the most effective support for both arches was obtained through triple arthrodesis [12]. The biomechanical stress caused by hindfoot arthrodesis on local bone and soft tissue structures was studied through a finite element model. It was observed that in situ talonavicular arthrodesis alone is superior to subtalar arthrodesis alone and equivalent to triple arthrodesis in relation to the biomechanical stress on bone and soft tissue structures supporting the plantar arch. Isolated subtalar arthrodesis was, among the isolated arthrodesis of the hindfoot, the one that contributed less to stress reduction in both the plantar fascia and the spring ligament and it was associated with higher stress in the forefoot and hindfoot. The triple arthrodesis is the one that has provided the most stress reduction in soft tissues and bones [13]. The blockage of the talonavicular joint, as in an arthrodesis, practically eliminates mobility of the subtalar joint. On the other hand, arthrodesis of the subtalar joint maintains 74% of mobility in the talonavicular joint and 44% of mobility in the calcaneocuboid joint [14].

6.2 Surgical Technique for Subtalar Arthrodesis

The procedure is usually performed under sedation and popliteal block or spine anesthesia. The use of tourniquet in the thigh or above the ankle, depending on the level of anesthesia, is practiced by most surgeons, after the limb is exsanguinated with Smarch band.

6.2.1 Approach

The subtalar joint approach is determined, among other factors, by the necessity or not of associated procedures. Subtalar arthrodesis by lateral approach is indicated for cases of primary or post-traumatic arthrosis of this joint and can be extended to the calcaneocuboid and even talonavicular joints. The incision starts at the fibula distal end and extends anteriorly parallel to the sole of the foot to the base of the fourth metatarsal. The subcutaneous tissue is dissected up to the subtalar joint protecting the sural nerve and moving the fibular tendons plantarly and the superficial fibular nerve dorsally. The capsule is incised exposing the joint and the cervical ligament, which is sectioned to facilitate access to all joint facets, using a bone spreader. This lateral approach, through the sinus tarsi, demonstrated in studies with cadavers to be adequate for exposure of the three facets of the subtalar joint [15, 16].

Subtalar arthrodesis performed in cases of talo-calcaneal coalition, a medial approach is used to remove the bone bridge and perform the arthrodesis. The incision is made following the upper edge of the posterior tibial tendon, extending from the medial malleolus to the navicular bone. Galli and collaborators studied the proximity of the neurovascular and tendon structures through this medial approach and observed that the distance from the medial facet to the flexor digitorum longus tendon was 5 mm, to the flexor hallucis longus was 19 mm and to the neurovascular bundle was 21 mm [17]. In the treatment of rigid flatfoot, common in advanced phases of posterior tibial tendon dysfunction, arthrodesis through a medial approach presents the advantages of easy facilitate incision closure, which is performed in the region of lower tension after correction of the deformity. Access to the joint is obtained by displacing the posterior tibial tendon plantarly or by resection of the diseased portion of it in cases of advanced tendinosis (Fig. 1). Double arthrodesis, subtalar and talonavicular, using a medial approach is an excellent alternative for the treatment of degenerative disorders of the hindfoot with or without deformity. The ability to correct deformities with double arthrodesis is the same as triple arthrodesis, and the approach has proven to be safe regarding the risk of neurovascular injury [18, 19]. This approach allows access to 90% or more of the hindfoot joints [20]. In summary, besides being technically simpler, the medial approach for double arthrodesis of the hindfoot avoids lateral incision and its complications, maintains the calcaneocuboid mobility, with clinical results similar to triple arthrodesis [21].

The posterior approach, lateral to the Achilles tendon, is an alternative in cases of inadequate skin conditions or higher risks of incisional complications, as in diabetics and smokers. Patients who need arthrodesis to the ankle as well (tibio-talar

Fig. 1 Medial approach with exposure of the subtalar joint by dislocating the posterior tibial tendon plantarly

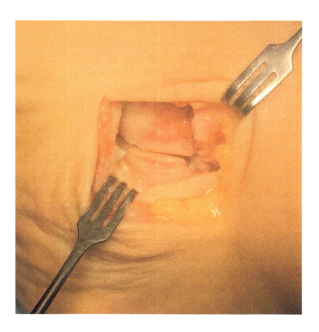

arthrodesis), with a previous lateral approach and/or poor skin conditions will also benefit from the posterior approach, since the implants are better protected in a deeper plane and the location of the incision facilitates the drainage of the hematoma in the postoperative period.

Regardless of the approach, we must keep in mind that joint preparation is one of the most important steps for the arthrodesis success. Using curette and osteotome, the joint cartilage is removed, the subchondral bone is exposed and perforated with a 1.5 mm Kirchner or with a narrow osteotome. The use of supplementary grafting in subtalar arthrodesis is debatable, but most authors agree that the main recommendation is restricted to cases of cysts, major bone defects and/or associated deformities.

The arthroscopic approach with lateral and/or posterior portals is described for the treatment of cartilage lesions, including subtalar joint arthrodesis [22, 23]. According to some studies, arthroscopic subtalar arthrodesis presents results comparable to open technique for in situ arthrodesis, but requires a longer learning curve and sophisticated equipment. In the lateral arthroscopic approach, the patient is positioned in lateral decubitus position, and the joint is accessed through the anterolateral portals; the anterior, 1 cm distal and 2 cm anterior to the tip of the fibula; the middle, at the sinus tarsus level 1 cm anterior to the tip of the fibula; and the posterolateral, 5 mm proximal to the tip of the fibula immediately lateral to the calcaneal tendon. In the posterior arthroscopic approach, with the patient in prone position and with the foot out of the operating table, two portals are performed. One immediately medial and another immediately lateral to the calcaneus tendon in line with the tip of the fibula. The posterolateral portal is performed first, and the trocar instrument is directed to the first intermetatarsal space. The posteromedial portal is performed following the path of the posterolateral portal to protect the medial structures, especially the neuro-vascular bundle. The most important reference point in this approach is the flexor hallucis longus tendon, which represents the medial limit of the working area. The subtalar joint is easily visualized through this approach, but distraction of the joint by introducing a 4.0 mm trocar instrument is necessary sometimes for proper access to the joint surface [22]. The average healing rate of arthroscopic subtalar arthrodesis is 93% [24]. Earlier return to work and sports activities is one of the advantages of the arthroscopic over the open approach, but it is important to observe that arthroscopic subtalar arthrodesis, although less invasive, presents more implant related complications [23–27]. Sural nerve lesion, which is located 4 mm anterior to the posterolateral portal, is described in 6% of the cases, as well as the tibial nerve bundle lesion, which is located 6.4 mm from the posteromedial portal [28].

Since bone block grafting cannot be performed arthroscopically, subtalar arthrosis with associated deformity should be approached openly [27, 29]. In these cases, the graft is preferably removed from the posterosuperior apophysis of the calcaneus through a longitudinal incision lateral to the Achilles tendon (Gallie approach)

Fig. 2 Longitudinal lateral para-Achilles approach for bone harvest from the posterosuperior apophysis of the calcaneus

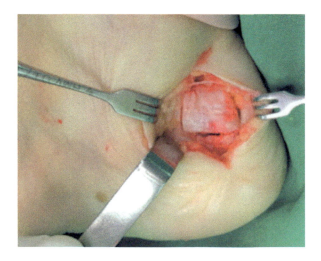

(Fig. 2). Alternatively, an extended L approach may be used in cases of calcaneus fracture sequelae, in which a block graft arthrodesis is programmed. This broad approach, allows lateral calcaneal wall removal, access to the graft donor area and wide view of the subtalar joint (Fig. 3) [30, 31].

6.2.2 Fixation of the Subtalar Arthrodesis

The internal fixation of the subtalar arthrodesis is one of the most important factors for successful consolidation. Although staple fixation is employed in some centers, fixation with screws of at least 6.5 mm in diameter is employed by most authors [7, 18, 22, 32].

6.2.3 Number of Screws

Single screw fixation distributes stress better at the subtalar joint, but has lower rotational and inversion/version stress resistance than double screw fixation [33]. Double screw fixation has higher compression, torsional stiffness and strength than single screw fixation [34]. Jastifer et al. demonstrated that torsional stiffness and maximum torque are higher with two screws compared to a single screw fixation, and that the more divergent these screws are introduced the better the stability obtained [35]. Subtalar fixation with two angled screws was superior to fixation with two parallel screws also in a biomechanical study applying cyclic loads in the three main mobility planes of the subtalar joint [36]. Wirth and collaborators observed a higher rate of nonunion, 35% versus 14%, when the fixation was performed with two compared to the fixation with three screws. The third screw can be

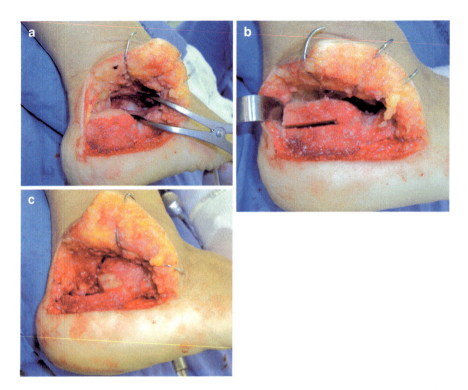

Fig. 3 (**a**) Extended L-shaped approach for removal of the enlarged portion of the calcaneus lateral wall, exposure of the subtalar joint, and use of the retractor blade to estimate the size of the block graft needed; (**b**) removal of the block graft from the posterosuperior apophysis of the calcaneus; (**c**) placement of the block graft from the posterior superior region of the calcaneus on the posterior facet of the subtalar

added depending on the position of the two screws initially introduced and the need to improve stability due to higher risk of nonunion, as in diabetics and smokers [37, 38].

6.2.4   Direction of Screws

Although the bone density of the neck of the talus and the tuberosity of the calcaneus are not the same, the direction of the screws from plantar to dorsal or from dorsal to plantar has not shown any biomechanical difference. From the clinical point of view the introduction of the screws from dorsal to plantar increases the risk of neurovasular injury [36, 39–41]. The disadvantages of the plantar to dorsal screw is that at least one of the screws must be short threaded to promote compression between the fragments and the risk of re-interventions to remove the implants is greater, especially in cases where a washer is added [38]. The use of headless screws can minimize this complication, but the cost of the procedure could rise [42].

6.2.5 Technical Considerations

Regardless of the fixation method chosen, it is very important to correct the subtalar alignment before fixation, especially the correction of talo-calcaneal divergence. It is of utmost importance to correct the alignment of the hindfoot when performing the arthrodesis, since the varus fixation leads to overload of the lateral column and the valgus fixation overloads the deltoid ligament. Both possibilities may require revision of the arthrodesis.

It is essential to use fluoroscopy to insert and check the correct positioning of the implants. The fixation is done from plantar to dorsal with two 6.5 mm cancellous screws, one partially thread initially to promote compression and another fully thread for rotational stability. At the time of in situ arthrodesis fixation, however, it is important to insert one screw (cannulated or not) first and only then start the fixation with the second screw, because the compression of the initial fixation may be impaired by the presence of a guide wire or Kirchner [22]. After the screw length is determined, a 6.5 mm cancellous screw with a short thread of 16 mm is introduced, obtaining compression between the fragments. A second 6.5 mm cancellous screw with full thread must be inserted 1–2 cm below the entry point of the first screw, preferably in divergent direction, below the Achilles insertion and above the plantar contact point, for rotational control of the fixation. Alternatively, this second screw may be inserted at the lateral edge of the calcaneus, approximately 1 cm proximal to the calcaneocuboid joint towards the talus head, or it may be the third screw, inserted after the two described above. The position and depth of the screws are checked by fluoroscopy in the sagittal and frontal plane.

6.3 Results

Subtalar arthrodesis, is a procedure that presents high success and low complication rates [43–45].

Radnay demonstrated that subtalar arthrodesis in patients with a fractured calcaneus obtained better results than patients who had been conservatively treated, due to the improved anatomy of the first group [46]. Worse results were obtained in subtalar arthrodesis if smoking, high-energy trauma and concomitant same limb fracture were associated [47].

In the treatment of calcaneus malunion with height loss, subtalar arthrodesis with bone block grafting can be performed with iliac crest, tibia or even from the superior calcaneus apophysis (Haglund area). The latter is an excellent alternative being in the same surgical field (Fig. 4) [30, 31, 46].

Fig. 4 Schematic
representation of the bone
block graft removal of the
posterosuperior apophysis
of the calcaneus

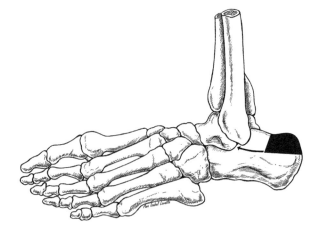

7 Talonavicular Osteoarthrosis

The talonavicular joint (TN) is considered the key articulation of the hindfoot. The arthrodesis of this joint leads to a limitation of 91% of the hindfoot mobility and eliminates 75% of the posterior tibial tendon excursion [14, 48]. To have an idea of its importance, the TN arthrodesis alone is as effective as double (talonavicular and calcaneocuboid) or triple arthrodesis to correct the deformity in the valgus plane [49].

The treatment of talonavicular osteoarthrosis mostly involves the arthrodesis of this joint, but good clinical and radiological results have been obtained with the use of calcaneus osteotomies in cases of localized talonavicular osteoarthrosis associated with Muller Weiss disorder [50].

7.1 Diagnosis

7.1.1 Clinical

Osteoarthrosis of the TN is often associated with degenerative conditions in other hindfoot joints. As described for the subtalar joint, the inspection of the alignment of the entire lower limb is paramount. Swelling in the dorsal medial aspect of the foot, associated or not with varus/valgus foot deviations and medial longitudinal arch colapse are frequently observed. During gait analysis claudication and antalgic position of the limb, as external rotation of the affected lower limb can be detected. Pain in the TN joint is common on palpation of the dorsal region, as well as with mobilization in adduction-abduction. During the physical examination is very important to identify the exact point of greatest pain, whether in the joint line or more distal, at the level of the navicular bone itself. The latter, suggests a navicular stress fracture.

7.1.2 Imaging

The image evaluation of the talonavicular joint involves a weight-bearing antero-posterior lateral and oblique view of the foot. Degenerative changes, with narrowing of the joint space, subchondral sclerosis with or without subchondral cysts are expected in cases of ostheoarthritis. Resonance magnetic imaging and computed tomography scan are useful in case of incipient desease.

7.2 Surgical Technique for Talonavicular Arthrodesis

Surgical procedures at the talonavicular joint level are performed under sedation and popliteal block anesthesia whenever possible. Tourniquet is used by most surgeons.

7.2.1 Approach

The most commonly used approach for talonavicular arthrodesis is the isolated medial approach, but the association of a lateral incision to stabilize the lateral portion of the joint is very useful biomechanically, and seems to promote better consolidation rates [51]. However, percutaneous fixation by lateral approach presents high rates of neuro-vascular injury, around 30–35% of cases [52, 53].

7.2.2 Internal Fixation

Through traditional medial exposure, the classical fixation of talonavicular arthrod-esis is performed with two or three retrograde screws from the medial region of the navicular to the lateral region of the talus. The technique does not stabilize the lateral portion of the talonavicular joint, allowing some local micromobility, with increased chance of nonunion. Jarrell et al. did not observe any significant biome-chanical difference when comparing fixation with medial screws and fixation with a medial plate and a dorsal screw in a study with cadavers [54]. In another similar study, however, Granata and collaborators observed that fixation with a locked dor-sal plate and a retrograde screw was more effective in blocking 3D mobility than fixation with two retrograde screws [55].

7.2.3 Technical Considerations

The crucial points for a successful talonavicular arthrodesis are joint preparation and internal fixation. Due to its concave shape, the exposure of joint surfaces and subchondral bone makes the talonavicular joint the most difficult to prepare among

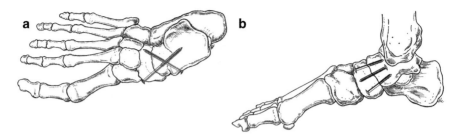

Fig. 5 Schematic representation of talonavicular fixation with two retrograde screws and one anterograde in anteroposterior (**a**) and lateral (**b**)

the hindfoot joints. The use of a bone spreader or Hintermann-type retractor is very useful to facilitate joint access, but care must be taken, especially in older patients, not to cause local bone sinking. Once the joint surface of the talus and navicular head is prepared, the joint is positioned in the desired position, provisionally fixing it with 1.5 mm Kirschner wires or guide wires. Once the adequate position of the joint is confirmed, fixation with three 4.5 mm cannulated screws is performed. The third screw can be partially threaded to confer additional compression to the lateral portion of the TN joint or fully thread, conferring rotational stability (Fig. 5). The direction and depth of the screws are controlled by fluoroscopy in the anteroposterior and lateral planes. To close the operative wound, meticulous hemostasis is performed to reduce bleeding, swelling and related complications (Fig. 6).

7.3 Results

Calcaneous osteotomy for TN osteoarthritis in Muller Weiss disease have shown good functional scores. This will be presented in another chapter [50].

Talonavicular arthrodesis is the most performed procedure and has a high rate of success in the treatment of arthrosis of this joint, as well as in the correction and stabilization of deformities of the hindfoot. Harper and collaborators published a study including 29 patients with talonavicular arthrodesis alone showing 86% of good results after 26 months of follow-up [56]. Chen and collaborators obtained fusion in 15 out of 16 patients submitted to arthrodesis using staples or screws after a mean follow-up of 51 months. Osteoarthrosis was observed in the neighboring joints of 5 of the 16 operated patients, but without symptoms and without affecting the clinical results obtained [57].

Through a minimally invasive dorsal approach and fixation by posterior approach, Carranza-Bencano et al. obtained healing in 10 cases of 11 performed, with significant improvement of clinical parameters evaluated, but patients with angular deformities were excluded in this study [58].

Lechler and collaborators obtained good and excellent results in 26 of 30 feet submitted to talonavicular arthrodesis fixed with a locked mini-plate [59].

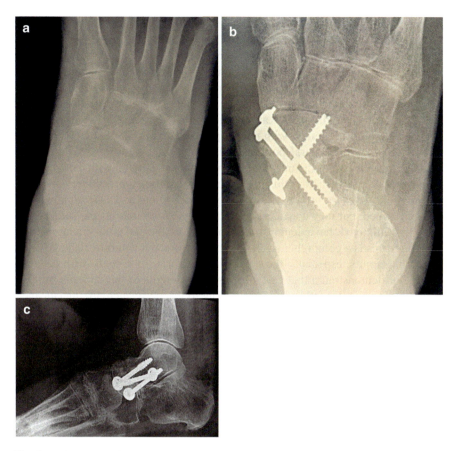

Fig. 6 (**a**) Anteroposterior X-ray with TN arthrosis; (**b** and **c**) anteroposterior and lateral image of the arthrodesis with triplanar fixation performed with two retrograde screws and one antero-grade screw

Harnroongroj and Chuckpaiwong obtained fusion in all 16 patients diagnosed with Muller-Weiss disorder submitted to isolated talonavicular arthrodesis. Improvement was also observed in the visual analog pain scale and in the Foot & Ankle Outcome Score (FAOSs) [60].

8   Treatment Complications

The most common complications of arthrodesis for surgical treatment of subtalar and talonavicular osteoarthrosis are delayed healing, nonunion, malunion, deep vein thrombosis, vasculo-nervous injury and infection [23, 43–45]. The occurrence of nonunion in the subtalar joint according to the literature varies from 2 to 30%, with higher rates reported in smokers and diabetic patients [39, 40]. Among the modifiable factors associated with the development of nonunion, possibly the joint preparation is one of the most important. The approach and the surgeon's experience are important as well. Although some authors recommend the use of bone grafting to decrease the chance of subtalar nonunion, this benefit is not fully proven.

Regarding the TN joint, due to its concave shape, its location in an area of great stress at the junction of the midfoot and the hindfoot, and the weak lateral stabilization with traditional fixation, this joint is the most prone to nonunion between the hindfoot joints, with rates reported between 3.8 and 29% [61]. The micromobility in the lateral portion of this joint after traditional fixation with medial screws is one of the most important factors associated with delayed or no unions [49, 62]. To decrease this micromobility, additional procedures involving the hindfoot, such as arthrodesis of neighboring joints and osteotomies, have been described, but they considerably increase the morbidity of the surgery [49, 62, 63]. Malik et al. have demonstrated that among the key points in talonavicular arthrodesis is a comprehensive and rigid fixation, but avoiding damage to the underlying joints, especially the naviculo-cuneiform. In a study with cadavers the author demonstrated that calcaneal osteotomy reduces the micromobility of isolated talonavicular arthrodesis. According to the study, medializing calcaneal osteotomy decreases the ground reaction forces medially by 57 to 91%, and recommends its addition step in patients at high risk of nonunion, like smokers, obese and diabetics patients [62]. Resnick, also in a study with cadavers, demonstrated that the association of triple arthrodesis with medializing calcaneal osteotomy decreases stress in the deltoid ligament by 56% compared to lateral tuberosity sliding [64].

As previously mentioned, one factor associated with the TN nonunion risk is the scarce fixation of the lateral joint region. Retrograde fixation with a lateral percutaneous screw through is recommended by some authors. In a cadaveric study, Lee et al, demonstrated that lateral percutaneous TN fixation was associated with nerve injury in 30% of cases and tibialis anterior tendon and extensor hallucis longus tendon injury in 20 and 30 % of the cases, respectively [53].

Other complications described in talonavicular arthrodesis are malunion and progressive osteoarthrosis of neighboring joints, described in up to 10% of cases.

9   Immobilization

The leg is immobilized with a well-padded splint and the patient must keep the foot elevated. Thromboprophylaxis is indicated in selected patients, and the risks and benefits of using anticoagulants should always be considered individually. When used, it is usually recommended during the whole period of immobilization and/or non weight bearing. 10 days postoperative, the first dressing change is performed and, with the operative wound with good signs of healing, the leg is casted and weight bearing as tolerated is allowed. Non weight bearing should be extended in patients with high risk of nonunion, such as diabetics and smokers. The cast removal is performed after joint fusion, usually between 8 and 12 weeks after surgery. CT scan is useful in cases of doubtful healing [65]. Another way of approaching the postoperative period, is not allowing weightbearing for 2 months until bone healing is shown by a CT scan. During these 2 months, a removable boot can be used.

10   Calcaneal-Cuboid Arthrosis

The calcaneocuboid joint integrates the lateral column of the foot. Its isolated arthrodesis is not common and is usually associated with other procedures in the foot [66, 67]. In this section we will discuss some particularities of this joint.

10.1   Anatomy and Biomechanics

It is a stable synovial joint formed by the anterior portion of the calcaneus and the proximal portion of the cuboid. Together with the talonavicular joint, it forms what we call the Chopart joint. In addition to the joint capsule, some ligaments confer stability, both dorsal and plantar (dorsal and palntar calcaneo-cuboid ligaments). The bifurcated ligament also aids in stability. This joint is not completely flat and has a sinuous shape [1].

During walking the calcaneocuboid joint, together with the talonavicular and talocalcaneal, plays a fundamental role in the accommodation of the foot on the ground and during the toe-off phase. These joints are responsible for making the foot a flexible structure in the beginning of stance phase and rigid one during the toe-off phase [1]. Therefore, any factor that leads to loss of mobility, whether by pathologies or surgeries, affects the biomechanical performance of the foot during walking. The calcaneocuboid arthrodesis alone seems to be the one that least affects the biomechanics of the foot [66]. Astion and collaborators [66], in study in anatomical pieces, found that talonavicular arthrodesis decreases about 98% of the inversion and eversion movement of the hindfoot. However, the calcaneocuboid movement blockade reduces about 33% of the talonavicular inversion and eversion movement. Apparently the talonavicular block significantly reduces the calcaneus-cuboid movement, but the reverse is not true.

10.2   Indications for Arthrodesis

Indications for calcaneocuboid arthrodesis are multiple [66, 68–71]. Fractures may lead to future osteoarthritis. Neurological diseases with loss of tendon function may require arthrodesis to stabilize the foot. The correction of deformities caused by congenital diseases, such as congenital clubfoot; or progressive collaspsing foot deformity are also part of the indications for calcaneocuboid arthrodesis. As mentioned above, arthrodesis of this isolated joint is not common, and is usually associated with some other procedure in the foot.

In 1961, Evans [70, 72] described calcaneocuboid arthrodesis as a procedure associated with the treatment of congenital clubfoot. Although currently this procedure is not routinely employed, the long-term result of calcaneocuboid arthrodesis in cases of congenital clubfoot with recurrent deformity, after failure of the initial treatment, still seems to be acceptable [68].

10.3 Surgical Technique

Surgical approach The approach employed is the dorsal-lateral, centered on the calcaneus-cuboid, extending between the anterior portion of the calcaneus and the proximal portion of the cuboid [69, 73]. When subtalar arthrodesis is also scheduled in the same procedure, the surgical access can be extended further proximal and the two joints exposed through the same approach. Partial detachment of the extensor digitorum brevis may be necessary. The fibular tendons are retracted to proximal and plantar [69, 74, 75]. This joint has a saddle shape [66], which should be taken into consideration when removing joint cartilage and subchondral bone.

Fixation Several fixation methods are described in the literature [66, 75–77]. One of the most used is the fixation with one or two oblique screws in the joint, performing compression. These screws can be inserted from the calcaneus to the cuboid or vice versa [75, 77, 78]. A 6.5 mm long screw, starting from the posterior process of the calcaneus to the cuboid is also described. In an anatomical study, Khann et al. [75] found that an axial screw provides better fixation than a screw inserted obliquely. Staple fixation is also a possibility [66, 77]. Milshteyn et al. [79], also in a study on cadavers, found that the fixation with locked plate is more rigid than the fixation with oblique screws.

10.4 Calcaneo-Cuboid Arthrodesis with Lateral Column Lengthening

Cuboid joint arthrodesis has been described as part of the surgical procedure for the treatment of progressive collaspsing foot deformity. When correction of the abduction deformity is necessary, one of the options is calcaneocuboid arthrodesis with bone grafting to lengthen the lateral column [69, 73, 76, 79–81]. Grunander and Thordarson [73] believe that the potential for correcting the deformity with this procedure is great. Deland et al. [69] observed that after calcaneocuboid arthrodesis with lengthening of the lateral column, the talonavicular preserves about 48% of its movement and the subtalar, about 70%. The surgical approach is the same used in arthrodesis. Thomas et al. [82] recommend for this procedure that the surfaces to be arthrodesed should be flat. Lateral column lengthening is performed through bone graft interposition in the space created. Bone graft size varies between 8 and 15 mm [69, 74, 82]. The intraoperative fluoroscopy helps measure the exact measurement of the graft by forefoot adduction. The source of the tricortical graft is usually the patient's own iliac crest. Despite the theoretical advantage of the autograft, this extra procedure increases the morbidity of the surgery [73]. Some authors report the use of allograft [73] or synthetic substitutes [76]. It is important that the lateral surface of the graft be molded to avoid peroneal tendons irritation [74]. In general, the healing time of this arthrodesis is about 12 weeks. The lateral column lengthening causes increased tension in the surgical scar, which may lead to dehiscence of the suture and lesion of the sural nerve more frequently. Care should be taken in the manipulation of soft tissues during surgery to reduce the incidence of these complications. The non-union of this arthrodesis varies from 11% to 20% in the literature [74, 83]. Proper preparation of joint surfaces and rigid fixation are tactics that help control non-union risk. Thomas et al. [82] recommend fixation with plate and screws. Immobilization and non-weightbearing should be kept por 8 weeks postoperatively (Figs. 7, 8, 9, and 10).

10.5 Results

CC fusion without lengthening the lateral column occurs in almost all cases. In literature, the possibility pseudoarthrosis varies from 0% to 11% [70, 71, 84], however, these studies are related to calcaneocuboid arthrodesis in triple arthrodesis. Grunander and Thordarson [73] described calcaneocuboid arthrodesis with

Fig. 7 Weightbearing radiography in lateral view of a triple arthrodesis demonstrating the fixation of the calcaneal-cuboid arthrodesis with a 6.5 mm screw from posterior to anterior

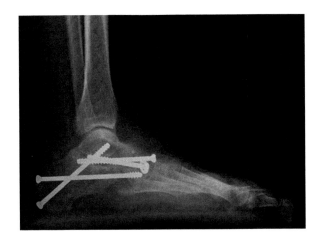

Fig. 8 Oblique view on X-ray showing bone graft in the calcaneal-cuboid joint

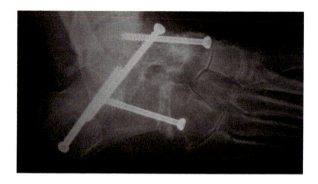

Fig. 9 Intraoperative photograph demonstrating the calcaneocuboid arthrodesis with the addition of a tricortical graft block for lateral column lengthening

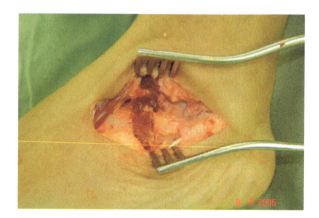

Fig. 10 Lateral X-ray of a case of triple arthrodesis in which lengthening of the lateral column with a tricortical graft block was employed in the calcaneus-cuboid arthrodesis

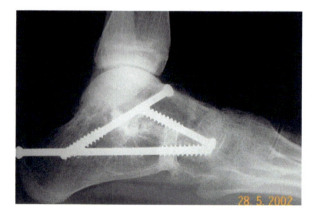

lengthening of the lateral column using an allograft (femoral head) associated with platelet-rich plasma and noted 7 cases of pseudoarthrosis in 16 patients. They considered the number of complications high and recommended against this technique. They commented that the use of the patient's own iliac graft and fixation with plate and screws should reduce the incidence of pseudoarthrosis.

However, as they observed good results with lateral column lengthening in the anterior part of the calcaneal bone (Evans procedure), they did not opt for calcaneocuboid arthrodesis anymore. Other possible complications are sural nerve injury, fibular tendon injuries, stress fractures [66], suture dehiscence, symptomatic harware and infection [73].

11 Tarso-Metatarsal Arthrosis

Although not widely cited in the literature, midfoot arthrosis can cause chronic pain with significant impact on daily life activities [84–86]. The intention of this chapter is to describe briefly the anatomy and biomechanics of this region the diagnosis and the possible treatments of this problem.

11.1 Anatomy and Biomechanics

The midfoot includes the tarso-metatarsal, intercuneiform and naviculo-cuneiform and cuboid-cuneiform joints. The Navicular has three articular facets that articulate with the three cuneiforms. We can also consider a joint between the cuboid and navicular, sometimes fibrous and more rarely even a synovial joint [85, 87].

In this section we will not address the talonavicular and calcaneal-cuboid joints, which are part of the hindfoot. The metatarsal tarsal joints can be divided into three columns [84, 85, 87, 88].

– Medial column: includes the medial cuneiform and the first metatarsal bone.
– Intermediate column: includes the intermediate and lateral cuneiform and the second and third metatarsal bone.
– Lateral column: includes the cuboid and the fourth and fifth metatarsal bone.

The stability of the region, which is important for the gait biomechanics, is given by the shape of the bone joints and the ligamentos strength [84, 87]. In a cross section, the midfoot bones are arranged in the shape of a Roman arch, giving intrinsic stability. The second metatarsal has a more proximal position, which also confers stability. The bones of this region are united by strong plantar, interosseous and dorsal ligaments [85]. However, there is no interosseous ligament between the first and second metatarsal bone. In fact, instead of a ligament between the base of the first and second metatarsal bone, there is a strong ligament between the base of the second metatarsal bone and the medial cuneiform, known as the Lisfranc ligament. This ligament plays a fundamental role in the stability and biomechanics of the region [84, 85]. The peroneos longus tendon, which runs from lateral to medial in the plantar region of the foot, also acts in the stabilization of the midfoot [84, 87].

With less mobility than other regions of the foot, the midfoot is the link between the forefoot and the hindfoot. It helps to keep the foot as a rigid structure during propulsive phase and flexible one in the stance phase [1, 85, 86]. The smallest movement occurs between the intermediate cuneiform and the second metatarsal, a place of greater stability and where most of the load passes during walking [84, 87]. This fact may explain these joints are the most frequent sites of midfoot osteoarthritis, even in the absence of a traumatic event [84, 87]. The loss of midfoot stability can be visualized with the collapse of the medial longitudinal plantar arch. This collapse compromises the foot function decreasing its mechanical efficiency [2, 6].

11.2   Diagnosis and Clinical Chart

History, physical examination and X-rays exams are key to midfoot osteoarthritis diagnosis.

Trauma is the most common cause of osteoarthritis in the Lisfranc region [84, 88, 90]. Patients with arthrosis of the midfoot usually report fractures or ligament injuries in the past. In some cases, these ligament injuries may have been subtle, having gone unnoticed [88, 90]. Primary arthrosis is not so common. Inflammatory arthritis, such as gout and rheumatoid arthritis [87], also cause joint degeneration in the midfoot and usually affects multiple joints. When the cause is suspected to be a rheumatic disease, blood tests and a rheumatologist's evaluation should be ordered. Overload caused by ankle and/or hindfoot arthrodesis can also lead to arthrosis in this region. Although it often does not cause painful symptoms, Charcot's arthropathy in insensitive foot can also lead to joint degeneration [84, 85, 87]. The progressive collaspsing foot deformity, in advanced phases, can also end up in tarso-metatarsal joint degeneration [85]. According to Nemec et al. [89], obesity is another factor that can lead to the appearance of arthrosis.

The patient with typical midfoot arthrosis has pain that worsens when walking on uneven ground [85]. There may be a feeling of instability [84]. In some cases, collapse of the plantar arch occurs [89, 90], associated with abduction deformity. Dorsal osteophytes, often painful, may appear on the dorsum of the foot [84, 85, 87]. Gastrosoleus shortening leads to loss of ankle and foot dorsiflexion, increasing the midfoot pressure when walking and is also a factor that may be involved in the appearance of arthrosis [86, 89].

Keiserman et al. [91] described the piano key test, which helps to better locate which joint is symptomatic. Although the injection of local anesthetic can also help identify which joint is symptomatic, these joints are small, making it difficult to inject in the correct place, which would hinder accurate diagnosis [84, 88, 90].

Weightbearing x-rays, in AP, lateral and obliques views are the first exams to order [84, 85, 87, 89]. In X-rays, correct alignment of the metatarsals with the cuneiform and cuboid bones has to be confirmed. Decreased joint space, presence of osteophytes, bone sclerosis and subchondral cysts are radiographic signs of osteoarthritis [90]. In the lateral X-ray observe whether the plantar arch has collapsed. The angles between the talus and the first metatarsal bone, both in the dorsal-plantar and lateral views, as well as the height from the medial cuneiform to the 5th metatarsal base are used to measure the deformity [89]. Both magnetic resonance imaging and computed tomography assist in mapping the severity and extent of arthrosis. It is important, when arthrodesis is considered as treatment, to evaluate signs of degeneration in neighboring joints [84].

11.3 Conservative Treatment

The conservative treatment should always be the first choice [87, 89, 92]. Analgesics and anti-inflammatory drugs, physiotherapy, local infiltrations, insoles, modifications in shoes and orthoses can be effective for pain relief [84, 87, 93]. The strategy must be focused on pain relief, increase of midfoot stability and load relief in the affected region [85].

Although analgesics and anti-inflammatory drugs can relieve the symptoms of affected joints, the chronic use of this type of medication should be viewed with caution due to the adverse effects of these medications, especially cardiovascular system [85, 90, 94].

As orthoses and insoles have little adverse effects, they are an attractive method in the initial approach to arthrosis of the midfoot [90]. Footwear with rigid soles (trekking shoes) tend to facilitate the transfer of load during walking, decreasing the overload in the midfoot and consequently relieving pain. The ankle foot orthosis (AFO) also relieves pain, however, it causes great restriction of movement both in the ankle and the foot, and they are not easily accepted by the patient [90]. Halstead et al. found that the use of orthosis for 12 weeks led to clinical and biomechanical improvements in patients with midfoot osteoarthritis [95].

Local injections with corticoids are also described in the treatment of arthrosis of the midfoot. They assist in pain relief and the correct location of painful joints for future arthrodesis [84]. However, the correct identification of the injection site can be difficult, and sometimes the assistance of ultrasound is necessary.

11.4 Surgical Treatment

The decision of surgical treatment should be guided by pain intensity, functional restriction and failure of conservative treatment [84, 87, 88, 90, 96]. Komenda et al., [88] as well as Gougoulias and Lampridis [86], recommend that the surgical treatment should only be chosen three to six months after the conservative treatment is initiated. When dorsal osteophytes are the cause of pain, exostectomy i.e. removal of these osteophytes, are effective for pain treatment. But the definitive treatment for this osteoarthritis is joint arthrodesis [84, 93], mainly of the medial and intermediate midfoot columns [85, 87]. One of the challenges of arthrodesis in the midfoot is the correct identification of which joints are painful, due to the large number of joints that may be involved in the genesis of pain [84, 85]. For this reason some authors advocate infiltration with local corticoid or anesthetic [87]. In the preoperative planning one should consider whether the correction of any deformity is necessary (modeling arthrodesis) or if the arthrodesis can be in situ [84, 88]. For Johnson and Johnson [97], the correction of the initial deformity did not seem to present advantages over in situ arthrodesis, and they do not recommend the correction of deformities in midfoot arthrodesis. Sangeorzan et al. [98], as well as Mann et al. [92], concluded that the reduction of joints with correction of deformities is an important factor for a good result. They also observed more than 90% of good results with midfoot arthrodesis, however, they noticed bad results when the initial deformity was not corrected. The choice of implant for fixation also be considered. There are several options, including Kirschner wires, cannulated screws, non-locking and locking plates, staples and hybrid systems [84, 86].

When the talo-medial cuneiform-first metatarsal (whole medial column) collapses, the fusion of the entire medial column, from the talus to the first metatarsal, can be an interesting option with satisfactory deformity correction and pain relief. According to Horton and Olney [99], and Mann et al. [92], it is important to correct residual deformities and restore the medial longitudinal arch.

Arthrodesis of the medial and intermediate columns is more frequent. It is important here to adequately prepare the joint surfaces and if possible, achieve a rigid stabilization [85]. Generally, a longitudinal approach is used between the base of the first and second metatarsals and another between the base of the third and fourth metatarsals. An adequate spacing between these two pathways is important to keep the viability of local soft tissues. Several materials are described for fixation, plates and screws or interfragmentary screws are the most employed [85, 90]. Nemec et al. [89], recommended the use of interfragmentary screws when there is good bone quality and the use of a plate with poor bone stock. Other studies report that there is no evidence favoring the use of one implant or another [85, 86]. Buddha et al. [96] found that the use of isolated dorsal plate, without the interfragmentary screw is associated with both delayed healing and pseudoarthrosis. They also call attention that the use of dorsal plates is associated with a greater possibility of skin problems. In a study in anatomical specimens, Cohen et al. [100] identified that the fixation with interfragmentary screws is also more rigid than the H-blocked plate. They affirmed that the plate does not achieve compression in the joint that has to be fused. This finding was the same of Baxter et al. [101], who also found in an anatomical study that the dorsomedial plate does not achieve the same compression at the site of the arthrodesis obtained with interfragmentary screws. Although interfragmentary screws are the preferred method of fixation of this arthrodesis, when there is bone gap or bone with poor quality (osteoporotic), some authors suggest the use of plates, with or without interfragmentary screws [102]. The use of bone graft helps with bone healing [89, 96] which generally takes around 12 weeks [3]. Gougoulias and Lampridis [86] do not recommend the use of routine bone grafting unless there is no bone contact. They reported 6.6% of pseudoarthrosis in 30 cases. Buddha and collaborators consider the use of bone graft essential in midfoot [96] arthrodesis. During the first 6 postoperative weeks, immobilization and non weightbearing is recommended (Figs. 11, 12, 13, 14, and 15) [89, 90].

Fig. 11 Planning of the access routes for medial and intermediate columns arthrodesis. The spacing between the pathways should be sufficient not to compromise the circulation of the local skin

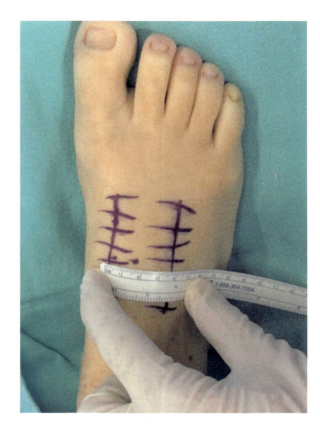

Fig. 12 Intermediate column exposure, with signs of osteoarthritis between the second and third metatarsals and cuneiforms. The plantar bending of the metatarsals facilitates the visualization of the surface to be prepared for arthrodesis

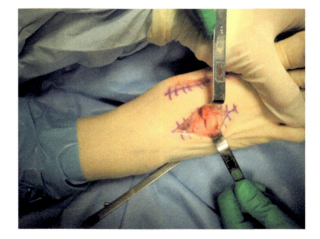

Fig. 13 Positioning of a dorsal H-plate for midline arthrodesis

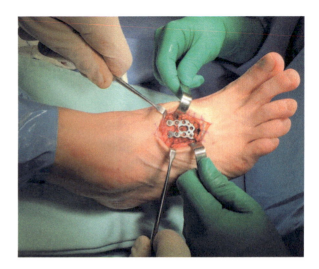

Fig. 14 X-ray showing arthrodesis of the medial and intermediate columns, consolidated, associated with arthrodesis of the intercuneiform and naviculo-cuneiform joints

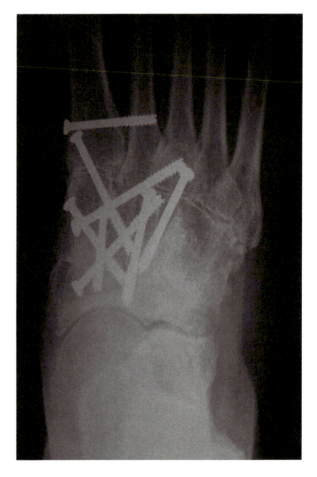

Fig. 15 Intraoperative
radiographic image of an
arthrodesis of the medial
and intermediate columns,
fixed with dorsomedial
plate and interfragmentary
screws

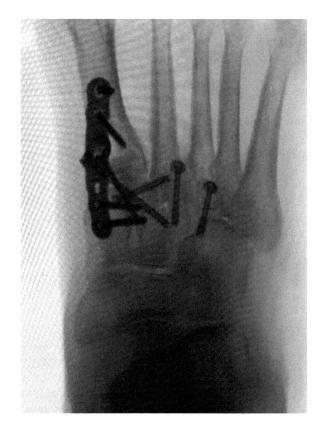

Complications of this arthrodesis range from non-union, neuroma, hardware related pain, metatarsalgia, stress fractures of the metatarsals [85, 89] and osteoarthritis of the adjacent joints. The incidence of non-union in the literature varies from 2% to 10% [89, 92, 96, 103]. Smoking [96] and obesity [89] have been associated with a higher possibility of pseudoarthrosis. Nemec et al. [89] observed, in a series of cases, that patients with body mass index (BMI) higher than 30 kg/m2, had worse clinical functional outcome according to the AOFAS score and more complications than patients with BMI < 30 kg/m2. Gougoulias and Lampridis [86] reported that despite a successful arthrodesis, 30% of the patients complain about pain in the neighboring joints and that 34% needed to wear insoles after surgery to relieve symptoms. The need for hardware removal varies in the literature between 9% and 25% [87, 89, 90].

The arthrodesis of the lateral column (lateral tarsus-metatarsal joints) is still controversial in the literature [85, 87, 93]. The mobility of these joints is important in the accommodation of the midfoot on the ground. The lateral column fusion has been associated with chronic lateral pain, pseudoarthrosis and stress fracture [84, 85, 93]. Raikin and Schon [93] stated that arthrodesis of the lateral column (cuboid - fourth and fifth metatarsal) can improve pain and function. However, in their study, most patients (22 arthrodesis) had deformity due to Charcot's arthropathy, which makes it difficult to evaluate the function and pain in the postoperative result, since these patients have insensitive feet and do not have the biomechanics of normal gait due to loss of proprioception. For this reason, although there is no formal contraindication for lateral column arthrodesis, there are descriptions in the literature of procedures that try to maintain the movement of the region [85]. Berlet et al. [104] retrospectively evaluated the results of joint resection of the lateral column and interposition of the peroneus tertius tendon. There are other studies that propose interposition of synthetic material in the region. Many authors recommend that surgery should be postponed as much as possible [84, 85]. Komenda et al. [88] affirm that the mobility of the lateral column is important for the function of the foot and many times, despite the radiographic images showing signs of joint degeneration, the patient is asymptomatic or has mild pain.

12 Summary

Arthrosis in the midfoot and hindfoot region are mostly post-traumatic or secondary to systemic inflammatory diseases, and usually cause significant pain and functional disability. Although conservative treatment is the first choice, it is often not effective, which makes surgery, especially arthrodesis, the best alternative in many cases. To achieve succesful results, the most important factors are joint preparation, patient selection and counseling, bone contact at the fusion site, rigid internal fixation and an adequate postoperative protocol including non weightbearing and immobilization.

References

1. Mann RA, Haskell A. Biomechanics of the foot and ankle. In: Coughlin MJ, Mann RA, Saltzmann CL, editors. Surgery of the foot and ankle. 8th ed. Philadelphia: Elsevier Health; 200. p. 3–45.
2. Silfverskiöld N. Reduction of the uncrossed two-joints muscles of the leg to one-joint muscles in spastic conditions. Acta Chir Scand. 1924;56:315–30.
3. Colin F, Lang TH, Zwicky L, et al. Subtalar joint configuration on weightbearing CT scan. Foot Ankle Int. 2014;35:1057–62.
4. Hirschmann A, Pfirrmann CWA, Klammer G, et al. Upright cone CT of the hindfoot: comparison of the non-weight-bearing with the upright weight-bearing position. Eur Radiol. 2014;24:553–8.
5. Krähebühl N, Tschuck M, Bollinger L, et al. Orientation of the subtalar joint. Foot Ankl Int. 2015;37:109–14.

6. Probasco W, Hallen AM, Yu J, et al. Assessment of coronal plane subtalar joint alignment in peritalar subluxation via weight-bearing multiplanar imaging. Foot Ankle Int. 2015;36:302–9.
7. Wirth SH, Zimmermann SM, Viehöfer AF. Open Technique for in situ subtalar fusion. Foot Ankle Clin N Am. 2018;23:461–74.
8. Mei-Dan O, Carmont M, Laver L, Mann G, Maffulli N, Nyska M. Intra-articular injections of hyaluronic acid in osteoarthritis of the subtalar joint: a pilot study. J Foot Ankle Surg. 2013;52(2):172–6.
9. Sadykov RI, Akhtyamov IF. Efficacy and safety of chondroitin sulfate therapy in patients with knee and hip osteoarthritis. Khirurgiia (Mosk). 2020;7:76–81.
10. Alekseeva LI, Kashevarova NG, Taskina EA, Sharapova EP, Anikin SG, Strebkovan EA, Raskina TA, Zonova EV, Otteva EN, Rodionova SS, Torgashin AN, Buklemishev UV, Shmidt EI, Shesternya PA, Naumov AV, Zagorodniy NV, Lila AM. The efficacy and safety of intra-articular application of a combination of sodium hyaluronate and chondroitin sulfate for osteoarthritis of the knee: a multicenter prospective study. Ter Arkh. 2020;92(5):46–54.
11. Fletcher AN, Lilies JL, Steele JJ, Pereira GF, Adams SB. Systematic review of subtalar distraction arthrodesis for the treatment of subtalar arthritis. Foot Ankle Int. 2020;41:437–48.
12. Chen Y, Zhang K, Quiang M, Hao Y. Maintenance of longitudinal foot arch after different mid/hindfoot arthrodesis procedures in a cadaveric model. Clin Biomech. 2014;29:170–6.
13. Cifuentes-De la Portilla C, Larrainzar-Garijo R, Bayod J. Analysis of biomechanical stresses caused by hindfoot joint arthrodesis in the treatment of adult acquired flatfoot deformity: A finite element study. Foot Ankle Surg. 2020;26:412–20.
14. Astion D, Deland J, Otis J, et al. Motion of the hindfoot after simulated arthrodesis. J Bone Joint Surg. 1997;79:241–6.
15. Patel NB, Blazek C, Scanlan R, Manway JM, Burns PR. Common pitfalls in subtalar joint preparation for arthrodesis via sinus tarsi approach. J Foot Ankle Surg. 2020;59(2):253–7.
16. Abyar E, McKissack HM, Pinto MC, Littlefield ZL, Moraes LV, Stefani K, Shah A. Subtalar fusion preparation: what are we really doing? A cadaver study. Foot Ankle Spec. 2020;13(3):201–6.
17. Galli MM, Scott RT, Bussewitz BW, Hyer CF. A retrospective comparison of cost and efficiency of the medial double and dual incision triple arthrodeses. Foot Ankle Spec. 2014;7:32–6.
18. Sammarco VJ, Magur EG, Sammarco GJ, Bagwe MR. Arthrodesis of the subtalar and talonavicular joints for correction of symptomatic hindfoot malalignment. Foot Ankle Int. 2006;27:661–6.
19. DeVries JG, Scharer B. Hindfoot deformity corrected with double versus triple arthrodesis: radiographic comparison. J Foot Ankle Surg. 2015;54:424–7.
20. Jeng CL, Tankson CJ, Myerson MS. The single medial approach to triple arthrodesis: a cadaver study. Foot Ankle Int. 2006;27:1122–5.
21. So E, Reb CW, Larson DR, Hyer CF. Medial double arthrodesis: technique guide and tips. J Foot Ankle Surg. 2018;57:364–9.
22. Wagner E, Melo R. Subtalar arthroscopic fusion. Foot Ankle Clin N Am. 2018;23:475–83.
23. Vilá-Rico J, Mellado Romero MA, Bravo-Giménez, Jiménez-Díaz V, Ojeda-Thies C. Subtalar arthroscopic arthrodesis: technique and outcomes. Foot Ankle Surg. 2017;23:9–15.
24. Dutra JMG, Barcelos VA, Prata SDS, Rizzo MAG, Filho RLR. Oliveira DB arthroscopic subtalar arthrodesis – results and complications. A systematic review. Journal of the. Foot and Ankle. 2020;14:205–10.
25. Rungprai C, Phisitkul P, Femino JE, Martin KD, Saltzman CL, Amendola A. Outcomes and complications after open versus posterior arthroscopic subtalar arthrodesis in 121 patients. J Bone Joint Surg Am. 2016;20(98):636–46.
26. Martín Oliva X, Falcão P, Fernandes Cerqueira R, Rodrigues-Pinto R. Posterior arthroscopic subtalar arthrodesis: clinical and radiologic review of 19 cases. J Foot Ankle Surg. 2017;56:543–6.

27. Albert A, Deleu PA, Leemrijse T, Maldague P, Devos BB. Posterior arthroscopic subtalar arthrodesis: ten cases at one-year follow-up. Orthop Traumatol Surg Res. 2011;97:401–5.
28. Beimers L, Frey C, van Dijk CN. Arthroscopy of the posterior subtalar joint. Foot Ankle Clin. 2006;11:369–90.
29. Mosca M, Caravelli S, Vannini F, Pungetti C, Catanese G, Massimi S, Fuiano M, Faldini C, Giannini S. Mini bone block distraction subtalar arthrodesis (SAMBB) in the management of acquired adult flatfoot with subtalar arthritis: a modification to the grice-green procedure. Joints. 2019;13(7):64–70.
30. Sanhudo JAV. Artrodese subtalar com enxerto em bloco de osso local. Revista ABTPé. 2012;6:37–8.
31. Sanhudo JAV. Bone block graft from calcaneus for foot and ankle reconstruction. Foot & Ankle Orthopaedics. 2016;1:1.
32. Herrera-Pérez M, Andarcia-Bañuelos C, Barg A, Wiewiorski M, Valderrabano V, Kapron AL, De Bergua-Domingo JM, Pais-Brito JL. Comparison of cannulated screws versus compression staples for subtalar arthrodesis fixation. Foot Ankle Int. 2015;36:203–10.
33. Yuan CS, Chen W, Chen C, Yang GH, Hu C, Tang KL. Effects on subtalar joint stress distribution after cannulated screw insertion at different positions and directions. J Foot Ankle Surg. 2015;54:920–6.
34. Chuckpaiwong B, Easley ME. Glisson RR screw placement in subtalar arthrodesis: A biomechanical study. Foot Ankle Int. 2010;30:133–41.
35. Jastifer JR, Alrafeek S, Howard P, Gustafson PA, Coughlin MJ. Biomechanical evaluation of strength and stiffness of subtalar joint arthrodesis screw constructs. Foot Ankle Int. 2016;37:419–26.
36. Eichinger M, Schmöiz W, Brunner A, Mayr R, Bölderl A. Subtalar arthrodesis stabilization with screws in an angulated configuration is superior to the parallel disposition: a biomechanical study. Int Orthop. 2015;39:2275–80.
37. Wirth SH, Viehöfer A, Fritz Y, Zimmermann SM, Rigling D, Urbanschitz L. How many screws are necessary for subtalar fusion? A retrospective study. Foot Ankle Surg. 2020;26:699–702.
38. Riedl M, Glisson RR, Matsumoto T, Hofstaetter SG, Easley ME. Torsional stiffness after subtalar arthrodesis using second generation headless compression screws: Biomechanical comparison of 2-screw and 3-screw fixation. Clin Biomech. 2017;45:32–7.
39. Tuijthof GJ, Beimers L, Kerkhoffs GM, Dankelman J, Dijk CN. Overview of subtalar arthrodesis techniques: options, pitfalls and solutions. Foot Ankle Surg. 2010;16:107–16.
40. Chaudhari N, Godoy-Santos AL, Netto CC, Rodriguez R, Dun S, He JK, McKissack H, Fleisig GS, Pires EA, Shah A. Biomechanical comparison of plantar-to-dorsal and dorsal-to-plantar screw fixation strength for subtalar arthrodesis. Einstein. 2020;18:1–6.
41. Pearce DH, Mongiardi CN, Fornasier VL, Daniels TR. Avascular necrosis of the talus: a pictorial essay. Radiographics. 2005;25:399–410.
42. Kunzler D, Shazadeh Safavi P, Jupiter D, Panchbhavi VK. A comparison of removal rates of headless screws versus headed screws in calcaneal osteotomy. Foot Ankle Spec. 2018;11:420–4.
43. Diezi C, Favre P, Vienne P. Primary isolated subtalar arthrodesis: outcome after 2 to 5 years Followup. Foot Ankle Int. 2008;29:1195–202.
44. Yildrin T, Sofu H, Çamurcu Y, et al. Isolated subtalar arthrodesis. Acta Orthop Belg. 2015;81:155–60.
45. Easley ME, Trnka H-J, Schon LC, et al. Isolated subtalar arthrodesis. J Bone Joint Surg Am. 2000;82:613–24.
46. Radnay CS, Clare MP, Sanders RW. Subtalar fusion after displaced intra-articular calcaneal fractures: does initial operative treatment matter? J Bone Joint Surg Am. 2009;91:541–6.
47. van der Vliet QMJ, Hietbrink F, Casari F, Leenen LPH, Heng M. Factors Influencing functional outcomes of subtalar fusion for posttraumatic arthritis after calcaneal fracture. Foot Ankle Int. 2018;39:1062–9.

48. Savory KM, Wulker N, Stukenborg C, Alfke D. Biomechanics of the hindfoot joints in response to degenerative hindfoot arthrodeses. Clin Biomech. 1998;13:62–70.
49. O'Malley MJ, Deland JT, Lee KT. Selective hindfoot arthrodesis for the treatment of adult acquired flatfoot deformity: an in vitro study. Foot Ankle Int. 1995;16:411–7.
50. Monteagudo M, Maceira E. Management of müller-weiss disease. Foot Ankle Clin. 2019;24:89–105.
51. Van den Broek M, Vandepitte G, Somville J. Dual window approach with two-side screw fixation for isolated talonavicular arthrodesis. J Foot Ankle Surg. 2017;56:171–5.
52. Miller SD, Schon LC, Melvani RT, Atwater LC, Aynardi M. Evaluating the safety of percutaneous dorsolateral talonavicular joint fixation in modified double arthrodesis: an anoatomic study. Foot & Ankle Orthopaedics. 1(1) https://doi.org/10.117 7/2473011416S00063.
53. Lee SR, Stibolt D, Patel H, Abyar E, Moon A, Naranje S, Shah A. Structures at risk during percutaneous screw fixation for talonavicular fusion. Foot Ankle Int. 2018;39:1502–8.
54. Jarrel SE, Owen JR, Wayne JS, Adelaar RS. Biomechanical comparison of screw versus plate/screw construct for talonavicular fusion. Foot Ankle Int. 2009;30(2):150–6.
55. Granata JD, Berlet GC, Ghotge R, Li Y, Kelly B, DiAngelo D. Talonavicular joint fixation: a biomechanical comparison of locking compression plates and lag screws. Foot Ankle Spec. 2014;7(1):20–31.
56. Harper MC. Talonavicular arthrodesis for the acquired flatfoot in adult. Clin Orthop Relat Res. 1999;65:8.
57. Chen C-H, Huang P-J, Chen T-B, Cheng Y-M, Lin S-Y, Chiang H-C, Chen L-C. Isolated talonavicular arthrodesis for talonavicular arthritis. Foot & Ankle Int. 2001;22:633–6.
58. Carranza-Bencano A, Tejero S, Fernández Torres JJ, Del Castillo-Blanco G, Alegrete-Parra A. Isolated talonavicular joint arthrodesis through minimal incision surgery. Foot Ankle Surg. 2015;21:171–7.
59. Lechler P, Graf S, Köck FX, Schaumburger J, Grifka J, Handel M. Arthrodesis of the talonavicular joint using angle-stable mini-plates: a prospective study. Int Orthop. 2012;36:2491–4.
60. Harnroongroj T, Chuckpaiwong B. Müller-weiss disease: three- to eight-year follow-up outcomes of isolated talonavicular arthrodesis. J Foot Ankle Surg. 2018;57:1014–9.
61. Xie M, Xia K, Zhang H, Cao H, Yang Z, Cui H, Gao S, Tang K. Individual headless compression screws fixed with three-dimensional image processing technology improves fusion rates of isolated talonavicular arthrodesis. J Orthop Surg Res. 2017;12:1–8.
62. Malik A, Grant E, Rhodenizer J. Analysis of micromotion in a talonavicular arthrodesis with and without a calcaneal displacement osteotomy in a cadaver model. J Foot Ankle Surg. 2020;59:91–4.
63. Lombardi CM, Dennis LN, Connoly FG, Silhanek AD. Talonavicular joint arthrodesis and Evans calcaneal osteotomy for treatment of posterior tibial tendon dysfunction. J Foot Ankle Surg. 1999;38:116–22.
64. Resnick RB, Jahss MH, Choueka J, Kummer F, Hersch JC, Okereke E. Deltoid ligament forces after tibialis posterior tendon rupture: effects of triple arthrodesis and calcaneal displacement osteotomies. Foot Ankle Int. 1995;16:14–20.
65. Coughlin MJ, Grimes JS, Traughber PD, Jones CP. Comparison of radiographs and CT scans in the prospective evaluation of the fusion of hindfoot arthrodesis. Foot Ankle Int. 2006;27:780–7.
66. Astion DJ, Deland JT, Otis JC, Kenneally S. Motion of the Hindfoot after simulated arthrodesis*. J Bone Jt Surg. 1997;79(2):241–6. https://doi.org/10.2106/00004623-199702000-00012.
67. Barmada M, Shapiro HS, Boc SF. Calcaneocuboid arthrodesis. Clin Podiatr Med Sur. 2012;29(1):77–89. https://doi.org/10.1016/j.cpm.2011.11.002.
68. Chu A, Chaudhry S, Sala DA, Atar D, Lehman WB. Calcaneocuboid arthrodesis for recurrent clubfeet: what is the outcome at 17-year follow-up? J Child Orthop. 2014;8(1):43–8. https://doi.org/10.1007/s11832-014-0557-4.

69. Deland JT, Otis JC, Lee K-T, Kenneally SM. Lateral column lengthening with calcaneocuboid fusion: range of motion in the triple joint complex. Foot Ankle Int. 1995;16(11):729–33. https://doi.org/10.1177/107110079501601111.
70. Evans D. Relapsed club foot. J Bone Jt Surg Br Volume. 1961;43-B(4):722–33. https://doi.org/10.1302/0301-620x.43b4.722.
71. Graves SC, Mann RA, Graves KO. Triple arthrodesis in older adults. Results after long-term follow-up. J Bone Jt Surg. 1993;75(3):355–62. https://doi.org/10.2106/00004623-199303000-00006.
72. Grier KM, Walling AK. The use of Tricortical autograft versus allograft in lateral column lengthening for adult acquired flatfoot deformity: an analysis of union rates and complications. Foot Ankle Int. 2010;31(9):760–9. https://doi.org/10.3113/fai.2010.0760.
73. Grunander TR, Thordarson DB. Results of calcaneocuboid distraction arthrodesis. Foot Ankle Surg. 2012;18(1):15–8. https://doi.org/10.1016/j.fas.2011.01.004.
74. Haeseker GA, Mureau MA, Faber FWM. Lateral column lengthening for acquired adult flatfoot deformity caused by posterior Tibial tendon dysfunction stage II: a retrospective comparison of calcaneus osteotomy with calcaneocuboid distraction arthrodesis. J Foot Ankle Surg. 2010;49(4):380–4. https://doi.org/10.1053/j.jfas.2010.04.023.
75. Kann NJ, Parks BG, Schon LC. Biomechanical evaluation of two different screw positions for fusion of the calcaneocuboid joint. Foot Ankle Int. 1999;20(1):33–6. https://doi.org/10.1177/107110079902000107.
76. Kobayashi H, Kageyama Y, Shido Y. Calcaneocuboid distraction arthrodesis with synthetic bone grafts: preliminary results of an innovative bone grafting procedure in 13 patients. J Foot Ankle Surg. 2017;56(6):1223–31. https://doi.org/10.1053/j.jfas.2017.07.003.
77. Van Der KA, Louwerens JWK, Anderson P. Adult acquired flexible flatfoot, treated by calcaneo-cuboid distraction arthrodesis, posterior tibial tendon augmentation, and percutaneous Achilles tendon lengthening: a prospective outcome study of 20 patients. Acta Orthop. 2009;77(1):156–63. https://doi.org/10.1080/17453670610045858.
78. Meyer MS, Alvarez BE, Njus GO, Bennett GL. Triple arthrodesis: a biomechanical evaluation of screw versus staple fixation. Foot Ankle Int. 1996;17(12):764–7. https://doi.org/10.1177/107110079601701209.
79. Milshteyn MA, Dwyer M, Andrecovich C, Bir C, Needleman RL. Comparison of two fixation methods for arthrodesis of the calcaneocuboid joint: a biomechanical study. Foot Ankle Int. 2014;36(1):98–102. https://doi.org/10.1177/1071100714552479.
80. Pell RF, Myerson MS, Schon LC. Clinical outcome after primary triple arthrodesis*†. J Bone Jt Surgery-american Volume. 2000;82(1):47–57. https://doi.org/10.2106/00004623-200001000-00006.
81. Sangeorzan BJ, Smith D, Veith R, Hansen ST. Triple arthrodesis using internal fixation in treatment of adult foot disorders. Clin Orthop Relat R. 1993;294(NA):299–307. https://doi.org/10.1097/00003086-199309000-00044.
82. Thomas RL, Wells BC, Garrison RL, Prada SA. Preliminary results comparing two methods of lateral column lengthening. Foot Ankle Int. 2001;22(2):107–19. https://doi.org/10.1177/107110070102200205.
83. Toolan BC, Sangerozan BJ, Hansen ST. Complex reconstruction for the treatment of dorsolateral Peritalar subluxation of the foot. Early results after distraction arthrodesis of the calcaneocuboid joint in conjunction with stabilization of, and transfer of the flexor Digitorum longus tendon to, the midfoot to treat acquired pes Planovalgus in adults*. J Bone Jt Surg. 1999;81(11):1545–60. https://doi.org/10.2106/00004623-199911000-00006.
84. Kurup H, Vasukutty N. Midfoot arthritis- current concepts review. J Clin Orthop Trauma. 2020;11:399–405.
85. Patel A, Rao S, Nawoczenski D, Flemister AS, DiGiovanni B, Baumhauer JF. Midfoot arthritis. Am Acad. Orthop Surg. 2010;18:417–25.
86. Gougoulias N, Lampridis V. Midfoot arthrodesis. Foot Ankle Surg. 2016;22:17–25.
87. Sayeed SA, Khan FA, Turner NS, Kitaoka HB. Midfoot arthritis. Am J Orthop. 2008;5:251–6.

88. Komenda GA, Myerson MS, Biddinger KR. Results of arthrodesis of the Tarsometatarsal joints after traumatic injury*†. J Bone Jt Surg. 1996;78:1665–76.
89. Nemec SA, Habbu RA, Anderson JG, Bohay DR. Outcomes following midfoot arthrodesis for primary arthritis. Foot Ankle Int. 2011;32:355–61.
90. Rao S, Nawoczenski DA, Baumhauer JF. Midfoot arthritis. Techniques. Foot Ankle Surg. 2008;7:188–95.
91. Keiserman LS, Cassandra J, Amis JA. The piano key test: a clinical sign for the identification of subtle Tarsometatarsal pathology. Foot Ankle Int. 2003;24:437–8.
92. Mann RA, Prieskorn D, Sobel M. Mid-tarsal and Tarsometatarsal arthrodesis for primary degenerative osteoarthrosis or osteoarthrosis after trauma*. J Bone Jt Surg. 1996;78:1376–85.
93. Raikin SM, Schon LC. Arthrodesis of the fourth and fifth Tarsometatarsal joints of the midfoot. Foot Ankle Int. 2003;24:584–90.
94. Da Costa BR, Reichenbach S, Keller N, Nartey L, Wandel S, Jüni P, et al. Retracted: effectiveness of non-steroidal anti-inflammatory drugs for the treatment of pain in knee and hip osteoarthritis: a network meta-analysis. Lancet. 2016;387:2093–105.
95. Halstead J, Chapman GJ, Gray JC, Grainger AJ, Brown S, Wilkins RA, et al. Foot orthoses in the treatment of symptomatic midfoot osteoarthritis using clinical and biomechanical outcomes: a randomised feasibility study. Clin Rheumatol. 2016;35:987–96.
96. Buda M, Hagemeijer NC, Kink S, Johnson AH, Guss D, DiGiovanni CW. Effect of fixation type and bone graft on Tarsometatarsal fusion. Foot Ankle Int. 2018;39:1394–402.
97. Johnson JE, Johnson KA. Dowel arthrodesis for degenerative arthritis of the Tarsometatarsal (Lisfranc) joints*. Foot Ankle Int. 1986;6:243–53.
98. Sangeorzan BJ, Verth RG, Hansen ST. Salvage of Lisfranc's Tarsometatarsal joint by arthrodesis. Foot Ankle Int. 1990;10:193–200.
99. Horton GA, Olney BW. Deformity correction and arthrodesis of the midfoot with a medial plate*. Foot Ankle Int. 1993;14:493–9.
100. Cohen DA, Parks BG, Schon LC. Screw fixation compared to H-locking plate fixation for first Metatarsocuneiform arthrodesis: a biomechanical study. Foot Ankle Int. 2005;26:984–9.
101. Baxter JR, Mani SB, Chan JY, Vulcano E, Ellis SJ. Crossed-screws provide greater Tarsometatarsal fusion stability compared to compression plates. Foot Ankle Specialist. 2015;8:95–100.
102. Filippi J, Myerson MS, Scioli MW, Hartog BDD, Kay DB, Bennett GL, et al. Midfoot arthrodesis following multi-joint stabilization with a novel hybrid plating system. Foot Ankle Int. 2012;33:220–5.
103. Jung HG, Myerson MS, Schon LC. Spectrum of operative treatments and clinical outcomes for atraumatic osteoarthritis of the Tarsometatarsal joints. Foot Ankle Int. 2007;28:482–9.
104. Berlet GC, Anderson RB. Tendon arthroplasty for basal fourth and fifth metatarsal arthritis. Foot Ankle Int. 2002;23:440–6.

Forefoot-Driven Hindfoot Deformity: Coupled Deformity

Norman Espinosa and Georg Klammer

1 Introduction

The foot and ankle are fascinating and complex biomechanical structures of the human body. They are composed of a multitude of bones, ligaments and tendons, which shape various joints [1, 2]. The smooth interplay of those kinematic chains allow a perfect bipedal gait.

Even in the presence of biomechanical alterations within this system, the foot and ankle is able to compensate for them. All of them – of course – being three dimensional and dynamic corrections. Sometimes those compensations may last for a long time before they start to fail.

The talonavicular joint represents the link between hind- and mid-to forefoot. It is crucial for the transfer of vertical forces into horizontal load distribution. Its cardan-style construction and function categorizes it as one of the most important joints in the foot and ankle [3–6].

The subtalar joint offers a large potential for corrections in patients suffering from flatfeet, while its potential in varus hindfeet is quite more limited [7–14]. However, both joints are connected to each other and act in concert to adapt to any motion and alteration within the system.

In this chapter the problem of forefoot-driven hindfoot deformities and pathologies will be discussed. To understand those mechanical abnormalities, it is mandatory to distinguish between forefoot-driven hindfoot valgus and forefoot-driven hindfoot varus deformities.

Whereas many scientific literature is available regarding the forefoot-driven hindfoot varus deformity, almost nothing is found for the forefoot-driven hindfoot

N. Espinosa (✉) · G. Klammer
Institute for Foot and Ankle Reconstruction Zurich, FussInstitut Zurich, Zurich, Switzerland
e-mail: espinosa@fussinstitut.ch; klammer@fussinstitut.ch

© The Author(s), under exclusive license to Springer Nature 669
Switzerland AG 2022
E. Wagner Hitschfeld, P. Wagner Hitschfeld (eds.), *Foot and Ankle Disorders*,
https://doi.org/10.1007/978-3-030-95738-4_30

valgus deformity [15, 16]. To the opinion of the author the latter does exist as well and could pose more challenging demands for any surgeon when treatment is needed.

2   Definition of Forefoot-Driven Hindfoot Deformity

Any biomechanical alteration of kinematics within the fore-and midfoot can result in compensatory misalignment of the hindfoot. Important to know is, that all hindfoot deformities, which are provoked by the forefoot, are flexible.

The cause can either be static (e.g. plantarflexed first ray) or dynamic (e.g. hyperactivity of the peroneus longus muscle). It is therefore crucial to properly identify the origin of pathology to formulate an adequate treatment strategy.

3   Etiologies of Forefoot-Driven Hindfoot Deformities

The causes for any forefoot-driven hindfoot deformity are variable and require correct clinical and intellectual judgement. Sometimes, combinations of causes could be responsible for the development of those pathologies and need therefore more complex or expanded treatment strategies. If only one of those causes goes mis- or undiagnosed the result of treatment may be unsatisfactory for the patient.

3.1   Forefoot-Driven Hindfoot Varus

The underlying causes should be classified into dynamic, static and combined forms [16].

One of the most discussed etiologies of a dynamically forefoot-driven hindfoot varus is a neurologic disorder resulting in an imbalance between agonists and antagonists. The peroneus longus, peroneus brevis, tibialis anterior and tibialis posterior play an essential role [17].

Weakness of the tibialis anterior and peroneus brevis muscle group in combination with an overpowering peroneus longus and strong tibialis posterior muscle lead to the characteristic deformation of the fore-, hind- and midfoot [16]: Pronation of forefoot, supination of midfoot and elevation of longitudinal arch. To compensate for the plantarflexed first ray the hindfoot needs to swing into varus.

In contrast, static plantarflexion of the first ray causing structural rigidity of the forefoot forces the flexible hindfoot also to push into varus [18]. The reason for a static plantarflexion might be congenital, traumatic or iatrogenic (i.e. after surgical interventions).

3.2 Forefoot-Driven Hindfoot Valgus

In contrast to forefoot-driven hindfoot varus, forefoot-driven hindfoot valgus [19, 20] encompasses a completely different etiology.

The most important cause for a forefoot-driven hindfoot valgus is the instability of the first ray [21–23]. Any excessive motion at the first tarsometatarsal, naviculo-cuneiform or talonavicular joint can result in a hyper-supination of the forefoot and midfoot [24, 25]. Other reasons encompass iatrogenically or traumatically induced elevation of the first ray forcing the forefoot to rotate into malposition.

Therefore, the pattern of forefoot-driven hindfoot valgus is: Supination of the forefoot, ± midfoot and decrease of the longitudinal arch. Consequently, the hindfoot compensates for this abnormal motion by turning into valgus.

4 General Aspects of Clinical Assessment

Any patient should be examined in a barefoot situation during walking and in a standing position. The bilateral evaluation of both legs and hindfeet helps to obtain a detailed appreciation of the deformity type. Leg, hindfoot, midfoot, and forefoot deformities should be identified, and the rigidity and corrective potential estimated.

Of course, throughout the clinical evaluation attention is paid to signs of other pathologic conditions such as peroneal tendinopathy and lateral as well as medial instability, osteochondral lesions, osteoarthritis including ankle impingement, occult fractures, and neuropathy of the superficial peroneal nerve. At some times it might be necessary to correct them to achieve a proper overall result.

4.1 Inspection

Hindfoot alignment is observed during stance and includes inspection of soft-tissue conditions. Measurement of hindfoot alignment is performed while inspecting the patient from posterior. The angle between long axis of the leg and axis of the calcaneus is measured. Normal values range from 0° neutral to 5° valgus. Any varus is pathologic. Valgus hindfoot deformities that exceed 10° can be seen as abnormal.

4.2 Palpation

Specific attention is paid to tender spots at the level of the ankle, subtalar, Chopart- and Lisfranc joints. In addition, palpation should be continued along the course of the medial and lateral ligament complexes around the ankle as well as along the joint lines of the ankle, subtalar, and Chopart joints. Tenderness along the peroneal tendons may indicate tendinopathy or partial rupture and needs specific imaging, for example, magnetic resonance imaging (MRI). Occasionally a prominent osteophyte formation points toward arthritic disorders. If local swelling is observed, palpation allows identification of joint effusion, tenosynovitis, or ganglion formation. Besides this, any tender spot at the site of the posterior tibial tendon insertion is important because it may hint onto the existence of insertional tendinopathy as well as a Spring-ligament insufficiency/- rupture.

4.3 Functional Testing

Range of motion (ROM) at the ankle, subtalar, and Chopart joints is assessed. Reduced ROM at any of those joints helps to identify the locus of rigidity and deformity.

An impaired ROM at the level of the ankle with associated equinus may be the result of a short gastrocnemius-soleus muscle complex [19]. The contracture of a short gastrocnemius-soleus complex, is best examined by means of the Silfverskjöld test [26]. It is important to distinguish shortening of the Achilles tendon from contractures of the triceps surae. Those structures may play a crucial role in correcting the hindfoot and in determining whether additional surgery should be performed.

A proper neurologic assessment is mandatory to rule out any muscular imbalance in the foot and ankle. Despite this vascular status should be checked (i.e. Aa. popliteal, tibialis posterior, dorsalis pedis).

• *Specific tests in forefoot-driven hindfoot valgus deformity*

In patients suffering from forefoot-driven hindfoot valgus the so-called reversed Coleman-block can be used (Fig. 1) [27, 28]. In addition to the reversed Coleman-block Test any hypermobility of the first ray should be evaluated [21–23, 29–32].

Testing of hypermobility of the first ray can be done as reported by Glasoe and Michaud [33].

• *Specific tests in forefoot-driven hindfoot varus deformity*

The most important functional test to assess the flexibility of hindfoot varus—in case of a forefoot-driven hindfoot varus—is the Coleman block test [27, 28, 34].

One of the most debated pathologies or causes of a forefoot-driven hindfoot varus is the hyperactivity of the peroneus longus. However, it can be functionally tested as follows: The patient sits in front of the examiner and is asked to forcefully dorsiflex at the ankle joint with the knee in full extension. In this position the examiner places one thumb underneath the first metatarsal head and the other thumb underneath the second, third, and fourth metatarsal heads. The patient then plantarflexes the foot maximally against resistance of the examiner hand. The combined pronation of the forefoot with a strong plantarisation of the first ray indicates the presence of a hyperactivity of the peroneus longus muscle. In contrast, patients who plantarflex their foot without pronation of the forefoot are considered to have a normal activity of the peroneus longus muscle [15, 17, 35].

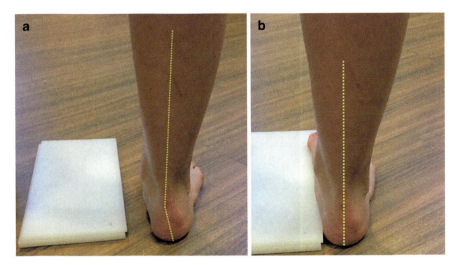

Fig. 1 (**a**) The image depicts a patient with a forefoot-driven hindfoot valgus on her right foot. Please note the remarkable valgus hindfoot deformity. (**b**) The reversed-Coleman-Block Test corrects the hindfoot valgus in neutral when the block is put underneath the greater toe joint

5   Imaging

Usually, surgeons start to analyse the deformities and pathologies of the foot and ankle by using conventional radiography.

In general, conventional radiography includes the following techniques:

5.1   Conventional Imaging

Normally, standard weightbearing radiographs, including anteroposterior, lateral views of the ankle and dorsoplantar, oblique and lateral views of the foot are performed. To assess the hindfoot alignment, the author recommends hindfoot alignment or long axial views to measure the amount of varus deformity. Any arthritic change around the foot and ankle should be identified. On the mortise view, the congruency of the ankle joint can be judged, and the lateral distal tibial angle (LDTA) measured (normal value 88°).

- *Specific alterations in forefoot-driven hindfoot varus feet*

On the lateral view of the foot, the deformity can be measured. In cavus feet most commonly the talus–first metatarsal (Meary [36]) and talocalcaneal angles as well as the calcaneal pitch angles are assessed to describe the deformity [37].

Usually, the slope of the first metatarsal bone is steep, indicating the driving-force of the deformity. The sinus tarsi represents wide open and circular in shape on lateral views of the ankle (Fig. 2).

- *Specific alterations in forefoot-driven hindfoot valgus feet*

Fig. 2 This image depicts
a cavus foot provoked by
the forefoot. The sinus tarsi
is wide open and the
angulation of the
metatarsals quite steep.
The Meary-angle is
positive

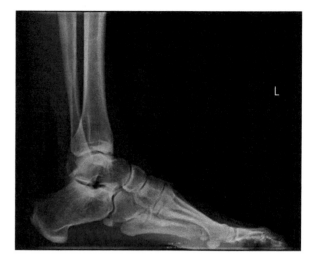

In flatfeet the Meary-angle [38, 39] serves to measure the deformity and to identify the sag of medial column. In valgus feet the sinus tarsi becomes almost not
visible or completely obliterated.

In patients with hypermobility of the first ray, it might be possible to see a plantar
gaping of the first tarsometatarsal joint and loss of parallelism between the dorsal
cortices of the first and second metatarsal bone (Fig. 3) [32, 33, 40].

5.2   Hindfoot Alignment

The classic radiographic hindfoot alignment view, as described by Saltzman and
el-Khoury, has been introduced to reduce the flaws as for example obtained from the
Cobey-view [41, 42].

Nowadays, there is quite a lot of scientific evidence revealing the usefulness of
the hindfoot view for visual judgment of the hindfoot alignment. In addition, the
hindfoot view shows good-to-excellent intraobserver reliability. However, interobserver reliability is very low and is clearly surpassed when using the classic long
axial view only (Fig. 4) [43–45]. One of the major drawbacks of the hindfoot view
is its susceptibility to rotatory malpositioning of the foot. Thus, the measurements
obtained with the hindfoot view need to be interpreted with caution.

A far more reliable angle measurement can be done using the long axial view or
the medial and lateral borders of the calcaneus [43, 46].

Whereas preoperative assessment of hindfoot alignment under weight-bearing
conditions is done in a standardised fashion, there is not yet a technique available to
do so under non–weight-bearing conditions, for example, during surgery. More
recently, Min and Sanders described varus-valgus referencing relative to the medial
process of the posterior calcaneal tuberosity in the unloaded Mortise view. Its usefulness and feasibility will be subject of future research [47].

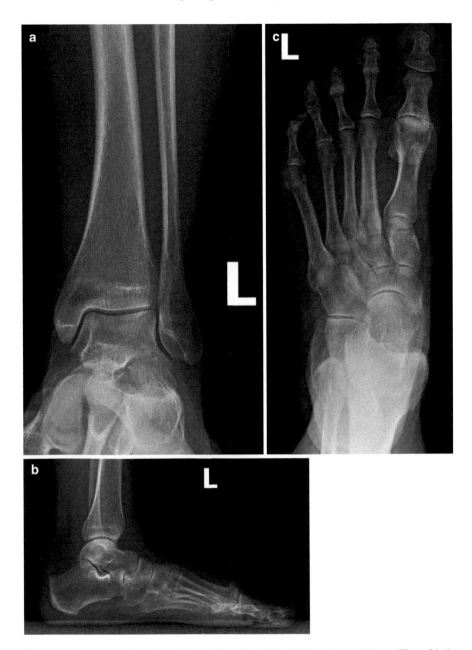

Fig. 3 (**a**) Anteroposterior view of the ankle under full-weightbearing conditions. The ankle is absolutely fine. (**b**) On the lateral view the sinus tarsi depicts itself as slightly obliterated while the first metatarsal is elevated. Please note a slight sag within the naviculocuneiform joint. Diagnosis: Forefoot-driven hindfoot valgus. (**c**) The dorsoplantar view of the foot in the same patient as under Fig. 1b does not reveal any major forefoot abduction

Fig. 4 This is the long-axial view of the same patient's hindfoot as reported in Figs. 3a–c. The valgus moment is clearly visible

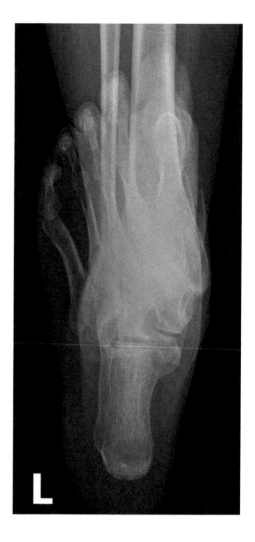

Full-length radiographs of both legs including the pelvis and hips are considered when complex reconstructions are planned.

5.3   Computed Tomography and MRI

MRI and computed tomography (CT) allow precise three-dimensional depiction of the bones and soft tissues. Both technologies are mainly indicated for evaluation of the lateral ligamentous complex and concomitant pathologic conditions such as peroneal tendinopathy, osteochondral lesions, and/or osteoarthritis.

MRI has been found to be highly specific in detecting lesions of the anterior talofibular and calcaneofibular ligaments; however, sensitivity is poor [48].

Because of its superiority when compared with a simple arthro-CT examination the authors perform CT only in selective cases, for example, to estimate the amount of fibular malrotation; to measure the true extent of osteochondral lesions of the talus or to evaluate presence of a tarsal coalition.

Weightbearing-CT has become a novel tool for the assessment of hindfoot deformities [49]. Burssens et al. presented a method of measuring the angular deformities [50]. And it seems to work well [51]. WBCT allows a clear depiction of where the apex of the deformity is and how fore- and hindfoot interact. This helps surgeons to plan the intervention as precise as possible. Recently, a consensus group defined the following parameters in the assessment of the foot and ankle: If available, a hindfoot alignment view is strongly recommended. 'If available, WEIGHTBEARING computed tomography is strongly recommended for surgical planning. When WEIGHTBEARING CT is obtained, important findings to be assessed are sinus tarsi impingement, subfibular impingement, increased valgus inclination of the posterior facet of the subtalar joint, and subluxation of the subtalar joint at the posterior and/or middle facet' [51].

6   Conservative Treatment

Conservative treatment has always had its place in the treatment of foot and ankle pathologies. While in the flexible forefoot-driven hindfoot deformity insoles and shoe modification may have a certain benefit, they might not be very useful in the presence of postural abnormalities or fixed mechanical deformities because they are not effective enough to correct those rigid anatomical alterations. Thus, they might fail very soon.

However, there will always be a group of individuals who do not qualify for any operation due to their comorbidities, which increase health risks and outweigh the benefits of surgery. This group encompasses elderly patients and those with inadequately adjusted diabetes mellitus, advanced peripheral vascular disease or cardiovascular disease, specific neurologic disorders, or respiratory disease.

Conservative treatment might not be able to address the underlying cause of a mechanically induced hindfoot deformity but could be beneficial in cases of flexible varus deformity.

Conservative treatment should be followed up for at least 6 months. If after a standardised nonoperative protocol there is no improvement, surgery may be considered.

6.1   Physical Therapy

Physical therapy has shown to influence functional instability by improving proprioception, peroneal muscle preactivation, and eversion strength. This is mainly useful in patients suffering from hindfoot varus associated with variable degrees of hindfoot instability [52].

Aggressive stretching protocols maybe performed to lengthen the gastrocnemius-soleus unit and to reduce tension exerted through the Achilles tendon. By so doing, the inversion moment can be reduced, and stability improved [53].

6.2   Braces

Braces can decrease severity and frequency of ankle sprains in patients with chronic instability. Laced braces have been shown to be most effective [54].

In addition, improved stability can be achieved by taping. Although the inversion moments at the ankle are reduced by means of taping, the true mechanical stabilising effect of taping is limited. It has been shown that almost 50% of the stabilising effect is gone after 10 minutes of exercise [55–59].

However, proprioception might remain improved due to other reflex mechanisms. Braces may also help to stretch the gastrocnemius-soleus unit.

6.3   Shoe Modifications and Insoles

Equalisation of pressure distribution and offloading of painful areas are the primary goals of insoles and orthoses.

Lateral wedging may partially correct flexible hindfoot varus and decrease subjective instability [37]. In flexible hindfoot valgus medial arch supports may be indicated to try to correct the deformity to some extent.

Prefabricated products are available, but custom-made devices have advantages, especially in patients with rigid deformity. Additional support may be achieved with specific shoe modifications, for example increased width of the heel sole. In case of secondary degenerative changes, rocker-bottom soles could alleviate pain by reducing the propulsive work at the ankle joint.

The OSSA-orthosis is a very specific tool to stop rotation at the talonavicular joint. In certain patients who are dealing with a forefoot-driven hindfoot valgus, this treatment modality could be a valuable option to treat the condition. However, due to the rigidity of the OSSA-orthosis, patients may complain about pain and stop continuation of the treatment.

7   Surgical Treatment

Surgical treatment is always warranted when conservative measures have failed. This may specifically apply for postural, i.e. anatomically rigid, deformities. The selection of treatment varies between forefoot-driven hindfoot varus and forefoot-driven hindfoot valgus deformities. The goal of any of those treatments is to create an equilibrium between fore-, mid- and hindfoot.

The surgeon needs to identify the origin of deforming force and restore anatomy and biomechanics where needed. The primary goal is to strive for joint-preserving surgery. However, in certain cases it might not be possible, and fusions should be considered the better option.

7.1 Forefoot-Driven Hindfoot Varus

Goal of treatment: To unload the first ray and to restore an equilibrium between fore- and hindfoot through the midfoot.

7.1.1 The Plantarflexed First Ray

A *flexible plantarflexed first ray* may arise from hyperactivity of the peroneus longus, which can be decreased by means of a peroneus longus to brevis transfer [17, 35]. The transfer is performed with a lateral incision between the cuboid tunnel and the peroneal tubercle on the lateral calcaneal wall. The sheaths of the peroneal tendons are opened and a side-to-side tenodesis achieved suturing the peroneus longus to the peroneus brevis tendon with the foot in neutral position. Pretensioning of the peroneus longus tendon in case of its hyperactivity is not necessary. Side-to-side tenodesis may be continued more proximally in case of a peroneus brevis degeneration or tear. After tenodesis the peroneus longus tendon is cut at the cuboid groove and if present an os peroneal excised. The peroneal tubercle may be removed to avoid impingement of the tendons [60].

Otherwise *fixed plantarflexion of the metatarsals*, for example as seen in idiopathic cavovarus foot, can be addressed by a dorsiflexion osteotomy. Dorsiflexion osteotomies, first described by Swanson et al., may involve a single metatarsal or more metatarsals [61]. In forefoot-driven hindfoot varus, the deformity is caused by a rigid and massively plantarflexed first ray. In such a situation a dorsiflexion osteotomy of the proximal first metatarsal bone is recommended. We approach the metatarsal bone with a dorsal incision. The dorsally based closing wedge osteotomy is started 2–3 cm distal to the tarsometatarsal joint and angled 60° distally. Fixation with a 2-hole plate is considered sufficient, as under weight-bearing the osteotomy with a preserved plantar hinge is compressed and stable (Fig. 5) [62]. Larger plantarflexion deformities might be better addressed using a fusion of the first tarsometatarsal joint [63]. Correction of the 2nd and 3rd ray is considered when simulated weightbearing indicates overload of the metatarsal heads.

7.1.2 Calcaneal Osteotomy

A *lateralising calcaneal osteotomy* is added if after soft tissue balancing by means of the peroneal tendon transfer and/or metatarsal osteotomies the hindfoot varus persists. Preoperatively this may be anticipated if hindfoot varus is incompletely corrected with the Coleman block test.

Vienne and colleagues published the results of a consecutive series of patients with cavo-varus deformity and recurrent ankle instability. All patients revealed a failed

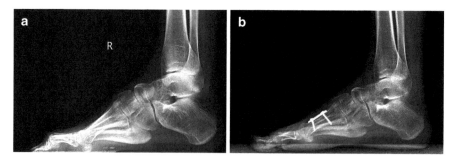

Fig. 5 (**a**) Lateral view of a patient with a forefoot-driven hindfoot varus. Note the wide sinus tarsi and the steep course of the metatarsal bones. (**b**) Lateral view of the same patient as mentioned in (**a**) after correction through a metatarsal elevation osteotomy. It is interesting how the hindfoot corrects as seen on the sinus tarsi

prior ligament stabilisation surgery. The plantarflexed first ray and hindfoot varus were flexible. Each patient was clinically detected to have a hyperactivity of the peroneus longus muscle. All were successfully treated by means of a lateralising calcaneal osteotomy and peroneus longus to brevis transfer. In half of the patients, a Broström procedure was added to address lateral ligament insufficiency. All patients showed good results with subjective and objective lateral stability [64]. Similar results were achieved by Fortin et al. adding dorsiflexion osteotomy in patients with flexible hindfoot deformities [65].

8   Forefoot-Driven Hindfoot Valgus

Goal of treatment: To increase the competence of the medial column and thus to restore an equilibrium between fore- and hindfoot through the midfoot.

8.1   Elevated First Ray Due to Traumatic or Iatrogenic Origin

Trauma or surgery can result in anatomical alterations of the first metatarsal bone. In those cases, the elevation of the bone itself can force the forefoot to turn into supination, which in turn accelerates the development of a flexible hindfoot valgus deformity. In such cases it is needed to correct the deformity at its apex and to straighten the first metatarsal bone in an anatomical manner.

8.2   Instability of the Medial Column

The stabilisation of the medial column is essential in patients who suffer from forefoot-driven hindfoot valgus. The treatment should be chosen as efficient as possible to achieve minimal loss of joints but maximum secondary correction at the hindfoot.

While the concept seems easy to understand, the treatment itself can pose significant problems to the surgeons. The difficulty lies in the assessment of instability and where it may occur. The first tarsometatarsal-, naviculocuneiform- and talonavicular joints are three different articulations, which can reveal isolated or combined instabilities. It is therefore mandatory to evaluate the potential apex of deformity on weightbearing lateral views of the foot.

Plantar gaping at the first tarsometatarsal joint, or a sag at the level of the naviculocuneiform and/or talonavicular joint indicate instability [32, 33]. In chronic forefoot-driven hindfoot valgus deformities, even the deltoid and spring ligament complex can become altered and insufficient [66–70].

By means of the reversed- Coleman-Block Test the amount of correction can be anticipated. However, until today it is not yet clear whether based on this test a simple stabilisation of the medial column would be sufficient or if other means (e.g. calcaneal osteotomies, medial deltoid ligament repair, etc.) should be added. Thus, the authors think that intraoperative judgment of the correction should always be done and where needed liberal use of the forementioned techniques applied.

- Fusion of the first tarsometatarsal joint [71–73].
  This is a very effective treatment to treat a forefoot-driven hindfoot valgus associated with an isolated but severe hypermobility at the first tarsometatarsal joint. Fusion of the first tarsometatarsal joint is done through a medial approach. It is in most cases an in-situ arthrodesis. In case of co-existing valgus deformities, it can also help to provide a correction. The subcutaneous tissues should be divided and then the distal margins of the retinaculum (lying over the tibialis anterior tendon) become visible. The retinaculum is cut, and the tibialis anterior tendon protected. Afterwards the first tarsometatarsal joint can be reached and the capsule of it is incised. The cartilage should be removed by means of osteotomes and curettes. The authors do not use a saw to prepare the joint surfaces to avoid any risk of over-shortening [73]. After this procedure the subchondral bone plate is freshened up using a 2.0 mm burr. The joint surfaces, i.e. their subchondral parts, are brought together and a K-wire (1.6–2.0 mm diameter) inserted to lock the joint in the position needed. First a laterally placed lag-screw that runs from distal-dorsal to proximal-plantar through the first tarsometatarsal joint is put in. After this a medially placed plate is laid over the first tarsometatarsal joint to secure the construct.
- Fusion of the naviculocuneiform joint [25, 39, 74–77]
  The approach is similar to that of the first tarsometatarsal joint fusion but more proximal. After subcutaneous preparation the retinaculum over the tibialis anterior tendon is incised and the tendon pulled distally by means of Langenbeck-hooks. The naviculocuneiform joint capsule should be opened up completely. By means of osteotomes and mini curettes, the cartilage is removed. It is essential not to remove too much of the subchondral bone because the larger the defect the more difficult to close the joint during fusion. If this situation occurs, the authors recommend adding autologous cancellous bone graft from the proximal and/or distal tibia. Fixation of the naviculocuneiform joint is tricky: According to

Hansen, the fusion can be achieved by means of 3.5 mm screws. However, contemporary plates and fixation systems allow even more stable means to achieve proper union.

- Fusion of the talonavicular joint [78–84].
  For this fusion, a medial approach is done right over the talar head and navicular tuberosity. The incision of the skin parallels with the course of the posterior tibial tendon. During subcutaneous preparation the surgeon needs to take care of the venous vessels and sometimes ligations of those structures are important. The capsule of the talonavicular joint should be opened without harming the insertion site of the posterior tibial tendon. The authors do not extend the preparation and separation of the capsule beyond the joint line. To the opinion of the authors, it is essential to preserve the vascular supply to the talar head. Therefore, any stripping of the capsule at the level of the talar neck is forbidden.

  By means of a curved osteotome and curettes the cartilage is removed. Sometimes specific distractors are needed to open up the talonavicular joint. As with every other joint the subchondral bone is freshened up using a 2.0 mm drill. The authors usually reduce the hindfoot through the so-called 'Myerson'-reduction-maneuver. Fixation can be done by means of 5.5 and/or 3.5 mm screws. The medially placed screw represents a true lag-screw while the other two function as positioning screws.

- Combined fusions of the medial column [85, 86]
  Sometimes, when the instability cannot be precisely found at one of the aforementioned joints, it is necessary to fuse the tarsometatarsal ± naviculocuneiform ± the talonavicular joint. The combination of fusion enhances the medial stability and provides a powerful tool to restore the longitudinal arch by ensuring durable correction at the hindfoot (Fig. 6).

- Calcaneal osteotomy [3, 87–93]
  The authors are quite liberal in terms of using a medialising calcaneal osteotomy. If there is a residual valgus found, during intraoperative evaluation, the medialising calcaneal osteotomy can help to correct the hindfoot, while turning it into neutral. The surgeon should be cautious not to overcorrect the hindfoot into varus. Thus, intraoperative judgement by help of an axial calcaneal view is recommended.

  The simplest way to perform is the medial sliding calcaneal osteotomy, which is performed by an oblique cut of the calcaneus. The approach is chosen laterally over the calcaneal tuberosity. The line of skin incision can be straight or slightly curved (preferred by the authors). After meticulous subcutaneous preparation two Hohmann-hooks are placed over the dorsum of the calcaneus tuberosity and plantar to the insertion site of the aponeurosis. The surgeon should hold the calcaneus in one hand to control the depth of cut during the osteotomy (which is performed by means of an oscillating saw). Holding the knee in 90° of flexion and the ankle in full plantarflexion the calcaneal tuberosity can be shifted easily to the medial side. Once the planned shift is reached the foot and knee are straightened up to neutral. By so doing, the tuberosity gets temporarily secured until final fixation is done by means of screws, which are inserted from posteriorly.

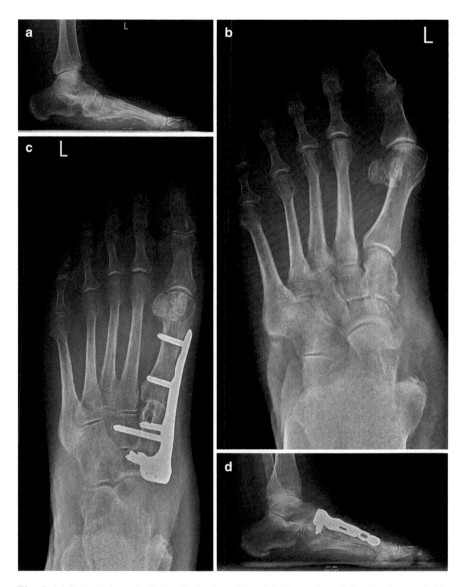

Fig. 6 (**a**) Lateral view of a foot with forefoot-driven hindfoot valgus deformity. A remarkable plantar gaping at the first tarsometatarsal joint and sag at the naviculocuneiform can be appreciated. The sinus tarsi is not visible anymore. (**b**) The dorsoplantar view of the foot demonstrates a small forefoot abduction and presence of a hallux valgus deformity. (**c**) Dorsoplantar view of the same foot after medial column fusion. The plate expands from the first tarsometatarsal over the naviculocuneiform joint. Note the correction of the forefoot. (**d**) On the lateral view of the foot the sinus tarsi has opened and the midfoot has been put in line with the forefoot and talar axis

In patients who require a more three-dimensional correction a so-called z-shaped osteotomy could be performed [94–96]. This type of calcaneal osteotomy allows correction in all three planes including medial shift, transversal and coronal rotation. It is a very powerful osteotomy. However, fixation can be somewhat difficult due to the course of the osteotomy-lines. It can also be used together with a talonavicular fusion (in the literature an Evans-osteotomy has been used for this purpose) [97].

- Deltoid and Spring-Ligament-reconstruction [98, 99]
  In patients who suffer from chronic forefoot-driven hindfoot valgus deformity the medial collateral ligament complex can become insufficient. This is specifically the case when a decompensation takes place at the talonavicular joint. In those cases, the forefoot starts to rotate and shift laterally while increasing stretch onto the deltoid and spring ligament is exerted. The diagnosis of a medial deltoid and spring ligament insufficiency can best be made using an MRI.

The authors adopted and modified the techniques described by Haddad et al. [99] and Nery et al. [98] Both techniques base on anatomic reconstruction of the deltoid ligament including the option to repair the Spring-ligament where needed. While in their original papers the techniques have been performed using tendon grafts the current method can be performed utilising non-resorbable fiber sutures.

A posteromedial approach is chosen for this specific technique. Skin incision follows the course of the posterior tibial tendon and is placed slightly dorsal to it. The posterior tibial tendon sheath is exposed and incised. The posterior tibial tendon should then be moved plantarly using a Langenbeck-hook. This maneuver allows direct inspection of both, the deltoid and Spring ligament. Two essential anatomical regions need now to be exposed: First the part dorsal to the insertion of the posterior tibial tendon at the navicular tuberosity and second the sustentaculum tali. Both loci are important for the suture anchor placement. When exposing the sustentaculum tali, it is important not to injure the tendon of the flexor digitorum longus or flexor hallucis longus. In addition, the anterior and medial part of the calcaneus as well as the tip of the medial malleolus needs to be exposed. Two drill holes are made in the medial malleolus (close to its tip). The reconstruction needs two autologous or allografts (minor morbidity). Alternatively, new tools, e.g. the InternalBrace™ (Arthrex Inc.; Naples, FL, USA) can be used. Additional drill holes are made in the navicular tuberosity, the anteromedial part of the calcaneus (underneath the anteromedial facet of the subtalar joint) and sustentaculum tali.

The first graft is inserted with its one end into the medial surface of the talus and secured with an interference screw. The foot is hold in neutral position. Afterwards the graft is brought close to the inferior drill hole in the medial malleolus and its limb secured by means of another interference screw. This reconstructs the *tibiotalar ligament*. Afterwards the distal graft limb is inserted into the drill hole, which has been made in the anteromedial portion of the calcaneus and passed from medial to lateral to achieve proper tension. The graft is then secured by means of an additional interference screw. This part reconstructs the *tibiospring-ligament*.

The second graft will then be inserted with its one end into the sustentaculum tali and secured with an interference screw. The distal part of the graft is then inserted into the anterior drill hole of the medial malleolus and secured. This reconstruction creates a band that connects the tibia and calcaneus. It corresponds to the *tibiocalcaneal ligament* and enhances the construct. Now the rest of the graft can be inserted, under tension, within the navicular tuberosity and fixed with an interference screw. This last step reconstructs the *tibionavicular ligament.*

By so doing, the surgical technique allows the reconstruction of 4 ligaments. In case of a complete rupture of the spring-ligament an additional graft/suture might be used, which is driven from the navicular tuberosity to the sustentaculum tali.

Nery et al. [98] described their technique and evaluated 10 consecutive patients with flatfoot deformity and insufficient ankle and midfoot ligaments. No postoperative complications, stiffness, or loss of correction were found. Therefore, the group stated that the novel technique to reconstruct the failed deltoid and spring ligament during flatfoot correction could have merit.

In contrast to Nery et al. [98], Haddad and co-workers [99] investigated their technique on six pairs of fresh frozen cadaveric lower extremities. As a result of the biomechanical testing angular displacement at a 2 Nm level torque was significantly greater in the sectioned group compared to the deltoid reconstruction group in external rotation and eversion ($p = 0.006$ and $p = 0.017$, respectively). The authors did not find a statistical difference in angular displacement between the deltoid intact and reconstructed group in external rotation and eversion when tested at 2 Nm of torque ($p = 0.865$ and $p = 0.470$, respectively). The stiffness of the reconstruction was $136.4 \pm 40.2\%$ compared to the intact ligament. Stiffness data were statistically insignificant in both plantar flexion and dorsiflexion between the reconstructed and sectioned groups ($p = 0.050$ and $p = 0.126$). As a final result the authors were able to demonstrate that the described reconstruction technique under low torque was able to restore eversion and external rotation stability to the talus, which was statistically similar to the intact deltoid ligament [100].

All those techniques, which have been described and discussed in brief help to correct the entire foot and ankle and can – if properly planned – be highly successful.

9   Summary

Forefoot-driven hindfoot deformities represent a highly interesting field in foot and ankle surgery. The most amazing fact is, that the hindfoot deformity itself is mainly corrected at the level of the fore- and midfoot.

The causes for each type are different and therefore the distinction into varus and valgus deformities is important. The same applies for the general rules of surgical treatment: Varus hindfoot corrections can be achieved by unloading the first ray, while valgus hindfoot corrections can reliably be achieved through stabilisation of the medial column.

The surgical armamentarium to correct those deformities has already been published for other pathologies and can be applied in the current types of pathology. Thus, a surgeon should feel quite familiar with those techniques. The main discrepancy, however, lies in the clinical and radiographic assessment of those patients and to identify the underlying cause and apex of deformity.

Once these basics are appreciated, it will be easy to treat any of those patients while ensuring a high probability for a good outcome.

References

1. Golano P, et al. Ankle anatomy for the arthroscopist. Part II: role of the ankle ligaments in soft tissue impingement. Foot Ankle Clin. 2006;11(2):275–96. v-vi
2. Golano P, et al. Ankle anatomy for the arthroscopist. Part I: the portals. Foot Ankle Clin. 2006;11(2):253–73. v
3. Sizensky JA, Marks RM. Medial-sided bony procedures: why, what, and how? Foot Ankle Clin. 2003;8(3):539–62.
4. Knupp M, Stufkens SA, Hintermann B. Triple arthrodesis. Foot Ankle Clin. 2011;16(1):61–7.
5. Amaha K, et al. Anatomic study of the medial side of the ankle base on the joint capsule: an alternative description of the deltoid and spring ligament. J Exp Orthop. 2019;6(1):2.
6. MacDonald, A. et al., Peritalar kinematics with combined deltoid-spring ligament reconstruction in simulated advanced adult acquired flatfoot deformity. Foot Ankle Int, 2020: p. 1071100720929004.
7. Noguchi K. Biomechanical analysis for osteoarthritis of the ankle. Nihon Seikeigeka Gakkai Zasshi. 1985;59(2):215–22.
8. Karlsson J, Eriksson BI, Renstrom P. Subtalar instability of the foot. A review and results after surgical treatment. Scand J Med Sci Sports. 1998;8(4):191–7.
9. Mittlmeier T, Rammelt S. Update on subtalar joint instability. Foot Ankle Clin. 2018;23(3):397–413.
10. Sangeorzan BJ, et al. Contact characteristics of the subtalar joint: the effect of talar neck misalignment. J Orthop Res. 1992;10(4):544–51.
11. Wagner UA, et al. Contact characteristics of the subtalar joint: load distribution between the anterior and posterior facets. J Orthop Res. 1992;10(4):535–43.
12. Sangeorzan BJ, Ananthakrishnan D, Tencer AF. Contact characteristics of the subtalar joint after a simulated calcaneus fracture. J Orthop Trauma. 1995;9(3):251–8.
13. Sangeorzan A, Sangeorzan B. Subtalar joint biomechanics: from normal to pathologic. Foot Ankle Clin. 2018;23(3):341–52.
14. Krahenbuhl N, et al. The subtalar joint: a complex mechanism. EFORT Open Rev. 2017;2(7):309–16.
15. Klammer G, Benninger E, Espinosa N. The varus ankle and instability. Foot Ankle Clin. 2012;17(1):57–82.
16. Krahenbuhl N, Weinberg MW. Anatomy and biomechanics of cavovarus deformity. Foot Ankle Clin. 2019;24(2):173–81.
17. Vienne P, et al. Hindfoot instability in cavovarus deformity: static and dynamic balancing. Foot Ankle Int. 2007;28(1):96–102.
18. Seaman TJ, Ball TA. Pes Cavus. Treasure Island: StatPearls; 2020.
19. Espinosa N, Brodsky JW, Maceira E. Metatarsalgia. J Am Acad Orthop Surg. 2010;18(8):474–85.
20. Maceira E, Monteagudo M. Mechanical basis of metatarsalgia. Foot Ankle Clin. 2019;24(4):571–84.

21. Myerson MS, Badekas A. Hypermobility of the first ray. Foot Ankle Clin. 2000;5(3):469–84.
22. Roukis TS, Landsman AS. Hypermobility of the first ray: a critical review of the literature. J Foot Ankle Surg. 2003;42(6):377–90.
23. Cowie S, et al. Hypermobility of the first ray in patients with planovalgus feet and tarsometatarsal osteoarthritis. Foot Ankle Surg. 2012;18(4):237–40.
24. Kadakia AR, et al. Did failure occur because of medial column instability that was not recognized, or did it develop after surgery? Foot Ankle Clin. 2017;22(3):545–62.
25. Metzl JA. Naviculocuneiform sag in the acquired flatfoot: what to do. Foot Ankle Clin. 2017;22(3):529–44.
26. Strayer LM Jr. Recession of the gastrocnemius; an operation to relieve spastic contracture of the calf muscles. J Bone Joint Surg Am. 1950;32-A(3):671–6.
27. Fortin PT, Guettler J, Manoli A 2nd. Idiopathic cavovarus and lateral ankle instability: recognition and treatment implications relating to ankle arthritis. Foot Ankle Int. 2002;23(11):1031–7.
28. Younger AS, Hansen ST Jr. Adult cavovarus foot. J Am Acad Orthop Surg. 2005;13(5):302–15.
29. Klaue K, Hansen ST, Masquelet AC. Clinical, quantitative assessment of first tarsometatarsal mobility in the sagittal plane and its relation to hallux valgus deformity. Foot Ankle Int. 1994;15(1):9–13.
30. Prieskorn DW, Mann RA, Fritz G. Radiographic assessment of the second metatarsal: measure of first ray hypermobility. Foot Ankle Int. 1996;17(6):331–3.
31. Bierman RA, Christensen JC, Johnson CH. Biomechanics of the first ray. Part III. Consequences of Lapidus arthrodesis on peroneus longus function: a three-dimensional kinematic analysis in a cadaver model. J Foot Ankle Surg. 2001;40(3):125–31.
32. King DM, Toolan BC. Associated deformities and hypermobility in hallux valgus: an investigation with weightbearing radiographs. Foot Ankle Int. 2004;25(4):251–5.
33. Glasoe WM, Michaud TC. Measurement of dorsal first ray mobility: a topical historical review and commentary. Foot Ankle Int. 2019;40(5):603–10.
34. Coleman SS, Chesnut WJ. A simple test for hindfoot flexibility in the cavovarus foot. Clin Orthop Relat Res. 1977;123:60–2.
35. Ramseier LE, et al. Treatment of late recurring idiopathic clubfoot deformity in adults. Acta Orthop Belg. 2007;73(5):641–7.
36. Boffeli TJ, Schnell KR. Cotton osteotomy in flatfoot reconstruction: a review of consecutive cases. J Foot Ankle Surg. 2017;56(5):990–5.
37. Sammarco GJ, Taylor R. Cavovarus foot treated with combined calcaneus and metatarsal osteotomies. Foot Ankle Int. 2001;22(1):19–30.
38. Lin YC, et al. Imaging of adult flatfoot: correlation of radiographic measurements with MRI. AJR Am J Roentgenol. 2015;204(2):354–9.
39. Aiyer A, et al. Radiographic correction following reconstruction of adult acquired flat foot deformity using the cotton medial cuneiform osteotomy. Foot Ankle Int. 2016;37(5):508–13.
40. Koury K, et al. Radiographic assessment of first tarsometatarsal joint shape and orientation. Foot Ankle Int. 2019;40(12):1438–46.
41. Saltzman CL, el-Khoury GY. The hindfoot alignment view. Foot Ankle Int. 1995;16(9):572–6.
42. Cobey JC. Posterior roentgenogram of the foot. Clin Orthop Relat Res. 1976;118:202–7.
43. Buck FM, et al. Hindfoot alignment measurements: rotation-stability of measurement techniques on hindfoot alignment view and long axial view radiographs. AJR Am J Roentgenol. 2011;197(3):578–82.
44. Buck FM, et al. Diagnostic performance of MRI measurements to assess hindfoot malalignment. An assessment of four measurement techniques. Eur Radiol. 2013;23(9):2594–601.
45. Sutter R, et al. Three-dimensional hindfoot alignment measurements based on biplanar radiographs: comparison with standard radiographic measurements. Skelet Radiol. 2013;42(4):493–8.
46. Reilingh ML, et al. Measuring hindfoot alignment radiographically: the long axial view is more reliable than the hindfoot alignment view. Skelet Radiol. 2010;39(11):1103–8.

47. Min W, Sanders R. The use of the mortise view of the ankle to determine hindfoot alignment: technique tip. Foot Ankle Int. 2010;31(9):823–7.
48. Chandnani VP, et al. Chronic ankle instability: evaluation with MR arthrography, MR imaging, and stress radiography. Radiology. 1994;192(1):189–94.
49. Hirschmann A, et al. Upright cone CT of the hindfoot: comparison of the non-weight-bearing with the upright weight-bearing position. Eur Radiol. 2014;24(3):553–8.
50. Burssens ABM, et al. Is lower-limb alignment associated with hindfoot deformity in the coronal plane? A weightbearing CT analysis. Clin Orthop Relat Res. 2020;478(1):154–68.
51. de Cesar Netto C, et al. Consensus for the use of weightbearing CT in the assessment of progressive collapsing foot deformity. Foot Ankle Int. 2020;41(10):1277–82.
52. Tourne Y, et al. Chronic ankle instability. Which tests to assess the lesions? Which therapeutic options? Orthop Traumatol Surg Res. 2010;96(4):433–46.
53. Taddei UT, et al. Effects of a therapeutic foot exercise program on injury incidence, foot functionality and biomechanics in long-distance runners: feasibility study for a randomized controlled trial. Phys Ther Sport. 2018;34:216–26.
54. Lin YC, et al. The hindfoot arch: what role does the imager play? Radiol Clin N Am. 2016;54(5):951–68.
55. Cramer EA, Friedhoff K. Taping--a safe alternative in the early functional treatment of all ligament instabilities of the proximal ankle joint? Results of a prospective study. Unfallchirurg. 1990;93(6):275–83.
56. Jerosch J, Bischof M. The effect of proprioception on functional stability of the upper ankle joint with special reference to stabilizing aids. Sportverletz Sportschaden. 1994;8(3):111–21.
57. Jerosch J, et al. The influence of orthoses on the proprioception of the ankle joint. Knee Surg Sports Traumatol Arthrosc. 1995;3(1):39–46.
58. Jerosch J, et al. Is prophylactic bracing of the ankle cost effective? Orthopedics. 1996;19(5):405–14.
59. Callaghan MJ. Role of ankle taping and bracing in the athlete. Br J Sports Med. 1997;31(2):102–8.
60. Huber M. What is the role of tendon transfer in the cavus foot? Foot Ankle Clin. 2013;18(4):689–95.
61. Krause FG, Iselin LD. Hindfoot varus and neurologic disorders. Foot Ankle Clin. 2012;17(1):39–56.
62. Reddy VB. Metatarsal Osteotomies: Complications. Foot Ankle Clin. 2018;23(1):47–55.
63. Jung HG, Park JT, Lee SH. Joint-sparing correction for idiopathic cavus foot: correlation of clinical and radiographic results. Foot Ankle Clin. 2013;18(4):659–71.
64. Vienne P, Schöniger R, Helmy N, Espinosa N. Hindfoot instability in cavovarus deformity: static and dynamic balancing. Foot Ankle Int. 2007;28(1):96–102.
65. Fortin PT, Guettler J, Manoli A 2nd. Idiopathic cavovarus and lateral ankle instability: recognition and treatment implications relating to ankle arthritis. Foot Ankle Int. 2002;23(11):1031–7.
66. Alshalawi S, et al. Medial ankle instability: the deltoid dilemma. Foot Ankle Clin. 2018;23(4):639–57.
67. Bastias GF, et al. Spring Ligament Instability. Foot Ankle Clin. 2018;23(4):659–78.
68. Pellegrini MJ, et al. Chronic deltoid ligament insufficiency repair with internal brace augmentation. Foot Ankle Surg. 2019;25(6):812–8.
69. Brodell JD Jr, et al. Deltoid-spring ligament reconstruction in adult acquired flatfoot deformity with medial peritalar instability. Foot Ankle Int. 2019;40(7):753–61.
70. Guerra-Pinto F, et al. The tibiocalcaneal bundle of the deltoid ligament – prevalence and variations. Foot Ankle Surg. 2021;27:138–42.
71. Claassen L, et al. Surgical procedures for the correction and stabilization of pes planovalgus. Orthopade. 2020;49(11):968–75.
72. Conti MS, Garfinkel JH, Ellis SJ. Outcomes of reconstruction of the flexible adult-acquired flatfoot deformity. Orthop Clin North Am. 2020;51(1):109–20.
73. Dahlgren N, et al. First tarsometatarsal fusion using saw preparation vs. standard preparation of the joint: a cadaver study. Foot Ankle Surg. 2020;26(6):703–7.
74. Catanzariti AR. Modified medial column arthrodesis. J Foot Ankle Surg. 1993;32(2):180–8.

75. Budny AM, Grossman JP. Naviculocuneiform arthrodesis. Clin Podiatr Med Surg. 2007;24(4):753–63. ix-x

76. Rush SM, Jordan T. Naviculocuneiform arthrodesis for treatment of medial column instability associated with lateral peritalar subluxation. Clin Podiatr Med Surg. 2009;26(3):373–84.

77. Ajis A, Geary N. Surgical technique, fusion rates, and planovalgus foot deformity correction with naviculocuneiform fusion. Foot Ankle Int. 2014;35(3):232–7.

78. O'Malley MJ, Deland JT, Lee KT. Selective hindfoot arthrodesis for the treatment of adult acquired flatfoot deformity: an in vitro study. Foot Ankle Int. 1995;16(7):411–7.

79. Lombardi CM, et al. Talonavicular joint arthrodesis and Evans calcaneal osteotomy for treatment of posterior tibial tendon dysfunction. J Foot Ankle Surg. 1999;38(2):116–22.

80. Chen CH, et al. Isolated talonavicular arthrodesis for talonavicular arthritis. Foot Ankle Int. 2001;22(8):633–6.

81. Weinheimer D. Talonavicular arthrodesis. Clin Podiatr Med Surg. 2004;21(2):227–40. vi

82. Rammelt S, Marti RK, Zwipp H. Arthrodesis of the talonavicular joint. Orthopade. 2006;35(4):428–34.

83. Kiesau CD, et al. Talonavicular joint fixation using augmenting naviculocalcaneal screw in modified double hindfoot arthrodesis. Foot Ankle Int. 2011;32(3):244–9.

84. Ma S, Jin D. Isolated Talonavicular arthrodesis. Foot Ankle Int. 2016;37(8):905–8.

85. Cohen BE, Ogden F. Medial column procedures in the acquired flatfoot deformity. Foot Ankle Clin. 2007;12(2):287–99. vi

86. Yu G, et al. Fusion of talonavicular and naviculocuneiform joints for the treatment of Muller-Weiss disease. J Foot Ankle Surg. 2012;51(4):415–9.

87. Horton GA, et al. Effect of calcaneal osteotomy and lateral column lengthening on the plantar fascia: a biomechanical investigation. Foot Ankle Int. 1998;19(6):370–3.

88. Mosier-LaClair S, Pomeroy G, Manoli A 2nd. Operative treatment of the difficult stage 2 adult acquired flatfoot deformity. Foot Ankle Clin. 2001;6(1):95–119.

89. Catanzariti AR, et al. Double calcaneal osteotomy: realignment considerations in eight patients. J Am Podiatr Med Assoc. 2005;95(1):53–9.

90. Penney NT, et al. Double-calcaneal osteotomy with a unilateral rail external fixator for correction of pes planus: a case report. Foot Ankle Spec. 2009;2(4):194–9.

91. Guha AR, Perera AM. Calcaneal osteotomy in the treatment of adult acquired flatfoot deformity. Foot Ankle Clin. 2012;17(2):247–58.

92. Chan JY, et al. The contribution of medializing calcaneal osteotomy on hindfoot alignment in the reconstruction of the stage II adult acquired flatfoot deformity. Foot Ankle Int. 2013;34(2):159–66.

93. Toullec E. Adult flatfoot. Orthop Traumatol Surg Res. 2015;101(1 Suppl):S11–7.

94. Knupp M, et al. Osteotomies in varus malalignment of the ankle. Oper Orthop Traumatol. 2008;20(3):262–73.

95. Krause FG, et al. Ankle joint pressure changes in a pes cavovarus model after lateralizing calcaneal osteotomies. Foot Ankle Int. 2010;31(9):741–6.

96. Hamel J. Calcaneal Z osteotomy for correction of subtalar hindfoot varus deformity. Oper Orthop Traumatol. 2015;27(4):308–16.

97. Lombardi CM, et al. Talonavicular fusion and Evans calcaneal osteotomy for treatment of PTTD. J Foot Ankle Surg. 1999;38(5):372.

98. Nery C, et al. Combined spring and deltoid ligament repair in adult-acquired flatfoot. Foot Ankle Int. 2018;39(8):903–7.

99. Haddad SL, et al. Deltoid ligament reconstruction: a novel technique with biomechanical analysis. Foot Ankle Int. 2010;31(7):639–51.

100. Keefe DT, Haddad SL. Subtalar instability. Etiology, diagnosis, and management. Foot Ankle Clin. 2002;7(3):577–609.

Localized Osteoarthritis of the Ankle

Emilio Wagner Hitschfeld and Pablo Wagner Hitschfeld

1 Introduction

Arthrosis of the ankle causes pain, dysfunction, and alterations in mobility, limitating activities and functional evaluations. The classic treatment alternatives for osteoarthritis of the ankle consist in distraction arthroplasties, total arthroplasties or ankle arthrodesis. The outcome of distraction arthroplasty is mixed, with satisfaction reported at about 60%, depending on where the results are reported [1, 2]. Total arthroplasties present a successful outcome in 80% of cases at 10 years (with a high re-operation rate), so it is not a life-long solution, especially in young patients who present with post-traumatic arthrosis [3].

It should be remembered that in cases of slight, initial localized osteoarthritis, the only symptom present is pain at the ankle with no radiological sign of osteoarthritis. Pain at the ankle plus alterations in the load distribution in the ankle joint constitutes the diagnosis of localized osteoarthritis of the ankle. We will use this term (i.e., localized osteoarthritis of the ankle, LOA) to characterize the clinical picture of ankle pain associated with localized overloading for cases with or without visible joint wear.

Since post-traumatic etiology is the most frequent in ankle osteoarthritis, it is easy to understand the possibility of finding asymmetrical ankle wear in the area where the greatest damage or impact has occurred. In fact, up to two-thirds of patients with ankle arthrosis present asymmetrical wear and tear, and may present greater damage to the anterior, posterior, medial or lateral aspect of the tibiotalar joint. In the surgical treatment of localized ankle osteoarthritis, given its greater

E. Wagner Hitschfeld (✉)
Orthopedic Surgery Department, Clínica Alemana de Santiago - Universidad del Desarrollo, Santiago, RM - Santiago, Chile

P. Wagner Hitschfeld
Orthopedic Surgery Department, Clínica Alemana de Santiago - Universidad del Desarrollo, Hospital Militar de Santiago – Universidad de los Andes, Santiago, RM - Santiago, Chile

© The Author(s), under exclusive license to Springer Nature   691
Switzerland AG 2022
E. Wagner Hitschfeld, P. Wagner Hitschfeld (eds.), *Foot and Ankle Disorders*,
https://doi.org/10.1007/978-3-030-95738-4_31

prevalence in young patients, the use of periarticular osteotomies is the most recommended treatment method given its joint sparing nature [4]. Joint preserving surgeries should always include complete ankle and foot rebalancing, considering soft tissue surgeries such as ligament reconstruction, supra- and inframalleolar osteotomies, tendon transfers, and selective arthrodesis. In cases of failure of these alternatives (patients who persist with symptoms), the realignment surgery is still deemed beneficial, since a consequent total ankle arthroplasty has better postoperative results and is technically simpler if it is performed on an aligned ankle [5].

In this chapter, we will analyze in depth the use of periarticular osteotomies for localized ankle osteoarthritis.

2 Etiology – Pathophysiology

The ankle is formed by the junction of the tibia, talus and calcaneus through the ankle and subtalar joints. We must not forget the relationship between the ankle and the rest of the foot, since the talus, not having any tendon or muscle insertion, behaves as an intercalary segment in the foot. Its position and stability depend on the neighboring bones and joints, as well as on the stability and strength of the tendons that cross the area.

The etiology of ankle osteoarthritis is estimated to be 70% post-traumatic, 12% rheumatological and 7% of no demonstrable origin [6]. The post-traumatic etiology includes mainly ankle fractures, tibial pilon fractures and ankle sprains, as well as fibular malunions and chronic ankle instabilities. The physiopathology of localized ankle osteoarthritis (LOA) is easy to understand as the main cause is post-traumatic. Trauma to the ankle generates asymmetric damage to the joint (see Fig. 1). The bone resistance of the tibia and talus is not uniform on its surface, with the tibia showing greater subchondral resistance in its posteromedial aspect than the anterolateral one [7]. The presence of instability in the ankle is another aggravating factor in localized osteoarthritis, since subluxation movements and localized loads are produced that lead to asymmetric wear, which has been observed in biomechanical [8] and clinical studies [9]. Finally, it is important to note that the load distribution in the ankle is determined both by its static component, i.e., its skeletal alignment, and by its dynamic component, composed of the tendon structures. In particular, the Achilles tendon is an important deforming vector since in varus deformities it increases the torque in inversion and in valgus deformities it increases the torque in eversion [3].

3 Biomechanical Considerations

In LOA, we must analyze the origin of the joint overload. This is mostly due to limb malalignment and can be found at the supramalleolar level as in post-traumatic deformities of the tibia, at the intra-articular level as in cases of asymmetric

Fig. 1 Ankle radiograph of a 28-year-old patient with an asymmetric arthrosis of the ankle joint, due to a previous pilon fracture treated surgically. Note the valgus inclination of the pilon and of the talus

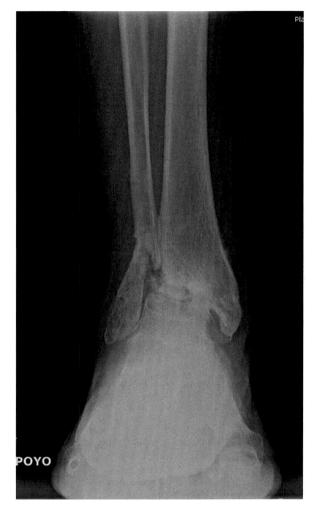

cartilage wear or inframalleolar level as in cases of pes cavus or valgus flatfoot in which joint instabilities or tendon imbalances of the midfoot and forefoot lead to overload and subsequent deformities within the ankle.

The alignment is studied with long leg radiographs, analyzing the anatomical and mechanical axes of the limb. It can also be analyzed by measuring the torque generated within the ankle, measuring the distance between the mechanical hip-calcaneal (or tibia-calcaneal) axis and the center of the ankle [10] (see Fig. 2). The published average distance is −3.2 mm (negative sign indicates varus of the hindfoot, 95% confidence interval between −18 mm and 12 mm). The hindfoot alignment is analyzed with Saltzman's rearfoot X-ray in which the contribution of the subtalar joint in the alignment of the hindfoot is discussed. The foot alignment is analyzed with weight bearing antero-posterior and lateral X-rays by measuring the angle between the talus and the first metatarsal, which helps to analyze the relative

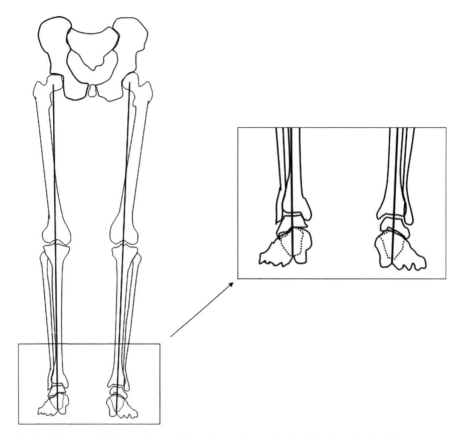

Fig. 2 Diagram of a bilateral lower limb radiograph, showing both limbs and pelvis. The mechanical axis of the extremities is represented with a line starting on the center of the femoral head and finishing distally where the calcaneus touches the floor. This line normally intersects the ankle joint in its middle. The distance between this mechanical axis and the middle of the talus represents the torque generated inside the ankle joint

abduction or adduction of the foot as well as any medial column insufficiency (see Fig. 3).

In cases of LOA, we must also differentiate the plane of space in which the osteoarthritis is occurring, which will lead to different manifestations in relation to the general alignment of the limb. Thus, in the coronal plane, when the wear is more pronounced in the lateral half of the joint, we will speak of valgus arthrosis (see Fig. 4), and when the wear is more pronounced in the medial half of the joint, we will speak of varus arthrosis. In the sagittal plane we can find more pronounced arthrosis in the anterior aspect of the joint which simulates recurvatum deformities and produces anterior subluxations of the talus. In the opposite case we can find more pronounced arthrosis in the posterior aspect of the ankle that simulates deformities in procurvatum and leads to posterior subluxations of the talus. The procurvatum is better tolerated despite being able to generate anterior ankle impingement.

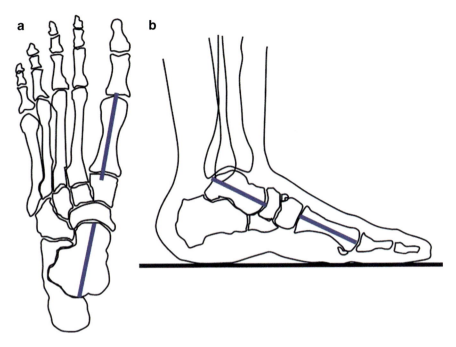

Fig. 3 Diagram of anteroposterior and lateral weight bearing foot radiographs. (**a**) shows the anteroposterior view of the foot, where a line was drawn representing the axis of the first metatarsal and another one was drawn representing the axis of the talus, allowing to measure the anteroposterior talo-first metatarsal angle. (**b**) shows the lateral view of the foot, where a line was drawn representing the axis of the first metatarsal and another one was drawn representing the axis of the talus, allowing to measure the lateral talo-first metatarsal angle

The recurvatum is more damaging to the joint as it leads to a larger "uncovered" talus surface and therefore a less constrained, unstable joint that is more susceptible to damage [3]. Supramalleolar alignment should therefore be evaluated in the coronal and sagittal plane using the lateral distal tibial angle or LDTA (average 90°, range 88–95°) and the anterior distal tibial angle or ADTA correspondingly (average 81°, range 78–82°) [11, 12]. These angles are measured between a line along the tibial axis and one tangential to the distal articular tibial joint surface, either in the coronal (LDTA) or sagittal (ADTA) plane (see Figs. 5 and 6). This measurement can only be made if the limb has no obvious deformity above the ankle. Intraarticular alignment can be evaluated with the talar tilt, which should not exceed 4°. The tilt angle is measured between the distal articular tibial surface and the talar dome line.

Peritalar stability must be analyzed since in cases of ankle osteoarthritis the talus loses intrinsic stability due to the decrease in cartilage thickness and consequent decrease in hindfoot height. The talus is "imprisoned" between the calcaneus and the tibia and therefore its position is controlled and manipulated by forces applied from proximal and distal segments (it is an intercalary or sesamoid bone without tendon attachments). Peritalar instability can manifest itself in various ways, either

Fig. 4 Radiograph of a
patient with a localized
ankle arthrosis, in this case
a valgus arthrosis, with a
lateral mechanical ankle
overload. It must be noted
that there is more
pronounced wear in the
lateral half of the joint
(decreased joint space in
the lateral half of the
ankle)

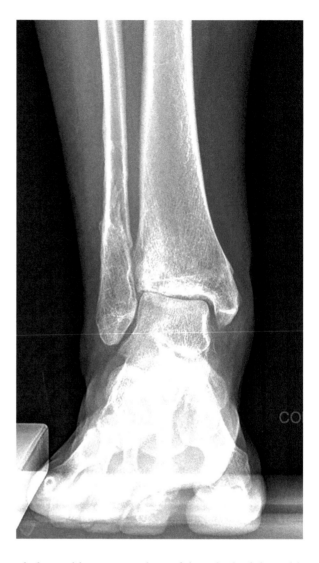

with deviations in the coronal plane with varus or valgus of the subtalar joint, with
talar external rotation, internal rotation, dorsiflexion, or plantar flexion. In cases of
peritalar instability the talus position should be evaluated using computed tomography (CT) under load (WBCT) as it is not predictable through a single radiological
projection [13]. Sometimes when the talus tilts into varus or valgus, the calcaneus
slightly tilts in the opposite direction, compensating the deviation. However, in
cases of peritalar instability, an exaggerated compensatory deviation of the calcaneus occurs. For example, in a varus ankle, an exaggerated valgus hindfoot is
observed. If a valgus calcaneal osteotomy (any) is performed in these cases (to
compensate the varus ankle), the hindfoot deviation may worsen with more varus at
the tibiotalar joint and no axis correction or symptomatic relief may be obtained. On

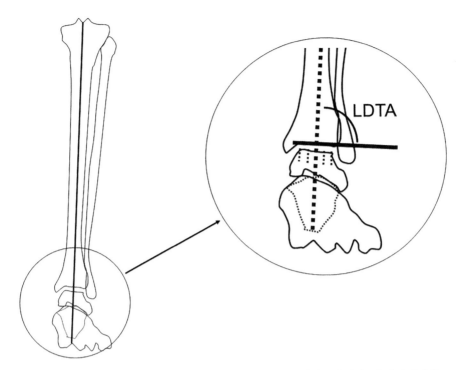

Fig. 5 Diagram of an anteroposterior radiograph of the ankle with the whole leg included. A line is drawn along the mechanical axis of the leg. In the inset picture provided, a magnification shows where the mechanical axis intersects the talus. The talus is subdivided in quarters with small vertical dotted lines. The alignment is measured by the distance in millimeters between the midpoint of the talus and the point where the mechanical axis of the leg intersects the talus. The alignment is measured also by the lateral distal tibial angle (LDTA) which is measured between the mechanical axis of the leg and a line tangential to the distal articular tibial joint surface

the other hand, a valgus of the ankle, will overcompensate with a varus subtalar joint. If a varus calcaneal osteotomy is performed, it will lead to an exaggeration of the ankle valgus due to peritalar instability [3]. In these cases, it is not useful to perform a calcaneal osteotomy, but a distractive subtalar arthrodesis is recommended instead [14]. It should be remembered that the subtalar joint more likely will compensate for deviations in the coronal plane when it is found without osteoarthritis, i.e., with preserved mobility [15].

Another important point to analyze is the foot, considering its function as a tripod, with the calcaneus, first and fifth metatarsals resting on the floor in static phase. In valgus deformities, an insufficiency of the medial column leads to a valgus inclination of the hindfoot (called "forefoot-driven hindfoot valgus"). This factor leads to asymmetrical lateral wear of the ankle cartilage due to overloading of the lateral aspect of the ankle. The wear of the cartilage leads to a loss of height of the hindfoot, which secondarily may end in a deltoid insufficiency, which in turn leads to a talar rotational instability. The talar rotational instability increases the asymmetric wear of the ankle. In forefoot-driven hindfoot valgus cases, the loading capability of

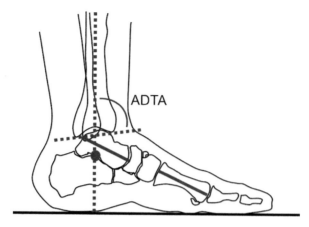

Fig. 6 Diagram of a lateral radiograph of the ankle. A line is drawn along the mechanical axis of the leg. This line normally intersects the talocalcaneal joint at the anterolateral process of the talus (represented by a circle). The alignment is measured by the distance in millimeters between the mechanical axis of the leg and the anterolateral process of the talus (along an imaginary line parallel to the floor). The alignment is measured also by the anterior distal tibial angle (ADTA) which is measured between the mechanical axis of the leg and a line tangential to the distal articular tibial joint surface

the medial column must be restored. The correction of the medial column insufficiency should be performed at the apex of the deformity. If the apex corresponds to an unstable or arthritic joint, a fusion is recommended. If no diseased joint is evident, a plantar flexion osteotomy of the medial column is one option (frequently of the medial cuneiform or cotton osteotomy), which will reduce the lateral ankle overload. In cavo-varus deformities, the varus hindfoot is tilted due to the medial column depression (called forefoot-driven hindfoot varus). In these cases, lateral and medial ankle instability can be found, as well as a torque increase in inversion due to the medialized Achilles pull which leads to greater load on the medial aspect of the ankle. This added to the relative weakness of the peroneal tendons increases the lateral instability and consequently the asymmetric ankle wear. Treatment for forefoot-driven hindfoot varus should include medial column elevation to decrease the inversion and load on the medial aspect of the ankle, for example, through a metatarsal elevation osteotomy [3].

4   Diagnosis and Analysis

4.1   Clinical Analysis

Patients with LOA initially present with ankle pain associated with changes in physical activity, changes in the surface where they develop their activity, differences in footwear, changes in body weight, etc. In other words, any variable that leads to an increase in the impact or torque that the ankle supports can cause this clinical picture. The pain may begin immediately after physical activity and subside in the following hours or persist for hours or days after completing the physical activity. In more advanced stages of arthrosis, pain may be present even at night [6].

The study of patients with osteoarthritis of the ankle should consider standing long leg radiographs, in addition to ankle X-rays. Alignment should be analyzed and evaluated at 3 levels, supramalleolar, intra-articular and infra-malleolar. As already mentioned, not only should we analyze the maintenance or alteration of the radiological indices (lateral distal angle of the tibia, talar tilt, anterior distal angle of the tibia), but we should also measure the leverage generated at the ankle level by measuring the distance between the calcaneal-hip mechanical axis and the center of the talus. Patients in early stages of the disease may have joint angles within normal, but will have ankle pain in the area affected by previous trauma (e.g., a pilon fracture with lateral joint damage) or alterations only visible within the joint on MRI or nuclear medicine tests such as Single Photon Emission Computed Tomography (SPECT-CT) (see Fig. 7). In more advanced stages of localized osteoarthritis, radiological alterations will already be seen consisting in changes in the joint space, angulation of the joint line, sclerosis or osteophytes, bone cysts or already formally advanced osteoarthritis.

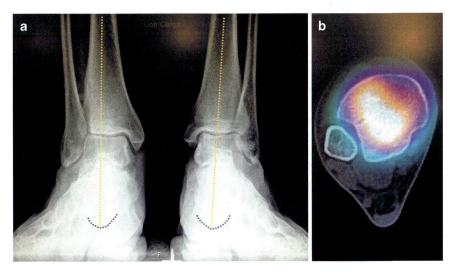

Fig. 7 Images from a patient with right ankle articular pain. (**a**) shows a bilateral ankle weight bearing radiograph, where the right ankle side is at the left of the image. Gross normal alignment can be observed. However, when drawing the mechanical axis of each leg, represented by the vertical dotted yellow line, a lateral overload of the right ankle joint can be suspected, represented by an increased distance between the midpoint of the talus and the intersection of the mechanical axis with the talus. (**b**) shows a SPECT-CT image of the right ankle joint of the same patient, where a clear increase in marker activity can be seen in the lateral half of the ankle pilon, confirming the lateral overload of the joint

In the analysis of patients with LOA, we must detect in the radiological study the apices of deformity. Once the apices are located, preservation surgery can be planned. It is accepted that the limit for attempting joint preservation surgery is determined by the amount of remaining cartilage, with up to 50% of the cartilage present in the ankle being accepted as adequate for joint preservation surgery. This theoretical limit for indicating joint preservation surgery can be inferred from the wear and tear on the ankle joint on loaded radiographs. If subchondral tibia-talus contact is already observed in the medial or lateral space of the ankle joint (gutters), in addition to subchondral tibia-talus contact being observed in the upper medial or lateral ankle space, it is no longer considered a candidate for joint preservating surgery. Formal contraindications for this approach are the presence of diffuse osteoarthritis, unreliable patients, bone infection, neurological deficit and neuroarthropathic disorders.

In terms of classifications, there are no generally accepted classifications for valgus arthrosis, but there are for varus osteoarthritis. For the latter cases, the Takakura classification is used, which uses load-bearing AP ankle X-rays, in which symptomatic ankle osteoarthritis without joint narrowing is considered a type 1; a type 2 presents with medial tibiotalar joint narrowing; a type 3A considers subchondral bone contact between the medial malleolus of the tibia and the corresponding talus; type 3B adds subchondral bone contact between the upper surface of the dome of the talus and the corresponding tibia (see Fig. 8); finally a diffuse osteoarthritis corresponds to a type 4 [16]. There is also the Knupp classification which can be used for valgus or varus osteoarthritis, in which stage 1 is diffuse osteoarthritis; stage 2 is localized osteoarthritis with tilt greater than 4° which is subdivided into: 2A if LOA has no subchondral bone contact; 2B if there is subchondral bone contact; 2C if there is talus protrusion through the tibial subchondral bone; and stage 3 is there is an isolated medial ankle osteoarthritis. This classification also considers whether there is correct alignment in the sagittal plane or whether there is an anterior extrusion of the talus, by adding to the main group a letter C (centered) or E (extruded) [17]. With respect to the use of other imaging modalities, the use of SPECT CT has been useful since it has been associated with failure of joint preservation treatment when cystic joint lesions, bipolar lesions, anterocentral tibial, anterocentral and medial talar uptake are detected on the exam. In isolation, the presence of bipolar lesions on SPECT CT is significantly associated with failure of joint preservation surgery [18].

4.2   Mechanical Analysis

The authors find the use of pre-operative planning extremely useful, for which several computer applications are available (e.g., Bone ninja app). With these applications, the necessary correction can be more adequately estimated at both the supra- and infra-malleolar levels and allows for better preparation of supplies and surgical time. When facing a patient with symptomatic LOA, we must analyze the type of mechanical overload of the ankle with or without radiological ankle wear, the talar tilt, the ankle joint congruency or symmetry, the subtalar joint and the foot alignment. We will analyze each of these characteristics in the following paragraphs.

Fig. 8 Anteroposterior weight bearing ankle radiograph of a 52-year-old patient. Moderate arthrosis can be seen at the ankle joint, with tilting of the talus into varus, and decreased joint space in the medial tibio-talar space and in the upper tibio-talar space. This can be classified as a varus ankle arthrosis Takakura type 3B

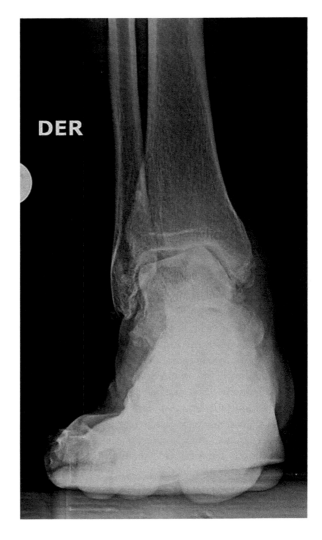

4.2.1 Type of Mechanical Overload of the Ankle

We must differentiate whether the patient presents a radiological consequence of his or her joint overload, that is, a skeletal malalignment with asymmetry of the ankle joint space. In this way, the following mechanical situations can occur: patients without radiological wear (without articular asymmetry of the ankle) but with medial, lateral, anterior or posterior mechanical overload (cavus feet, flat feet, metatarsal adductus, etc.) which we will call neutral ankles; patients with medial or lateral radiological wear of the ankle (medial or lateral overload), which we will call varus or valgus ankles; and patients with anterior or posterior wear of the ankle (anterior or posterior overload) that can generate anterior or posterior subluxated ankles.

Neutral Ankles

It should be considered that there are cases with medial, lateral, anterior or posterior overload of the ankle that, being initial, do not yet present visible wear and deformity in ankle X-rays. In these cases, a long leg mechanical axis deviation could be observed (congenital limb deformity), associated with ankle symptoms such as periodic synovitis according to the level of activity of the patient. These cases can be treated with joint preservation surgery, but it is not always needed to perform supramalleolar corrections, since the ankle is still preserved. In these cases, we must plan corrections at the apex of the deformity (called inframalleolar in cases of foot deformities), either at a subtalar level in isolation or combined with a correction at a medial column level (flatfoot or pes cavus surgery, for example). In valgus deviations of the hindfoot, if an apex of deformity is found at the medial column (i.e., a loss of the Meary's angle or "sag" at a particular joint) an osteotomy or arthrodesis of the involved joint should be considered to achieve medial column plantar flexion. The Cotton osteotomy is the most frequently used. In cases of severe subtalar deformities with talonavicular subluxation, peritalar instability cannot be resolved by medial column plantar flexion. Procedures that attempt to align the talus over the calcaneus are recommended [19]. This can be achieved through a calcaneal lengthening osteotomy, with or without a medializing posterior calcaneal osteotomy, procedures that can be associated or not with a reconstruction of the medial ligament complex of the ankle (intraoperative decision depending on the resulting alignment of the hindfoot) [14]. In hindfoot varus cases, it is frequent to find a midfoot cavus with an increased first metatarsal load, leading to medial ankle overload (forefoot contribution to the hindfoot varus). In addition, there is a muscular imbalance that often accompanies cavo-varus feet, with lateral instability and selective loss of strength (peroneal muscle paresis). The Coleman test is often used to determine the contribution of the forefoot to the hindfoot varus. It helps to decide whether to perform surgery to elevate the medial column if the deformity is flexible (positive Coleman test). With a negative Coleman test (i.e., none or minimal forefoot contribution to hindfoot varus) a calcaneal osteotomy should be added to a first metatarsal elevating osteotomy. In more severe cases there is significant equinus and forefoot adductus. Midfoot osteotomies are recommended for these cases, where the entire midfoot can be derotated in relation to the hindfoot.

Varus or Valgus Ankles

When analyzing the radiological deformity, we will analyze the deviation of the extremity mechanical axis (from hip to calcaneus) using the projection called long leg ray or teleradiography of lower extremities. In addition to the LDTA angle (lateral distal tibial angle) and the talar tilt, importance has been given to the torque or moment generated at the ankle. The latter is calculated measuring the distance (in mm) between the hip – calcaneus mechanical axis and the center of the ankle. For varus ankles with medial osteoarthritis, the load bearing axis will traverse the ankle joint through its medial half. The opposite will occur for valgus ankles with lateral LOA. To achieve symptomatic relief, the aim is to unload the diseased half of the ankle joint and overload the healthier tibiotalar cartilage. This should be performed by means of a supramalleolar osteotomy (SMOT) that moves the extremity mechanical axis to the healthier joint half. If the talar dome is divided into four quarters in an anteroposterior radiographic ankle projection, our aim will be to position the "new" weight bearing axis on the contralateral quarter (see Fig. 5). This mechanical axis correction corresponds to an LDTA overcorrection of approximately 5° [20].

Ankles with Talar Anterior or Posterior Subluxation

This type of deformity is visible on a lateral ankle or foot X-ray. Generally, the tibial weight bearing axis intersects the anterolateral process of the talus. The angle measured is the anterior distal tibial angle (ADTA) with a normal value of 81° on average. In cases of post-traumatic deformities in which there are supramalleolar malunions with shortening of the anterior pilon column or anterior ankle wear, the tibial load axis intersects the talus posterior to the anterolateral process. In these cases, the ADTA decreases below 80°. The resulting joint load is increased in the anterior half of the distal tibial joint surface (anterior ankle overload) (see Fig. 9).

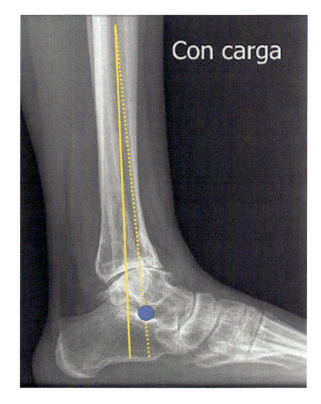

Fig. 9 Lateral weight bearing ankle radiograph showing posttraumatic localized arthrosis at the anterior aspect of the ankle joint. Please see the osteophytes on the anterior aspect of the ankle joint, besides the decrease in joint space. The mechanical axis of the leg is drawn as a yellow line, and it can be observed how the line intersects the subtalar joint posterior to the anterolateral process of the talus, representing an anterior displacement of the talus and therefore an anterior overload of the ankle joint

This constitutes an ankle with anterior talus subluxation simulating recurvatum deformities that are poorly tolerated, as previously discussed. In cases of post-traumatic deformities in which there are supramalleolar malunions with shortening of the posterior pilon column or posterior wear of the ankle cartilage, the load axis of the tibia intersects the talus anterior to its anterolateral process. In these cases, the ADTA increases above 81°. The resulting load is increased in the posterior ankle half (posterior ankle overload). This deformity presents clinically as an anterior ankle impingement and is better tolerated than the previously mentioned deformity. The treatment of both previous situations generally consists of a SMOT that corrects the anterior distal tibial angle as well as the ankle mechanical alignment.

4.2.2 Analysis of the Talar Tilt

Frequently the deformity is intra-articular, either because of a post-traumatic intra-articular deformity (for example, after a pilon fracture), or because of an extremity mal alignment that evolved into localized ankle osteoarthritis. In these cases, there is a pathological inclination of the talus within its mortise, which leads to an increased talar tilt. It is important to measure the talar tilt since it has been seen that in SMOT for localized osteoarthritis in varus ankles, the clinical results are better if the tilt is less than 10° [21]. In cases where the tilt already exceeds 5°, it is recommended that when performing the SMOT, check under fluoroscopy if the tilt is manually correctable within its mortise. This is done by stabilizing the distal end of the tibia with one hand and forcing the hindfoot to the opposite attempting to correct the talar tilt. If the tilt is corrected, the supramalleolar osteotomy can be performed in isolation. If the talus persists misaligned, and preoperatively or intraoperatively it has been detected that there is a severe pilon joint collapse that explains the tilt, an articular osteotomy or "plafondplasty" can be done. Studies at six years of follow-up show good results with this technique in which the talar tilt in varus improved from 19° to 7° [22]. Evidently this surgery is more demanding and needs the use of double plates for fixation. Another alternative to treat varus talar tilt over 5° that does not correct with intraoperative manual maneuvers, is to intraoperatively use a medial or lateral pin distractor (Hintermann's distractor) or external fixator (should be positioned depending on where the soft tissue retraction is). This helps reduce the talar tilt. Good results have been reported with this technique, but with a low number of cases, with a follow-up of five years [23]. This technique is indicated when retracted soft tissues are responsible for the talar tilt and not an intra-articular bone deformity.

4.2.3 Symmetry of the Ankle Join

The purpose of ankle preservation surgery should be to achieve the best possible alignment, improving balance and load distribution within the ankle. We should be able to decrease the loads in the damaged or arthritic sector of the ankle, increasing relatively the load in the healthier segment of the ankle. The final goal is to achieve symptomatic improvement and prolong the life of the ankle to the maximum. Joint symmetry means a uniform joint space is present throughout the joint with no (or minimum) talar tilt. This is very uncommon in cases of LOA, in which a joint asymmetry is present most of the time. Cadaveric studies have found that SMOT improves joint congruency and load distribution within the ankle in a more predictable way when performed in conjunction with a fibula osteotomy [24]. Fibular osteotomies allow the talus to be repositioned as symmetrically as possible within its mortise after a SMOT. A relative fibular shortening (together with a valgizing SMOT) helps in cases of varus deformities [3] (in addition to a medial gutter debridement) by "pulling" the talus into valgus. In cases of valgus deformities, a fibular lengthening osteotomy is indicated, working as a lateral talar buttress. The authors always consider adding a fibular osteotomy to a SMOT to obtain better correction of joint symmetry.

4.2.4 Subtalar Joint

We should try to differentiate how much the subtalar joint is involved in the ankle overload. In cases of ankle valgus osteoarthritis (lateral LOA), if the subtalar joint is also in valgus, it will be increasing and worsening the intra-articular overload of the ankle. The opposite will occur in varus deformities. For the hindfoot alignment evaluation, a Saltzman axial X-ray or a WBCT is recommended. The WBCT will help to measure the Foot and Ankle Offset (FAO) as well. The FAO analyzes the foot as if it were a tripod in which the head of the first metatarsal, the head of the fifth metatarsal and the point of contact of the calcaneus with the floor form a triangle. The center of the talar dome is then determined. If the talar dome center lies medial to the triangle axis, the foot is considered to be aligned in valgus. On the contrary, if the talus center is lateral to the triangle axis, the foot is considered to be aligned in varus (FAO is expressed as a percentage relative to the foot length, normal values FAO: 2.3%, varus feet: −11.6%, valgus feet: 11.4%) [25].

Calcaneal osteotomies or subtalar arthrodesis help to increase the SMOT correction power regarding weight bearing axis location. If the subtalar joint is healthy (no signs of osteoarthritis), a displacement calcaneal osteotomy can be considered (valgus producing for varus ankle osteoarthritis, and varus producing for valgus ankle osteoarthritis) to improve load distribution at the ankle level (see Fig. 10). The amount of calcaneal displacement depends directly on the distance in millimeters that we want to move the limb load axis (see commentary in paragraph entitled "Type of mechanical overload of the ankle"). When comparing different type of calcaneal osteotomies, no biomechanical advantage has been found in studies of varus ankles in terms of decreasing medial intra-articular pressure when doing a lateralizing calcaneal osteotomy versus a z-osteotomy or a lateralizing osteotomy plus wedge resection. In varus deformities, a pure lateralizing osteotomy can be sufficient and is technically simpler [26].

Peritalar instability should be ruled out using a CT or WBCT ensuring that peritalar joint relationships are maintained. If this is not the case and peritalar instability is suspected (a common condition in valgus flat feet), a calcaneal osteotomy is not recommended, and a subtalar arthrodesis would be more reliable.

Fig. 10 Lateral weight
bearing ankle radiograph
showing a calcaneal
osteotomy performed in a
medial ankle overload
case. The ankle presented a
varus localized arthrosis,
and therefore a valgizating
calcaneal osteotomy to
improve load distribution
at the ankle joint was
performed and fixed with
two screws

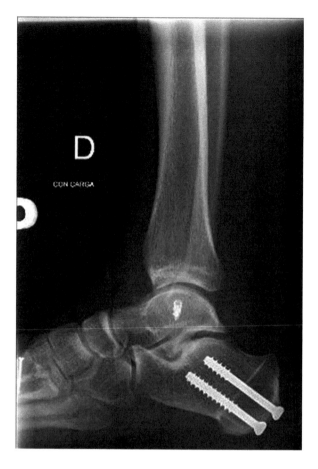

4.2.5 Alignment of the Foot

Finally, we must consider the alignment of the foot. If there is an instability of the medial column of the foot, characteristic of valgus plane deformities, we must analyze the foot with concepts of acquired flatfoot. For cases of varus hindfoot with medial ankle overload, we will analyze the contribution of the foot to the varus hindfoot using concepts of cavo-varus foot (see commentary in paragraph entitled "Type of mechanical overload of the ankle").

5 Treatment

Any treatment that seeks to lessen the symptoms for localized osteoarthritis of the ankle should decrease the load and impact on the joint. Therefore, weight management, physical fitness and healthy living should be promoted. Impact activities should be avoided as well. The use of insoles and shoes that have cushioning help decrease ankle joint impact. The use of intra-articular injections with corticoids or hyaluronic acid achieved partial and temporary symptomatic improvement. They are helpful but not a lasting option. The use of analgesics and oral anti-inflammatories is indicated in an intermittent manner for pain crisis. Failure of conservative treatment means that a more radical treatment is needed. A surgical procedure will have to include actions determined by the previous mechanical analysis. We will analyze the surgical procedures depending on the type of mechanical overload of the ankle.

5.1 Lateral Mechanical Ankle Overload

5.1.1 Arthroscopy

In general, arthroscopy is the initial procedure used to diagnose medial or lateral instabilities that may have been in doubt, remove free bodies, remove exostoses that may be impeding ankle mobility, or perform bone marrow stimulation procedures on osteochondral lesions which are not validated in the literature but may favor the SMOT outcome. When removing anterior exostoses of the tibia, the surgeon should remember that they are part of a biomechanical response to instability and osteoarthritis. The surgeon should not be aggressive in removing these exostoses since they can destabilize the ankle [3]. It should also be confirmed that there is remaining cartilage in the joint (at least 50%), so that a SMOT is likely to be successful.

5.1.2 Osteotomy Depending on Type of Radiological Wear

1. Neutral ankle

   If no alteration is found in the extremity alignment study (hip-calcaneus), the axis alteration is probably in the foot. In these cases, it is not necessary to perform supramalleolar osteotomies (SMOT) as already mentioned before. The foot should be corrected accordingly depending on where the apex of the deformity is located (go to Sect. 5.1.4 and 5.1.5 of this surgical technique).

2. Ankle with valgus arthritic deviation

   In these cases, the hip-calcaneus mechanical load axis intersects the talar dome through its lateral half. The ankle will have an articular asymmetry (intra-articular valgus) with alteration of the LDTA (under 90°) and probably an altered talar tilt (see Fig. 11). The correction should be planned to move the load axis to the medial half of the ankle joint, which corresponds to an overcorrection of the LTDA by 5°. This correction should be made through a varus producing SMOT. With a digital planning app (e.g., Bone ninja), it is easy to evaluate how much supramalleolar correction is needed to move the mechanical load axis to the desired position. If you do

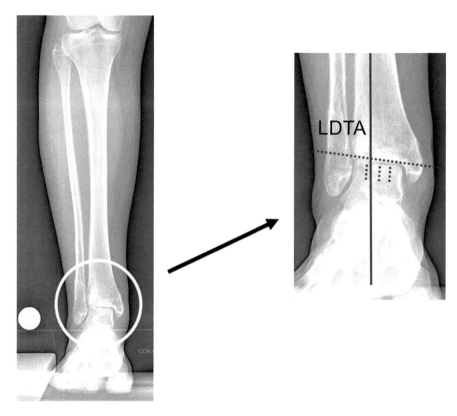

Fig. 11 Anteroposterior weight bearing ankle radiograph, where a lateral ankle overload can be suspected. Please see the augmented image on the right side of the figure, where the mechanical axis is represented by a vertical continuous line. The talus is subdivided in quarters by small, dashed lines. Please note that the mechanical axis of the leg intersects the talus through its lateral quarter, representing a lateral mechanical overload. The angle that can be measured is the LDTA or lateral distal tibial angle, which will measure less than 90°

not have a planning app, the recommendation is to calculate the osteotomy with respect to the LDTA. If the LDTA is 85° (5° of valgus), it should be brought to 95° (5° of varus) to achieve the desired overcorrection.

Most of these cases present with an intra-articular apex of deformity and not a supramalleolar one, because the deformity is generated by a posttraumatic localized joint arthrosis, rather than by a bone deformity. Cases of malunited tibia fracture or a long standing congenital tibial deformity (tibia valga) could present with both a supramalleolar deformity (at the tibial deformity) and an intraarticular deformity (at the degenerated joint). To avoid overlooking these findings, always start the ankle evaluation with a long leg x-ray to rule out other causes for the LOA.

The ankle radiological study is performed by drawing the mechanical axis of the tibia (from center of tibial spines to center of tibial plafond) and a line parallel to the tibial pilon. The resulting angle is the LDTA and should be 90° in a normal ankle. For valgus ankles LDTA will be <90°.

When a SMOT is performed for LOA with an intraarticular deformity apex, since the tibial osteotomy is performed outside the apex, the so-called third rule of osteotomies occurs. This rule mandates that when angular misalignment is corrected through an osteotomy outside the deformity apex, a secondary translation of the distal segment occurs [27]. This secondary translation occurs in the direction of correction (a SMOT in varus medializes the distal segment). This third rule is desirable in arthritic cases since it further helps with mechanical axis medialization. The most frequently used tibial osteotomy is medial wedge resection. As already mentioned, the authors recommend always adding a lengthening fibular osteotomy, which favors adequate replacement of the talus in its mortise. If a supramalleolar angular correction greater than 10° is necessary, dome osteotomies are preferred.

Supramalleolar Osteotomy Technique: Wedge Osteotomy

Tibial wedge resection uses a trigonometric equation or formula for planning: the height of the wedge should measure: $H = \tan \alpha * W$, with H being the wedge height to be resected, α the degrees to be corrected, and W the tibial width at the height of the osteotomy (32 mm in average). If we take an ankle valgus with an LDTA of 83°, it has an intra-articular deformity of 7° of valgus (difference to reach 90° of LDTA). An 5° overcorrection must be achieved in arthritic cases, so the target LDTA is 95°. In this hypothetical case, a 12° correction must be calculated. Applying the formula previously shown, a 7 mm wedge should be resected to correct 12°. Because this formula is easy to forget, there is a simpler rule of thumb which can be followed. If there is an LDTA of 83°, the difference with a normal LDTA is calculated, e.g., 7° (difference between 90 and 83° LDTA). Then, the wedge to be resected should be a 7 mm wedge (number of mms equivalent to number of degrees).

A longitudinal medial approach is made at the distal tibial end. The osteotomy is located under radiographs according to the preoperative planning. In general, the osteotomy is performed in metaphyseal bone, 3–4 cm proximal to the tibiotalar joint, in the metaphyseal area where the tibia is concave in its medial aspect. The osteotomy trajectory should be oblique from proximal medial to distal lateral, so that it ends at the tibiofibular syndesmosis (about 2 cm proximal to the ankle joint). This makes the lateral osteotomy exit more stable thanks to the syndesmotic ligaments in that area. Two K-wires are used marking the proximal and distal limits of the wedge to be resected. The wedge height has already been calculated in the preoperative planning. The two Kirschner wires must be placed from the medial side, converging towards the lateral side. An oscillating saw of adequate length is used to resect the wedge, using frequent cooling and intermittent power (avoiding thermal osteonecrosis). If we use the previously mentioned example with an LDTA of 83°, this wedge demarcated by the wires should be of 7 mm height. Once the bone wedge is resected, the osteotomy should be closed and a Kirschner wire is used for temporary fixation (see Fig. 12). If correction is adequate, a small fragment locking plate is used. If talar correction is not adequate, check for calcifications on the

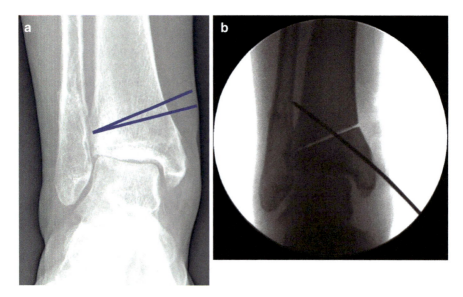

Fig. 12 Anteroposterior ankle radiograph of the same patient shown in Fig. 11. (**a**) shows the planned resection of a supramalleolar medial closing wedge, to achieve a varizating effect. (**b**) shows the bone wedge already resected, and the osteotomy closed and fixed temporarily with K wires

anteromedial tibial rim that could prevent talus correction. The position and length of the fibula should also be monitored (see Sect. 5.1.3 of this surgical technique).

Supramalleolar Technique: Dome Osteotomy

An anterior ankle approach is performed, over the distal metaphysis of the tibia. Subperiosteal dissection is performed, and the osteotomy site is marked according to preoperative planning, usually 3–4 cm proximal to the ankle joint line. It is recommended that the osteotomy be planned using a third tube plate by fixing one end of the plate as subchondral as possible to the distal tibia and rotating the other end of the plate, using it as a compass. In the third or fourth hole (coinciding with 3–4 cm proximal to the articular surface), multiple drill holes are made to "draw" the osteotomy at the distal tibial metaphysis. The fibula should always be included in these cases performing an oblique osteotomy at the same level of the tibial osteotomy (through the same approach or through a separate lateral approach). The tibial dome osteotomy is completed with a small osteotome uniting the drill holes previously made.

The amount of rotation needed at the osteotomy should be confirmed with fluoroscopy until adequate correction is achieved. An alternative way of estimating correction is to measure the mms of step formed at the osteotomy level medially; 10 mm is equivalent to 20° of correction / [28]. A Hintermann's distractor (pin distractor) is of great help when performing the rotation. Once the osteotomy has been sufficiently rotated, it is temporarily fixed with Kirschner wires. If the desired correction has been achieved, 2 anterior locking plates are recommended for definitive fixation.

5.1.3   Ankle Symmetry

In cases where SMOT has been performed through a medial closing tibial wedge osteotomy, the general recommendation is to perform a fibular osteotomy when it prevents adequate correction of the talus in its mortise. This is measured by evaluating the talar tilt after the SMOT correction. When the desired correction is greater than 10° or the ankle is congruent (no increased talar tilt, such as in initial LOA with minimum cartilage wear), fibular osteotomy is necessary to avoid paradoxical load shifts in the joint [24]. In general, the authors recommend always performing a long oblique fibular osteotomy, at the level of the tibia osteotomy, through a direct lateral approach to ensure adequate tibiotalar load transfer, both in cases of varus and valgus osteoarthritis. The fibula should always be fixed in the position that allows an adequate reduction of the mortise, usually by lengthening it minimally. In some cases (severe valgus) it is necessary to lengthen the fibula by 1 cm or more. For these cases, a Z osteotomy is recommended, which is very stable and easy to fix (resembles a "scarf osteotomy")(see Fig. 13). In cases of valgus LOA, with a preoperative tilt greater than 10° in valgus, a plafondplasty or even grafting in the area of lateral collapse should be considered (see alternative to plafondplasty for osteoarthritis varus below).

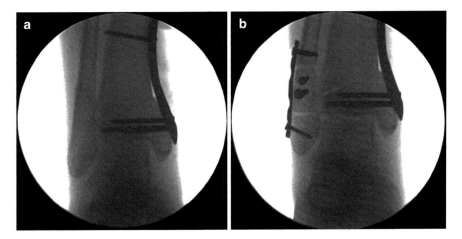

Fig. 13 Anteroposterior ankle radiograph of the same patient shown in Fig. 12. (**a**) shows a distal tibial plate fixing the supramalleolar osteotomy. Please note the slightly shortened fibula, represented by an increased space between the talus and the distal end of the fibula. (**b**) shows a lengthening fibular osteotomy, performed in a "z" fashion, and stabilized by two interfragmentary screws and a small third tubular plate

5.1.4 Inframalleolar Correction

As noted in the biomechanics paragraph, there are cases of lateral ankle overload without extremity malalignment. In these cases, the alignment should be analyzed at the inframalleolar and midfoot level. If there are no signs of subtalar instability, we will decide whether to add a medializing calcaneal osteotomy. In cases where a SMOT was performed, it is important to have a complete preoperative planning to be prepared to add a calcaneal osteotomy if necessary. We must clinically evaluate the hindfoot axis after completion of the SMOT to assess whether it is slightly varus or neutral (which is the objective). If the SMOT did not completely correct the lever arm described above as much as necessary, a medializing calcaneal osteotomy should be added. The medializing osteotomy of the calcaneus or Koutsogiannis technique, is performed through a direct lateral approach on the calcaneus, oblique in 45° from proximal cephalic to distal caudal, accessing the lateral surface of the calcaneus. After careful dissection two Hohmann-type retractors are placed, one in the proximal cephalic concave part of the calcaneus, and another is placed in the lower concave part of the calcaneus. The osteotomy is initiated with an oscillating saw (with frequent cooling) until it touches the medial cortex of the calcaneus. A narrow chisel is then used to carefully breach numerous areas of the medial calcaneal cortex and then completed with a wider osteotome (1 cm or more). This ensures that no damage is done to the medial neurovascular bundle. The ankle is brought into plantar flexion to relax the Achilles tendon and the posterior tuberosity is then moved medially according to preoperative planning. Two axial screws are recommended for fixation (4 mm or more in diameter).

5.1.5 Foot Deformity - Stability of the Medial Column

In cases of valgus LOA, it is common to find instabilities of the medial column associated with flatfoot. In these cases, the joints that may be unstable include the talo-navicular, naviculocuneiform, and cuneometatarsal joints. It is beyond the scope of this chapter to analyze a flatfoot deformity, but a medially unstable foot should be addressed as an unstable flatfoot and the apex of the medial column should be located through clinical analysis and AP and lateral X-ray of the patient's foot. If an apex is identified in which the medial column presents a plantar sag or deformity, plantar flexion osteotomies (cotton osteotomy) are recommended in young patients without arthrosis. If there is severe instability with evident subluxation of a medial column joint, or older patients with associated osteoarthritis, an arthrodesis of the involved joints is recommended. If there is a symptomatic hallux valgus, we recommend performing plantar flexion of the first metatarsal through a cuneometatarsal fusion, thus correcting the medial column insufficiency and the first metatarsal varus.

5.1.6 Ligament Reconstruction

In a valgus deformity we must consider repairing medial hindfoot-midfoot ligaments. Radiographs under varus or valgus stress can help identify these cases. If ankle instability is identified, bone anchored sutures may be added to the medial or lateral side of the ankle. Continuing distally, the spring ligament may be damaged as well as the entire tibiocalcaneonavicular component. In cases of severe instability, allograft or synthetic graft reconstruction may be considered.

5.2 Medial Ankle Mechanical Overload

5.2.1 Arthroscopy

As in the case of lateral overloads or ankle valgus, we must begin with an arthroscopy to confirm there is at least a 50% of remaining cartilage. Intra-articular free bodies are removed and any exostosis that is believed to be participating in ankle motion restriction is resected.

5.2.2 Osteotomy Depending on Type of Radiological Wear

1. Neutral ankle

   As discussed in the biomechanics paragraph, it is possible to find patients with ankle pain and clinical ankle synovitis due to medial ankle overload, without yet presenting with osteoarthritis or loss of cartilage thickness on the medial side of the ankle. These patients benefit from ankle-sparing surgeries that realign the limb to correct the medial overload and should be treated as cavo-varus deformities. As such, osteotomies or arthrodesis that correct the varus hindfoot and medial column elevations allowing a more plantigrade foot are recommended. These procedures decrease medial ankle pressure (see Chap. 26 on cavarus feet). It is the authors preference to correct pronation of the forefoot in relation to the hindfoot through midfoot osteotomies rather than isolated osteotomies of the first metatarsal.

2. Ankle with varus arthritic deviation

   In cases of varus LOA (LDTA>90°), as we discussed in the biomechanics section, there is information that suggests that the more lateral we move the weight bearing axis, the better functional results can be obtained. The current preference is to perform a SMOT that moves the weight bearing axis to the lateral central talar dome quarter [20]. To perform this, the ankle should end up in a slight valgus (LDTA <90°). As with ankle valgus deviations, most of these cases present an intra-articular deformity apex, due to ankle cartilage wear. This apex can be evaluated by drawing the mechanical axis of the tibia and a line parallel to the surface of the tibial pilon (this resulting angle is the LDTA and should be 90° in a normal ankle). In these cases, since the tibial SMOT is performed proximal to the apex, the so-called third rule of osteotomies occurs. This rule means that when an angular correction is performed outside the deformity apex, a secondary translation of the distal segment occurs [27]. This secondary translation in cases of valgus SMOT, means there is a distal segment lateralization. Lateral translation is desired since it favors and strengthens the correction into valgus of the mechanical axis.

The most frequently recommended osteotomy is the opening medial tibial wedge plus fibular shortening. If the correction needed is greater than 10°, dome osteotomies are preferred.

For medial tibial opening wedge, the same formula already presented is used (H = tan α * W). The only difference is that the height delivered by the formula corresponds to the height of the opening wedge, instead of the wedge to be resected. The authors use the same rules discussed for closing wedge osteotomies. An easier technique is to open the wedge the number of mm corresponding to the number of degrees of deformity (if LDTA = 95°, then open 5 mm).

In cases where the talar tilt exceeds 10°, soft tissue retraction and/or medial tibial plafond erosion must be suspected. In those cases, some procedure should be added to improve the talar tilt. Recommended procedures include aggressive releases of the medial ankle ligament, medial malleolus osteotomy, medial soft tissue distraction through an external fixator or performing an intra-articular osteotomy - plafondplasty. For cases with tilt under 5° that persist after SMOT, an aggressive deltoid ligament release is sufficient. In cases where the tilt exceeds 5° after SMOT, and a change in the curvature of the tibial plafond is observed, the authors recommend adding the previously mentioned intra-articular osteotomy (plafondplasty) to the supramalleolar osteotomy.

Intraarticular Ankle Osteotomy (Plafondplasty) Technique

This technique is recommended in cases where the talar tilt is over 5° and there are significant erosions on the medial tibial plafond. Normally, the tibial joint line is straight. If there is a depression or change in curvature medially at the joint, an intra-articular osteotomy may be indicated.

The same medial approach is used as for supramalleolar osteotomy. A Kirschner wire is used to plan the osteotomy. It starts 2 to 2.5 cm proximal to the ankle joint line. The exit point of the osteotomy should be planned just lateral to the erosion site or change in the tibial plafond curvature. After placing and confirming under fluoroscopy the position of the guide wire, 2 to 3 one mm Kirchner wires are placed parallel to the tibiotalar joint, in a subchondral position from medial to lateral. These thin wires help avoiding the osteotomy completion so that the cartilage is not violated when the osteotomy is performed. The osteotomy is then performed with an oscillating saw. Check the AP image to make sure that the cut plane is straight. A distractor or osteotome is then used to open the osteotomy until a straight joint line is obtained, thus eliminating the joint incongruence. This position is secured with a structured graft and fully threaded screws. After completing the intra-articular osteotomy, the supramalleolar osteotomy is performed [29].

Supramalleolar Osteotomy Technique: Opening Tibial Wedge Osteotomy

This technique is simpler than the closing wedge resection seen previously. A medial approach is used on the distal tibia. The apex where the osteotomy is to be performed must be located and marked with a single Kirschner wire. Following the wire, the osteotomy is performed with an oscillating saw. Then, the osteotomy is opened, thus correcting the arthritic varus malalignment (see Fig. 14). The calculations for performing this medial tibial opening are the same as those explained for the medial tibial closure. If there is a varus deformity with a 97° LDTA (7° deformity), the tibial opening wedge should overcorrect the LDTA to 85° (12° of total correction). Using the previously explained rule, we would just equal the opening wedge to the number of degrees of the deformity, which equals 7 mm. It is recommended to use a structural graft to fill the gap, being the authors preference a structural iliac crest allograft. For fixation, a locking medial tibial plate is recommended. A very frequent finding for opening tibial wedges of 5 mm or more, is that the lateral tibial cortex does not open as a hinge and distracts. This decreases the angular correction power and increases the limb length. If this distraction occurs, a lateral non locking plate should be placed at the lateral tibial osteotomy exit. One screw above the osteotomy and one below is enough to avoid osteotomy distraction allowing osteotomy angular opening.

Fig. 14 Anteroposterior ankle fluoroscopic image, where a medial opening wedge supramalleolar osteotomy was performed, besides a fibular closing wedge osteotomy. The tibial osteotomy is shown being opened with a lamina spreader, correcting the ankle varus

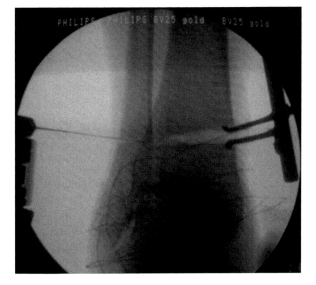

Supramalleolar Osteotomy Technique: Dome Osteotomy

A technique similar to the one mentioned for lateral ankle overload is performed for medial ankle overloads. The difference occurs when the osteotomy is rotated or moved as it is turned in the opposite direction, valgizing the distal bone segment. The amount of rotation needed at the osteotomy should be confirmed with fluoroscopy until adequate correction is achieved. An alternative way of estimating correction is to measure the mms of step formed at the osteotomy level medially; 10 mm is equivalent to 20° of correction [28]. Once the osteotomy has been rotated, it is fixed with 1 or 2 anterior tibial locking plates.

5.2.3 Ankle Symmetry

It is the experience of the authors that a fibula osteotomy should almost always be performed, to allow an adequate correction of the talus. There are some cases in which due to dysplasia of the medial malleolus (longstanding varus) the literature does not recommend performing a fibula osteotomy, so that the medial malleolus pushes and closes the mortise thus reducing the talus. The authors believe that this is very uncommon and the cases reported that benefit from this alternative are scarce [30]. Usually, an oblique osteotomy is sufficient to shorten the fibula to pull the talus to its corrected position and not impede the varus correction. This osteotomy is usually fixed with a non-locking third tubular plate. It should be kept in mind that in ankles with medial malleolus dysplasia (in varus, short and rounded malleolus), an additional osteotomy of the medial malleolus can be considered to achieve medial tibiotalar space closure. If the preoperative tilt is greater than 10° in varus and there is a medial depression of the joint, a plafondplasty should be considered in cases of varus osteoarthritis.

5.2.4 Inframalleolar Correction

As noted in the biomechanics paragraph, there are cases of medial ankle overload without evident ankle malalignment, but it should be noted that this is much rarer than for lateral ankle overloads. The approach to these cases is seen in the chapter on cavovarus deformities, and consist of hindfoot valgizing procedures, medial column elevating techniques and soft tissue procedures to achieve a static (repair of lateral and/or medial ligaments) and dynamic balance (tendon transfers or tenodesis). After completion of the supra- and intra-articular phase, the alignment of the hindfoot should be in neutral or slight valgus, from 2 to 5°. If this is not achieved, consideration should be given to add an inframalleolar correction, consisting of a lateralizing calcaneal osteotomy or subtalar arthrodesis. The authors recommend always to combine both lateralizing (Koutsogiannis = translation) and valgus (Dwyer = wedge resection) methods for calcaneal correction to enhance the weight bearing axis lateralization. Performing midfoot or medial column elevation osteotomies should also be evaluated on a case-by-case basis. Lateralizing and valgus osteotomy of the calcaneus is performed in a similar way to the medializing osteotomy described in the previous section. The desired effect of the osteotomy is to lateralize the load axis. The posterior calcaneal tuberosity must be laterally translated in addition to a lateral calcaneal wall wedge resection of approximately 5 mm. This technique combination will enhance the valgus effect of the osteotomy. It is usually fixed with two axially placed screws.

5.2.5   Foot Deformity

In the case of cavovarus feet, we must consider whether the position of the forefoot can be fully corrected through an elevation osteotomy of the first metatarsal, or if a midfoot osteotomy is necessary to completely correct the foot. The latter type of osteotomies is preferred by the authors and have the greatest correction power. The first metatarsal elevation osteotomy and the midfoot osteotomy are described in detail in the cavovarus foot section.

5.2.6   Ligament Reconstruction

The lateral and medial ankle ligaments are frequently compromised and must be evaluated intra-operatively and aggressively reconstructed. The lateral side requires the use of anchors and sometimes even grafts since after the debridement (necessary to achieve a reduction of the talus in its mortise), the ligaments can be damaged. Medially, a deltoid imbrication is generally enough.

Since these are long-standing varus deformities, the peroneal tendons are usually damaged and must be examined and repaired if necessary. If complete ruptures are found, autograft or free allograft can be used to reconstruct the peroneus brevis or longus. If both tendons are completely ruptured, it is recommended to reconstruct one of them with an auto or allograft and to perform a tenodesis of the remnant (brevis to longus). It is preferable to keep the longus since it achieves greater eversion leverage in the forefoot.

5.3   Anterior or Posterior Mechanical Overload of the Ankle (Sagittal Plane)

Generally, the tibial load axis intersects the anterolateral talus process in the lateral ankle X-ray. The angle measured is the anterior distal angle of the tibia (ADTA, normal value 81°) which was mentioned in the mechanical analysis section. Deformities in the sagittal plane are usually associated with deformities in the coronal plane. Anterior ankle overload (with anterior talar subluxation) is usually corrected with a posterior tibial closing wedge; rarely anterior opening osteotomies are performed. In cases of posterior ankle overload (with posterior talar subluxations), correction is achieved through anterior tibial wedge resections. The correction is achieved through the same calculation commented before, that is, resecting a wedge that equals the number of degrees in mm. It is common to find fibular or syndesmotic malunions that contribute to ankle deformities in the sagittal plane. In these cases, fibular corrective osteotomies or tibiofibular arthrodesis are added to the SMOT to aid in the correction. When correcting sagittal deformities of more than 10°, a Dome osteotomy can be considered, and we recommend performing it from a medial approach.

5.3.1 Supramalleolar Osteotomy Technique: Wedge Osteotomy

In the case of combined coronal and sagittal plane deformities that are being corrected through tibial wedge osteotomies, it is quite simple to add a second plane to the resection. Through the same approach performed for the correction of varus or valgus, a second plane can be added to the resected wedge, that is, to perform a biplanar wedge osteotomy. A posterior wedge resection is added if we want to correct an anterior ankle overload. Vice-versa, an anterior wedge resection is added if we want to correct a posterior ankle overload. After performing the biplanar wedge, the tibial osteotomy is usually totally unstable, so it is recommended to add an anterior tibial plate in addition to the medial locking plate.

5.3.2 Supramalleolar Osteotomy Technique: Dome Osteotomy

In the case of dome osteotomies, it is difficult to correct the sagittal plane in addition to the coronal plane. When the dome osteotomy is done through an anterior approach and performed primarily to correct coronal plane deformities, only minor corrections in the sagittal plane can be achieved. In these cases, it is recommended to impact the cancellous bone (to achieve angulation correction) and to translate the osteotomy (anterior or posterior) to achieve sagittal plane weight bearing axis correction. If the sagittal plane deformity is more significant than the coronal plane deformity, or if the sagittal deformity to be corrected exceeds 10°, we recommend performing a dome osteotomy from a medial approach (see Figs. 15 and 16).

6 Published Results and Complications

The published results of ankle joint preservation surgery refer mainly to surgeries that correct deformities or malalignments in the coronal plane. The largest published series shows 189 patients with valgus LOA, 163 with good results at five years minimum [5]. In 2016, Krähenbühl published a series of the same group showing a five-year survival rate of 88%, reporting that patients over 60 years of age

Fig. 15 Lateral weight
bearing ankle radiograph,
showing a deformed distal
pilon with severely altered
LDTA. Note the anterior
talar subluxation relative to
the pilon, the osteophytes
in the anterior distal tibia
and the reduced joint
space. In this case, the
sagittal deformity to be
corrected exceeds 10° and
therefore we recommend
performing a dome
osteotomy from a medial
approach

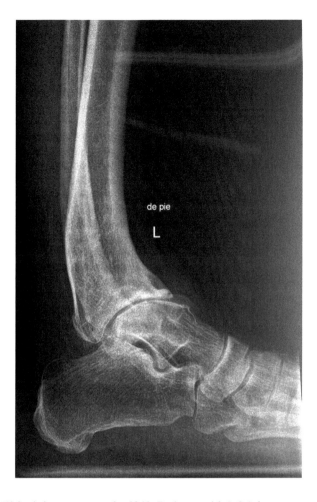

and with tilt greater than 7° had the worst results [31]. Patients with LOA in varus,
Takakura 2 and 3A show a five-year survival rate of 88% and 93% respectively. The
Takakura 3B group shows a 47% survival rate. If tilt is considered, survival for tilt
between 4 and 10° is 85%, and for more than 10° it is 65% [21]. Having said this,
there is recent information with a low number of cases that shows the possibility of
treating ankle arthrosis in stage Takakura 3b (varus) with SMOT plus distraction
with external fixation for three months, with follow-up at 3.2 years, with good
results. This information should be confirmed with a greater number of published
cases but could extend the indication for SMOT [32].

In terms of quality of life, patients who undergo joint preservation osteotomies
achieve quality of life scores comparable to healthy controls. In any case, they walk
slower, have less range of sagittal mobility of the hindfoot and have less dorsiflexion
torque in their affected ankle [33]. Bone healing has been reported in closing wedge
osteotomies at 2.3 months and in opening wedge osteotomies at 5.4 months [34].

Fig. 16 Intraoperative picture of same patient presented in Fig. 15. A medial distal tibia approach was performed. Please note the third tubular plate which was used to "draw" a dome osteotomy on the medial tibia using the plate as a hinge to guide the drilling

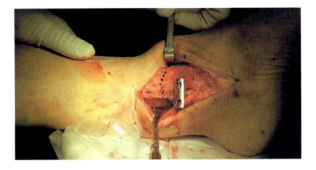

As far as complications are concerned, the percentages published are low, but considering infection, non-union, delayed consolidation, over- or under-correction, joint impingement, inadequate fixation or natural progression of the osteoarthritis, as a whole they can reach up to 22% [34]. In the largest series of osteotomies published so far, the most frequent complication reported is progression of osteoarthritis by 10% [35, 36]. The prognostic factors for loss of alignment correction have been identified as male gender, BMI >26.4 and lateral tibial cortex violation when performing the opening tibial wedge osteotomies [37].

Finally, in relation to fixation plates, no mechanical differences have been demonstrated between different plates models (anatomical and non-anatomical), but there are currently no dedicated plates for SMOT [38].

References

1. Wynes J, Kaikis AC. Current advancements in ankle Arthrodiastasis. Clin Podiatr Med Surg. 2018;35(4):467–79. https://doi.org/10.1016/j.cpm.2018.05.006.
2. Nguyen MP, Pedersen DR, Gao Y, Saltzman CL, Amendola A. Intermediate-term follow-up after ankle distraction for treatment of end-stage osteoarthritis. J Bone Joint Surg Am. 2015;97(7):590–6. https://doi.org/10.2106/JBJS.N.00901.
3. Knupp M. The use of osteotomies in the treatment of asymmetric ankle joint arthritis. Foot Ankle Int. 2017;38(2):220–9. https://doi.org/10.1177/1071100716679190.
4. Barg A, Saltzman CL. Single-stage supramalleolar osteotomy for coronal plane deformity. Curr Rev Musculoskelet Med. 2014;7(4):277–91. https://doi.org/10.1007/s12178-014-9231-1.
5. Valderrabano V, Paul J, Monika H, Pagenstert GI, Henninger HB, Barg A. Joint-preserving surgery of valgus ankle osteoarthritis. Foot Ankle Clin. 2013;18(3):481–502. https://doi.org/10.1016/j.fcl.2013.06.008. Review. PubMed PMID: 24008214.
6. Barg A, Pagenstert G, Hugle T, Gloyer M, Wiewiorski M, Henninger H, Valderrabano V. Ankle osteoarthritis etiology, diagnostics, and classification. Foot Ankle Clin N Am. 2013;18:411–26.
7. Jensen, N; Krmer, K; Hvid, I. Distribution of bone strength at the distal tibia and fibula. Clin Biomech. 1989;4(4):228–31.
8. McKinley TO, Tochigi Y, Rudert MJ, Brown TD. Instability-associated changes in contact stress and contact stress rates near a step-off incongruity. J Bone Joint Surg Am. 2008;90(2):375–83. https://doi.org/10.2106/JBJS.G.00127.
9. Sugimoto K, Takakura Y, Okahashi K, Samoto N, Kawate K, Iwai M. Chondral injuries of the ankle with recurrent lateral instability: an arthroscopic study. J Bone Joint Surg Am. 2009;91(1):99–106. https://doi.org/10.2106/JBJS.G.00087.

10. Saltzman C, El-Khoury G. The Hindfoot alignment view. Foot Ankle Int. 1995;16:572.
11. Paley, D; Herzenberg, J; Tetsworth, K; McKie, J; Bhave, A. Deformity planning for frontal and sagital plane corrective osteotomies. Orthoped Clin North Am. 1994;25(3):425–65.
12. Lopez M, Wagner P. Analisis y Plan quirúrgico de deformidades en tobillo y retropié del adulto. Rev Chil Ortop Traumatol, abril. 2019; https://doi.org/10.1055/s-0039-3400508.
13. Nosewicz TL, Knupp M, Bolliger L, Henninger HB, Barg A, Hintermann B. Radiological morphology of peritalar instability in varus and valgus tilted ankles. Foot Ankle Int. 2014;35(5):453–62. https://doi.org/10.1177/1071100714523589.
14. Hintermann B, Knupp M, Barg A. Joint-preserving surgery of asymmetric ankle osteoarthritis with peritalar instability. Foot Ankle Clin. 2013;18(3):503–16. https://doi.org/10.1016/j.fcl.2013.06.010.
15. Wang B, Saltzman CL, Chalayon O, Barg A. Does the subtalar joint compensate for ankle malalignment in end-stage ankle arthritis? Clin Orthop Relat Res. 2015;473(1):318–25. https://doi.org/10.1007/s11999-014-3960-8.
16. Tanaka Y, Takakura Y, Hayashi K, et al. Low tibial osteotomy for varus-type osteoarthritis of the ankle. J Bone Joint Surg Br. 2006;88(7):909–13.
17. Knupp M, Stufkens SA, Bolliger L, et al. Classification and treatment of supramalleolar deformities. Foot Ankle Int. 2011;32(11):1023–31.
18. Gross CE, Barfield W, Schweizer C, Rasch H, Hirschmann MT, Hintermann B, Knupp M. The utility of the ankle SPECT/CT scan to predict functional and clinical outcomes in supramalleolar osteotomy patients. J Orthop Res. 2018;36(7):2015–21. https://doi.org/10.1002/jor.23860.
19. Hintermann B, Knupp M, Barg A. Peritalar instability. Foot Ankle Int. 2012;33(5):450–4. https://doi.org/10.3113/FAI.2012.0450. PubMed PMID: 22735291.
20. Haraguchi N, Ota K, Tsunoda N, Seike K, Kanetake Y, Tsutaya A. Weight-bearing-line analysis in supramalleolar osteotomy for varus-type osteoarthritis of the ankle. J Bone Joint Surg Am. 2015;97(4):333–9. https://doi.org/10.2106/JBJS.M.01327.
21. Krähenbühl N, Akkaya M, Deforth M, Zwicky L, Barg A, Hintermann B. Extraarticular Supramalleolar osteotomy in asymmetric Varus ankle osteoarthritis. Foot Ankle Int. 2019;40(8):936–47. https://doi.org/10.1177/1071100719845928.
22. Hintermann B, Ruiz R, Barg A. Novel double osteotomy technique of distal tibia for correction of asymmetric Varus osteoarthritic ankle. Foot Ankle Int. 2017;38(9):970–81. https://doi.org/10.1177/1071100717712543. Epub 2017 Jul 1. PubMed PMID:28670918.
23. Zhao HM, Wen XD, Zhang Y, Liang JQ, Liu PL, Li Y, Lu J, Liang XJ. Supramalleolar osteotomy with medial distraction arthroplasty for ankle osteoarthritis with talar tilt. J Orthop Surg Res. 2019;14(1):120. https://doi.org/10.1186/s13018-019-1168-z.
24. Knupp M, Stufkens SA, van Bergen CJ, et al. Effect of supramalleolar varus and valgus deformities on the tibiotalar joint: a cadaveric study. Foot Ankle Int. 2011;32(6):609–15. https://doi.org/10.3113/FAI.2011.0609.
25. Lintz F, Welck M, Bernasconi A, Thornton J, Cullen NP, Singh D, Goldberg A. 3D biometrics for Hindfoot alignment using Weightbearing CT. Foot Ankle Int. 2017;38(6):684–9. https://doi.org/10.1177/1071100717690806.
26. Krause FG, Sutter D, Waehnert D, Windolf M, Schwieger K, Weber M. Ankle joint pressure changes in a pes cavovarus model after lateralizing calcaneal osteotomies. Foot Ankle Int. 2010;31(9):741–6. https://doi.org/10.3113/FAI.2010.0741.
27. Paley D, Herzenberg JE. Principles of deformity correction. In: Chapter 5, Osteotomy concepts and frontal plane realignment. Berlin: Springer-Verlag; 2002. p. 102–9.
28. Wagner P, Colin F, Hintermann B. Distal tibia dome osteotomy. Techniques in Foot & Ankle Surgery June. 2014;13(2):103–7.
29. Al-Nammari SS, Myerson MS. The use of Tibial osteotomy (ankle Plafondplasty) for joint preservation of ankle deformity and early arthritis. Foot Ankle Clin. 2016;21(1):15–26. https://doi.org/10.1016/j.fcl.2015.09.009.
30. Ahn TK, Yi Y, Cho JH, Lee WC. A cohort study of patients undergoing distal tibial osteotomy without fibular osteotomy for medial ankle arthritis with mortise widening. J Bone Joint Surg Am. 2015;97(5):381–8. https://doi.org/10.2106/JBJS.M.01360.

31. Krähenbühl N, Zwicky L, Bolliger L, Schädelin S, Hinterman B, Knupp M. Mid- to long-term results of Supramalleolar osteotomy. Foot Ankle Int. 2016; https://doi.org/10.1177/1071100716673416.
32. Nozaka K, Miyakoshi N, Kashiwagura T, Kasukawa Y, Saito H, Kijima H, Chida S, Tsuchie H, Shimada Y. Effectiveness of distal tibial osteotomy with distraction arthroplasty in varus ankle osteoarthritis. BMC Musculoskelet Disord. 2020;21(1):31. https://doi.org/10.1186/s12891-020-3061-7.
33. Nüesch C, Huber C, Paul J, Henninger HB, Pagenstert G, Valderrabano V, Barg A. Mid- to long-term clinical outcome and gait biomechanics after realignment surgery in asymmetric ankle osteoarthritis. Foot Ankle Int. 2015;36(8):908–18. https://doi.org/10.1177/1071100715577371.
34. Barg A, Saltzman CL. Joint-preserving procedures in patients with Varus deformity: role of Supramalleolar osteotomies. Foot Ankle Clin. 2019;24(2):239–64. https://doi.org/10.1016/j.fcl.2019.02.004.
35. Knupp M, Stufkens SA, Bolliger L, et al. Classification and treatment of supramalleolar deformities. Foot Ankle Int. 2011;32:1023–31.
36. Espinosa N. What leads to failure of joint-preserving surgery for ankle osteoarthritis?: when this surgery fails, what next? Foot Ankle Clin. 2013;18(3):555–69. https://doi.org/10.1016/j.fcl.2013.06.014.
37. Kim YS, Kim YB, Koh YG. Prognostic factors affecting correction angle changes after Supramalleolar osteotomy using an opening wedge plate for Varus ankle osteoarthritis. J Foot Ankle Surg. 2019;58(3):417–22. https://doi.org/10.1053/j.jfas.2018.09.003.
38. Ettinger S, Schwarze M, Yao D, Ettinger M, Claassen L, Stukenborg-Colsman C, Thermann H, Plaass C. Stability of supramalleolar osteotomies using different implants in a sawbone model. Arch Orthop Trauma Surg. 2018;138(10):1359–63. https://doi.org/10.1007/s00402-018-2981-2.

Diffuse Ankle Osteoarthritis

Markus Knupp

1 Introduction

Arthritis of the ankle joint is common and found in 1% of the world's population. In contrast to arthritis of the hip or knee (mainly primary arthritis), the etiology at the ankle is posttraumatic in a large majority of patients. As a result, the patients become symptomatic 12–15 years earlier than arthritic hip or knee patients. This underlines the importance of long-lasting treatment options for this patient group [1].

Surgical treatments for ankle joint arthritis are divided into two categories: procedures that preserve the joint and those that do not.

This chapter focuses on conservative treatment and joint distraction arthroplasty for joint preservation and non-joint-preserving treatments, e.g., arthrodesis and total ankle replacement.

2 Etiology

The ankle joint is less commonly affected by degenerative wear than the hip and the knee. The reasons for this are the high resistance towards wear of the ankle cartilage, the well guided joint motion during flexion/extension (see below), and the susceptibility of the ankle cartilage to inflammatory mediators [2]. The most common cause for ankle joint arthritis is trauma (70%). Inflammatory arthritis accounts for approximately 12% of all cases and primary arthritis for the rest [3].

M. Knupp (✉)
University of Basel, Mein Fusszentrum Basel, Basel, Switzerland
e-mail: markus.knupp@meinfusszentum.ch

3 Anatomy

The ankle joint is a very congruent joint and comprises the tibia, the fibula, the talus, the collateral ligaments, the syndesmosis, and the joint bridging tendons. Stability of the joint is provided by the bony configuration and the surrounding soft tissue mantle (tendons and ligaments).

3.1 Bony Elements

The talus articulates with the malleolar fork on three articulating surfaces: the talar dome articulates with the pilon and the medial and the lateral gutter. The articulating surfaces of the gutters are opened anteriorly creating the gutter angle.

3.1.1 Talus

The talus has a conical shape with the radius of the medial shoulder being smaller than the radius of the lateral talar shoulder. Sixty percent of the surface is covered by cartilage and there are no tendons inserting into the talus. The width of the talus is wider anteriorly than posteriorly, making the bone wedge-shaped in the transverse plane. The radius of the talar dome is slightly smaller than the corresponding radius of the tibia, which allows for some sagittal motion in the ankle joint.

3.1.2 Tibia

The tibia shares two articulating surfaces with the talus: the pilon and the medial gutter. In the Caucasian population the angle of the distal tibial articulating surface is in slight valgus, when measuring it in relation to an axis drawn from the tibial tuberosity to the center of the ankle joint [1, 4]. Radiologically women tend to have a joint surface in more varus than men [4].

The strength of the tibia decreases with increasing distance from the joint line: the bone in the metaphyseal area is 70–90% weaker than in the subchondral area [5]. The subchondral bone is strongest posteromedially and weakest anterolaterally.

3.1.3 Fibula

The fibula is dynamically attached to the tibia (syndesmosis complex). This allows for a slight diastasis in the distal tibio-fibular joint, proximalization and endorotation of the fibula during dorsiflexion of the ankle. During plantarflexion, the fibula moves distally and rotates externally [6].

3.2   Ligaments

The lateral ankle ligaments comprise the calcaneofibular, the anterior and the posterior talofibular ligament. These three ligaments stabilize the ankle joint in different positions of the ankle; in dorsiflexion the posterior talofibular ligament is tight whereas in plantarflexion the anterior talofibular ligament is tight.

The deltoid ligament on the medial side has a superficial portion which stabilizes the ankle, the subtalar and the talonavicular joint with their fibers running from the medial malleolus to the navicular, the calcaneus and the spring ligament. The deep portion of the deltoid bridges the ankle joint with stabilizing fibers running from the medial malleolus to the talus. In its entirety, the deltoid ligament provides ankle stability against exorotation, lateral translation and valgus forces on the ankle joint.

4   Biomechanical Considerations

Anatomical and biomechanical studies have shown that the ankle joint is not just a simple hinge but much more, it provides motion in the sagittal, coronal and the transverse plane [7–10] with a rotational axis of the talus that varies during flexion and extension.

4.1   Rotational Axis

The ankle joint is part of a kinematic chain containing the tibiofibular joint, the tibiotalar joint, the subtalar joint and Choparts jointline. Dorsiflexion of the ankle leads to internal rotation of the lower leg, eversion/valgization of the hindfoot and pronation of the mid-/forefoot. Plantarflexion leads to external rotation of the lower leg, inversion/varization of the hindfoot and supination of the mid-/forefoot.

4.2   Range of Motion

The normal range of motion of the ankle joint varies from 23–56° in plantarflexion and 13–33° in dorsiflexion. Walking on even surface requires 10–15° plantarflexion and 10° dorsiflexion. Climbing stairs has been found to require 37° (upstairs) and 56° (downstairs). For normal daily activities (without climbing of stairs) a range of motion of 15° in the ankle joint has been described to be sufficient.

4.3   Load Transfer at the Ankle Joint

Walking on even surfaces creates axial forces up to 5.2 times body weight at the ankle joint. These forces result from ground reaction forces, gravitation and forces resulting from the muscles/tendons and the ligaments. These forces are transmitted over the articular surface which is 7 cm^2 in size.

5   Diagnosis

A thorough *history* includes questions on all joints of the lower extremity, a history of trauma (fractures, osteochondral lesions, ligament/tendon tears), disorders during childhood, history of inflammatory or infectious arthropathies, gout, hemophilia, metabolic diseases (diabetes), or neuropathy.

Physical examination includes observation of gait and the alignment when standing. Assessment of hindfoot alignment is done in standing and while standing and in tip toe position (heel rise). A thorough neurovascular examination is mandatory, not only to assess the nature of the arthritic process in the ankle joint but also to determine the necessity of further investigations (angiological and neurological workup). Motion and stability of the ankle and subtalar joint should be assessed. The function of the joint bridging tendons is noted.

Radiographic examination includes a full set of weight-bearing radiographs of the foot and ankle. For the planning of ankle replacement and ankle fusion, a whole leg length radiograph is recommended. Additional alignment views, as described by Saltzman, may provide further information in case of deformity [11]. These examinations can be completed with CT and/or Spect-CT in selected cases, e.g., involvement of multiple joints, altered bone quality such as osteonecrosis.

6   Conservative Management

Conservative therapy of ankle osteoarthritis is symptomatic and not curative. Nonsurgical treatment of ankle arthritis focuses on reduction of inflammation and pain control. Options include NSAIDs, nutritional supplementation, joint injections, and bracing/shoe modifications. Indications for conservative therapy include: initial treatment before surgery, end-stage OA to buy time in the young and active patient, severe vascular or neurologic deficiency, neuropathic disorders, unstable soft tissues and ongoing infection of soft tissue, bone or joint [12].

6.1   Viscosupplementation

Viscosupplementation injections in the ankle are discussed controversially. Some studies showed significant improvement in the short term, however, after 1 year no difference was found when comparing viscosupplementation with saline injection [13].

6.2 Platelet-Rich Plasma/Corticosteroids Injections

Platelet-rich plasma (PRP) has gained increasing popularity in the treatment of a multitude of disorders. While intraarticular injections have shown to be beneficial in mild to moderate knee osteoarthritis, the literature for the ankle remains controversial.

Corticosteroids can provide pain relief for a limited amount of time. However, repetitive injections are not without risks. Corticosteroids can cause damage to the soft tissue and there are reports on serious deleterious effects on the articular cartilage in repeated corticosteroids injections.

6.3 Physical Therapy

Keeping patients with osteoarthritis active has been shown to slow down the degenerative wear in the joint with the potential to postpone surgery. The focus is set on local anti-inflammatory measures, muscle strengthening, ankle and hindfoot joint mobilization to prevent joint stiffness and gait educations.

6.4 Orthoses and Shoe Modification

Orthoses can provide effective pain reduction and postpone ankle replacement/ankle fusion in patients with ankle arthritis. The orthoses/shoe modifications aim to absorb shock, cushion the heel, decrease the peak joint forces (for example corrective wedges in cases with a deformity) and stabilize the affected joints.

7 Surgical Treatment

Surgical treatment of ankle arthritis is divided into joint preserving surgery (corrective osteotomies, open/arthroscopically debridement, distraction arthroplasty) and non-preserving options (ankle fusion and arthroplasty).

7.1 Distraction Arthroplasty

The author has only very limited experience with this technique and has not used it in the last 14 years. Distraction arthroplasty unloads the ankle joint with an external fixator. Distraction is performed in conjunction with osteophyte removal, microfracture, soft tissue release and deformity correction, where needed. Decreasing the load on the joint surface for a certain time potentially promotes cartilage repair. The external fixator is used to mechanically unload the ankle to halt or even partially reverse the arthritic process in the ankle joint. Patient selection is crucial for success of distraction arthroplasty. Inclusion criteria are a congruent joint with a preserved motion of >20° [14].

Distraction is maintained for at least 8 weeks. No added benefit has been seen beyond 12 weeks [15]. The frames can provide distraction with or without a hinge. In a randomized study the patients with a hinged framed showed a better outcome 2 years after frame removal [16]. However, with a longer follow up the same authors reported on better outcomes in the fixed frame group in the same cohort. Some authors have tried to stimulate hyaline cartilage regeneration by injection of autologous bone marrow aspirate into the ankle joint. However, no clinical evidence for this method has been presented.

Considering that most recruited patients in the studies were classified as candidates for ankle arthroplasty or ankle fusion, it is not surprising that the survivorship analysis of this method shows a high failure rate. Fusion rates within the first year after frame removal range from 24% to 27% [17, 18]. Long-term follow-up studies reported fusion rates of 45% at 8 years [16] and 44% at 12 years [19].

7.2 Ankle Fusion

Ankle fusion has for many years been the most reliable treatment in end-stage ankle arthritis. In contrast to the hip and the knee, which are now rarely fused, ankle arthrodesis will never be completely replaced by arthroplasty of the ankle joint. Despite the very promising development of the newest technology in ankle replacement, ankle fusion will remain an important tool in the armamentarium of a foot and ankle surgeon- not only as a salvage procedure but also as a primary treatment option.

For the indications, please refer to the section "fusion versus ankle replacement."

Ankle fusion can be done through an anterior, lateral (transfibular or anterolateral), posterior approach or arthroscopically. Traditionally most authors preferred the lateral approach. In recent years many surgeons increasingly use the same anterior approach for isolated ankle fusions as for ankle arthroplasty.

7.2.1 Anterior Approach

An incision of 10–12 cm is placed anteriorly to the ankle joint, extending to the level of the talonavicular joint. The extensor retinaculum is exposed and split between the anterior tibial tendon and the extensor hallucis longus tendon. The distal tibia is approached through a longitudinal incision along the lateral border of anterior tendon and exposed subperiosteally. After arthrotomy and partial resection of the capsule, the exposure is extended to the talar neck. To improve visualization of the joint, a self-retaining retractor can be used, e.g., Hintermann distractor.

In primary ankle fusion, osteophytes are removed and the tibial and talar joint surfaces, including the gutters, are cleared from cartilage, fibrous and necrotic material. Cartilage removal will lead to a mismatch of the joint surfaces; the radius of the tibial surface will increase whereas the talar radius decreases. Therefore, the joint surfaces need to be feathered with a chisel to increase bony contact.

In cases of failed arthroplasty or ankle fusion, the implants are removed, preserving as much bone stock as possible. Any necrotic bone is removed until healthy, viable bone is exposed. The void is filled with autologous bone graft from the iliac bone crest, allograft (e.g., Tutoplast®, Tutogen Medical GmbH, Neunkirchen a.B, Germany) or – in large defects – vascularized bone grafts from the medial femoral condyle, pelvis or scapula. Orthobiologics, such as demineralized bone matrix (DBX®, Synthes, Oberdorf, Switzerland) can be added to stimulate bone healing.

Fixation is done with screws and/or plates. Different techniques for the placement of the screws have been suggested. In primary fusion, two or three cannulated screws are used. If the screws (for example cannulated 7.0 mm screws) are placed strictly parallel (usually from the medial tibia into the talus), partially threaded screws can be used to create compression across the fusion site. If the screws are not placed parallel (for example one screw from the medial tibia and one screw from the lateral tibia) only one screw should be used as a compression screw while the second screw should be a fully threaded one. An additional third screw can be placed; however, this has not shown to increase the union rate.

Different plating systems can be used for the anterior approach. When choosing a plating system, the surgeon must plan the positioning of the plates carefully. In a primary ankle fusion, the main fusion sites are the two articulating surfaces of the tibiotalar joint (talar dome/medial gutter). Therefore, the plate(s) should create compression on the talar dome and in the medial gutter. When using compression devices with anterior plating systems, the surgeon must avoid anterior subluxation of the talus. This is prevented by attaching the plates to the talus first, also using a spacer temporarily between the proximal end of the plate and the anterior tibia, which will shift the talus posteriorly when the tibial screws are tightened (Fig. 1).

Positioning of the fusion is usually neutral in flexion/extension, neutral or slight exorotation in the transverse plane and neutral to slight valgus in the coronal plane. However, the positioning can vary in special indications, e.g., patients with quadriceps weakness, for example in post-polio syndrome, benefit from an ankle fusion in equinus to stabilize their knee joint.

7.2.2 Lateral Approach

The patient is placed in a lateral decubitus or supine position on the operating table. An incision is made over the fibula and soft tissue dissection to the bone is directed anteriorly. With a sagittal saw, an osteotomy of the fibula is created about 10 cm proximal from the tip of the fibula. Distally, the anterior syndesmosis and the anterior talofibular ligaments are detached to allow for the fibula to be reflected posteriorly. Care is taken to preserve the posterior soft tissue. The articular surfaces between the tibia, the fibula and the talus are removed. The bone is prepared with multiple drill holes in the subchondral bone und feathered to encourage fusion. The talus is then reduced and either fixed with as above or a lateral plate. If a plate is chosen, care is taken not to violate the subtalar joint. Finally, the fibula is reduced and secured with screws into the tibia/fibula. The retromalleolar groove must be maintained to preserve peroneal tendon function.

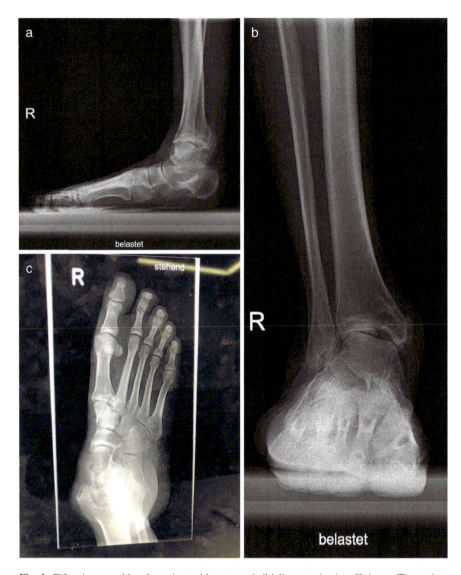

Fig. 1 Fifty-six-year-old male patient with a stage 4 tibialis posterior insufficiency. The patient has been advised against a total ankle replacement because of a complete incompetence of all medial soft tissues. (**a–c**) show the preoperative weight bearing radiographs. (**d–f**) the postoperative images 9 months after the ankle fusion and a medial displacement calcaneal osteotomy

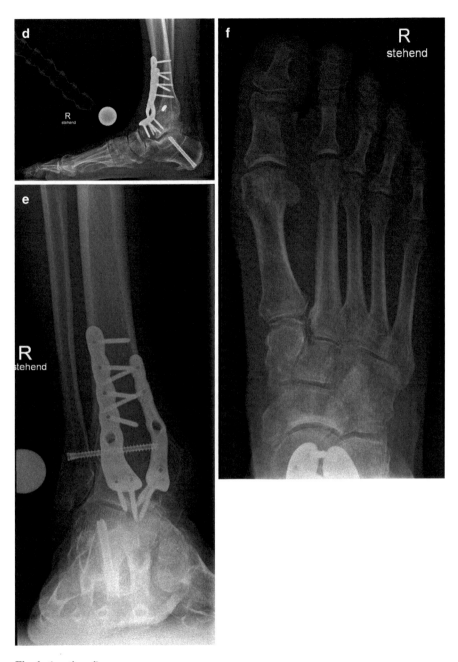

Fig. 1 (continued)

7.2.3 Posterior Approach

The ankle can be approached through a posteromedial or a posterolateral approach. The posterolateral approach uses a skin incision posterior to the fibula. To enable deep dissection, the peroneus longus and brevis muscles/tendons are pulled anteriorly. The interval between the flexor hallucis longus tendon and the peroneal tendons is split bluntly to access the posterior aspect of the ankle. For the posteromedial approach, the skin incision is made 1 cm medial to the Achilles tendon, extending from the calcaneal insertion proximally for a length of 10 cm. The Achilles tendon is retracted laterally, and blunt dissection used to expose the transverse intramuscular septum. This is opened sharply to expose the FHL muscle belly. The interval between the FHL and neurovascular bundle is then developed and the FHL is elevated from the posterior tibia using a periosteal elevator. Hohman retractors are then placed over the medial and lateral borders of the tibia to fully expose the posterior aspect of the ankle. Thereafter the ankle joint is freed from the remaining cartilage and prepared for the fusion analogously to the description above. Fixation usually is achieved with two cannulated screws entering the tibia dorsally and aiming to the talar neck. Alternatively, a plate can be used: either a blade-plate, which is inserted posteriorly into the talar body and then secured to the tibia, or with a standard plate (Fig. 2).

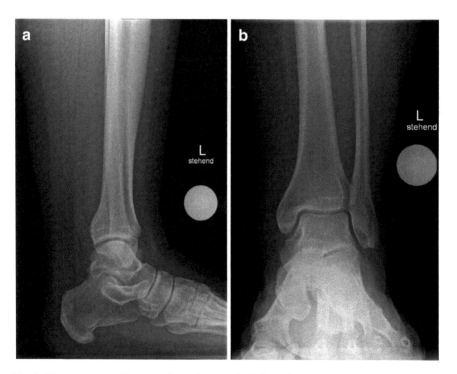

Fig. 2 Sixty-two-year-old male patient with a paralytic foot after spinal surgery. The dorsal plate was chosen to act as a tension banding device. The images (**a**, **b**) show the preoperativeand the images (**c**–**f**) the 6 months postoperative radiographic presentation (**g**)

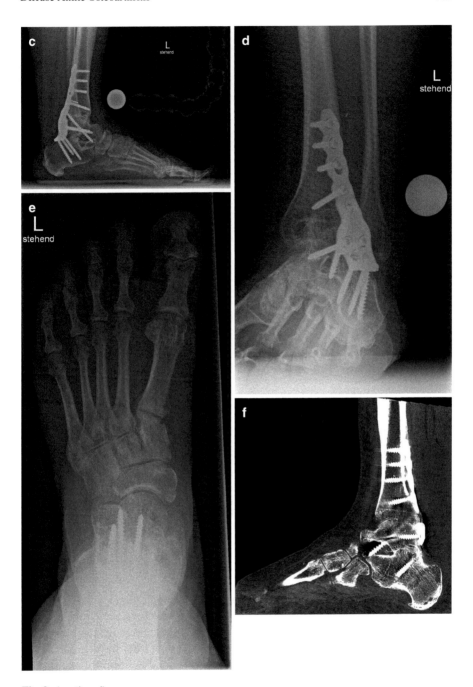

Fig. 2 (continued)

Fig. 2 (continued)

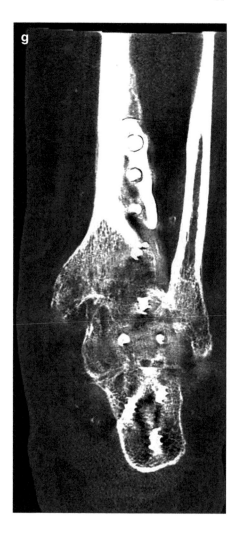

7.2.4   Arthroscopic Ankle Fusion

Arthroscopic joint preparation can be achieved through either anterior portals with the patient in a supine position or posterior portals in a prone position. An abrader is used to remove the cartilage. Care is taken to remove as little of the subchondral bone as possible while maintaining the joint's normal contour. A burr is then used to make multiple holes through the subchondral bone to maximize the bleeding surface, giving the joint the aspect of a 'golf ball'. Thereafter the talus is reduced, and percutaneous cannulated screws used for fixation in the above-described manner.

7.2.5 Postoperative Treatment

Once the wounds have healed and the swelling has decreased, the preliminary post-operative splint is replaced by either a below-knee cast or a walker. Patients who did not receive bone grafting are allowed weight bearing as tolerated after 4 weeks, whereas patients who receive a bone graft for interposition are allowed only partial weight bearing during the first 8 weeks after surgery and full weight bearing thereafter.

7.2.6 Outcomes of Ankle Fusion

Union rates vary from 60% to 100% with larger studies showing 90% union rates [20]. The nonunion rate dramatically increases in patients with previous subtalar joint fusion and in varus deformity.

    The clinical impact of the altered gait after ankle fusion has not been fully eluci-dated. While the effect on the knee seems to be very minor, the compensatory increase of motion in the talonavicular and the subtalar joint increases the risk for adjacent joint arthritis in these joints [21].

7.3 Ankle Arthroplasty

Total ankle replacement was first attempted in the early 1970s. The initial implants lead to very poor outcomes with catastrophic failures. The interest was then renewed in the 1980s and 1990s with new designs. With increasing understanding of the hindfoot kinematics the surgical techniques and implants for total ankle replace-ment improved and became more reliable in mimicking the physiological mechan-ics. This led to more consistent clinical results making ankle arthroplasty a valuable alternative to ankle fusion.

    For the indications, please refer to the section "fusion versus ankle replace-ment" below.

7.3.1 Technique

All but one implant design (Zimmer TM) use an anterior approach (see above) as described in the fusion section.

    After exposure of the ankle joint as described above, removal of the osteophytes, synovial tissue and excessive capsule is carried out. In *congruent ankles* the surgeon can directly move on to the bony resection. This is carried out with the aim to posi-tion the tibial and talar components perpendicular to the plumb line of the body. In *tilted ankles (incongruent ankles)* two different subgroups need to be distinguished. In the first group the tilt of the talus results from the loss of joint height and subsequently leads to slack ligaments. In these cases, intraoperative distraction of the tibiotalar joint allows for gapping/correction of the joint space. In the second subgroup, the tilt of the talus results from contract intraarticular deformity and passive correction of the talus is not possible through traction. While the first subgroup can be addressed by joint line distalization, using the ankle arthroplasty as a spacer. Patients in the second subgroup with contract intraarticular deformities a thorough soft tissue balancing is mandatory. In most cases the latter comprises (cavo-) varus feet. These are addressed with a medial soft tissue release including the deltoid, the posterior tibial tendon and the spring ligament (Fig. 3). In rare cases an osteotomy of the medial malleolus is necessary to balance the joint.

The bony preparation is then continued according to the guidelines of the implant manufacturer. After implantation of the components the alignment, the ligament balancing, and the range of motion is reassessed. In case of ligamentous instability, the ligaments need to be tightened/augmented. In case of lack of dorsiflexion the posterior joint capsule is resected, and the Achilles' tendon lengthened.

7.3.2 Postoperative Treatment

The post-operative treatment protocol is determined by the combined bony procedures (fusions, osteotomies) or soft tissue procedures. In isolated ankle arthroplasties most authors immobilize the patients in a cast or walker boot for 6 weeks and allow for early weight bearing as tolerated.

7.3.3 Outcomes of Ankle Arthroplasty

Reports on the survivorship of the implants vary widely in the literature. Data from the Cochrane collaborations found an 89% survivorship after 10 years with an annual failure rate of 1.2% after reviewing 7942 total ankles [22]. This is consistent with a few multicenter studies showing survivorship rates of 96% at 5 years and 90% at 10 years [23]. Some of the register data from Europe, New Zealand and Australia show lower survivorships. It is important to note that comparisons of international registries are very difficult because the implants differ from country to country. Furthermore, a large majority of the surgeons in these registries implant less than 20 ankle arthroplasties per year, which has been shown to be a major factor for a worse outcome [24].

While diabetes (with a good glycemic control), weight and etiology (primary-rheumatoid-posttraumatic) does not seem to affect the outcome, smoking has been found to significantly increase the risk for wound complications and a worse outcome [25].

One of the most feared early complications is an infection. In our own case-control study we reported an infection rate of 4.7%. This is significantly higher than in the reported data on ankle arthrodesis. The most common pathogen was a Staphylococcus aureus, followed by coagulase-negative staphylococci. Risk factors

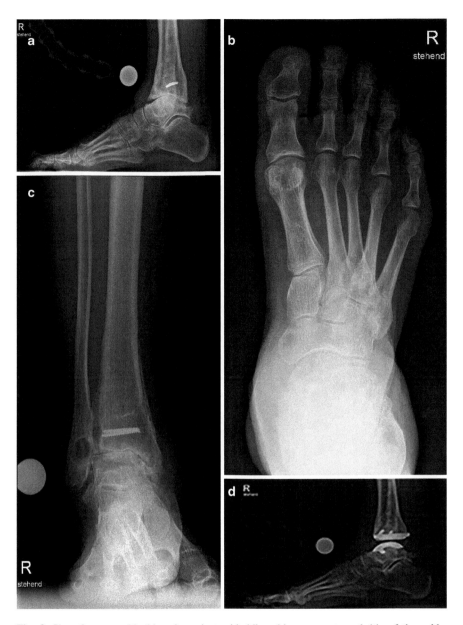

Fig. 3 Sixty-five-year-old old male patient with idiopathic varus osteoarthritis of the ankle. Previously attempted supramalleolar osteotomy did not give a lasting effect. The ankle was addressed with a total ankle replacement. The tight soft tissues on the medial side were released (superficial deltoid ligament, lengthening of the tibialis posterior tendon and release of the spring ligament). Preoperative images: (**a**–**c**), 4 months postoperative images: (**d**–**f**)

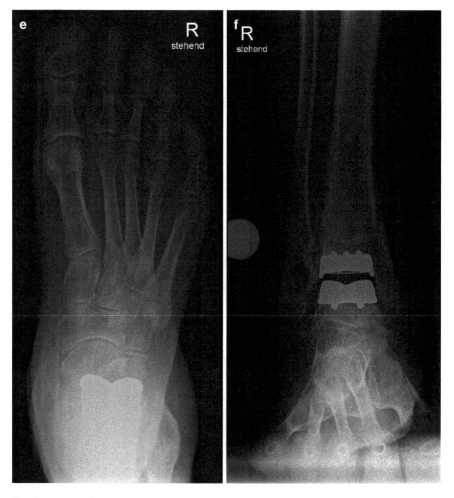

Fig. 3 (continued)

for periprosthetic joint infection included previous surgery at the ankle, a long operative time, and secondary wound-healing problems [26].

7.4 Fusion Versus Arthroplasty

The indication for both, fusion, and ankle arthroplasty, is end-stage ankle arthritis. Although patient selection has been described to be critical for the outcome, particularly for ankle arthroplasty, the recommendations in the literature remain controversial. High volume ankle arthroplasty surgeons simplify the indication for ankle fusion; all cases that do not qualify for joint replacement are fused. The primary requirements for ankle arthroplasty are a stable joint, a correct alignment and a sufficient bone stock to guarantee stable implant fixation. If these factors cannot be established prior or during the implantation of an ankle prothesis, a fusion should be chosen.

There is an agreement on absolute contraindications for ankle arthroplasty: inadequate soft-tissue envelope, Charcot neuroarthropathy, severe malalignment involving several segments (ankle, midfoot, forefoot), uncorrectable ankle instability/severe sensomotoric deficits and osteonecrosis of the talus and active infections. For patients with active infections, a majority of authors recommend ankle fusion after the infection has been treated.

In the following paragraphs some factors are discussed that help to decide over one or the other procedure.

7.4.1 Age and Weight

Earlier recommendations stated that the patients subjected to joint replacement surgery should be older than 50 years, non-obese and with low physical demands. The recent literature shows no difference in the outcome in younger patients or obese patients. Patients with higher expectations do better with an ankle arthroplasty.

7.4.2 Multiple Joint Involvement

It is generally agreed that the presence of degenerative changes in other joints, such as the subtalar, midtarsal, knee and the contra-lateral ankle, must be considered when choosing between ankle arthroplasty and ankle fusion. Patients with multiple joint involvement show better outcomes with an ankle arthroplasty than with an ankle fusion. The reason is that an ankle fusion increases the loads in the neighboring joints and therefore makes them prone to degeneration. It has been shown that 8 years after ankle fusion half of the patients present with hindfoot arthritis [27] and after 22 years all patients developed hindfoot arthritis [21].The treatment of secondary arthritis of the subtalar joint after ankle fusion is demanding. Surgical treatment options of secondary subtalar joint osteoarthritis are subtalar joint fusion with or without a takedown of the ankle fusion (desarthrodesis). In isolated subtalar joint fusions after ankle fusion the non-union rates have been reported to be as high as 38.5%. This is a significantly higher nonunion rate than in the isolated subtalar joint fusion (8.7%) [28]. The alternative is to combine the subtalar joint fusion with a conversion of the ankle fusion into an ankle arthroplasty (desarthrodesis). The latter is a technically demanding procedure with high complication rates and should be only offered to very selected cases [29].

The concerns about secondary adjacent joint involvement are also true for patients with systemic diseases, such as rheumatoid arthritis and hemochromatosis. These patients carry the risk of multiple joint involvement and are prone to develop adjacent joint arthritis. This is in accordance with observations on rheumatoid patients who underwent ankle fusion. Cracchiolo et al. reported on 14 fusions in patients with rheumatoid arthritis with only one patient reporting a functional improvement [30].

7.4.3 Deformity

Malalignment increases the risk for early implant failure in ankle arthroplasty. While earlier recommendations limited ankle arthroplasty to patients with less than 10° deformity in any planes, recent publications have shown no difference in the outcome in patients with greater deformity when comparing them to preoperatively well aligned ankles, provided the deformity is corrected during or before the replacement surgery [31]. Deformities of less than 10° can be corrected with the tibial cut. Larger deformities usually require osteotomies. It is mandatory to eliminate all deforming forces during the time of implantation of an ankle arthroplasty: the ligaments and the joint crossing tendons must be balanced and deforming forces resulting from mid-/forefoot must be addressed. If the deformity cannot be corrected in all planes, the surgeon should choose ankle fusion.

To date all studies comparing ankle arthroplasty versus fusion have been observational and randomized data is sparse. A randomized study has been launched but the data not yet published [32]. In a meta-analysis by Haddad, TAR and fusions had a similar intermediate term outcome in terms of clinical scores, patients' satisfaction and revision rate [33]. The functional scores are higher in the ankle arthroplasty group than in the ankle fusion [34], however, the risk for a major a complication in the arthroplasty group is higher than in the fusion group [35, 36].

Acknowledgments The author wishes to thank Jennifer Anderson, M. D. for her support in the preparation of this chapter.

References

1. Sammarco J. Biomechanics of the ankle: surface velocity and instant centre of rotation in the sagittal plane. Am J Sports Med. 1977;5:231–4.
2. Huch K, Kuettner KE, Dieppe P. Osteoarthritis in ankle and knee joints. Semin Arthritis Rheum. 1997;26(4):667–74.
3. Saltzman CL, Salamon ML, Blanchard GM, et al. Epidemiology of ankle arthritis: report of a consecutive series of 639 patients from a tertiary orthopaedic center. Iowa Orthop J. 2005;25:44–6.
4. Knupp M, Ledermann HP, Magerkurth O, Hintermann B. The surgical tibiotalar angle: a radiological study. Foot Ankle Int. 2005;26:713–5.
5. Hvid I, Rasmussen O, Jensen NC, Nielsen S. Trabecular bone strength profiles at the ankle joint. Clin Orthop Relat Res. 1985;199:306–12.
6. Kapandji IA. Das obere Sprunggelenk. In: Kapandji IA, editor. Funktionelle Anatomie der Gelenke, Band 47. Enke Verlag; 1987. pp. 150–63.

7. Michelson JD, Schmidt GR, Mizel MS. Kinematics of a total arthroplasty of the ankle: comparison to normal ankle motion. Foot Ankle Int. 2000;21:278–84.

8. Rasmussen O, Tovberg-Jensen I. Mobility of the ankle joint: recording of rotatory movements in the talocrural joint in vitro with and without the lateral collateral ligaments of the ankle. Acta Orthop Scand. 1982;53:155–60.

9. Lundberg A, Goldie I, Kalin B, Selvik G. Kinematics of the ankle / foot complex, part 1: plantar flexion and dorsiflexion. Foot Ankle. 1989;9:194–200.

10. Lundberg A, Svennson OK, Nemeth G, Selvik G. The axis of rotation of the ankle joint. J Bone Joint Surg Br. 1989;71:94–9.

11. Saltzman CL, el-Khoury GY. The hindfoot alignment view. Foot Ankle Int. 1995;16(9):572–6.

12. Schmid T, Krause FG. Conservative treatment of asymmetric ankle osteoarthritis. Foot Ankle Clin. 2013;18(3):437–48.

13. Karatosun V, Unver B, Ozden A, Ozay Z, Gunal I. Intra-articular hyaluronic acid compared to exercise therapy in osteoarthritis of the ankle. A prospective randomized trial with long-term follow-up. Clin Exp Rheumatol. 2008;26(2):288–94.

14. Saltzman CL, Hillis SL, Stolley MP, Anderson DD, Amendola A. Motion versus fixed distraction of the joint in the treatment of ankle osteoarthritis: a prospective randomized controlled trial. J Bone Joint Surg. 2012;94(11):961–70.

15. van Valburg AA, van Roermund PM, Marijnissen AC, et al. Joint distraction in treatment of osteoarthritis (II): effects on cartilage in a canine model. Osteoarthr Cartil. 2000;8(1):1–8.

16. Nguyen MP, Pedersen DR, Gao Y, Saltzman CL, Amendola A. Intermediate term follow-up after ankle distraction for treatment of end-stage osteoarthritis. J Bone Joint Surg. 2015;97(7):590–6.

17. Marijnissen AC, Van Roermund PM, Van Melkebeek J, et al. Clinical benefit of joint distraction in the treatment of severe osteoarthritis of the ankle: proof of concept in an open prospective study and in a randomized controlled study. Arthritis Rheum. 2002;46(11):2893–902.

18. Ploegmakers JJ, van Roermund PM, van Melkebeek J, et al. Prolonged clinical benefit from joint distraction in the treatment of ankle osteoarthritis. Osteoarthr Cartil. 2005;13(7):582–8.

19. Marijnissen AC, Hoekstra MC, Pré BC, et al. Patient characteristics as predictors of clinical outcome of distraction in treatment of severe ankle osteoarthritis. J Orthop Res. 2014;32(1):96–101.

20. Chalayon O, Wang B, Blankenhorn B, et al. Factors affecting the outcomes of uncomplicated primary open ankle arthrodesis. Foot Ankle Int. 2015;36(10):1170–9.

21. Coester LM, Saltzman CL, Leupold J, et al. Long-term results following ankle arthrodesis for post-traumatic arthritis. J Bone Joint Surg. 2001;83A(2):219–28.

22. Zaidi R, Cro S, Gurusamy K, et al. The outcome of total ankle replacement: a systematic review and meta-analysis. Bone Joint J. 2013;95B(11):1500–7.

23. Mann JA, Mann RA, Horton E. STARankle: long-term results. Foot Ankle Int. 2011;32(05):473–84.

24. Basques BA, Bitterman A, Campbell KJ, Haughom BD, Lin J, Lee S. Influence of surgeon volume on inpatient complications, cost, and length of stay following total ankle arthroplasty. Foot Ankle Int. 1987;37(10):1046–51. https://doi.org/10.1177/1071100716664871.

25. Lampley A, Gross CE, Green CL, et al. Association of cigarette use and complication rates and outcomes following total ankle arthroplasty. Foot Ankle Int. 2016. https://doi.org/10.1177/1071100716655435.

26. Kessler B, Knupp M, Graber P, Zwicky L, Hintermann B, Zimmerli W, Sendi P. The treatment and outcome of peri-prosthetic infection of the ankle: a single cohort-centre experience of 34 cases. Bone Joint J. 2014;96-B(6):772–7. https://doi.org/10.1302/0301-620X.96B6.33298.

27. Easley ME, Vertullo CJ, Urban WC, Nunley JA. Review total ankle arthroplasty. J Am Acad Orthop Surg. 2002;10(3):157–67.

28. Zanolli D, Nunley J, Easley M. Subtalar fusion rate in patients with previous ipsilateral ankle arthrodesis. Foot Ankle Int. 2015;36(9):1025–8. https://doi.org/10.1177/1071100715584014.

29. Hintermann B, Barg A, Knupp M, Valderrabano V. Conversion of painful ankle arthrodesis to total ankle arthroplasty. J Bone Joint Surg. 2009;91(4):850–8. https://doi.org/10.2106/JBJS.H.00229.

30. Cracchiolo A III, Cimino WR, Lian G. Arthrodesis of the ankle in patients who have rheumatoid arthritis. J Bone Joint Surg. 1992;74(6):903–9.

31. Hobson SA, Karantana A, Dhar S. Total ankle replacement in patients with significant preoperative deformity of the hindfoot. J Bone Joint Surg Br. 2009;91(4):481–6.

32. Goldberg A, Zaidi R, Thomson C, Doré CJ, Skene SS, Cro S, Round J, Molloy A, Davies M, Karski M, Kim L, Cooke P, TARVA study group. Total ankle replacement versus arthrodesis (TARVA): protocol for a multicentre randomised controlled trial. BMJ Open. 2016;6(9):e012716. https://doi.org/10.1136/bmjopen-2016-012716.

33. Haddad SL, Coetzee JC, Estok R, et al. Intermediate and long-term outcomes of total ankle arthroplasty and ankle arthrodesis. A systematic review of the literature. J Bone Joint Surg Am. 2007;89:1899–905.

34. Saltzman CL, Mann RA, Ahrens JE, et al. Prospective controlled trial of STAR total ankle replacement versus ankle fusion: initial results. Foot Ankle Int. 2009;30(7):579–96.

35. Daniels TR, Younger ASE, Penner M, et al. Intermediate-term results of total ankle replacement and ankle arthrodesis: a COFAS multicenter study. J Bone Joint Surg. 2014;96(2):135–42.

36. Kim BS, Choi WJ, Kim YS, Lee JW. Total ankle replacement in moderate to severe varus deformity of the ankle. J Bone Joint Surg Br. 2009;91(9):1183–90.